Dentistry, Dental Practice,
and the
Community

Sixth 6 Edition

Dentistry, Dental Practice,

and the

Community

Brian A. Burt, BDS, MPH, PhD
Program in Dental Public Health
School of Public Health
The University of Michigan
Ann Arbor, Michigan

Stephen A. Eklund, DDS, MHSA, DrPH
Program in Dental Public Health
School of Public Health
The University of Michigan
Ann Arbor, Michigan

ELSEVIER
SAUNDERS

PENSACOLA STATE-PEN LIBRARY

ELSEVIER
SAUNDERS

11830 Westline Industrial Drive
St. Louis, Missouri 63146

DENTISTRY, DENTAL PRACTICE, AND
THE COMMUNITY
Copyright © 2005, 1999, 1992, 1983, 1969, 1964 by Elsevier Inc.
All rights reserved.

0-7216-0515-X

NOTICE

Dentistry is an ever-changing field. Standard safety precautions must be followed, but as new research and clinical experience broaden our knowledge, changes in treatment and drug therapy become necessary or appropriate. Readers are advised to check the product information currently provided by the manufacturer of each drug to be administered to verify the recommended dose, the method and duration of administration, and the contradictions. It is the responsibility of the treating physican, relying on experience and knowledge of the patient, to determine dosages and the best treatment for the patient. Neither the publisher nor the editor assumes any responsibility for any injury and/or damage to persons or property.

International Standard Book Number

0-7216-0515-X

Publishing Director: Linda Duncan
Executive Editor: Penny Rudolph
Developmental Editors: Courtney Sprehe and Jaime Pendill
Publishing Services Manager: Deborah Vogel
Senior Project Manager: Mary Drone
Senior Designer: Kathi Gosche

Printed in the United States of America

Transferred to Digital Printing, 2013

To Lizzie and Sue

and to the memory of Dr. Keith Heller, a dear friend and dedicated colleague

PREFACE TO THE SIXTH EDITION

Change is the only true constant in our uncertain world, and this sixth edition comes into a world that is very different from that which greeted the fifth edition in 1999. The budget surpluses of that time have plunged to become record deficits, and as a nation we are ambivalent about a war that may bring democracy to a troubled land or may drag us into a morass. Most of all, our national mindset is dominated by the horrors and heroism of September 11, 2001. And what has unpredictable social change got to do with dentistry? The answer is a great deal, for the dental world, like any other institution, is part of the overall pattern. If the world is an ecosystem, then changes in population, income, employment, inflation, and just about everything else will affect dentistry to some extent.

The purpose of this book is to present dentistry and dental practice against the backdrop of social events: economic, technological, and demographic trends, as well as the distribution of the oral diseases that dental professionals treat and prevent. The pace of change in these areas can be bewildering, and substantial rewriting of many parts of this book has thus been required. Since the 1999 edition came out, we have seen our health system, based on something called managed care, become less and less workable. Dentistry in Medicaid is barely visible, "access" has emerged as a major health issue, and the corporate burden of providing health care for employees is threatening our national economy. Dentistry cannot be a bystander as these issues continue to demand public attention. Rather, dentistry needs to understand them as best we can and take its place at the table as a leader in setting health care policy.

Our guiding principle in this sixth edition is that we lay out the facts on all matters discussed and interpret them as we see them. We express our opinions, taking care to distinguish opinion from fact, and leave the reader to develop his or her own views. We subscribe to the view that health is a major contributor to a higher quality of life rather than an end in itself. We have no doubt that good oral health significantly improves the quality of life and that the constant improvement of the public's oral health is a worthy goal.

The lineage of this book can be traced from the landmark work of Pelton and Wisan's *Dentistry in Public Health*, first published in 1949, up to our fifth edition in 1999. We carry on the tradition in this sixth edition, which has 30 chapters in five parts, more than ever before. That growth reflects the expansion of the issues with which dentistry is involved. The first part looks at the dental professions and the public they serve and deals with ethics, the public-private partnership, public health practice, and health promotion. Part II deals with the structure and financing of dental practice, types of personnel in the dental workforce, infection control and mercury safety, and a new chapter on access to dental care. The chapter on reading the literature is now joined by a new chapter on evidence-based dentistry. Part III is the nitty-gritty of oral epidemiology, from research designs and survey methods to the various indexes used to measure oral disease, and Part IV looks at the distribution of these diseases in the population and the various risk factors associated with them. In conclusion, Part V deals with the prevention of oral diseases and conditions.

In matters of style, we favor liberal referencing. This gives readers a chance to pursue further the issues that interest them, and the references give the basis for our interpretation of the more contentious issues. We list more references with potentially contentious issues than with the more straightforward ones. Although most references reflect current work, we have retained a lot of older ones to illustrate how issues have developed over time and to show the richness of the dental literature. We should never forget our roots. As would be expected, a growing number of references are to sites on the Internet, although we all have mixed feelings about the growing dominance of the Internet as a source of basic information. On the one hand, it makes information more immediately available than ever: if knowledge is power, we are all more powerful. On the other hand, Internet material can be startlingly temporary. Even during the production of this edition, a number of websites we were using as reference sources simply disappeared. Citing full websites can be extremely awkward, with URLs running on for two or three lines. When just the home page or second-level main page is cited in the quest for a stable reference, readers need enough familiarity with the Internet to be able to go to the other one or two levels to find the precise table or text statement. We know the Internet will continue to develop rapidly, although what it will look like in 10 years' time is anybody's guess.

We have continued our method of dealing with the gender-specific personal pronoun by making it feminine in the odd-numbered chapters, masculine in the even-numbered. The "her" of Chapter 1 thus becomes the "his" of Chapter 2. In our frequent use of the term *dental professionals*, we include both dental hygienists and dentists as colleagues working together.

Contrasts have to be made at times between how things are done in the richer parts of the world compared to the poorer. We use the term *developed countries*, or sometimes *industrialized* or the World Bank term of *high-income* countries, to refer to nations such as the United States, Canada, most European countries, Australia, New Zealand, and Japan, which have industrial and service-based economies, high levels of literacy, a large middle class, sophisticated transport systems, and mass distribution of goods far from their point of origin. By contrast, the *developing* or *low-income* nations are those in which those factors are just beginning to be seen or in which they do not exist at all. In addition, there are many nations that don't clearly fit either category but lie somewhere between the two: well-developed in some areas and less so in others. Without going into details of world economics, we occasionally use those oversimplified categories of "developed" and "developing" to illustrate broad differences.

We owe a debt of gratitude to those who have helped us with materials and other information for this book. In alphabetical order, we thank Patricia Anderson, Pilar Baca, Eugenio Beltrán-Aguilar, Robert (Skip) Collins, Steve Levy, Thom Marthaler, Kevin O'Brien, Jim Pittman, Scott Presson, Woosung Sohn, Scott Tomar, and Helen Whelton. All of these people made our task a little easier, although we emphasize that responsibility for every word in this book lies with us, and with us alone.

So who knows what lies ahead for the twenty-first century? We certainly don't pretend to have the answers, other than to state the obvious: it will be a challenging and exciting time for dentistry. To thrive and progress, dental professionals require a mindset that permits them to adapt to changing circumstances. We hope that this book will help readers to develop that mindset.

Brian A. Burt, BDS, MPH, PhD

Stephen A. Eklund, DDS, MHSA, DrPH

CONTENTS

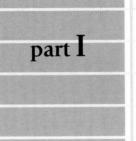

part I Dentistry and the Community

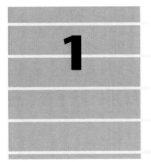

1 The Professions of Dentistry and Dental Hygiene

Dental practice has existed in some form since the dawn of time, but it is only in comparatively recent years that its practitioners in the economically developed nations have achieved the status of a profession. In most of the low-income world, dental practice is still more of a craft. In countries with a moderate level of economic development, dentistry exhibits some aspects of a profession, but not all.

Webster's dictionary defines a *profession* as "a calling requiring specialized knowledge and often long and intensive academic preparation" and "the whole body of persons engaged in a calling." The definition of *professionalism* is "the conduct, aims, or qualities that characterize or mark a profession or professional person." These terse dictionary definitions, however, do not fully capture the essence of a profession or of professionalism: commitment to patient welfare, ethics, and other professional ideals are not included. Nor are all aspects of professionalism necessarily high-minded or noble. Admission to some professional groups can be based on self-perpetuation rather than public good, and aspects of "closed shop" practices in professions have not been uncommon.[30]

Three models of professionalism have been described,[25] none of which by itself fully characterizes dentistry, although collectively they may do so. The first is the *commercial model*, in which dental care is viewed as a commodity sold by the practitioner. The services are thus not based primarily on the client's needs, but rather on what the client is able or willing to buy. This rather crass view is distasteful to many, although there are aspects of it in dental practice. The second is the *guild model*, in which dental care is seen as a privilege with the professional dominant in practitioner-patient relations. In the guild model the professional is the repository of all knowledge and wisdom, the patient is a passive recipient, and the practitioner has an ethical trust to provide the best-quality care. This model has probably been dominant in the United States, although it may be slowly merging with the third model, the *interactive model*, in which dental care is considered a partnership of equals. In this model, practitioner and patient jointly determine care provided through a combination of professional expertise and patient values.

What are the criteria that characterize a profession, and how can a profession be distinguished from, say, a trade union? The first is the criterion given in the dictionary definition, a substantial body of knowledge, a corollary of which is the obligation to keep that knowledge up to date through continuing education. The

3

second is self-regulation, a tradition whereby society delegates to professional groups the legal responsibility for determining who shall join them in serving the public and for disciplining those members who do not meet the profession's requirements. A third and perhaps the main distinguishing criterion of a profession is a code of ethics, guidelines for professional conduct that are rooted in a moral imperative rather than in law or regulation (see Chapter 3). A profession sets its own code of ethics and its own procedures for dealing with infringements. Taking the various criteria mentioned, one can distinguish a profession by the features listed in Box 1-1.

A health profession can then be defined by paraphrasing Webster's definition given earlier: a calling in the health sciences requiring specialized knowledge, and one that meets the other criteria listed. Dentistry meets all the requirements of a profession. Dental hygiene is usually considered a profession within dentistry, although for the most part it is not self-regulating.

DEVELOPMENT OF THE DENTAL PROFESSIONS
Dentistry

Dental diseases have afflicted the human race since the dawn of recorded history.[22,29] Dentistry, however, has existed as a vocation only in recent years, historically speaking, and it was not until modern times that any sort of scientific basis was developed for the care of oral diseases. One landmark event was the 1728 publication of Pierre Fauchard, *Le Chirurgien Dentiste, ou Traite des Dents*, a two-volume book of more than 800 pages. Fauchard, a Frenchman, is looked upon as a seminal figure in the evolution of the dental profession. His work was the first complete treatise on dentistry published in the Western world, and it remained an authoritative document for over 100 years. Fauchard, despite the lack of formal training, was clearly a first-class empiricist with keen powers of observation.

Aspiring dentists of the time served as apprentices. It is worth noting that even the formal education of G. V. Black, one of the profession's most notable nineteenth-century pioneers, did not exceed 20 months. His introduction to dentistry consisted of "a few weeks" with one Dr. Speers, who was not considered a particularly good dentist and whose dental library consisted of one book.[9] Fortunately, Dr. Black was a true professional and followed the precept that "a professional person has no choice other than to be a continuous student."

The first American dental school was the Baltimore College of Dental Surgery, later part of the University of Maryland, established in 1840. The course was 16 weeks in length after a year or more of apprenticeship. The initial enrollment was five, of whom two graduated. At about the same time, the first national professional dental journal appeared, the *American Journal of Dental Science*, and the first national dental organization, the American Society of Dental Surgeons, was established. The genesis of the dental profession in the United States can thus be dated fairly precisely to the 1840 period. The path of professional progress was not entirely smooth, however, for the emergence of dentistry as a fledgling profession was followed by an undignified scramble to open proprietary dental schools. In the best American

---

BOX 1-1   Characteristics of a Profession

- A body of knowledge exists that is constantly being expanded, updated, and archived in a literature record. The purpose is constant improvement of the quality of the profession's service to individuals and to the public.
- Academic preparation is required, carried out in specialized institutions.
- The profession and its members accept a lifelong commitment to continuing education.

- Society awards the profession the privilege of self-regulation, which means determining the requirements for entering and remaining in the profession, and dealing with those members who do not meet the requirements.
- Its members subscribe to a code of ethics drawn up by the profession itself.
- The members form organized societies to enhance the development of the group and its societal mission, and to serve its individual members.

traditions of free enterprise and entrepreneurship, most of these places were run strictly for profit. In the years before public and professional regulation, the proprietary schools turned out thousands of graduates whose professional abilities covered the spectrum from respectable to dreadful.

The anarchic events of the time, however, led to dentistry's development in the United States as a profession separate from medicine, a position that has been maintained to the present day. This separate development actually occurred more by chance than by deliberate policy, for it was originally intended that the Baltimore dental school be established within the medical school. It was not, but only because of lack of space and internal friction among medical school faculty. The separation of dentistry from medicine was standard in the English-speaking world, Scandinavia, and some other European countries, but in central and southern Europe, by contrast, there was a division between stomatologists (physicians with specialty training in clinical dentistry) and dentists, who in this context were second-level providers. This division of labor is thought not to have benefited oral health in most of the countries concerned[13] and has been abandoned in most of them as the European Community moves toward standardization of professional training. On the other hand, whether American dentistry benefited from its evolution on a branch that grew out of the main medical trunk, rather than being more closely allied to medicine during its formative years, can be debated. By the early twenty-first century, there were signs that dentistry might be evolving into something closer to the medical model.

Dentistry in the Twentieth Century

The era of modern dentistry could be said to date from the closing of the last proprietary school in 1929, which came shortly after the landmark Gies report on dental education. Gies collected information from the dental schools of the time and concluded that the dental profession would only progress when dental education became university based and subject to the maintenance of high standards through accreditation. Despite the adoption of Gies's recommendations, however, dental practice during the economic depression of the 1930s was

largely a matter of survival, with few patients able to afford dental care. World War II followed, during which dentists, along with other health professionals, were drafted into the armed forces. As part of the national mobilization for the war effort, American dental schools compressed the curriculum of four academic years into three calendar years. This expedient was dropped when the war ended in 1945, although it was flirted with again for a short time in the 1970s.

The 1930s and 1940s were a hard time for dental education. The teaching of basic science was often perfunctory and the emphasis in the clinical sciences was almost entirely on restorative dentistry and prosthetics. Subjects such as radiology, oral diagnosis, endodontics, periodontics, and pediatric dentistry were neglected in many dental schools, and full-time faculty were the exception rather than the rule. There were few educational programs for the preparation of specialists, and the few that did exist varied in quality and length.[20] One of the few bright spots during this difficult period was the beginning of the first controlled water fluoridation projects in 1945 (see Chapter 25).

With a rapidly expanding postwar economy and population, added to accelerating technologic growth and a spirit of optimism, dentistry entered what some saw as a golden age during the 1950s. New dental materials expanded treatment horizons, and the arrival of the high-speed air-turbine engine in 1957 revolutionized dental practice. Dental research, stimulated by the establishment of the National Institute of Dental Research (now the National Institute of Dental and Craniofacial Research) in 1948, grew rapidly, and the publication of *The Survey of Dentistry* in 1961[18] led to improvements in education and practice. Stagnating dental schools were revitalized with the passage of the Health Professions Educational Assistance Act in 1963. This act authorized federal funds for construction and student aid. Later renewals in 1971 and 1976 included per capita funding to support the basic instructional program. In the 15 years from 1963 to 1978, the addition of federal monies to state, local, and private sources spurred the reconstruction of the entire physical plant of dental education.[16] New schools were built too; the 39 dental schools in 1930 had increased to 59 by 1980.[1]

The 1960s and 1970s saw the emergence of comprehensive care, growth in use of auxiliaries, the beginnings of prepaid dental insurance, and the development of a community outlook in dentistry. Growth in the number of dentists and in dental business was sharp, in retrospect perhaps too sharp. The economic downturn following the Vietnam War (1964–75), added to the decline in dental caries among children (see Chapter 20), led to a growing perception of an oversupply of dentists, despite increasing public utilization of services (see Chapter 2) and continued growth of dental insurance (see Chapter 7). During the 1980s, enrollment in dental schools dropped substantially from its peak during 1977–79 and rose only a little from these levels through the mid-1990s (see Chapter 8). In response, seven dental schools closed during this period (Emory, Fairleigh Dickinson, Georgetown, Loyola of Chicago, Northwestern, Oral Roberts, Washington University). Applications to dental schools picked up again in the late 1990s, and new dental schools opened in Arizona, Florida, and Nevada. In the early twenty-first century there were 56 dental schools in the United States.[6]

In the new century, the major oral diseases are better controlled than ever, and dental practice will evolve accordingly. Research in molecular biology is promising a new understanding of many diseases, including those oral diseases that currently are poorly understood and that to date have not been treated in dental practice. Other features that will shape dental practice in the new century are the changing demographic profile (see Chapter 2), disease patterns (see Chapters 19-23), developments in dental insurance (see Chapter 7), and new restorative materials. Infection-control procedures and their associated regulations had become standard practice by the 1990s (see Chapter 10).

Dental Hygiene

Dr. Alfred Fones, an 1890 graduate of the New York College of Dentistry, developed a technique for scaling and polishing teeth and also taught his patients to carry out home-care procedures. By 1906, acting under the preventive dictum that "a clean tooth never decays," Dr. Fones was sure that the oral health of his patients was improved through his oral prophylactic practices. He trained his assistant to practice dental hygiene, and in 1907 he was instrumental in having dental hygiene legally recognized in Connecticut as an adjunct to dental practice. Fones went on to establish the first school of dental hygiene in 1913. Accepting only "young ladies of good character," the school was located in a carriage house on the grounds of the Fones residence.[23] Connecticut passed legislation specifically describing the practice of dental hygiene in 1916. Ten states had similar legislation in place by 1920, and the total rose to 34 in 1935. Not until 1951, however, did the practice acts of all states, the District of Columbia, and the Commonwealth of Puerto Rico include provisions for the practice of dental hygiene.[14]

This leisurely development of dental hygiene was largely tied to the development of dental schools. In 1945, of the 16 dental hygiene programs then in existence, 13 were associated with schools of dentistry. By 1974, however, only 37 of 158 were so affiliated. The explosive growth after 1960 mostly took place in junior and community colleges,[14] stimulated by federal funds for vocational-technical education in health occupation training centers. The numbers of training programs, especially the 2-year programs, fluctuated with demand for hygienists and the availability of federal funding. By 1980 the number of programs was 204; it was down to 190 by the end of the 1980s and back over 250 again early in the new century (see Chapter 8).

During the first 30 years of dental hygiene education, there was no uniformity in either prerequisites or curriculum. These variations were due to differences in state licensing acts, problems of integrating a 2-year clinical program into a 4-year baccalaureate degree curriculum, and the lack of nationally approved standards. The latter problem was remedied in 1947, when the Council on Dental Education of the American Dental Association (ADA) adopted the first accreditation requirements for dental hygiene schools. In 1952, the council began an active program in accreditation of dental hygiene schools. The requirements developed then still essentially stand today.

For training in dental hygiene, a 2-year curriculum must meet the standards of the ADA's Commission on Dental Accreditation. In all states except Alabama, which recognizes preceptorship, the completion of an accredited

2-year curriculum is the minimum requirement for admittance to licensure examination by a state dental board. An individual enrolled in a 4-year baccalaureate degree program must also meet university standards for that degree. Many dental hygienists earn advanced degrees (MS, MPH, PhD, DrPH), for which the requirements of the university's graduate school also must be met.

ORGANIZATION OF THE DENTAL PROFESSIONS IN THE UNITED STATES

The legal basis for dental practice in the United States is the dental practice act in each state. It is not a federal matter. The effect of these acts on dental practice is discussed more fully in Chapter 8. Here we look at the professional organizations in dentistry.

American Dental Association

The ADA was founded in 1859 by 26 dentists meeting at Niagara Falls. Today it claims some 147,000 members,[2] about 70% of the nation's dentists. It is easily the largest and most influential dental organization in the country. It operates on a tripartite basis, meaning that members must join the local society (a component), the state or territorial society (a constituent), and the national ADA; they cannot be members of just one or two (with the exception of students and dentists in the federal services). There are 53 constituent societies and 545 components.[3]

The tripartite system has been in place since 1913, when it was modeled on the structure of the American Medical Association. The purpose of adopting the tripartite structure was to unify a profession that at the time was highly fragmented and to improve efficiency through avoiding duplication of effort. The tripartite structure was challenged in 1972 by four Arizona dentists, who argued that by requiring membership at all levels the ADA had instituted an illegal arrangement. The district court ruled against the dentists in 1980, stating that the membership requirement did not suppress competition between dentists, and it also disagreed with the charge that the associations or their members held a monopoly on the practice of dentistry in Arizona. The decision was upheld in the court of appeals in 1982,[21] and subsequent challenges to the tripartite structure have been similarly unsuccessful.

Dentists apply for membership in a component society, which represents a county, a group of counties, or a large city. If accepted at this local level, the dentist automatically becomes a member of the state dental society and of the ADA. Traditionally membership standards have included graduation from an accredited dental school, a license to practice in the jurisdiction, and "good moral standing," a vague term that has been interpreted in various ways.

ADA membership provides access to a number of fringe benefits that are important to a self-employed practitioner, such as group insurance plans and the availability of expert consultative services. It also serves its members, and indirectly the public, by the activities shown in Box 1-2.

The ADA is cohesive and well organized. Its ultimate governing body is the 427-member

---

BOX 1-2 Three Primary Areas in Which the American Dental Association Serves Its Members and, Indirectly, the Public

1. Facilitating the growth and dissemination of scientific information. This is done by holding scientific meetings at the local, state, and national levels and is enhanced by the publication of a variety of scientific journals. The Internet continues to emerge as an ever more important medium of information exchange.
2. Establishing standards, such as accreditation of professional schools for dentists, dental hygienists, dental assistants, and dental laboratory technicians.

Standards are also established for materials, drugs, and devices used by dentists in practice and for some products offered for sale to the public. These standards are established by having experts in specialized fields serve as members of reviewing councils and committees.
3. Obtaining a consensus among the profession on major issues and transmitting this consensus to government agencies and others concerned with establishing policies for public health.

House of Delegates, which comprises elected representatives from the 50 states, the District of Columbia, the Commonwealth of Puerto Rico, the Virgin Islands, five federal dental services (Air Force, Army, Navy, U.S. Public Health Service, Department of Veterans Affairs), and the American Student Dental Association.[3] As in the U.S. House of Representatives, state delegations are proportional to state dental populations; they range from 1 delegate (the Virgin Islands) to California's 47.

The Board of Trustees, charged with day-to-day responsibility for the ADA's operations, is made up of a trustee from each of 17 geographic districts of roughly equal numbers of dentists, plus the president, president-elect, and first and second vice-presidents. The Board reports on its activities to the House of Delegates. It also reviews most resolutions on their way to the House and recommends what action should be taken on them.[7]

The House of Delegates conducts business once a year for 5 days during the annual session. Resolutions may be introduced by the Board of Trustees, the ADA's commissions and councils, the trustee districts, constituent and component societies, or directly by delegates. Resolutions, along with supporting documentation, are referred for hearing to one of seven reference committees. Depending on the issues in any given year, special (generally single-issue) committees may be established to study particular questions in depth. The hearings of the reference committees are open to all members of the association. At these meetings members are encouraged to speak their minds and advise the House of Delegates of their positions on specific issues or on the status of the association as a whole. The reference committees prepare reports that are transmitted to the House of Delegates. As the House considers the issues, it usually has the original resolution and background report, the comments and recommendations of the Board of Trustees, and the report and recommendations of the reference committee. On the basis of this information, the House acts to adopt, defeat, amend, substitute, or refer.

The ADA has long been keenly aware of the public image of dentistry and has conducted many campaigns to promote it. Children's Dental Health Month, which grew from an original 1-week campaign and is held in February each year, is the oldest annual public relations exercise. The ADA notes that on its Give Kids a Smile! Day in February 2003 thousands of children received needed dental treatment from dentists who donated their services.[4] The impact of these campaigns is discussed in Chapter 5.

Dentistry just might be a bit overly preoccupied with its image, for many public opinion polls show that the public consistently ranks dentists high in terms of professional trust.[12] The sometimes prickly sensitivity of dentistry to its image is seen in the chorus of complaints when dentists are portrayed in movies or TV as bumbling, obsessive, or sadistic, or when newscasters refer to "doctors and dentists." (One that gets under our skin is reference to "medical treatment" and "dental work.") These things can grate at times, but they seem to be part of the territory. When they are viewed in the perspective of how all professions are treated in the media, it is doubtful if any real harm is done by media imagery.

National Dental Association

In past years, rigid attitudes on racial separation meant that most component dental societies of the ADA did not accept dentists of African-American origin. African-American dentists therefore went their own way and in 1913 established the National Dental Association (NDA). Those days of nonacceptance are now happily gone; in recent years both the ADA and the NDA have stated that their objective is complete integration of the dental profession. White dentists now belong to the NDA and African-American dentists belong to the ADA, and there is a good cooperative relationship between the two organizations. They continue to exist separately, however, for traditional reasons. Today the NDA has some 7000 dentist members, and it also has acted as the umbrella organization for the National Dental Hygienists' Association since 1963.[24]

Perhaps more so than the ADA, the NDA has been a consistent champion of efforts to improve the health status of those in our society who are most often underserved by the health care system. Such groups include racial and ethnic minorities, children, the indigent, the elderly, and the disabled.

Hispanic Dental Association

Established in 1990, the Hispanic Dental Association (HDA) represents the interests of both Hispanic professionals and patients.[17] This active organization already has some 15,000 members, a well-established organizational structure, and a number of affiliated groups throughout the country. The mission of the HDA is to improve the oral health of the Hispanic community, and to that end it sponsors continuing education and oral health promotional activities directed at the Hispanic population. Since Hispanics are the fastest-growing ethnic minority in the United States (see Chapter 2), the HDA is confidently looking forward to increased growth.

Other Groups in Dentistry

Beyond the major national organizations and their constituent and component societies, each specialty group has its own organization: the American Academy of Periodontology, the American Association of Oral and Maxillofacial Surgeons, the American Association of Public Health Dentistry, and so on. These specialty organizations serve as sponsors of the specialty-certifying bodies whose role is discussed in Chapter 8. At another level still, there are myriad study clubs and groups of dentists brought together by common interests.

FDI World Dental Federation

Practically every country with a recognizable dental profession has a working national organization, an equivalent of the ADA, although no other national dental association has resources as extensive as those of the ADA. On the international scene, the FDI World Dental Federation is an organization of national dental associations. The name needs some explanation. Formed in the early twentieth century as a loose grouping of several European national associations, the organization was first known as the Fédération Dentaire Internationale (French for International Dental Federation, hence the acronym FDI). In its early years it was a distinctly European organization, but with global expansion it changed its name to the World Dental Federation. The acronym FDI was so well known by that time, however, that it was kept as part of the title of the organization. FDI now represents over 150 national dental organizations and 35 other international organizations, encompassing altogether over 700,000 dentists.[15] Headquartered in London for years, the FDI is now based at Ferney-Voltaire, France, the same city where the World Medical Association[31] is located and close to the World Health Organization's home in Geneva, Switzerland. The FDI has a full-time executive secretary, a large staff, and a structure that resembles that of the United Nations. Its work is both scientific and political. Its technical committees bring international experts together to develop state-of-the-art reports and recommendations for further action. Politically, the FDI has been helpful in the development of the dental professions and dental care services in many countries where the local profession has little political clout. It publishes the *International Dental Journal*, a respected journal in the dental literature.

American Dental Hygienists' Association

In 1923, 46 dental hygienists from 11 states met in Cleveland, Ohio, to organize the American Dental Hygienists' Association (ADHA). They received strong support from the dental profession. While early growth was not spectacular, in the 1925–45 period, active membership went from several hundred to about 2000. In the next 10 years (1945–55) membership more than doubled to nearly 4400, and growth has been spectacular since then. In 2003 the ADHA represented the interests of more than 120,000 registered dental hygienists.[8]

The organization of the ADHA closely parallels that of the ADA. There are seven classifications of membership (including student membership for a modest fee), but the basic category of "active" membership must be held through constituent and component associations if such exist. There are 375 component (local) associations. The House of Delegates meets once a year and has all legislative and policy-making powers for the association. The Board of Trustees is composed of the elective officers (except the Speaker of the House), 12 trustees, and the immediate past president, and has responsibility for supervising the day-to-day operations. It reviews reports and makes recommendations and relates all of its activities to the House. The *Journal of the American Dental Hygienists' Association* was established in 1927 and became the *Journal of Dental Hygiene* in 1988.

CAREERS IN DENTISTRY AND DENTAL HYGIENE

Private Practice

Private practice, in which the dentist invests capital into land, buildings, equipment, and furnishings and in turn seeks to attract patients who will pay for dental services, is the primary career choice for most dentists in the United States. Private practice is a small business, and so from the career perspective it has all the advantages and disadvantages of small business operation.

The advantages are considerable. A dentist has an almost unlimited choice of where to locate a practice (provided of course that she is licensed to practice in the chosen state). Other advantages are usually a good income, high status in the community, and the freedom that comes from being one's own boss. Autonomy, in work practices as well as in selection of treatment options, continues to be the bedrock value of private practice.[10] This is to be expected, since it fits well with American cultural values.[11] Private practice also brings the satisfaction of knowing that the profession is generally held in high esteem by the public.

Disadvantages of private practice also relate to the small business aspects: overhead costs for utilities, malpractice insurance, disability insurance, staff benefits, equipment maintenance; retirement planning. The need to adhere to various government regulations also absorbs some effort. Dental practice is highly physical in nature, and conditions that are only an inconvenience in many occupations, such as mild arthritis, a bad back, or failing eyesight, can be career threatening for a dental practitioner.

An associate in an established practice is usually paid by salary, or salary plus percentage of gross production. These arrangements allow skills to be sharpened before the practitioner establishes her own practice and can lead to buying into an established practice. Partnership too can ease the financial burden of starting practice, and so can entering a group practice. Partnerships can provide more flexibility in practice patterns than does solo practice, but partners setting out together should be sure that they are of the right temperament to make joint decisions and that the personalities involved are mutually compatible. An unhappy business partnership can be as emotionally traumatic and financially devastating as a broken marriage.

Dental specialists generally earn higher incomes than generalists. Achievement of specialist status requires at least an extra 2 years of education beyond dental school, followed by specialty board examinations (see Chapter 8). For specialists, the process of choosing a practice location parallels that for general practitioners, with two important exceptions. First, the choice usually is limited to the larger population centers; second, the referral potential of the practitioners in the area, as well as the number of specialists located there, must be assessed. In a specialty practice, the supply of patients is dependent primarily on referrals from general practitioners. When the general practitioners are all mature dentists with busy, established practices, they will usually refer patients more readily than will younger generalists attempting to establish their own practices. In the latter instance, referrals may be few and limited to the most extreme problems. The choices for the two types of specialists who usually work only in salaried positions, oral pathologists and public health dentists, are limited by positions available.

Colorado is the only state that permits independent practice of dental hygiene, although only a few hygienists established their own practices there after the 1986 law that permitted independent practice. Most hygienists, in Colorado as elsewhere, begin their careers treating patients in the offices of private dental practitioners. They are either reimbursed on a straight salaried basis or paid a combination of salary and commission.

Salaried Practice

The advantages and disadvantages of salaried practice, like those of private practice, are most related to whether the dentist is temperamentally comfortable in an organization as opposed to being a private entrepreneur. Even if a new graduate does not wish to stay in salaried service permanently, it is often a good place to start. Advantages include the opportunity to reduce dental school debts before incurring more, an immediate specified income, a chance to improve clinical skills, and time to think about careers before becoming "locked in" to a practice.

However, for some dentists salaried practice appeals as a life career. A reasonably good salary (although not as high as peak earnings in private practice), fringe benefits such as health and disability insurance, liability coverage, a retirement plan, paid vacation time, and freedom from the overhead costs and day-to-day worries of private practice can combine to make the long-term financial prospects of salaried employment attractive. Some organizations employing dentists provide opportunities for continuing education.

For the new dentist interested in general practice, a general practice residency offers a form of short-term salaried practice that combines advanced educational opportunities with the ability to earn. There are over 300 general practice residencies and advanced general dentistry programs accredited by the ADA, all lasting 12 or 24 months and offering adequate stipends. They generally include rotations through such areas as medicine, emergency care, anesthesia, and various special areas of clinical dentistry. This excellent clinical experience is broadened even further when general practice residencies include some public health perspectives (see Chapter 4).

U.S. Public Health Service

Dentists in the U.S. Public Health Service (USPHS), a component of the Department of Health and Human Services, serve as commissioned officers of the federal government and enjoy essentially the same pay, rank, and privileges as their counterparts in the armed services. The USPHS's broad mission relates to the health of the entire nation, in recognition of which its chief officer is commissioned as Surgeon General of the United States. The USPHS carries out major responsibilities in health research (principally through the National Institutes of Health) and in the promotion of health through public health efforts. Clinical care is provided primarily to merchant seamen, the Coast Guard, American Indians and Alaska Natives, and residents of federal prisons. USPHS dental officers serve in a wide variety of assignments in all states. The clinics of the Indian Health Service, for example, extend

from Point Barrow, Alaska (the farthest northern point of the United States above the Arctic Circle), to Arizona just north of the Mexican border. Although the USPHS is the oldest health service of the federal government, beginning as the Marine Hospital Service in 1798 and with its Commissioned Corps dating from 1873, it remained relatively unknown to the public before Surgeon General C. Everett Koop gave it high visibility during his campaigns against smoking and in favor of education on acquired immunodeficiency syndrome during the 1980s.[19] In more recent years, the release of the Surgeon General's report on oral health in America[26] and the subsequent call to action[27] has thrust the USPHS into an unaccustomed position of prominence in dentistry.

Other major federal dental services are the dental corps of the Army, Navy (which also serves the Marine Corps), and Air Force. Availability of positions varies with the degree of military activity, although some openings are usually present at any given time. The dentist in the armed services receives all the advantages of a service career: a reasonably good income, generous fringe benefits, usually excellent clinical facilities, and a chance to receive graduate education funded by the service. Dentists serve on military bases in the United States and overseas. In the Navy, duty is also available on some ships.

Another major federal dental service, that in the Department of Veterans Affairs (previously the Veterans Administration, and hence still referred to as the VA), was established in 1920 to improve services to veterans of American wars. It is a major participant in postdoctoral dental education and it offers, in addition to specialty programs, more than half of the general practice residencies available in the federal services. Many VA institutions are affiliated with dental schools. Care is provided in VA hospitals and outpatient clinics. Occasionally it is purchased from private practitioners. Like all federal dental programs, the VA program offers equal employment opportunities for male and female dentists. Sometimes the VA has been able to accommodate married couples when both are health professionals.

For hygienists, expanded opportunities in the federal service are available for those with a degree of MPH (Master of Public Health). A number of hygienists with this degree have advanced into leadership positions. Civilian hygienists are employed in the Army, Navy, and Air Force, although a major share of clinical procedures ordinarily performed by hygienists are carried out by specially trained enlisted personnel.

Outside of the federal dental services there are other opportunities for salaried employment. Although the number of state dental directorships has declined in the twenty-first century, usually falling victim to state budget crunches, most states still maintain this post. Most are filled by a dentist or hygienist with advanced training in public health, most commonly the MPH degree. Dentists and dental hygienists without advanced training are also employed by state and local health departments, group dental practices, prepaid dental programs, industry-sponsored clinics, and institutions such as hospitals, prisons, schools for the mentally retarded, and homes for the mentally ill. These positions may involve public health and administrative activities, clinical practice, or a combination of both.

Academia: Dental Education and Research

Dental schools, as noted earlier in this chapter, used to be staffed largely by part-time faculty whose primary task was to grade students' clinical treatment. Academic careers have evolved, however, and the emphasis now is on full-time teachers and researchers. The ability to conduct independent research has become a major criterion for an academic career because research grant funds increasingly form an important part of a school's budget.

An advanced degree is more or less mandatory for the new dentist or hygienist who is thinking of an academic career. The most common is the MS (Master of Science), the usual 2-year degree taken to fulfill specialty training requirements, which mixes advanced clinical training with some research training. Those who want to make their careers in research need doctoral-level training in the philosophy and methods of research through the degrees of PhD (Doctor of Philosophy), DrPH (Doctor of Public Health), or ScD (Doctor of Science). The National Institute of Dental and Craniofacial Research in Bethesda, Maryland, has information on research training programs that it supports.[28]

Academic positions for dental professionals with advanced degrees have attractive salaries and fringe benefits. They can be intellectually demanding, and university politics can be just as vigorous as politics anywhere else. The future of dentistry rests with its dental education institutions and research institutes, and in the early twenty-first century the shortage of dental faculty was becoming an issue of some concern.[5] Those employed in these institutions have the rewards and challenges of being on the cutting edge of new developments, of interacting with talented fellow faculty members, and of relating to students who represent the future.

REFERENCES

1. American Dental Association. Summary of the 1979–1980 annual report on dental education. J Am Dent Assoc 1980;100:926-30.
2. American Dental Association. About the ADA, website: http://www.ada.org/ada/about/index.asp. Accessed October 26, 2003.
3. American Dental Association. Background on the American Dental Association, website: http://www.ada.org/ada/about/ada_background.asp. Accessed October 26, 2003.
4. American Dental Association. Give Kids a Smile!, website: http://www.ada.org/prof/events/featured/gkas/gkas_background.asp. Accessed October 26, 2003.
5. American Dental Education Association. Faculty shortages challenge dental education, and, thus, dentistry: What is being done?, website: https://www2.adea.org/adcn/FacultyShortages.pdf. Accessed October 26, 2003.
6. American Dental Education Association. Links to dental schools and allied education programs, website: http://www.adea.org/links/default.htm. Accessed October 26, 2003.
7. American Dental Association, House of Delegates. Structure and function of the ADA's policy-making body. J Am Dent Assoc 1976;93:708-12.
8. American Dental Hygienists' Association, website: http://www.adha.org/aboutadha/profile.htm. Accessed September 5, 2003.
9. Bremner MDK. The story of dentistry; from the dawn of civilization to the present. 3rd ed. Brooklyn NY: Dental Items of Interest, 1954.
10. Burgess K, Ruesch JD, Mikkelsen MC, Wagner KS. ADA members weigh in on critical issues. J Am Dent Assoc 2003;134:103-7.
11. Chambers DW. Work. J Am Coll Dentists 2002; 69:38-41.
12. DiMatteo MR, McBride CA, Shugars DA, O'Neill EH. Public attitudes towards dentists: A U.S. household survey. J Am Dent Assoc 1995;126:1563-70.
13. Ennis J. The story of the Fédération Dentaire Internationale. London: The Federation, 1967.

14. Fales MJH. History of dental hygiene education in the United States, 1913 to 1975 [dissertation]. Ann Arbor MI: University of Michigan, 1975.
15. FDI World Dental Federation, website: http://www.fdiworldental.org. Accessed September 5, 2003.
16. Galagan DJ. Back from the brink: How and why U.S. dental schools were rebuilt. Dent Surv 1978;54:14-8.
17. Hispanic Dental Association, website: http://www.hdassoc.org/site/epage/8138_351.htm. Accessed September 4, 2003.
18. Hollinshead BS. The survey of dentistry: The final report. Washington DC: American Council on Education, 1961.
19. Koop CE, Ginzburg HM. The revitalization of the Public Health Service Commissioned Corps. Public Health Rep 1989;104:105-10.
20. Mann WR. Dental education. In: Hollinshead BS. The survey of dentistry; the final report. Washington DC: American Council on Education, 1961:239–422.
21. McCann D. Tripartite system: Working together for a common goal. J Am Dent Assoc 1989;119:241–7.
22. Moore WJ, Corbett ME. The distribution of dental caries in ancient British populations. II. Iron Age, Romano-British and mediaeval periods. Caries Res 1973;7:139-53.
23. Motley WE. Ethics, jurisprudence, and history for the dental hygienist. 3rd ed. Philadelphia PA: Lea and Febiger, 1976.
24. National Dental Association. About us, website: http://www.ndaonline.org/aboutus.htm. Accessed September 4, 2003.
25. Ozar DT. Three models of professionalism and professional obligation in dentistry. J Am Dent Assoc 1985;110:173-7.
26. US Public Health Service. Oral health in America: A report of the Surgeon General. Rockville MD: National Institutes of Health, 2000.
27. US Public Health Service. A national call to action to promote oral health. NIH Publication No. 03-5303. Rockville MD: National Institutes of Health, 2003.
28. US Public Health Service, National Institute of Dental and Craniofacial Research. Research, website: http://www.nidr.nih.gov/research/. Accessed October 26, 2003.
29. Weinberger BH. An introduction to the history of dentistry, with medical and dental chronology and bibliographic data. St. Louis: Mosby, 1948.
30. Wolfenden. What makes a profession? Br Dent J 1975;139:61-5.
31. World Medical Association. Policy: Introduction and history, website: http://www.wma.net/e/policy/index.htm. Accessed November 6, 2003.

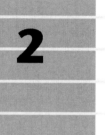

2   The Public Served by Dentistry

Dentistry exists to serve the public. Many aspects of that broad statement will be examined throughout this book, and in this chapter we start by looking at the structure of the U.S. population. The age distribution of the population, its ethnic makeup, and its geographic distribution within the country all profoundly affect the practice of dentistry. We then look at the public's use of dental services and the factors that affect that use.

POPULATION OF THE UNITED STATES
Population Size and Growth

In the decennial census of 2000, the population of the United States was over 281 million, about 4.6% of the world's population. By 2004 the population had exceeded 292 million.[10] Life expectancy around the beginning of the twenty-first century reached 76.5 years. Women live longer than men on average, and the highest life expectancy was among white women, at 79.9 years. They were followed by African-American women at 74.7 years, white men at 74.3 years, and African-American men at 67.2 years.[12] Life expectancy continues to increase steadily and is expected to keep on increasing, although the disparities between whites and African-Americans are likely to persist. Those interracial disparities reflect social problems, whereas the fact that women usually live longer than men is likely to be genetically determined.

Fig. 2-1 features the population pyramid, a graphic method of showing age distribution, to demonstrate some population dynamics in the United States. The pyramid in Fig. 2-1, *A*, is from the 1990 census[14] and the pyramid in Fig. 2-1, *B*, is from the 2000 census.[15] The bulge of the baby-boomer generation, the large number of children born between 1946 and 1964 in the aftermath of World War II (1939–45), is clearly evident in the 25-39 age-groups in 1990 and the 35-49 age-groups in 2000. Of interest to dental practitioners is the aging of the population and the predominance of women in the oldest age-groups. As time goes by, the population pyramid for the United States will come to look more like a rectangle. Average age will continue to increase for the foreseeable future, and an ever-increasing proportion of the population will be in the older age-groups.

Fig. 2-1 illustrates two areas of important population change. One is the growth in the

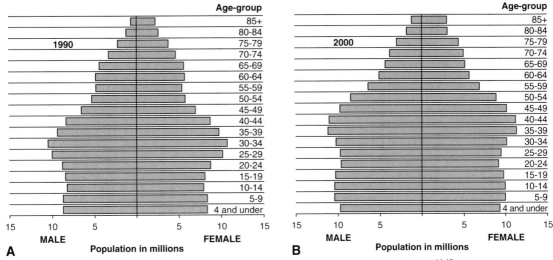

Fig. 2-1 Population pyramids for the United States, 1990 (**A**) and 2000 (**B**).[14,15]

middle years, the inexorable upward movement of the baby-boomer bulge toward the older years. Less obvious, and less publicized, is the increase in the population 10-24 years old between 1990 and 2000. These bars are noticeably longer in 2000 than in 1990, and the fact that the numbers were not present in the birth to 14 years groups in 1990 means that immigration is making its mark.

The Census Bureau estimates that the total population of the United States in the year 2020, when many of today's dental students will be practicing, will be 325 million.[16] The rate of population increase during the 1980-95 period was generally around 0.9% per year, which does not sound a lot but is still more than 2 million people per year. To provide a global perspective, the contrast between current and projected population growth rates in some high-income countries and low-income countries is shown in Fig. 2-2. The highest rates of population growth are clearly occurring in the low-income world. In the year 2000, the population of the high-income countries was about one-fifth of the world's total.

Age Distribution

Low fertility rates since the late 1960s have combined with increasing life expectancy to produce the "graying of America," the term often used to describe to the nation's constantly increasing average age. Those ages 65 years and older were 11.2% of the population in 1979[6]

and 12.6% in 2000,[12] and are estimated to be 13.4% by 2010 and 18.5% by 2025 as the last of the baby boomers approach 65 years.[12] Fig. 2-3 shows the change in age distribution of the U.S. population between 1980 and 2000, with Census Bureau projections to the year 2020. The main points to note are the continuing shrinkage of the 29 years and under group as a proportion of the total and the continuing growth in the 65 years and older group. The elderly population is not spread evenly around the country. Although the proportion of persons aged 65 years and older in the United States was 12.6% in 2000, it ranged from 18.1% in Florida to 5.1% in Alaska.

As noted, the U.S. population will continue to get older in future years, with profound social ramifications (e.g., for Social Security, housing, medical care). This aging trend, already well recognized in dentistry by greater attention to geriatric dentistry, will clearly affect the types and distribution of dental services in future years. For example, population trends alone indicate that there is likely to be a greater emphasis on periodontic and maintenance care than on treatment for children, even apart from trends in the oral diseases (see Chapters 19-23).

Geographic Distribution

Extensive migration of people from one region to another has long been a characteristic of the United States. It still is, with 15% of the population changing their address in 1998-99.[13]

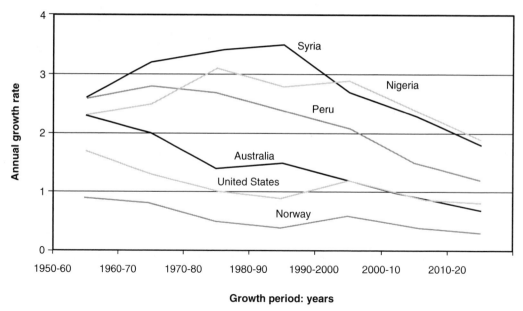

Fig. 2-2 Rates of population growth, actual and projected, in six countries, 1950–60 to 2010–20.[11]

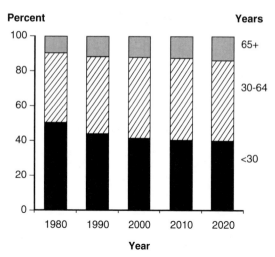

Fig. 2-3 Projected population distribution by age-group in the United States, 1980–2020.[7]

A major trend since 1970 has been population movement from the Northeastern, North Central, and Midwest regions to the South and West, with the rate of population growth in recent years being most pronounced in the mountain states. Fig. 2-4 shows the percentage of total population by region for 2000. In the decade of the 1990s, Nevada's population grew by 66%, Arizona's by 40%, and Colorado's by 30%. By comparison, the population of

Rhode Island grew by only 4.5% and that of Pennsylvania by 3.4%.[17] Since interregional migrants tend to be younger people, the median age in the South, the mountains, and the West is already lower than it is in the Northeast, and the interregional differences are expected to remain or even increase in the years ahead.

Reasons for the "Sun Belt" migration since 1970 are primarily economic. The nation's economic base, once concentrated in the industries of the Northeast and Midwest, has become more spread out, and businesses in the computer age have greater flexibility in choice of location than they used to have. The importance of the Pacific Rim nations in the American

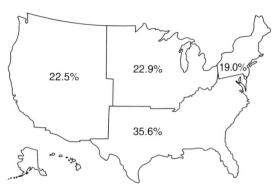

Fig. 2-4 Population distribution by geographic regions in the United States, 2000.[17]

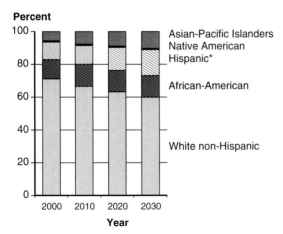

Percent

Asian-Pacific Islanders
Native American
Hispanic*

African-American

White non-Hispanic

Year

Fig. 2-5 Distribution of the U.S. population by race and ethnicity, 2000–30. (*In these data, Hispanics can be of any race.)[17]

economy ensures that the West Coast will remain a leading business area, as well as a stopping place for immigrants from Asia. However, some potential constraints to this pattern of growth could change things. The main one concerns access to limited water supplies, already a major political issue in California. If the rapidly growing cities in the region also develop the social problems of the older northern cities, they could become less attractive places to live.

At a different level, big cities continue to lose population to suburbs and small towns and are financially troubled as job opportunities move out. The provision of dental services in these inner city areas is one of many functions that are adversely affected by these population movements.

Racial and Ethnic Composition

The 2000 census of the United States listed 35.3 million African-Americans, which is 12.8% of the total population. Persons of Hispanic descent numbered 32.4 million, 11.8% of the total, and the number is increasing rapidly.[17] Because the racial and ethnic groups now considered "minorities" are growing rapidly, the term *minority groups* will lose much of its current meaning during the twenty-first century. Fig. 2-5 shows the percentages of various racial and ethnic groups in the United States in 2000 and compares that distribution with the projected distribution over the next three decades. The main features of Fig. 2-5 are the expansion

of the Asian–Pacific Islander population from 4% to 7%, the growth in the Hispanic population from 12% to 19%, and the decrease in the proportion of non-Hispanic whites from 71% to 60% of all Americans.

By 2003 Hispanics had become the largest minority group in the United States. *Hispanic* is a generic term for Spanish-speaking persons and covers a variety of cultures and even races. Most of the Hispanic population is of Mexican heritage, and many live in the Southwest. The large New York Hispanic population is predominantly Puerto Rican, and Cubans are centered in Miami. One third of the Hispanic population in the 2000 census was from other countries in South or Central America or the Caribbean.[17]

Economic Distribution

The federal definition of poverty changes with inflation and in 2003 was set as an annual income of $18,400 for a nonfarm four-person family in the contiguous United States. It is higher in Alaska and Hawaii.[18]

A disturbing trend that became evident during the 1980s, and has continued into the new century, is the increase in the proportion of Americans living in poverty. The proportion of Americans in poverty through the 1980s was 13%-15%.[8] There was some improvement during the 1990s, but by 2002 the poverty rate was 12.1%, up from 11.7% in 2001.[9] The problem of poverty is especially pronounced among America's children and minority populations. The proportion of the nation's children ages 5-17 years living in poverty was 16.7% in 2002, higher than the overall rate. Poverty is also far more pronounced in minority groups: 8% of the non-Hispanic white population, 24% of African-Americans, and 22% of Hispanics were in poverty in 2002.[9]

This heavy burden of poverty has implications for the provision of dental care, because the problem of untreated oral disease is considerably greater among people of low income and education. This issue will be touched on frequently throughout the book.

Summary of Population Trends

The American population is aging, and the so-called minority groups comprise an ever-growing proportion of it. The polarization between richer and poorer segments is showing no signs of ending, and the population continues to shift south and west. Some implications for dentistry are that patients in their eighties and nineties, and even some over 100 years of age, will become common in dental practice, and all dental personnel will need training in the special needs of the older patient. The dental professions will need to face the problems of providing care for the 35 million people in poverty, because the lack of access to dental care among these groups is already a major public health problem and will only grow further in the absence of programmatic action. Adequate provision of dental care for the growing minority populations may require more dentists from those groups, and all dental professionals will need to be culturally competent if they are to be both effective and comfortable working with minorities. These adaptations will all be basic necessities if dental care for minorities is ever to achieve the status in their lives that it has in the lives of the majority.

UTILIZATION OF DENTAL SERVICES

The need for dental care can be defined as that quantity of dental treatment that expert opinion judges ought to be consumed over a certain period for people to achieve the status of being dentally healthy.[4] This professionally determined dental need is sometimes called *normative* need. Need for an individual or population can be expressed as (1) individual items of care required, such as those entered on a patient's chart; (2) total professional time needed for treatment; (3) the numbers of professionals needed for a particular time; or (4) the total cost of such care. *Perceived* need, also referred to as *subjective* or *felt* need, is need for dental care as determined by a patient or the public. Perceived need can often differ considerably from normative need. For example, a dentist might judge that a patient needs a root canal treatment followed by a crown whereas the patient wants the tooth extracted. Demand for dental care is the expression by a patient or the public of a desire to receive dental care to attend to their perceived needs.[3] Related terms are *potential* or *latent* demand, meaning a desire for care that is not being met for some reason.

Utilization is the actual attendance by members of the public at dental treatment facilities to receive dental care. Utilization is expressed as (1) the proportion of a population who visited a dentist within a given time, usually a year, or (2) the average number of visits per person made during a year. The latter measure generally uses the whole population as denominator, so it is weighted by people who did not visit the dentist at all over the time in question.

Annual Dental Attendance

Information on the use of dental services, in addition to a lot of other health-related information, comes from the continuing series of household interviews conducted by the National Center for Health Statistics, an agency within the U.S. Department of Health and Human Services. In 2001, 65.6% of people in the United States reported that they had visited a dentist within the previous year, the highest proportion ever to do so.[19] By way of contrast with utilization some 30 years earlier, only 37% reported visiting a dentist within the previous year in 1957-58.[22]

Utilization of dental services in the United States, as measured by those who reported making at least one dental visit over the previous year, rose modestly during the 1960s, plateaued at about 50% during the 1970s, and then rose noticeably during the 1980s. The upward trend continues. At all times, more women than men reported visiting the dentist. The trend of increasing annual utilization over recent years, for both men and women, is shown in Fig. 2-6.

FACTORS ASSOCIATED WITH THE USE OF DENTAL SERVICES

The profile of the most frequent user of dental services is a white, female, college-educated suburbanite in a higher income bracket, who enjoys good general health and has dental insurance. The profile of the chronic nonuser is a minority male, poorly educated, with little money and certainly no dental insurance. The variations in dental service utilization by demographic and other variables provide some basis for predicting how dental services may be used in the future.

Gender

As seen in Fig. 2-6, women report using dental services more than men do. This finding is so

Percent

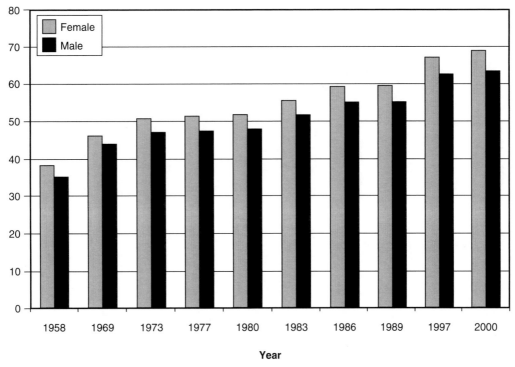

Fig. 2-6 Proportion of the U.S. population who reported having visited a dentist within the previous year, by gender, 1958–2000.[20,22–25]

consistent over time, and so constant in all countries that have studied the issue,[1] that it seems virtually universal—one of the few trends of which we can say it "always" happens. No one really knows why; numerous attempts to explore the issue have not come up with convincing explanations. In the past, vanity has been suggested as a reason, but are women really more vain than men? Unspecified "cultural factors" is another suggestion, but the trend is seen across a wide variety of cultures. It has also been hypothesized that the largely male composition of the dental profession is part of the answer, but that proposition breaks down with evidence from countries such as Finland, where dental professionals are predominantly female.[5] Women also make more physician contacts than do men,[21] so perhaps it is just in the nature of things.

Age

The peak ages for dental visits have traditionally been school age and the late teenage years, with a gradual tailing off with increasing age. Service use has traditionally been low in preschool years, and although it is improving, more than 50% of children aged 2-4 years had still never visited a dentist in 1999.[26] The distribution of dental service use is also the polar opposite of that for physician services, because use of physician services is highest among the youngest and the oldest age-groups, in which use of dental services is the lowest. The utilization curve for medical care services has traditionally been U-shaped, although as Fig. 2-7 shows it is approaching a straight line. The dental services utilization curve is still an inverted U shape. The contrast between use of medical and dental services is particularly important for administration of managed care plans (see Chapter 7).

The traditional tailing off of dental service use with increasing age is changing quite rapidly, however, as tooth retention among older adults increases. Fig. 2-8 shows utilization by age in 1969 compared with that in 1989; the marked increase in the oldest and youngest age-groups is obvious. As Fig. 2-6 shows, overall utilization has increased even further since 1989.

Percent

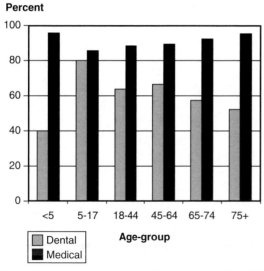

Fig. 2-7 Contrasting patterns in the proportion of the U.S. population using medical and dental services, by age, 1999.[26,27]

Percent

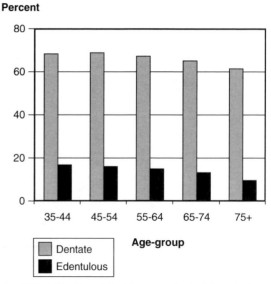

Fig. 2-9 Utilization of dental services by dentate and edentulous persons in the United States, 1989.[25]

Percent

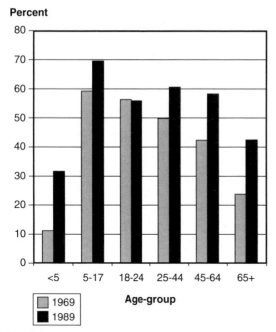

Fig. 2-8 Increases in the utilization of dental services in the United States, 1969–89.[23,25]

Low use of dental services by older adults was once thought to be caused by loss of interest in dental health with age, but in fact is more related to loss of teeth than loss of interest. The difference was first pointed out in an analysis of 1983 data from the National Health Interview Survey, in which it was found that among den-

tate people, there was little decrease in use of dental services with increasing age.[2] That analysis showed that 59.5% of dentate persons ages 65-74 years reported a dental visit within the previous year, which was actually more than the 58.4% utilization among dentate persons ages 25-34 years. Among edentulous persons of all ages, however, annual utilization was only 12.6%. The distribution of annual dental visits for American adults ages 35 years or older in the 1989 National Health Interview Survey, by age and dentate-edentulous status, is shown in Fig. 2-9. When the data are viewed in this way, it is remarkable how uniform dental utilization remains with increasing age when people retain their teeth.

Socioeconomic Status

Socioeconomic status (SES) in the United States is usually measured by years of education and annual income, which not surprisingly are closely correlated. SES is directly related to use of dental services: the higher the SES, the greater the use of dental services. As with gender differences, this relationship is found consistently in all countries, even in those where the cost barrier for dental care has been reduced by public financing. This pattern is illustrated by data for the United States from 1989 presented in Fig. 2-10, which shows utilization for adults 22

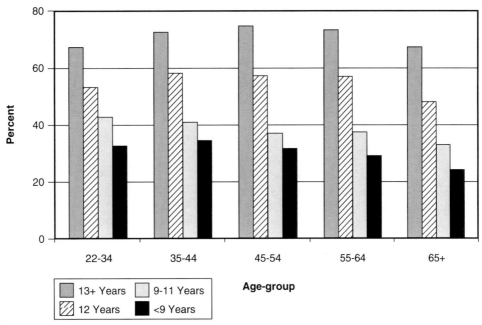

Fig. 2-10 Utilization of dental services by U.S. adults, by years of education received, 1999.[26,27]

years or older, by age, for four different educational levels. The close association between use of dental services and educational levels is obvious, and the difference in the older age-groups is especially marked. The majority of edentulous people, and those without dental insurance, are in the lower educational attainment groups, so those factors would influence the data seen in Fig. 2-10. Once again, it is remarkable how uniform is the use of dental services with increasing age among college-educated people (13+ years of education). Persons with higher incomes also visit the dentist more frequently than do persons with lower incomes, and as noted earlier, income and educational level are tightly correlated in the United States.

The pattern in 1999 was the same: dental visits within the previous year were reported by 38.2% of those with less than a high school diploma and by 80.2% of those with a college degree.[27]

The reasons for this consistent relationship between SES and use of dental services are more complicated than they might appear. It is easy to say that people of lower SES are less interested in oral health or less aware of the value of dental care, but that often-heard assertion is oversimplified. Values, attitudes, and expectations naturally vary among people with differ-

ent income and educational levels. Many lesser-educated people are from backgrounds in which dental care was virtually nonexistent, so they have none of the middle-class culture of which dental care is a part. More obviously, lower SES groups are less able to afford care when it does exist, and they are less likely to have dental insurance. There are fewer dentists in lower SES areas (see Chapter 8), so dental care is less available; people just adapt to living without dental care. Dental insurance has made some difference to the problem of affording care, but experience in a number of countries has long shown that even when the cost barrier is completely removed, clear disparities are still seen in use of dental services among the different socioeconomic groups.

Race and Ethnicity

In 2000 70.2% of white non-Hispanic Americans reported visiting a dentist, compared with 57.5% of non-Hispanic African-Americans and 51.4% of Hispanic Americans.[27] As noted earlier, utilization data are not easy to interpret because race and ethnicity in the United States are inextricably related to wealth and poverty, education, cultural values, and residential location. Hispanics and African-Americans have also suffered historically from deliberate

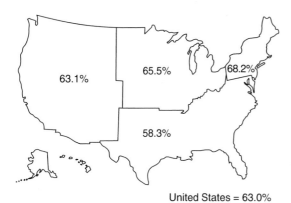

United States = 63.0%

Fig. 2-11 Proportion of the U.S. adult population reporting a dental visit within the previous year, by geographic region, 1999.[27]

exclusion from many care facilities, and there are relatively few dental providers from these groups. The National Health Interview Survey data for 2000 also show that 54.6% of Native Americans and Alaskan natives reported a dental visit, as did 66.3% of Asians.[27] As noted earlier, race and ethnicity are inextricably bound into SES, geographic location, and availability of dental care, so the disparity between whites and minorities in dental visits again reflects all of these factors.

Geographic Location

There are variations in frequency of dental visits by region of the country, as shown in Fig. 2-11. The Northeast, Midwest, and West show similar usage patterns, but the South has a lower level of utilization. The South has the lowest SES ranking of the four regions, as well as the most unfavorable dentist/population ratio, which probably are major factors in explaining these variations.

General Health

People who consider themselves in excellent health visit a dentist more often than those who see themselves as in good or only fair health. Among those who considered themselves to be in "excellent" health, 61.9% reported a visit during 1989 compared with 51.5% who thought their health was "good" and 39.8% who thought it was "fair or poor."[25] Distributions of a similar nature were found among those who had no restriction of activity compared with those whose activity was limited to some degree.

These findings are hardly unexpected, because people whose mobility is restricted quite naturally would find getting to a dentist more difficult. Those in poor general health may be too preoccupied, or too restricted generally, to face going to the dentist. These distributions also are likely to be related to age and to SES.

Dental Insurance

People with dental insurance visit a dentist more often than do people without insurance. The 1999 data showed that 71.9% of adults aged 18–64 years with private dental insurance visited a dentist within the previous year, compared with only 38% of those without.[27] The contrast for all age-groups, using 1989 data, is shown in Fig. 2-12.

These differences are to be expected because dental insurance can substantially reduce the financial burden of dental care. It was mentioned earlier that cost is not as much of a barrier to receiving dental care as is often thought. Even among groups for whom there is no direct charge for dental treatment, the association between utilization of care and SES is still seen. To explain the role of dental insurance, we must look at who has it: professionals, white-collar workers, and members of the larger labor unions who receive group dental care as a fringe benefit of employment. So again, there is likely to be an association with SES as well as some financial incentive for these groups.

FUTURE USE OF DENTAL SERVICES

Should we expect the trend of steadily increasing dental utilization to continue? If so, how far before it hits a ceiling? These questions are of fundamental importance to students and new graduates, and the data presented give us a basis for making estimates.

Apart from gender, the data show that the most powerful correlates of dental utilization are SES, dentate status, and the extent of dental insurance. Overall economic conditions are also a major factor. Prosperity provides more disposable income for people to afford dental care, permits employers to offer more generous dental insurance plans, and leads to a feeling of optimism. If economic conditions in the United States decline over the long term, how-

Percent

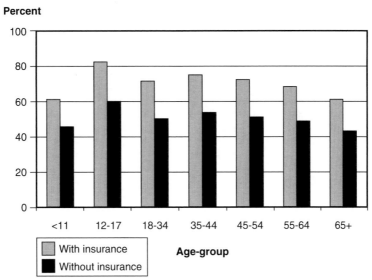

Fig. 2-12 Proportion of U.S. adults reporting a dental visit within the previous year, by age and status of dental insurance, 1989.[25]

ever, more people will be forced out of the middle classes and use of dental services will decline. Poor economic conditions would force many corporations to drop dental insurance, which would also reduce the use of dental services.

Increasing tooth retention (see Chapter 7), especially among the elderly, is reason for optimism about an increase in the use of dental services by the next generation of older Americans. The data clearly show that when people are dentate, they go to the dentist; when they are edentulous, they do not.

As stated earlier, population growth in the United States in recent years has been greatest in the lower SES groups, among African-Americans and Hispanics, groups with relatively low use of dental services. Immigration is a major force in population growth, and many of the new immigrants from the Spanish-speaking world live in deep poverty. Because these groups make up a larger proportion of the population (see Fig. 2-5), rigid adherence to current methods of providing dental care will lead to a decline in utilization. People in these social strata are largely outside the usual dental insurance groups, and the cuts in public health programs through the 1980s left many of them with little opportunity to receive dental care at all, let alone to adopt habits of regular attendance. Growth in the population utilizing dental services will require the introduction of the lower SES population to dental care, which in turn will require more resources in the public health sector to provide the necessary education and acculturation.

SUMMARY

The use of dental services is tied closely to economic developments and demography, neither of which dental personnel can do much to influence. Increasing tooth retention is one factor that tends to increase utilization among older Americans. The utilization patterns of younger generations are harder to predict, and overall utilization could remain at current levels, but with a distributional shift away from younger toward older patients. Specific programs aimed at bringing today's minority groups into the dental care system will also be a major step toward improvement of the nation's oral health. Without such action, utilization of dental services could go into long-term decline.

REFERENCES

1. Gift HC. Utilization of professional dental services. In: Cohen LK, Bryant PS, eds: Social sciences and dentistry: A critical bibliography. Vol II. London: Quintessence/Fédération Dentaire Internationale, 1984:202–66.
2. Ismail AI, Burt BA, Hendershot GE, et al. Findings from the dental care supplement of the National Health Interview Survey, 1983. J Am Dent Assoc 1987; 114:617–21.

3. Jeffers JR, Bognanno MF, Bartlett JC. On the demand versus need for medical services and the concept of "shortage." Am J Public Health 1971;61:46-63.
4. Spencer AJ. The estimation of need for dental care. J Public Health Dent 1980;40:311-27.
5. Tala H. Oral health in Finland. Helsinki: Finnish National Board of Health, 1989.
6. US Department of Commerce, Bureau of the Census. Current population reports: Estimates of the population of the states by age; 1971 to 1979. Series P-25 No. 875. Washington DC: Government Printing Office, 1980.
7. US Department of Commerce, Bureau of the Census. U.S. population estimates by age, sex, race, and Hispanic origin: 1993 to 2050. Series P-25 No. 1104. Washington DC: Government Printing Office, 1994.
8. US Department of Commerce, Bureau of the Census. Measuring the effect of benefits and taxes on income and poverty. Series P-60 No. 186RD. Washington DC: Government Printing Office, 1994.
9. US Department of Commerce, Bureau of the Census. Poverty: 2002 highlights, website: http://www.census.gov/hhes/poverty/poverty02/pov02hi.html. Accessed September 27, 2003.
10. US Department of Commerce, Bureau of the Census. Population clocks, website: http://www.census.gov. Accessed September 12, 2003.
11. US Department of Commerce, Bureau of the Census. IDB summary demographic data, website: http://www.census.gov/ipc/www/idbsum.html. Accessed September 12, 2003.
12. US Department of Commerce, Bureau of the Census. Statistical abstract of the United States, website: http://www.census.gov/prod/2001pubs/statab/sec02.pdf. Accessed September 12, 2003.
13. US Department of Commerce, Bureau of the Census. Statistical abstract of the United States, website: http://www.census.gov/prod/2001pubs/statab/sec01.pdf. Accessed September 18, 2003.
14. US Department of Commerce, Bureau of the Census. 1990 Census lookup server, website: http://homer.ssd.census.gov/cdrom/lookup/1063328204. Accessed September 11, 2003.
15. U.S. Department of Commerce, Bureau of the Census. 2000 Census lookup server, website: http://factfinder.census.gov/servlet/SAFFpeople?_sse=on. Accessed July 31, 2003.
16. US Department of Commerce, Bureau of the Census. Statistical abstract of the United States, website: http://www.census.gov/prod/2001pubs/statab/sec01.pdf. Accessed September 12, 2003.
17. US Department of Commerce, Bureau of the Census. Statistical abstract of the United States, website: http://www.census.gov/prod/2002pubs/01statab/pop.pdf. Accessed September 18, 2003.
18. US Department of Health and Human Services. The 2003 HHS poverty guidelines, website: http://aspe.hhs.gov/poverty/03poverty.htm. Accessed September 27, 2003.
19. US Public Health Service, National Center for Health Statistics. Dental attendance, website: http://www.cdc.gov/nchs/data/hus/tables/2002/02hus080.pdf. Accessed September 18, 2003.
20. US Public Health Service, National Center for Health Statistics. Dental visits in the past year according to certain characteristics. United States selected years 1997–2001, website: http://www.cdc.gov/nchs/data/Tables/2003/03hus078.pdf. Accessed October 27, 2003.
21. US Public Health Service, National Center for Health Statistics. Current estimates from the National Health Interview Survey, 1993. DHHS Publication No. (PHS) 95-1518, Series 10 No. 190. Washington DC: Government Printing Office, 1994.
22. US Public Health Service, National Center for Health Statistics. Dental care: Interval and frequency of visits. United States, June 1957–June 1959. PHS Publication No. 584-B14, Series B No. 14. Washington DC: Government Printing Office, 1960.
23. US Public Health Service, National Center for Health Statistics. Dental visits: Volume and interval since last visit. United States—1969. DHEW Publication No. (HSM) 72-1066, Series 10 No. 76. Washington DC: Government Printing Office, 1972.
24. US Public Health Service, National Center for Health Statistics. Use of dental services and dental health. United States, 1986. DHHS Publication No. (PHS) 88-1593, Series 10 No. 165. Washington DC: Government Printing Office, 1988.
25. US Public Health Service, National Center for Health Statistics. US Health: United States, 1989. DHHS Publication No. (PHS) 93-1511, Series 10 No. 183. Washington DC: Government Printing Office, 1992.
26. US Public Health Service, National Center for Health Statistics. Summary health statistics for U.S. children: National Health Interview Survey 1999. DHHS Publication No. (PHS) 2003-1538, Series 10 No. 210. Washington DC: Government Printing Office, 2003.
27. US Public Health Service, National Center for Health Statistics. Summary health statistics for U.S. adults: National Health Interview Survey 1999. DHHS Publication No. (PHS) 2003-1540, Series 10 No. 212. Washington DC: Government Printing Office, 2003.

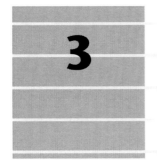

3   Ethics and Responsibility in Dental Care

As noted in Chapter 1, professionalism brings with it the responsibility to adhere to the highest ethical standards. Public trust is the greatest asset that the dental professions possess, and that trust has been hard-earned by the professions' willingness to adhere to ethical practice and to follow through if there has been a breach. Even the most conscientious practitioner will find that ethical dilemmas arise frequently. For example, how does a practitioner respond to a patient who wants all her amalgam restorations removed because she believes they are the cause of her chronic fatigue? What is the practitioner's obligation in treating a patient who is mentally unable to provide his own informed consent? Straight answers are not always easy to find, although ethical codes are intended to give the practitioner guidelines to follow.

This chapter discusses the place of professional ethics in dental care. We discuss the framework for ethical codes, the social and cultural background against which our ethical standards have evolved, ethics in patient care and research, and the role of the professional associations in defining ethical codes.

FRAMEWORK FOR ETHICAL STANDARDS

Ethics, a branch of philosophy and theology, is the systematic study of what is right and good with respect to conduct and character.[27] *Ethics*

has also been used as a generic term for various ways of understanding and examining the moral life.[8] Our understanding of ethics can also be helped by defining some things that ethics is not: it is not a set of rules or restrictions, it is not religion, and it is neither relative nor subjective.[24]

The very nature of moral decisions means that much of the ethics literature asks questions rather than provides answers, and this lack of a "formula" to solve problems can be frustrating for some. Because ethics is the study of both the general nature of morals and of specific moral choices, ethical decisions can vary over time and between locations when cultural standards differ. This means, as noted earlier, that a formula for finding what is the right thing to do in specific circumstances cannot always be provided, only guidelines.

The dictum "First, do no harm" has been around since Hippocrates, around 400 BC, and from that point ethical principles have developed slowly over the centuries. Today there are four basic principles (Box 3-1) that have become widely accepted as guidelines for decision making in biomedical ethical dilemmas and that apply to dental professionals as they do to physicians and nurses.

For a professional organization, these principles then need to be formulated as ethical standards. Standards can take the following forms:

- *Aspirational*, a broadly worded statement of ideals. No precise definitions of right or wrong behavior are given.

BOX 3-1 Summary of Ethical Guidelines for Biomedical Decision Making[8]

1. *Respect for autonomy*, which is respect for all persons and all points of view, and for the decision-making capacities of autonomous persons.
2. *Nonmaleficence*, which basically means to do no harm.
3. *Beneficence*, which encourages one to promote good for others and provides norms for balancing benefits against risks and costs.
4. *Justice;* distributive justice is the fair distribution of social benefits, risks, and costs in the community, an issue that makes up the core of much of our political debate.

- *Educational*, which combine the principles with explicit guidelines that can assist decision making in morally ambiguous situations.
- *Regulatory*, which go a step further and include a set of detailed rules to govern professional conduct and which serve as a basis for adjudicating grievances. Such rules are assumed to be enforceable, with a range of sanctions imposed by the profession if the rules are contravened.[14]

Professions adopt ethical standards because that is part of the professional charge. A patient's trust in a professional comes in part from the expectation that the professional's behavior is governed by norms prescribed by the group.[14] It is also a public expectation that ethical standards be developed and enforced by any profession, a requirement that comes with the privilege of self-regulation.

It was stated earlier that ethical standards are shaped in part by cultural forces, so it is well to examine briefly some of the social and cultural forces that underlie ethical expectations in the United States.

INDIVIDUAL VERSUS SOCIAL RESPONSIBILITY

Who is responsible for health? Is it society as a whole, or is health each individual's responsibility? That is a broad question, to which the answer can only be, "Some of both."

It is well understood today that individual lifestyle choices are a major factor in determining a person's health status. Every educated person knows the basic rules: don't smoke, drink in moderation, eat lots of fresh fruit and vegetables and a varied diet low in saturated fats, get enough sleep, exercise regularly, fasten the car's seatbelt, maintain friendships and social contacts. But what about those individuals who are unfortunate enough to have genetic predispositions to disease or are mentally or physically handicapped? Or those who live in rundown neighborhoods where food choices are limited and there is little opportunity to practice a healthy lifestyle? Many people became addicted to cigarettes at a time when such addiction was not understood, and some became alcoholic or drug-addicted in response to social or personal pressures. The problems these conditions present can be compounded by the individual's inability to pay for necessary medical care. What are the professions' ethical obligations in these and related instances?

If we believed that health is solely an individual responsibility, we would shrug our shoulders, say "Bad luck," and be thankful that these bad things weren't happening to us. But we don't do that. All high-income nations accept some degree of public responsibility through health and social support systems for sick people. In many European countries, Canada, Australia, and New Zealand these systems can be extensive, usually more so than their counterparts in the United States. Arguments in the United States can turn toward whether such programs should exist at all, although most balk at suggestions that the last vestiges of a "safety net" should be removed. There is ongoing vigorous debate, however, about the extent of and eligibility criteria for public financing of health and welfare, and about the right division between public and personal financing for them. American attitudes toward publicly financed social systems are generally not as positive as those in other developed countries, so it is worth looking at how American cultural attitudes toward individualism and social responsibility have evolved.

INDIVIDUALISM IN THE UNITED STATES

Americans rightly cherish their individual rights and freedoms; individualism has been a more powerful cultural force in the United States than in other countries.[9] Many of the settlers who first immigrated to America (voluntary settlers at least) were leaving rigid social, religious, or political systems to seek a new life where they and their children could prosper in an environment that was free of the constraints they had left behind, and where hard work would create its own opportunities and yield its own rewards. An abundance of natural resources and a seemingly limitless frontier gave rise to the attitude that in America people could mold their own destinies largely by their own efforts. Although historical evidence shows that this belief is at best only partly true,[9] it still remains a powerful cultural perception and is still the magnet attracting today's immigrants.

The high point of unfettered laissez-faire capitalism occurred in western Europe around the mid-nineteenth century and in the United States a generation or so later. By the early years of the twentieth century, however, philosophies in Europe were turning away from individualism toward more shared responsibility for basics like housing, education, social security, and health care. Programs grew slowly, but by the 1970s, a network of national state-sponsored social programs was the norm in Europe, less so in the United States. Why the more hesitant growth in America? One reason suggested for the slower development in the United States is that America's relative isolation from external political turbulence during its formative years allowed the development of a more introspective national character than was the case in Europe.[28] Another reason, given that catastrophic events have a way of hastening social change, is that the social devastation wrought by two major wars in the first half of the twentieth century hastened the development of social welfare programs in Europe. The United States largely escaped the social devastation of those wars. It should be remembered, however, that the first Social Security Act in the United States was passed in 1935 in the midst of the Great Depression, which was a catastrophe by any measure.

Another major contribution to the individualist culture in America comes from what is referred to as the *puritan ethic*, which historians consider to have arrived with the first English colonists.[11] Many of these and other pioneers were members of nonconformist religious groups who brought their rigid beliefs about human nature to the new land. These attitudes became part of the American national character, and as such they remain prominent today. Essentially, the puritan ethic is a set of beliefs and attitudes which holds that God rewards people for their honest toil in this life as well as in the next, and that individual wealth or poverty is justified and largely controllable by one's own efforts. It follows that under the puritan ethic the accumulation of great personal wealth can be seen as a reward for virtue and hard work, just as poverty can be seen as a punishment for immorality or laziness. It logically follows that the puritan ethic also involves a strong aversion to paying taxes, especially when the funds can be "wasted" for social programs aimed at helping the "undeserving" poor.

The first serious questioning of individualism in the United States came during the widespread social distress caused by the Great Depression of the 1930s. Many people at that time lost everything through what was clearly no fault of their own, and the response of the federal government was a series of emergency relief measures aimed at avoiding total societal collapse. Most of these no longer exist, although Social Security has not only survived but has become institutionalized as a major entitlement that figures prominently in current political debate. World War II (1939–45) followed the depression, after which the next wave of social activity followed the revelations about the extent and consequences of poverty in the United States during the early 1960s. The Eighty-ninth Congress (1964–65) passed a series of legislative measures intended to improve social equity, the main ones being the Medicare and Medicaid health programs (see Chapter 8), the Voting Rights Act, the Economic Opportunity Act, the Model Cities Act, and the Elementary and Secondary Education Act. This trend was slowed, and in some cases reversed, by the more conservative mood that set in during the 1980s and continues today. This public mood was also affected by a growing awareness of limited resources and a loss of faith in government's ability to solve complex social problems.

RIGHT TO HEALTH CARE

American attitudes, historically shaped by individualism and the puritan ethic, are evolving only slowly to the belief that access to health care is a right rather than a privilege.[7] The "right to health care" is an emotional and often misunderstood concept, one frequently interpreted as "the right to health." Of course, no one has a right to health. Health, an elusive entity to define, is a dynamic state influenced by genetic endowment, nutrition, housing, physical and social environment, life habits, personal attitudes and beliefs, and medical care received, quite possibly in that order of importance. Although medical care has probably been overvalued as a determinant of health,[7,16,18] most individuals at some time in their lives have a need for it, sometimes an urgent need.

Health care has always been rationed in one way or another. The traditional rationing method has been fee for service, meaning that those who can afford care get it, whereas those who cannot afford it do not. The method is simple enough, and it conforms with the puritan ethic, although there is an untold cost in wasted human resources. This philosophy was challenged in the United States during the 1960s, when access to health care was extended to millions of poorer citizens through Medicaid and to the elderly through Medicare (see Chapter 7). As would be expected, one result of better access to care was that public expenditures on medical care increased substantially. When the public mood later swung toward controlling medical care expenditures as the first priority, "managed care" emerged in the 1980s and grew rapidly in the 1990s (see Chapter 7). Managed care appeared to reduce the rate of increase of medical expenditures, although it did so by introducing other forms of rationing (e.g., restricting services and which physicians may be consulted). The ethical problems have multiplied as a result.

PROFESSIONAL ETHICS AND SELF-REGULATION

The American Dental Association (ADA) maintains a code of ethics, which is reviewed and amended periodically by the association's Council on Ethics, Bylaws, and Judicial Affairs.

The current version of the code of ethics can be found on the ADA's website.[4] It has three sections: Principles of Ethics, Code of Professional Conduct, and Advisory Opinions. This code is classified as *aspirational* by the ADA, meaning that it is made up of broad principles, though parts of it seem to be more *educational*, as defined by the standards listed earlier. It is primarily concerned with issues related to the care of patients, though it also deals with the handling of fees, referrals, criticism of colleagues, advertising, and specialty practice. The code has been modified over the years as new issues arise and as societal views on particular issues evolve. It is also influenced by judicial outcomes, which presumably represent social values, as evidenced by growth in the legal advisory opinions in the code. As an example, the 1982 statement on patient selection stated the following:

While dentists, in serving the public, may exercise reasonable discretion in selecting patients for their practices, dentists shall not refuse to accept patients into their practice or deny dental service to patients because of the patient's race, creed, color, sex or national origin.[2]

That statement was unchanged in later versions of the code, but there was an advisory opinion appended after 1988 that dealt primarily with treating infected patients. This opinion stated the following:

A dentist has the general obligation to provide care to those in need. A decision not to provide treatment to an individual because the individual has AIDS or is HIV seropositive, based solely on that fact, is unethical. Decisions with regard to the type of dental treatment provided or referrals made or suggested, in such instances, should be made on the same basis as they are made with other patients, that is, whether the individual dentist believes he or she has need of another's skills, knowledge, equipment or experience and whether the dentist believes, after consultation with the patient's physician if appropriate, the patient's health status would be significantly compromised by the provision of dental treatment.[3]

This advisory opinion, maintained in the 2003 version of the code, is an example of an issue that causes misgivings among some practitioners who do not feel it unethical to turn away a patient who has tested positive for human immunodeficiency virus on the grounds that the health of the dentist and staff would be unduly at risk if treatment were offered. (Note: not only is such behavior unethical, it is also illegal.[12]) By the new century, this issue had advanced to the point where the code in Section 2.E stated the following:

All dentists, regardless of their bloodborne pathogen status, have an ethical obligation to immediately inform any patient who may have been exposed to blood or other potentially infectious material in the dental office of the need for post exposure evaluation and follow-up and to immediately refer the patient to a qualified health care practitioner who can provide postexposure services.[4]

Another area in which professional viewpoints have changed is in reporting bad treatment by other dentists. Not very long ago those in the biomedical professions considered it unethical to report poor treatment by a colleague that they observed. The response to seeing substandard care was very much to close ranks. By the new century, this had turned around, so that Section 4.C reads:

Dentists shall be obliged to report to the appropriate reviewing agency as determined by the local component or constituent society instances of gross or continual faulty treatment by other dentists. Patients should be informed of their present oral health status without disparaging comment about prior services. Dentists issuing a public statement with respect to the profession shall have a reasonable basis to believe that the comments made are true.[4]

Not all aspects of practice are covered by the ADA code of ethics. For example, the obligation to keep current through continuing education and reading the literature, a prime ethical responsibility,[22] is nonetheless given only cursory mention in the ADA code. Although some think that this issue could be stated more strongly, perhaps it is being overtaken by events. Minnesota was the first state to introduce mandatory continuing education as a requirement for dental relicensure in 1969, and by the mid-1990s almost every state had such a requirement in place. It could be argued that continuing education is therefore no longer an ethical responsibility but a legal one. It would be a pity, however, if continuing education came to be interpreted solely as a legal requirement, for uncaring practitioners can always fulfill the requirements on paper without transferring the knowledge to practice. Regulations

aside, the ethical responsibility still remains for practitioners to do their best to keep themselves current.

Community service is also dealt with rather vaguely in the ADA code. Section 3.A of the code states the following:

Since dentists have an obligation to use their skills, knowledge, and experience for the improvement of the dental health of the public and are encouraged to be leaders in their community, dentists in such service shall conduct themselves in such a manner as to maintain or elevate the esteem of the profession.[4]

Some dentists working for a fluoridation campaign in the community, for example, have felt that an appearance on local television may contravene the spirit of the ethical constraint on false and misleading advertising, even if such an appearance would help the campaign. This unduly cautious interpretation has to be respected, though the statement in the code was never intended to preclude such obviously public-spirited activity. Some would like to see Section 3.A of the code strengthened to encourage dentists to work cooperatively with public health authorities for the benefit of the whole community.

Dental hygienists should all be familiar with the code of ethics adopted by the American Dental Hygienists' Association (ADHA).[5] Aspects dealing with professional conduct and patient care are generally similar to those in the ADA code. The ADHA lists as "basic beliefs" that all people should have access to health care and to oral health care, and that people are responsible for their own health and entitled to make choices regarding their health. No such statement about access to health care can be found in the ADA code.

Dentists may not give much thought to the ethical problems of hygienists, but a national survey of ADHA members in the late 1980s disclosed that the three most frequent ethical issues faced by hygienists were (1) observation of a dentist's behavior in conflict with standard infection control procedures; (2) failure of the dentist to refer patients to specialists, such as periodontists; and (3) nondiagnosis of oral disease by the dentist.[17] Although 86% of those responding said that they had some instruction in ethical theory, only 51% reported that they had received instruction in how to cope with these ethical problems. It is noted that the current ADHA code of ethics includes a requirement in the section To the Community and Society for a hygienist to report inappropriate, inadequate, or substandard care to the proper authorities. In the same section there is an item that states, "Recognize and uphold our obligation to provide pro bono service."[5] In general, the ADHA code mixes some assertive statements about dental hygiene practice with a stronger community outlook than is found in the ADA code.

The social climate of recent times has led many professional organizations to develop their own codes of ethics. There are of course some overlaps; ethical conduct for an orthodontist is basically no different than that for a periodontist. But these codes also address matters specific to the discipline. The code of ethics of the American Public Health Association, for example, provides a statement of the key values and beliefs inherent to the public health perspective on which the ethical principles are based.[6] The preamble goes on to say:

The code is neither a new nor an exhaustive system of health ethics. Rather, it highlights the ethical principles that follow from the distinctive characteristics of public health. A key belief worth highlighting, and which underlies several of the ethical principles, is the interdependence of people. This interdependence is the essence of community. Public health not only seeks the health of whole communities but also recognizes that the health of individuals is tied to their life in the community.[6]

The emphasis on community is a keystone of public health (see Chapter 4) and is somewhat at odds with the individualist tradition described earlier. Likewise, the ethical code of the American Association of Public Health Dentistry emphasizes community action and care.[1]

Ethics in Patient Care

The world was jolted by the atrocities, in the name of medical experimentation, committed by Nazi Germany on prisoners in concentration camps during World War II. In a reaction against these appalling crimes, the World Medical Association, a group of national medical associations rather like the FDI (see Chapter 1), adopted the Declaration of Geneva in 1948.[29] The principles of the declaration are in the form of a physician's oath, to be taken at the time of graduation, and the oath itself is shown in Box 3-2. Written in idealistic terms in a time of postwar optimism, its emphasis is on the primacy of patient care, a natural response to the horrors of the war.

Society's bestowing of self-government upon the dental profession comes from its recognition that the profession conducts itself in a fair and honorable manner in its contacts with patients. As discussed in Chapter 1, this is one of the cornerstones of professionalism. The ADA states that "the ADA Code is, in effect, a written expression of the obligations arising from the implied contract between the dental profession and society."[4]

Because the professional has knowledge that the patient does not and is usually in a position to evaluate likely treatment outcomes better than the patient, the professional carries the burden of avoiding paternalism

---

BOX 3-2 Declaration of Geneva, Adopted in 1948 by the World Medical Association[29]

Physician's oath, taken at the time of being admitted as a member of the medical profession:
- I solemnly pledge myself to consecrate my life to the service of humanity.
- I will give to my teachers the respect and gratitude which is their due.
- I will practice my profession with conscience and dignity; the health of my patient will be my first consideration.
- I will maintain by all the means in my power, the honor and the noble traditions of the medical profession; my colleagues will be my brothers.

- I will not permit considerations of religion, nationality, race, party politics or social standing to intervene between my duty and my patient.
- I will maintain the utmost respect for human life from the time of conception, even under threat, I will not use my medical knowledge contrary to the laws of humanity.
- I make these promises solemnly, freely and upon my honor.

and sharing her knowledge and experience with the patient in such a way that the patient can make informed choices.[22] Even with the best of intentions this is frequently difficult to do, especially when a patient yearns to put unqualified trust in the professional:

> *Although intellectually patients—including doctors when they become patients—know that doctors are not infallible, emotionally we want to believe that they are, that they know what they are doing and are capable of doing it. The most skeptical of us longs to leave such skepticism in the waiting room.*[15]

This situation can force the professional to take a paternalistic role, no matter how reluctantly, and it can sharpen the conflict between professional and proprietary values that frequently arises in dental practice.[21] Some have argued that dentistry needs well-defined standards of care to fall back on in such circumstances,[15] but the profession has never been comfortable about defining such standards because of its reluctance to take action that might be seen as infringing upon professional judgment. The ADA took a hesitant step in the direction of standards with its Dental Practice Parameters, adopted by the House of Delegates in 1994–95, in which the broad descriptions of what constitutes acceptable procedures are preceded by statements that the clinical judgment of the dentist comes first. These parameters might have added that dentists have the obligation to form their clinical judgments based on the best available science, rather than a personal preference or unfounded belief, which is the essence of "evidence-based dentistry" (see Chapter 12). Discharging this professional obligation requires dentists to have a good grasp of what constitutes scientific study (see Chapter 13) and to keep up with the literature and with continuing education. Regardless of what framework for studying ethics is used, the requirement to maintain professional competence is a prime ethical responsibility.[22]

Ethics in Research

Researchers bear the responsibility for identifying and propagating truth in matters of science. Much research involves studies with humans and human tissues, as well as with animals, and there are strict rules governing research with both. As with patient care, the first detailed research codes were developed in the shadow of World War II. The revulsion that followed the disclosure of Nazi "experiments" brought serious public scrutiny to patients' rights in research studies and resulted in the 1947 Nuremberg Code,[20] which introduced the requirements that research subjects be able to exercise choice and have the legal and intellectual capacity to give consent, and be able to understand to what they are consenting.[19] Over the years since then, the Nuremberg Code has served as the basis for the extensive legal requirements that many countries have developed to govern the participation of humans in research. In addition to drafting the Declaration of Geneva (see Box 3-2), which was aimed at patient care, the World Medical Association has further refined the subject of the rights of human participants in research through the Declaration of Helsinki in 1964, its subsequent amendments,[30] and a host of national and professional codes since then.

The Declaration of Helsinki uses forthright language: "considerations related to the well-being of the human subject should take precedence over the interests of science and society." For example, with respect to the role of placebos in clinical trials (see Chapter 13), the declaration stated the following in 2000:

> *The benefits, risks, burdens and effectiveness of a new method should be tested against those of the best current prophylactic, diagnostic, and therapeutic methods. This does not exclude the use of placebo, or no treatment, in studies where no proven prophylactic, diagnostic or therapeutic method exists.*[30]

This statement was expanded in the 2002 meeting of the World Medical Association to say:

> *The WMA hereby reaffirms its position that extreme care must be taken in making use of a placebo-controlled trial and that in general this methodology should only be used in the absence of existing proven therapy. However, a placebo-controlled trial may be ethically acceptable, even if proven therapy is available, under the following circumstances:*
>
> • *Where for compelling and scientifically sound methodological reasons its use is necessary to determine the efficacy or safety of a prophylactic, diagnostic or therapeutic method; or*

- *Where a prophylactic, diagnostic or therapeutic method is being investigated for a minor condition and the patients who receive placebo will not be subject to any additional risk of serious or irreversible harm.*[30]

Legal requirements aside, researchers always have the ethical obligation to treat all human research volunteers with respect and dignity. Codes for treatment of animals in research are also now well developed.

In the United States, formulation of codes of ethics in research is now mostly based on the Belmont Report.[25] The National Research Act of 1974 (Public Law 93-348) brought into being the National Commission for the Protection of Human Subjects of Biomedical and Behavioral Research. The commission identified the basic ethical principles intended to underlie the conduct of biomedical and behavioral research involving human subjects, and it developed guidelines to be followed to ensure that such research is so conducted. The report is a statement of basic ethical principles and guidelines to assist in resolving the ethical problems that surround the conduct of research with human subjects.

The International Association for Dental Research (IADR) is the umbrella organization for dental research activities around the world. The IADR approached the ethical issue by adopting a preamble and principles for a code of ethics.[23,24] Given the range of cultural values of those involved in research, the IADR considered that trying to set a single ethical

code for the whole world would seem too authoritarian and would lack local buy-in. Instead, the intent is that its divisions (usually individual countries or groups of countries) will use the preamble and principles, plus other parts of the comprehensive report on ethics,[23] to develop their own codes. Despite periodic encouragement through the IADR and periodic symposia on ethics in research at IADR annual meetings, progress toward this goal has been slow. The IADR's statement of research principles directed at its members, shown in Box 3-3, is clearly *aspirational* in nature. The principles applying specifically to research with human subjects (Box 3-4), included in the IADR's report in 1994 but never formally adopted, are more specifically *educational*. Indeed, parts of these principles have become *regulatory* in the United States and other countries.

The trend in the United States is toward ever-expanding regulations governing research with human subjects, especially documentation of informed consent. Every institution in which research involving human subjects takes place is required to have an institutional review board, whose task it is to review all research proposals before the research actually starts to ensure that regulations for the protection of human subjects have been followed. Punishment for not complying with these regulations can be strict— several major research universities have had all research funding cut off until alleged human subjects' transgressions have been corrected.

BOX 3-4 Ethical Principles for Research Involving Human Subjects[23]

- The research must be scientifically sound, with an identifiable prospect of benefit.
- Human subjects must be selected equitably.
- Risks to humans, and the numbers of humans involved, must both be minimized.
- Voluntary informed consent must be obtained from all human subjects, or from their proxies, before any research is started.
- Human research subjects must be permitted to withdraw from the research at any time and to be assured that such withdrawal will not prejudice any ordinary treatment, if they are receiving any.
- Human subjects must be removed from the research project as soon as there is any indication of possible harm, whether physical or psychological, being done to them as a consequence of their being research subjects.
- The privacy of human subjects and the confidentiality of the data about them must be protected.
- Research results must be written honestly and accurately.

Although some researchers look on institutional review board requirements as a burden, it is better to look on them as just one of the basic requirements of a complete research protocol.

It has been suggested that codes of research ethics need to distinguish between two types of problematic practices: those that are clearly misconduct because they undermine the trustworthiness of science (e.g., data falsification) and those that are unethical but are better described as disrespectful of the work of others. An example of the latter kind is plagiarism, which is unethical but rarely undermines the trustworthiness of science.[10] Plagiarism, which is circumventing attribution to represent the works or ideas of others as one's own, has always been around, but the Internet is highlighting the issue more than ever. Some who would never lift a paragraph from a book or journal without attribution have no such qualms about lifting Internet material without attribution, even though the principles are the same.

DENTISTRY'S ETHICAL CHALLENGE: ACCESS TO CARE FOR EVERYONE

An overriding ethical challenge to the dental professions is to meet their stated aims of bringing oral health care to all members of the public. This commendable goal can only be reached with the right mix of public and private care.

The vast majority of the dentist-attending public receives its dental care from private practitioners. Private practice in the United States is well suited to the healthy, employed, dentally conscious, compliant, middle-class patient for whom accessibility to private care is rarely a problem and who can generally afford necessary treatment (frequently assisted by insurance). Private practice has adapted readily to dental insurance since that payment mechanism began to grow in the 1960s, and this serves to make private practice even more attractive. The oft-used expression "the best dental care in the world" is accurate enough in these circumstances.

Not every prospective dental patient in the United States, however, fits the category just described. As discussed in Chapter 2, some 12% of Americans exist below the federal poverty line, and millions of others live on the fringe of poverty. It is a major challenge for the nation to find ways of making health care accessible to the steady proportion of Americans without health insurance of any kind. This proportion has been around 16%-17% of the population for years, and despite all the hand wringing that goes on it is not getting any lower.[26] (This figure is for general health insurance, not dental insurance. The proportion without dental insurance is around 40%.) Intertwined with the world of poverty are the homeless, the unemployed and unemployable, and the homebound and chronically ill. The marginally mentally retarded, who used to reside in institutions, can have the capacity and the will to work but need social supports to do so. When these are not available, these individuals can drift off into dependency again. For those who remain institutionalized for mental and physical disabilities, dental care is sporadically available at best. Then there is a virtual army of working poor, usually uninsured and in minimum-wage positions, who can find the typical private practice not only expensive but also intimidating.

It is really a cultural matter, for these are groups for whom regular visits to the dentist occupy no place in their lives. Not only is such care financially out of reach for the people concerned, but also many practitioners can signal the message, often inadvertently, that they would prefer not to have to treat such patients. Private practice is most efficient when patients understand the need for care, know how to behave while receiving treatment, and are from the same socioeconomic level as the dentist. But handicapped people take longer to treat and often require special equipment and training to be treated satisfactorily, and the circumstances of poverty mean that the poor are often interested only in minimal care and frequently skip appointments. As a consequence, dental care for many of these groups can only be delivered effectively with public assistance.

Although the need for dental public health services is self-evident, there are still formidable practical problems in making them available. Public services in the United States, in contrast to their counterparts in Canada and Europe, are chronically underfunded. This is partly an offshoot of the individualist culture described earlier, which leads to public services' being held in low esteem. The problem was exacerbated by the severe cuts in public spending for social services during the 1980s,[13] cuts that have gone even deeper since then and are causing new lows in funding as states endure their financial crises of the new century. Even when resources are adequate, treatment for these special groups is usually less efficient than it is for patients in private practice. Oral health needs are often greater, appointments can be missed if a patient has a chance to earn some money instead of going to the dentist, and the mentally or physically disabled just take more time to treat. Many poor people change their place of residence frequently in search of jobs, which makes continuity of care impossible.

There is no simple answer to these problems, though adequate funding of public health departments would enable most of them to be dealt with in time. Continuation of funding would permit adequate staffing and equipment levels, acceptable clinical facilities, special transport where necessary, and community outreach programs to educate the special groups on the benefits of dental care. Adequate funding for public services would assist more dentists and hygienists to receive special training than is possible at present, so that in time the care received by these diverse groups would approach that received by mainstream America. Public treatment programs do not present a threat to private practice, for they aim to care for a different patient.

REFERENCES

1. American Association of Public Health Dentistry. Code of ethics and standards of professional conduct, website: http://www.aaphd.org/prof/prac/law/code/index.asp. Accessed October 10, 2003.
2. American Dental Association, Council on Bylaws and Judicial Affairs. Principles of ethics and code of professional conduct. J Am Dent Assoc 1982;105:493-5.
3. American Dental Association, Council on Ethics, Bylaws, and Judicial Affairs. Principles of ethics and code of professional conduct. J Am Dent Assoc 1988;117:657-61.
4. American Dental Association, Council on Ethics, Bylaws, and Judicial Affairs. ADA Principles of Ethics and Code of Professional Conduct, website: http://www.ada.org/prof/prac/law/code/index.asp. Accessed September 26, 2003.
5. American Dental Hygienists' Association. Code of ethics for dental hygienists, website: http://www.adha.org/aboutadha/codeofethics.htm. Accessed September 26, 2003.
6. American Public Health Association. Public health code of ethics, website: http://www.apha.org/code-ofethics/ethics.htm. Accessed October 10, 2003.
7. Banta D. What is health care? In: Jonas S, ed: Health care delivery in the United States. 1st ed. New York: Springer, 1977:12-39.
8. Beauchamp TL, Childress JF. Principles of biomedical ethics. 5th ed. New York: OUP, 2001.
9. Billington RA. Frontiers. In: Woodward CV, ed: The comparative approach to American history. New York: Basic Books, 1968:75-90.
10. Camenisch PF. The moral foundations of scientific ethics and responsibility. J Dent Res 1996;75:825-31.
11. Cooke A. America. New York: Knopf, 1974.
12. Dentist must pay $100,000 to settle HIV case. ADA News, 1994:Oct 3.
13. Evans CA. A national survey of public health dental services in local health departments. J Public Health Dent 1984;44:112-9.
14. Frankel MS. Developing ethical standards for responsible research. J Dent Res 1996;75:832-5.
15. Friedman JW, Atchison KA. The standard of care: an ethical responsibility of public health dentistry. J Public Health Dent 1993;53:165-9.
16. Fuchs V. Who shall live? Health, economics, and social choice. New York: Basic Books, 1974.

17. Gaston MA, Brown DM, Waring MB. Survey of ethical issues in dental hygiene. J Dent Hyg 1990;64:216-23.
18. Illich I. Medical nemesis: The expropriation of health. New York: Bantam Books, 1976.
19. McCarthy CR. Legal and regulatory considerations concerning research involving human subjects. J Dent Res 1980;59(Spec Issue C):1228-34.
20. Mitscherlich A, Mielke F. Doctors of infamy: The story of the Nazi medical crimes. New York: Schuman, 1949.
21. Nash DA. A tension between two cultures. Dentistry as a profession and dentistry as a proprietary. J Dent Educ 1994;58:301-6.
22. Ozar DT. A framework for studying professional ethics. J Am Coll Dent 1991;58:4,6-9.
23. Proceedings of the IADR Council meeting. J Dent Res 1994;73:1289-94.
24. Shah RM. Introduction: Proceedings of a symposium, Ethics in dental research. J Dent Res 1994;74:1757-8.
25. US Department of Health, Education, and Welfare, National Commission for the Protection of Human Subjects of Biomedical and Behavioral Research. The Belmont Report, April 18, 1979, website: http://www.dhhs.gov/ohrp/humansubjects/guidance/belmont.htm. Accessed February 15, 2004.
26. US Public Health Service, National Center for Health Statistics. Population without health insurance, 1984–2001, website: http://www.cdc.gov/nchs/data/hus/tables/2003/03hus129.pdf. Accessed October 10, 2003.
27. Weinstein BD. Ethics and its role in dentistry. Gen Dent 1992;40:414-7.
28. Woodward CV. The comparability of American history. In: Woodward CV, ed: The comparative approach to American history. New York: Basic Books, 1968: 3-17.
29. World Medical Association. Declaration of Geneva (1948), website: http://www.cirp.org/library/ethics/geneva/. Accessed September 26, 2003.
30. World Medical Association. Policy: World Medical Association Declaration of Helsinki, 1964, with amendments to 2002, website: http://www.wma.net/e/policy/b3.htm. Accessed November 6, 2003.

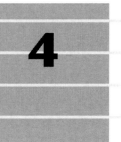

4

The Practice of Dental Public Health

Public health is one of those aspects of life that most people take for granted, or more likely don't think about at all. We take for granted that we can drink a glass of water without thinking about cholera, choose a restaurant without concern about rats in the kitchen, and buy a can of vegetables without worrying about botulism. The source of the occasional outbreak of food poisoning is rapidly identified by the authorities, and thoughts of scarlet fever, typhoid, and poliomyelitis simply never enter our heads. To many of the younger generations, dental caries is almost as distant as those infectious diseases of the past. But this happy state of affairs has not just happened; rather, it is the end point of years of public health research and practice.

The low profile of public health has both good and bad aspects. Although it is good that mostly invisible basics like drains, sewage treatment, fluoridated drinking water, and immunizations against infectious diseases are part of the accepted institutions of modern life, it is not good that most people have so little grasp of how public health functions. It is not good because, without a constituency to press for it, funding and legislation for public health can be eroded, with subsequent threats to health and the quality of life. By way of contrast, everyone is acutely conscious of access, or lack of it, to personal health services, and that subject is a constant political issue. As is described later, development of the public health infrastructure has taken a long time and has required some painful lessons in lifting our quality of life to its present level.

The purpose of this chapter is to examine the structure and practice of dental public health in the United States and to develop the theme that dental public health and private dental practice need to work together for the good of the community's oral health.

WHAT IS PUBLIC HEALTH?

Health is an elusive concept to define. The World Health Organization (WHO) definition[64] is often quoted. It states that "health comprises complete physical, mental, and social well-being and is not merely the absence of disease." Noble indeed, but too idealistic to be of much practical value. A sociologist's more pragmatic definition is that health is "a state of optimum capacity for the performance of valued tasks."[37] This is a more useful definition in that it presents health as a means to an end, that of maximizing the quality of life, rather than as an end in itself.

Public health, too, does not lend itself to easy definition. Among the many definitions that have been formulated, Winslow's is the most widely accepted and quoted. Winslow defined public health as "the science and art of preventing disease, prolonging life, and promoting physical health and efficiency through organized community efforts."[63] The generality of Winslow's definition has much to do with its widespread acceptance; however, it still provides little working knowledge of public health. A more businesslike definition is "the organization and application of public resources to prevent dependency which would otherwise result from disease or injury."[39] In this context, *dependency* is defined as a condition in which external resources, such as an attendant or medication, are required for the individual to carry out the routine activities of daily living. Just as some definitions of public health can be vague and idealistic, however, this one might go too far in viewing dependency as the only outcome to be avoided. Public health should deal with quality-of-life conditions, rather than just those that result in death or dependency, when it is economically reasonable to do so.

A more useful definition of the public health mission, one that accepts health as a means rather than an end, is "fulfilling society's interest in assuring conditions in which people can be healthy."[23] That seems to encompass everything from maintaining the stratospheric ozone layer to picking up the garbage to providing recreational facilities, decent housing, or dental care where needed. This definition might have been ahead of its time in stressing the public responsibility for a healthy physical and social environment, while still leaving some room for personal choices ("... in which people *can* be healthy").

The landmark 1988 report of the Institute of Medicine (IOM), from which the last definition came, went on to describe the functions of public health agencies as the following:
- *Assessment.* The regular collection and dissemination of data on health status, community health needs, and epidemiologic issues.
- *Policy development.* Promotion of the use of the base of scientific knowledge in decision making on policy matters affecting the public's health.
- *Assurance.* The provision of services necessary to achieve mutually agreed-upon goals, either directly, by encouraging other entities to supply them, or by regulation.[23]

These three domains have become the foundation for evaluating many aspects of the public health mission. The 1988 IOM report concentrated primarily on the role of governmental agencies in public health, and it came up with the somber conclusion that the public health system in the United States was "in disarray," deficient in many areas: availability of trained personnel, communications, networking, and of course funding. The IOM's follow-up assessment in 2002 found that too many of those problems were still present.[24]

This 2002 IOM report incorporated the broader, more inclusive view of public health that emerged with the new century. This view states that, although governmental agencies remain the backbone of the public health system, they cannot and should not do the job alone.[24] The IOM report goes beyond the traditional view of individual responsibility for health and bases its recommendations on the concept of *population health*, alluded to in the 1988 IOM definition but not clearly spelled out. *Population health* is defined as "the health of a population as measured by health status indicators and as influenced by social, economic, and physical environments, personal health practices, individual capacity and coping skills, human biology, early childhood development and health services."[24]

The essence of understanding population health is grasping that people's health is a function of more than just biology and other individual clinical factors. People influence, and are influenced by, the values and beliefs of the broader community in which they live and work. To illustrate, exhorting a person to stop smoking is likely to be fruitless if everyone in that individual's world smokes and smoking is an important part of the person's social interactions. Attempts to persuade a person to eat more vegetables will fail when the social environment calls for a diet of deep-fried foods or when local food stores do not stock the needed items. All of this means that, in the promotion of public health, the governmental public health agencies need to coordinate with community-based organizations, the health care delivery system, academia, business, and the media if good population health is to be achieved. A shift of the mindset more toward population health and away from purely individual health could help the United States reduce anomalies such as expenditure of 95% of health care dollars on medical care and biomedical research when there is evidence that behavior and environment are responsible for 70% or more of avoidable mortality.[24] The United States is easily the world leader in health care expenditures, but its scores on health status measures are well down in the list. A shift in where we invest our health care resources would help redress that imbalance, though this is not easy in a society in which individualism is dominant (see Chapter 3).

The core of public health practice is shown in Box 4-1, which presents a succinct definition of the mission and essential services that only public health can provide. This statement, developed by the American Public Health Association in 1994, has since received virtually universal acceptance.

Identifying a Public Health Problem

Ask people in the street whether they consider human immunodeficiency virus (HIV) or West Nile virus a public health problem, and most will give a resoundingly affirmative reply. What about deaths from traffic accidents? There will be more equivocation, even though the number of deaths from road accidents in 2000 was three times higher than that from HIV-related disease.[58] Substance abuse similarly is seen by

most as a major social and public health problem, but fewer would view infant mortality as such a problem, even though the United States had only the twenty-eighth lowest infant mortality rate globally in 1999.[59] So, given that handling a public health problem demands some allocation of resources and some opportunity costs, how is a public health problem determined?

Over the years some criteria have emerged for its definition. Blackerby, for example, listed them as the following: (1) a condition or situation that is a widespread cause of morbidity or mortality, (2) there is a body of knowledge that could be applied to relieve the situation, and (3) this body of knowledge is not being applied.[10] However, these criteria seem unduly restrictive. For example, the Black Death in the fourteenth century killed off one third of the population of Europe in 3 years. There is no question that it was a public health problem, even though there was no body of knowledge on how to deal with it. Subsequent epidemics of typhoid, cholera, yellow fever, and other infectious diseases were also public health problems before there were effective means to deal with them, and the same

---

BOX 4-1   Essential Public Health Services in the United States[3]

Vision: Healthy people in healthy communities.
Mission: Promote physical and mental health and prevent disease, injury, and disability.

What Public Health Does: The *Purpose* of Public Health
- Prevents epidemics and the spread of disease.
- Protects against environmental hazards.
- Prevents injuries.
- Promotes and encourages healthy behaviors and mental health.
- Responds to disasters and assists communities in recovery.
- Assures the quality and accessibility of health services.

How Public Health Serves: The *Practice* of Public Health
- Monitors health status to identify and solve community problems.

- Diagnoses and investigates health problems and health hazards in the community.
- Informs, educates, and empowers people about health issues.
- Mobilizes community partnerships and action to identify and solve health problems.
- Develops policies and plans that support individual and community health efforts.
- Enforces laws and regulations that protect health and ensure safety.
- Links people to needed personal health services and assures the provision of health care when otherwise unavailable.
- Assures a competent public and personal health care workforce.
- Evaluates effectiveness, accessibility, and quality of personal and population-based health services.
- Researches for new insights and innovative solutions to health problems.

can be said for some viral infections today. The nonapplication of effective treatment for a problem, as suggested by Blackerby,[10] is more a breakdown in public organization, funding and personnel resources, or political will.

Additional criteria can broaden the scope of what constitutes a public health problem. Public perception is one, as in the earlier example of the HIV epidemic. If enough of the public perceive a public health problem, then the mandate exists to allocate resources to deal with it. HIV is in that category (even though the only means to prevent its spread, apart from the barrier precautions in medical and dental practice, are behavioral modifications). Not only public perception, but governmental perception, goes far toward defining a public health problem. When a government assigns a problem to its public health agency for attention, virtually by definition it is a public health problem. If a president, governor, or mayor defines a public health problem by decree, then a public health problem it is, whether or not public health professionals agree. These latter two types of decision, legislative mandate and executive order, can have the advantage of ensuring immediate action as well as the potential disadvantage of disturbing the orderly process of program planning and operation.

Today, we can define a public health problem as an issue that meets the following criteria:

- A condition or situation is a widespread actual or potential cause of morbidity or mortality.
- There is a perception on the part of the public, government, or public health authorities that the condition is a public health problem.

To use cigarette smoking as an illustration, the first condition has been satisfied based on the first report of the Surgeon General of the United States in 1964,[53] and there is no question that the second condition has also been met. These criteria have also been met for the HIV epidemic. Allocation of public resources to deal with a recognized problem is a logical consequence, although not a criterion for problem recognition. In the case of cigarette smoking, there has been considerable action through widespread public education campaigns, advertising bans, and efforts to block the sale of cigarettes to minors. On the other hand, the public is divided about condom distribution and needle-exchange programs intended to inhibit the spread of HIV infection.[36]

DEVELOPMENT OF PUBLIC HEALTH IN THE UNITED STATES

Early public health practice in the colonies on the eastern seaboard naturally reflected the English experience. The first English Poor Laws, dating from the seventeenth century, put the burden of caring for the disadvantaged on the local community. This was rational enough in an agrarian society when people didn't move around. However, when the Industrial Revolution took hold in Britain during the late eighteenth century the Poor Laws broke down, for industrialization was really a massive social revolution.[51] Mass migration to the cities created overcrowding, disease, and epidemics, while the laissez-faire economic attitudes of the time led to great wealth for some, the emergence of a middle class, and appalling squalor for many. The Poor Laws, which dealt only with the relief of destitution, were not designed for these completely new kinds of social and health problems.

The ideology of laissez-faire economics in Victorian Britain, combined with an acceptance of Malthusian theories of population growth, led to only grudging action to improve the lot of the destitute. Malthus, a nineteenth-century English country clergyman, wrote that unrestricted growth of population would eventually exceed the expansion of the food supply.[32] The growth of population therefore needed to be checked, either by "moral restraint" or by the inroads of starvation, disease, or other disasters, which Malthus grouped under the cheerful heading of "misery and vice." Public attitudes at the time were such that Malthus struck a sympathetic chord with his views that terrible living conditions were not the result of uneven socioeconomic development but rather the consequence of necessary natural laws. Given these views, new public welfare programs that were degrading to their recipients were perceived as being in the public interest as well as morally justified.

Although British provision of health services subsequently turned full circle to the establishment of a National Health Service in 1948, these condescending views on public health and welfare were the norm when organized public health development began in the United States during the nineteenth century. It was an environment in which public health could not grow much beyond attempts to limit the spread of epidemics. Not surprisingly, nineteenth-century industrialization produced the same pattern of social turbulence in the United States that had occurred earlier in England.[13] At a local level, similar upheavals are seen today, when the abrupt closure of an industry can blight the vacated community. These disruptions take place now in a highly mobile society, in which the old Poor Law approach that local communities should be fully responsible for public assistance is clearly obsolete. In modern-day industrial and postindustrial society such problems are national in scope and should be treated that way.

One reason why the modern American approach to public health and welfare differs from the current British model is that the stern puritan views of the early European settlers have had a more sustained influence on public policy in the United States than they did in Britain and Europe. One expression of the puritan ethic in the United States was that general welfare relief and payment for health care services for the indigent remained linked together longer than they did in European countries, which compounded rather than disentangled the problems.[49] When this is added to the American culture of individualism and the relative freedom from the wartime cycle of social disruption and reform, we can see why communal attitudes toward health and environment have never really flourished in the United States (see Chapter 3).

Dentistry did not play a significant part in the early development of public health in the United States. Oral health was of little concern at a time when the population was decimated periodically by typhoid, diphtheria, cholera, smallpox, and gastroenteric diseases. Although a few public clinics were established on a voluntary basis by dentists as early as the mid-nineteenth century, public dental care facilities remained almost nonexistent for many years.[42] The U.S. Public Health Service, for example, did not employ dentists on a regular basis until 1919,[43] and philanthropic dental clinics such as

Eastman, Forsyth, Guggenheim, Mott, and Strong-Carter all opened between 1910 and 1930.

DENTAL PUBLIC HEALTH

Dental public health is one of the nine board-certified specialties of dentistry in the United States and was certified in 1950. The American Board of Dental Public Health adapted Winslow's definition to develop one subsequently approved by the American Association of Public Health Dentistry, the Oral Health section of the American Public Health Association, and the American Dental Association (ADA). That definition is as follows:

Dental public health is the science and art of preventing and controlling dental diseases and promoting dental health through organized community efforts. It is that form of dental practice which serves the community as a patient rather than the individual. It is concerned with the dental education of the public, with applied dental research, and with the administration of group dental care programs as well as the prevention and control of dental diseases on a community basis.[2]

Implicit in this definition is the requirement that the specialist have broad knowledge and skills in program administration, research methods, the prevention and control of oral diseases, and the methods of financing and providing dental care services. Box 4-2 is the dental corollary of the essential public health functions summarized in Box 4-1, a concise listing of the essential functions of dental public health (sometimes referred to as *core functions*) as adopted by the Association of State and Territorial Dental Directors (ASTDD).

Dentists and dental hygienists have entered the dental public health field when they are employed in the administration of public health programs (which can include health promotion, community prevention, and provision of dental care to specified groups); become faculty members in departments dealing with community-oriented dental practice; or become researchers in epidemiology, prevention, or provision of health services. Some researchers in the behavioral sciences related to dental health can also be considered public health personnel. Dentists become recognized specialists when, in addition to being employed full time

---

BOX 4-2 Essential Public Health Services to Promote Oral Health in the United States[4]

I. Assessment	**III. Assurance**
A. Assess oral health status and needs so that problems can be identified and addressed.	A. Inform, educate, and empower the public regarding oral health problems and solutions.
B. Analyze determinants of identified oral health needs, including resources.	B. Promote and enforce laws and regulations that protect and improve oral health, ensure safety, and ensure accountability for the public's well-being.
C. Assess the fluoridation status of water systems and other sources of fluoride.	C. Link people to needed population-based oral health services, personal oral health services, and support services, and ensure the availability, access, and acceptability of these services by enhancing system capacity, including directly supporting or providing services when necessary.
D. Implement an oral health surveillance system to identify, investigate, and monitor oral health problems and health hazards.	
II. Policy Development	D. Support services and implementation of programs that focus on primary and secondary prevention.
A. Develop plans and policies through a collaborative process that support individual and community oral health efforts to address oral health needs.	E. Ensure that the public health and personal health workforce has the capacity and expertise to address oral health needs effectively.
B. Provide leadership to address oral health problems by maintaining a strong oral health unit within the health agency.	F. Evaluate effectiveness, accessibility, and quality of population-based and personal oral health services.
C. Mobilize community partnerships between and among policy makers, professionals, organizations, groups, the public, and others to identify and implement solutions to oral health problems.	G. Conduct research and support demonstration projects to gain new insights and applications of innovative solutions to oral health problems.

---

in the fields mentioned, they achieve diplomate status with the American Board of Dental Public Health. Specialty certification first requires satisfaction of the educational requirements of the Council on Dental Education of the ADA (i.e., 2 years of accredited advanced graduate education in the specialty, plus fulfillment of a work experience requirement, and then completion of the specialty board examinations).

Although there are fewer than 200 board-certified specialists in dental public health, the specialty's influence on the oral health of the public is greater than those numbers would suggest.[1] Dental public health professionals are employed by federal, state, and local health departments, conduct research in universities and government agencies, and are administrators in professional organizations and various foundations. Dental public health practice gets away from the relative isolation of the dental office, for its programs require cooperative effort with other professionals such as physicians, nurses, engineers, social workers, and nutritionists. Among the rewards is the ability to bring about improvement of the oral health

status of whole populations rather than of single patients. Public health dentists serving in the Indian Health Service of the U.S. Public Health Service, for example, have demonstrated over the last generation their ability to upgrade dental care for several million Native Americans from a bare emergency service to comprehensive care for many, carried out in excellent clinical facilities. Similarly, a dental public health professional who institutes water fluoridation in a community has done more for its oral health than could be achieved in a lifetime of private dental practice.

Achievements of dental public health professionals include conducting the epidemiologic studies that established the basis for community water fluoridation, carrying out clinical trials to demonstrate the effectiveness of fluoride toothpastes and other products, and implementing the associated caries-control programs, which have been fundamental to the decline in caries among children.[1] Oral epidemiologists have also charted the natural progression of periodontal diseases[7] and are beginning to assess other oral conditions about which little is known. Administrators in dental public health pioneered the concept of providing regular dental care in a logical, sequential way for large population groups,[16,17,62] and they demonstrated the increased productivity that efficient use of dental auxiliaries brings to patient care.[31,38] Dental hygienists have proved their value in dental public health well beyond their traditional role as educators. Hygienists act as directors of sealant teams and members of epidemiologic survey teams, and serve in several capacities in the growing field of special programs for the elderly.

To round out this discussion of what dental public health is, it might be useful to state what it is not. It is not just "dentistry for the poor," although provision of care to persons who do not fit the private practice mode is part of it. It is not just "Medicaid dentistry," although improving that creaky and inefficient program is of concern to all health professionals. It is not just conducting surveys of oral health, although monitoring disease trends and collecting data for program planning and evaluation is an integral part of public health practice. It is not just fluoridation, though dental public health has always been in the front line with regard to that public health measure. Similarly, dental public health is not "socialized dentistry," health maintenance organizations, preferred provider organizations, Occupational Safety and Health Administration regulations, infection control, quality assurance, financial support (or lack of it) for dental education, or expansion of functions for dental auxiliaries. And public health is not just the provider of last resort. Its function goes well beyond filling the health care gaps for those whom the private sector cannot or will not treat.

Simply put, dental public health is concern for, and activity directed toward, the improvement and protection of the oral health of the whole population. Narrowing the role of dental public health only to groups defined as high risk or underserved would exclude such basic activities as the efforts to control tobacco exposure, infection control in dental practice, and water fluoridation.[14] Because organized dentistry also espouses the goal of optimum oral health for all, public and private sectors need to understand each other and work cooperatively if this worthy goal is to be achieved.

Collection and Use of Data in Dental Public Health

Information on health conditions is fundamental to public health practice, and the necessary data can be collected in different ways. Data on vital statistics, plus information on certain infections that could become epidemics, are gathered by a process known as *surveillance*. Surveillance in public health is the ongoing systematic collection, analysis, and interpretation of outcome-specific data for planning, implementation, and evaluation of public health practice.[50] It is an ongoing data collection system which uses methods that are quick, simple, and practical and are designed to put as little burden as possible on the busy health professionals who do the reporting. As a result, the data are usually not as accurate as those collected under a strict protocol in research projects, but they are seen as accurate enough for disease monitoring. This is a key concept in public health: data for planning and evaluation, although they must be valid, do not need to be as precise as data in clinical trials. Some data are always better than no data, and the collection of data for public health purposes needs a collection protocol that emphasizes practicality and reliability rather than total precision. One must remember that the main purpose of surveillance is to detect changes in trends or distribution of disease so that investigative or control measures can be initiated if needed. Surveillance is a finger on the pulse of the public's health.

In the United States, surveillance activities at the state and local level are coordinated by the Epidemiology Program Office at the Centers for Disease Control and Prevention (CDC) in Atlanta. Guidelines are available for evaluating surveillance systems.[57] Perhaps the best known of these surveillance systems is the Surveillance, Epidemiology, and End Results (SEER) program for cancer reporting. SEER is the source of virtually all cancer data in the United States (see Chapters 18 and 23), including oral cancer.

Data sources for surveillance activities include the following:
- Vital statistics (e.g., births, deaths)
- Information on reportable diseases (e.g., plague, cholera, yellow fever, and others designated by states)
- Registries (e.g., congential defects, cancer)

• Administrative data collection systems (e.g., hospital discharge data)

Information is mostly collected by *passive surveillance*, which means that, although physicians and hospitals are required to notify appropriate authorities whenever reportable conditions are encountered, the authorities themselves do not actively solicit such data. Some errors of omission undoubtedly occur as a result. On some occasions, health department staff go into the field to collect data, often on a specific disease, for a limited time. The staff people call physicians and hospitals, by arrangement, to obtain data on new cases and to get demographic and other relevant data. This process is known as *active surveillance* and is similar to investigating an outbreak of an infectious disease.

Until recently, the absence of a surveillance system for oral conditions (other than oral cancer, which is included in cancer registries, and cleft lip and palate, for which some states have registries) hampered the development of targeted approaches to improve oral health. Surveillance in dental public health had been largely restricted to surveys, in which samples of a defined population are examined clinically or assessed by questionnaire. Surveys, which have a lot in common with active surveillance, range in scope from large national surveys conducted by federal agencies (see Chapters 19–22), to statewide surveys,[41] to local community surveys conducted by a state or local public health agency.[46] Important though they are, surveys involving clinical examinations can be too expensive and logistically demanding for most state or local agencies. National surveys, conducted by the National Center for Health Statistics and in the past by the National Institute of Dental (and Craniofacial) Research, provide excellent clinical data for the whole nation, but state-level data cannot be pulled out because the sampling system is not so designed. A sampling system that permits extraction of state-level data is possible but would be too expensive for the budget of the National Center for Health Statistics. National data do not work well as a basis for local planning for the reasons given in Box 4-3, and the future of extensive clinical examinations in national surveys is uncertain because of time and cost. More reliance on true surveillance systems, in which

useful data can be collected fairly inexpensively, is needed.

A new approach came with the establishment in the mid-1990s of the National Oral Health Surveillance System, a joint venture of the CDC and ASTDD.[55] Although its full development will take time, this is a historic enterprise in that the traditional suspicion between the federal government and the states has now been replaced by a cooperative federal-state arrangement. States wanting to collect their own survey data can now turn to the CDC for help with financing and expertise, and quite a number have done so. The result is that, within a fairly short period, a number of states have collected valuable data for planning and evaluation that they otherwise would not have obtained. The main focus of the National Oral Health Surveillance System is on data for a set of eight oral health indicators: dental visits, teeth cleaning (professional), complete tooth loss, fluoridation status, caries experience, untreated caries, sealants, and oral cancer. The data themselves are mostly state specific and mostly come from several state-based surveys, of which the most used are the Behavioral Risk Factor Surveillance System (BRFSS)[56] and its companion Youth Risk Behavior Surveillance System (YRBSS). In these telephone surveys, the core questionnaire developed by the CDC can be adapted by a state health agency for its local needs. Use of chewing tobacco is one example of a topic about which some states want information when the habit is known to be a problem, whereas other states do not. The BRFSS telephone surveys began in the early 1980s, and by 1994 all states and territories were participating. These two surveys are the basis for current data on four of the oral health indicators: dental visits, teeth cleaning, complete tooth loss, and fluoridation status.[55]

Some state dental directors have already conducted statewide oral health surveys with CDC assistance; others are planning to do so. Having both statewide clinical data and BRFSS data gives a state an excellent view of conditions when preparing an oral health plan.

National surveys that include a clinical dental examination of the participants usually involve performance of a lengthy and detailed clinical examination, a type of examination that states could not handle because of the cost—time is money in dental public health as

BOX 4-3   Problems Related to the Use of National Surveys As a Type of Surveillance[9]

National surveys that include clinical dental examinations, such as those conducted by the National Center for Health Statistics, provide a superb data set on oral conditions. The data are collected by trained examiners, and the representative sampling ensures that the data are generalizable to the national population. National surveys are not true surveillance, however, and reliance on them as a type of surveillance brings its problems. These can be listed as follows:

- Reliance on primary data collection comes from the underlying view that only trained dental professionals can record oral disease. Experience with the use of death certificates, which are completed by all sorts of untrained persons following standard protocols, is just one example which implies that the traditional attitude has become a dinosaur.
- The protocol for national surveys was developed primarily to record dental caries. However, caries continues to decline, and other conditions are becoming of more concern. In addition, the recording of past disease (restorations and extracted teeth), rather than just present disease, does not fit the philosophy of surveillance and may even be invalid.

- Examination protocols record data at the surface level (caries) and at up to six sites per tooth (periodontitis). However, oral health objectives are stated with the individual person as the unit of measurement, so all that time and effort is probably not well spent.
- There is no good surveillance tool to measure periodontal diseases. Despite all the detailed indexes of periodontal diseases (see Chapter 16), we cannot yet identify a person with active progressing disease.
- Visual-tactile clinical examinations in national surveys consume a lot of resources—they are expensive.
- Public participation in surveys of representative samples of population is diminishing. This problem is severe enough in some instances to introduce response bias—the people who do participate are different in some way from those who do not. This weakens the generalizability of the results, one of the chief reasons for conducting such surveys.
- The sheer logistics of national surveys means that data are nearly always reported late, sometimes years late. More timely data are needed for public health authorities to plan and evaluate programs.

it is anywhere else. Hence, this increased activity in collecting state-level oral health data has been stimulated by the development of quick and simple data collection protocols—again we see the underlying principle of making surveillance as practical as possible, even at the expense of precision.

The first major step toward practical oral health surveillance came in the mid-1990s, when the ASTDD developed a seven-step model for state and local agencies for collecting dental data by choosing from a variety of approaches to best suit local needs.[45] This model includes the planning process, identification of partner organizations, determination of whether new data collection (clinical examinations, telephone surveys, questionnaires) is needed or whether existing data will do, and prioritization of the issues that arise from the collected information. For new data collection (step 4 in the seven-step program), a basic screening survey, plus a training program to use it effectively, has been developed by the ASTDD.[5] Again, the prin-

ciple behind the basic screening survey is to permit limited but valid clinical data to be collected as efficiently and unobtrusively as possible.

WHO has developed and systematized basic methods of data collection for surveillance of oral conditions in all parts of the world into an approach known as *Pathfinder.*[66] Although not all details of these methods have received universal acceptance (see Chapter 16), WHO has succeeded very well in promoting the collection and use of data in parts of the world where previously there was no information at all on oral conditions. The simplicity of the protocol for sampling and data collection permits it to be used by dental personnel with no previous training in survey methods. The country-specific data collected by Pathfinder and other survey methods are maintained in WHO's Global Oral Data Bank.[65]

By whatever method they are collected, dental data are used to identify needs and to plan programs to meet those needs. Functioning programs then need to be evaluated. The results of

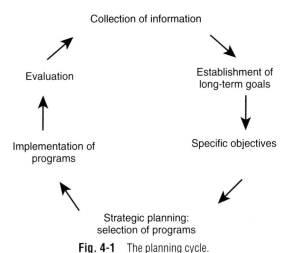

Collection of information

Evaluation

Establishment of
long-term goals

Implementation of
programs

Specific objectives

Strategic planning:
selection of programs

Fig. 4-1   The planning cycle.

evaluation can lead to plan modifications, and so the cycle continues. This ongoing process is known as the planning cycle and is illustrated in simplified form in Fig. 4-1.

Data from surveys or surveillance are part of the foundation on which public policy at federal, state, and local levels is built. Some federal funding programs for dental public health, such as the Maternal and Child Health block grants, require that needs assessment and planning data be submitted each year with a state's application for funds. Agencies and foundations that fund research use oral survey data to help establish their research priorities; dental schools use them when establishing curricula; state agencies can use them in regulating the activities of dentists and hygienists; and dental insurance companies consult them when establishing benefit packages.

We now look at two issues that are major concerns for all of dentistry in the early twenty-first century but that are of particular concern to public health dentistry.

Issues in Dental Public Health

Access to Care

The highest public health post in the country is that of Surgeon General of the United States. In 2000, the Surgeon General at the time, Dr. David Satcher, published a landmark report on oral health in America.[52] Although there had

been many previous Surgeon Generals' reports on various aspects of public health in the past, this was the first report devoted to oral health. This comprehensive and detailed review of all aspects of oral health hammered two principal themes throughout:

1. There are substantial disparities in oral health status between upper and lower socioeconomic groups; between the white mainstream and racial-ethnic minorities; between the insured and uninsured; and between suburban areas and inner city and rural areas.
2. Poor access to care is a major barrier in eliminating these disparities.

Access to care refers to whether or not a person can obtain needed care. In dental care, it involves the following:

- Is there a dental office physically available within a reasonable distance and open at reasonable times?
- Is there transportation to this dental office?
- Does the person have the financial resources, either on his own or through insurance, to pay for dental treatment?
- Can the person take the time to go to the dentist without jeopardizing his job?

If the answer to these four questions is not "yes," then the person has access to dental care that is restricted, at least to some degree.

Dentists in general, and public health dentists in particular, have been aware of the access problem for years. The federal government has also been involved in the issue for years, though not always with great success. Federal programs for Medicaid and designation of dental health professional shortage areas are discussed more fully in Chapters 7 and 8.

Health centers are an approach to improving dental care access for all people that is having some success. Some health centers have been around since the enabling legislation in 1965, and now federal funding assistance is available for community health centers, migrant health centers, programs providing health care for the homeless, and public housing primary care programs that meet federal requirements for their administration. Those that meet the requirements are known as federally qualified health centers (FQHCs). There are some 670 such centers in the United States that are supported by the Bureau of Primary Health Care in the federal

Health Resources and Services Administration.[54] These centers, often referred to as "safety-net" facilities, provide comprehensive care for some 11 million Americans. Care is not totally free, and the centers have some local funding sources and have community-based boards of directors. Nearly 1000 dentists are employed in FQHCs.[54]

Dentists in public health are highly supportive of FQHCs, for they go a long way to reducing access barriers for low-income people. Continuing support of FQHCs will reduce the access problem even further.

Should Preventive Strategies Be Targeted or Population Based?

The idea of predictively identifying caries-susceptible individuals was given renewed emphasis with the decline in caries experience that became evident during the 1980s (see Chapter 20). Most caries and severe periodontitis is now found to be concentrated in relatively small groups; that is, in statistical terms these problems have a *skewed distribution*, which logically leads to the concept of *targeting* these susceptible individuals in preventive programs. Simply put, *targeting* means that it is deemed more efficient for both practitioners and public health administrators to focus prevention efforts on the susceptible minority rather than apply them across the board, including to people who would not necessarily benefit (water fluoridation is an important exception to this philosophy). Targeted prevention is often assumed to be more cost effective than a whole-population strategy, although it has not yet been demonstrated to be so. When administrative costs and the costs of the predictive tests themselves are added, targeting may not always be the most efficient approach. The issue is still the subject of a spirited debate in dentistry, with arguments for[40] and against.[6,22] An interactive computerized approach (the "cariogram") to assess caries risk and demonstrate it graphically has been evaluated for children[21] and for an elderly group,[20] though how best to apply the cariogram remains uncertain.

Most research into caries prediction has been in microbiology, with tests based on the assumption that high counts of *Streptococcus mutans* and lactobacilli indicate high risk of subsequent caries.[28,44,48] Although the causative role of these bacteria in caries is unquestioned,[30] a direct association between bacterial counts and caries incidence is found only within groups, rather than for any one individual.[25] Bacteriologic tests, in general, are highly specific,[60] which means that a low *S. mutans* count accurately predicts low caries experience; however, they have less positive predictive value, that is, a lot of persons who test positive with high *S. mutans* counts will not develop caries (see Chapter 13).

Efforts have also been made to predict caries susceptibility in the permanent dentition from caries experience in the primary dentition. Although some researchers have found correlations, others have not, so this approach cannot be recommended.[61] The reason for the variable correlations is probably that the caries-causing factors during young childhood differ from those in later years.

As caries incidence continues to decline in the economically developed world, it becomes more difficult to predict the susceptible minority in a population.[26] It is also likely that the cost effectiveness of public health efforts to identify susceptible individuals will diminish as the proportion of such individuals decreases.[27] A combination of tests is more effective than any single test,[8] but the more tests used, the higher the cost. One rationale for identifying the highly susceptible individual is to improve cost effectiveness by focusing preventive programs; thus, if it becomes too expensive to identify susceptible persons, that rationale collapses. This is a vexing dilemma, and it inhibits targeting based on individual susceptibility. The philosophical basis for research that equates high disease status with high risk can also be debated, for outcome cannot be used to determine risk[34] and deterministic models do not allow for random effects.[33]

So what should be done about targeting, given that individual targeting is not efficient? There is always the social dimension, which has gained more attention in recent years. Caries is a social disease, given that it has been related to neighborhood characteristics such as the percentage who live in public rather than private housing, rates of poliomyelitis vaccination, car ownership rates, and degree of financial problems.[19] Evidence has long suggested that socioeconomic status is as good a predictor of group susceptibility to caries as any[12,15,18,35] for public health programs. This introduces the idea of *geographic targeting*.[11] In virtually any jurisdiction there is always some area with poor social conditions that can be selected for special attention. States that conduct sealant programs, for example, do not have the resources to go to all schools in a state, so they choose target areas based on the proportion of children eligible for free or subsidized lunch. In Ohio, one such state, the program does not attempt to select out individual "high-risk" children from these schools; all children in selected schools are eligible for treatment where indicated. This is an example of true geographic targeting—the whole population is eligible within specific geographic boundaries. And it works—evaluation results show that such programs have substantially reduced the disparity in sealant placement between children from low-income families and those from higher-income families.[47]

New York also selects geographic areas for its sealant program. The choice is based on socioeconomic status, demonstrated need, community interest, operational feasibility, and ability to comply with the health department's rules and regulations.[29] Evaluation showed that the criteria for selection of individual children and teeth were not well followed by the sealant teams. This finding did not mean that the sealant teams showed a cavalier disregard for the carefully designed criteria; rather, their behavior was a necessary response to pressures from parents and school personnel that the sealant teams found difficult to resist. It indicates yet again that targeting of individuals is just difficult to do in real-life situations.

DIFFERENCES BETWEEN PERSONAL AND COMMUNITY HEALTH CARE

In addition to the similarities between private and public health practice, there also are some notable differences. It is fair to say that most practitioners do not understand the goals of public health. That is unfortunate, because both privately and publicly employed dental professionals are working toward the same end: the oral health of the public. At the philosophic level, one major difference between personal care and public health is that the goals of public health are socially determined, whereas the priorities of private care are only coincidentally related to social goals. Another way of looking

at this distinction is to say that private care seeks to maximize the chance that the best outcome will occur, often unlimited by resource restraints. Public health, on the other hand, seeks to minimize the chance that the worst outcome will occur.[39]

The private practitioner works more or less alone. Decisions the dentist makes are in the context of his training, the legal framework for dental practice, and the dentist-patient relationship. Despite insurance carriers, quality assurance programs, and governmental requirements, the private practitioner is still a relatively independent health care provider. By contrast, the public health professional is a salaried employee who is accountable to both an immediate supervisor and to the taxpayers, represented in such forms as a board of health, a community advisory board, and a governing body. Rarely is a major decision in public health made on one's own.

The public health professional often works in communities with special characteristics of culture, language, socioeconomic status, and values. Public health workers often must care for those outside the mainstream, where those characteristics just mentioned make some groups of people more difficult and often more expensive to reach. The challenge in dental public health practice is that patients in these groups often do not share middle-class values with regard to brushing their teeth, keeping appointments, or making regular dental visits, but they still need care if the professional trust of working for the oral health of the public is to be preserved.

REFERENCES

1. American Association of Public Health Dentistry, American Board of Dental Public Health. Dental public health: the past, present, and future. J Am Dent Assoc 1988;117:171-76.
2. American Dental Association, Council on Dental Accreditation and Licensure. Definitions of special areas of dental practice, website: http://www.ada.org/prof/ed/specialties/definitions.asp. Accessed October 17, 2003.
3. American Public Health Association. The essential services of public health, 1994, website: http://www.apha.org/ppp/science/10ES.htm. Accessed October 16, 2003.
4. Association of State and Territorial Dental Directors. Guidelines for state dental public health programs: revised 2001, website: http://www.astdd.org/docs/ASTDDguidelines.pdf. Accessed October 17, 2003.

5. Association of State and Territorial Dental Directors. ASTDD 2003 Basic Screening Survey, website: http://www.astdd.org/docs/BSSPlanningguide.pdf. Accessed October 24, 2003.

6. Batchelor P, Sheiham A. The limitations of a high-risk approach for the prevention of dental caries. Community Dent Oral Epidemiol 2002;30:302-12.

7. Beck JD, Sharp T, Koch GG, Offenbacher S. A study of attachment loss patterns in survivor teeth at 18 months, 36 months, and 5 years in community-dwelling older adults. J Periodont Res 1997;32:497-505.

8. Beck JD, Weintraub JA, Disney JA, et al. University of North Carolina Caries Risk Assessment Study: comparisons of high risk prediction, any risk prediction, and any risk etiologic models. Community Dent Oral Epidemiol 1992;20:313-21.

9. Beltrán-Aguilar ED, Malvitz DM, Lockwood SA, et al. Oral health surveillance: past, present, and future challenges. J Public Health Dent 2003;63:141-9.

10. Blackerby PE, Jr. Treatment in public health dentistry. In: Pelton WJ, Wisan JM, eds: Dentistry in public health. Philadelphia: Saunders, 1949:187-221.

11. Burt BA. Prevention policies in light of the changed distribution of dental caries. Acta Odontol Scand 1998;56:179-86.

12. Clark BJ, Graves RC, Webster DB, Triol CW. Caries and treatment patterns in children related to school lunch eligibility. J Public Health Dent 1987;47:134-38.

13. Cooke A. America. New York: Knopf, 1974.

14. Corbin SB, Mecklenburg RE. Report on the future of dental public health. J Public Health Dent 1994;54:80-91.

15. Drury TF, Garcia I, Adesanya M. Socioeconomic disparities in adult oral health in the United States. Ann N Y Acad Sci 1999;896:322-4.

16. Freire PS. Planning and conducting an incremental care program. J Am Dent Assoc 1964;68:199-205.

17. Galagan DJ, Law FE, Waterman GE, Spitz GS. Dental health status of children 5 years after completing school care programs. Public Health Rep 1964;79:445-54.

18. Gillcrist JA, Brumley DE, Blackford JU. Community socioeconomic status and children's dental health. J Am Dent Assoc 2001;132:216-22.

19. Gratrix D, Holloway PJ. Factors of deprivation associated with dental caries in young children. Community Dent Health 1994;11:66-70.

20. Hansel Petersson G, Fure S, Bratthall D. Evaluation of a computer-based caries risk assessment program in an elderly group of individuals. Acta Odontol Scand 2003;61:164-71.

21. Hansel Petersson G, Twetman S, Bratthall D. Evaluation of a computer program for caries risk assessment in schoolchildren. Caries Res 2002;36:327-40.

22. Hausen H, Karkkainen S, Seppä L. Application of the high-risk strategy to control dental caries. Community Dent Oral Epidemiol 2000;28:26-34.

23. Institute of Medicine. The future of public health. Washington DC: National Academy Press, 1988.

24. Institute of Medicine. The future of the public's health in the 21st century, 2002, website: http://www.iom.edu/includes/DBFile.asp?id=4165. Accessed October 17, 2003.

25. Kingman A, Little W, Gomez I, et al. Salivary levels of *Streptococcus mutans* and lactobacilli and dental caries experiences in a US adolescent population. Community Dent Oral Epidemiol 1988;16:98-103.

26. Klock B, Emilson CG, Lind SO, et al. Prediction of caries activity in children with today's low caries scores. Community Dent Oral Epidemiol 1989;17:285-88.

27. Koch G. Importance of early determination of caries risk. Int Dent J 1988;38:203-10.

28. Krasse B. Biological factors as indicators of future caries. Int Dent J 1988;38:219-25.

29. Kumar JV, Wadhawan S. Targeting dental sealants in school-based programs: evaluation of an approach. Community Dent Oral Epidemiol 2002;30:210-5.

30. Loesche WJ. Role of *Streptococcus mutans* in human dental decay. Microbiol Rev 1986;50:353-80.

31. Lotzkar SJ, Johnson DW, Thompson MB. Experimental program in expanded functions for dental assistants. Phase 3: experiment with dental teams. J Am Dent Assoc 1971;82:1067-81.

32. Malthus TR. An essay on the principle of population. 7th ed. 1872. Reprint, New York: Kelley, 1971.

33. Manji F, Fejerskov O, Nagelkerke NJ, Baelum VA. Random effects model for some epidemiological features of dental caries. Community Dent Oral Epidemiol 1991;19:324-8.

34. Manji F, Nagelkerke N. What can variations in disease outcome tell us about risk? Community Dent Oral Epidemiol 1990;18:106-7.

35. Milen A. Role of social class in caries occurrence in primary teeth. Int J Epidemiol 1987;16:252-56.

36. Moss AR. Epidemiology and the politics of needle exchange. Am J Public Health 2000;90:1385-7.

37. Parsons T. Definitions of health and illness in light of American values and social structures. In: Jaco EG, ed: Patients, physicians, and illness. Glencoe IL: Free Press, 1958:165-87.

38. Pelton WJ, McNeal DR, Goggins JK. Student dental health program of the University of Alabama in Birmingham: VI. Chair time expended for the delivery of services. Ala J Med Sci 1971;8:373-77.

39. Pickett G, Hanlon JJ. Public health: administration and practice. 9th ed. St. Louis: Times Mirror/Mosby, 1990.

40. Pienihakkinen K, Jokela J. Clinical outcomes of risk-based caries prevention in preschool-aged children. Community Dent Oral Epidemiol 2002;30:143-50.

41. Rozier RG, Dudney GG, Spratt CJ. The 1986–87 North Carolina school oral health survey. Raleigh: North Carolina Department of Environment, Health, and Natural Resources, 1991.

42. Salzmann JA. Principles and practice of public health dentistry. Boston: Stratford, 1937.

43. Schmekebier LF. The Public Health Service. Baltimore: Johns Hopkins, 1923.

44. Seppä L, Pollanen L, Hausen H. *Streptococcus mutans* counts obtained by a dip-slide method in relation to caries frequency, sucrose intake and flow rate of saliva. Caries Res 1988;22:226-29.

45. Siegal MD, Kuthy RA. Assessing oral health needs; ASTDD seven-step model. Jefferson City MO:

Association of State and Territorial Dental Directors, 1995.

46. Siegal MD, Martin B, Kuthy RA. Usefulness of a local oral health survey in program development. J Public Health Dent 1988;48:121-24.

47. Siegal MD, Miller DL, Moffat D, et al. Impact of targeted, school-based dental sealant programs in reducing racial and economic disparities in sealant prevalence among schoolchildren—Ohio, 1998–1999. MMWR Morb Mortal Wkly Rep 2001;50:736-8.

48. Stecksen-Blicks C. Lactobacilli and *Streptococcus mutans* in saliva, diet and caries increment in 8- and 13-year-old children. Scand J Dent Res 1987;95:18-26.

49. Stevens R, Stevens R. Medicaid: Anatomy of a dilemma. Law Contemp Probl 1970;35:348–425.

50. Thacker SB, Berkelman RL. Public health surveillance in the United States. Epidemiol Rev 1988;10:164-90.

51. Trevelyan GM. English social history. 1942. Reprint, London: Pelican Books, 1967.

52. US Department of Health and Human Services. Oral health in America: A report of the Surgeon General. Rockville MD: National Institutes of Health, 2000.

53. US Public Health Service. Smoking and health. Report of the Advisory Committee to the Surgeon General of the Public Health Service. PHS Publication No. 1103. Washington DC: Government Printing Office, 1964.

54. US Public Health Service, Bureau of Primary Health Care. Home page, website: http://bphc.hrsa.gov/. Accessed October 17, 2003.

55. US Public Health Service, Centers for Disease Control and Prevention. National Oral Health Surveillance System (NOHSS), website: http://www.cdc.gov/nohss/index.htm. Accessed October 21, 2003.

56. US Public Health Service, Centers for Disease Control and Prevention. Behavioral Risk Factor Surveillance System, website: http://www.cdc.gov/brfss/about.htm. Accessed October 21, 2003.

57. US Public Health Service, Centers for Disease Control and Prevention. Updated guidelines for evaluating public health surveillance systems, website: http://www.cdc.gov/mmwr/preview/mmwrhtml/rr5013a1.htm. Accessed December 16, 2003.

58. US Public Health Service, National Center for Health Statistics. Age-adjusted death rates for selected causes of death, according to sex, race, and Hispanic origin: United States, selected years 1950-2001, website: http://www.cdc.gov/nchs/data/hus/tables/2003/03hus029.pdf. Accessed October 16, 2003.

59. US Public Health Service, National Center for Health Statistics. Infant mortality rates and international rankings: Selected countries, selected years, 1960–99, website: http://www.cdc.gov/nchs/data/hus/tables/2003/03hus025.pdf. Accessed October 16, 2003.

60. Van Houte J. Microbiological predictors of caries risk. Adv Dent Res 1993;7:87-96.

61. Van Palenstein Helderman WH, ter Pelkwijk L, Van Dijk JWE. Caries in fissures of permanent first molars as a predictor for caries increment. Community Dent Oral Epidemiol 1989;17:282-84.

62. Waterman GE. The Richmond-Woonsocket studies on dental care services for school children. J Am Dent Assoc 1956;52:676-84.

63. Winslow CEA. The untilled fields of public health. Mod Med 1920;2:183-91.

64. World Health Organization. Constitution of the World Health Organization. Geneva: WHO, 1946:3.

65. World Health Organization. WHO oral health country/area profile programme, website: http://www.whocollab.odont.lu.se/index.html. Accessed October 24, 2003.

66. World Health Organization. Oral health surveys; basic methods. 4th ed. Geneva: WHO, 1997.

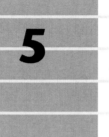

5 Oral Health Promotion

Is any individual's health status solely her own responsibility, or does society have some part to play in it? We discussed this issue when defining health in Chapter 4 and concluded that both were involved. Put concisely, the individual is responsible for the *conduct* of her life, but society is largely responsible for the *conditions* of her life.[5] The achievement of health requires a set of social conditions within which the individual can then take actions that enhance health.[85]

This chapter discusses the promotion of oral health in the community and among individual patients. Issues of public policy that permit people to maximize their oral health are considered and some examples of major community-based health promotional interventions are assessed. Because cultural values strongly influence health promotion, public and professional attitudes and beliefs are also examined. As an example of how health promotional principles might be applied at the community level, the role of health professionals in promoting water fluoridation is assessed. We do not go into details of educational theory in this chapter; a number of excellent texts provide such details.[39–41,83]

WHAT IS HEALTH PROMOTION?

Community health promotion is defined as any combination of educational, social, and environmental actions conducive to the health of a population of a geographically defined area.[39] Another definition is that health promotion is a set of processes that can be employed to change the conditions that affect health, so that targets are not always the people whose health is in question.[83] Yet another simply states that health promotion is the process of enabling people to increase control over, and to improve, their health.[101] These definitions all envision roles for the health professional, political leaders, society as a whole, and the individual in maximizing health status. Health education is an important part of health promotion, though it is just one part of the larger entity. Health education is defined as any combination of learning opportunities designed to facilitate voluntary adaptations of behavior that are conducive to health.[38] Health education and health promotion have been described as the mechanisms that connect prevention activities, policy development, and program implementation, maintenance, and evaluation.[31]

Although health is an elusive entity to define, we stated in Chapter 4 that it is more than the mere absence of disease and less than the idealistic definition of the World Health Organization (WHO). Greenberg refers to health as a quality of life with social, mental, emotional, spiritual, and physical functions,[41] and he points out that too much emphasis is usually given to the physical function at the expense of the others. In effect, Greenberg is arguing for a "holistic" view of health. He defines *wellness* as a positive state, the degree to which a person has reached her potential regarding each of the components of health.

Because it is the integration of social, mental, emotional, spiritual, and physical components at any level of health or illness, people can be healthy or ill and still possess a high degree of wellness.

At least among the better educated, the traditionally narrow view that equates health with the absence of disease has already given way to a broader, positive concept based on Greenberg's definition. In day-to-day terms, attainment and maintenance of health are no longer just a matter of an annual medical checkup, but also include engaging in regular exercise, making sensible food choices, getting sufficient sleep, having some form of spiritual belief, maintaining friendships, and indulging in a diversity of interests. Society is much less tolerant of destructive behaviors like smoking and drunken driving than it once was, and interest in healthy eating has never been higher.

It is recognized, however, that this positive view has not permeated all strata of society to the same extent.[33,95] There are good reasons why. At the individual level, education results in greater access to knowledge and information, and it develops information-seeking attitudes and skills. In addition, better-educated people usually lead lives that give them more opportunities to develop healthy lifestyles than do those who have to spend more time and energy in just making ends meet. At the community level, the characteristics of the neighborhood and communities in which people live and work have become recognized as prime determinants of health status.[50,51]

This concept of health promotion began to take root during the 1970s and was much influenced by a working paper put out by the Canadian Minister for Health at the time, Marc Lalonde. More of a visionary than many political leaders, Lalonde introduced the health field concept, a new idea at the time, as he tried to evaluate the impact of Canadian health policies.[57] Specifically, Canada had moved to a program of equal access to health care for all citizens through public financing, and Lalonde had observed that increased access to health care services did not by itself improve health status.

The health field concept, as Lalonde envisioned it, is a framework for the evaluation and analysis of community health needs that includes assessments of human biology, environment, lifestyle, and health care organization in more or less equal parts. Before Lalonde's analysis, such assessments had usually been dominated by health care organizations (i.e., the view was that health services equal health), but today we are much more aware of the importance of the other factors as well. The cohesion and functionality of a community is often expressed as its *social capital*, which consists of features of social organization such as trust between citizens, norms of reciprocity, and group membership, that facilitate collective action.[52] The wider concept of health promotion includes the investment of social capital, which can relate health status to availability of community amenities such as libraries, recreational facilities, biking and walking trails, public transportation, and employment opportunities, things that are provided by the community rather than by the individual. Factors that were seen by the influential Ottawa Charter as fundamental preconditions for health are shown in Box 5-1.

In an ideal world, governments would have policies in place that do not interfere with peoples' lives but that give them the freedom to make informed choices on their health behavior. As a negative example, homeless people are preoccupied with fundamentals of day-to-day survival and live in a world that is deficient in many of the preconditions for health listed in Box 5-1. As a result, they have little opportunity to make rational choices on matters affecting their health. The first step in promoting health among the homeless, therefore, is to provide

BOX 5-1 Fundamental Social Preconditions and Resources for the Achievement of Health, as Defined by the Ottawa Charter for Health Promotion[101]

- Peace
- Education
- Shelter
- Food
- Income
- A stable ecosystem
- Sustainable resources
- Social justice and equity

decent housing and adequate food, and do whatever else can be done to improve self-esteem. If we hark back to the definition of health promotion, we see that such steps represent the organizational, social-economic, and environmental supports that are basic to the development of healthy behaviors. Governmental action in this area often means legislation. In the high-income countries we are familiar with specific laws on matters like cigarette advertising, use of seatbelts and safety helmets, and immunizations for children. These laws, through which society accepts some constraints on absolute freedom in the interest of public health, are in addition to the public health codes covering water supplies, food preparation, and public accommodations. In the oral health area, legislation that mandates or permits water fluoridation, and the statutory basis in some countries for school dental programs, are both organizational aspects of oral health promotion.

COMMUNITY-BASED HEALTH PROMOTION

The principal community-based health promotion programs that have been conducted in the United States have been directed at reducing the risk for cardiovascular disease. Nothing on this scale has been carried out for oral health, though there are issues in these programs from which dentistry could well learn for implementation of its own health promotional programs.

Three major community-based programs aimed at reducing the risk factors for cardiovascular disease were implemented in the United States during the 1980s. All were focused on individual risk factors, because an appreciation of the role of social factors was still in its infancy at the time. These programs were conducted in Pawtucket, Rhode Island,[8] the state of Minnesota,[46] and five cities in central California.[27] These projects were completed by the 1990s, and in retrospect they were all modestly successful, though not as conclusive as had been hoped.[2,28,35] Certainly a great deal was learned about the benefits and limitations of large-scale health promotion programs.

The projects had some features in common:
- The extensive use of epidemiologic data in planning. Specific data on the frequency of

heart attacks in the communities concerned was added to research information on the major risk factors: hypertension, obesity, sedentary lifestyle, smoking, high-fat diets, and high blood cholesterol levels.
- Educational and interventional activities were based on currently accepted theories of health behavior.
- Clearly specified hypotheses, involving measurable exposures and outcomes, could be readily tested to evaluate the success of the projects.

To assess the impact of community-wide health promotion, it is worth looking at one of these projects in detail. The purpose of the Stanford Five-Cities study, as an example, was to seek reductions in the cardiovascular risk factors of smoking behavior, high blood cholesterol level, and hypertension. The project began as the Stanford Three-Community study in 1972,[23] and promising results led to its expansion to become the Five-Cities study. The project was designed to test whether a comprehensive program of community organization and health education would produce favorable changes in risk factors, morbidity, and mortality in two treatment cities compared to three control cities over a period of 6 years. The methods chosen for comparative study were mass media health education in one city, and mass media education plus personal instruction for those at highest risk in the second.

This 6-year intervention was influenced by Bandura's social learning theory.[4] This theory states that reciprocal relationships exist between an individual's behavior, cognitive processes, and the external environment, and that these relationships are mediated by self-efficacy: the individual's belief in her competence to carry out specific actions. In practical terms, this theory states that the professional office environment is not conducive to learning and maintaining good health behavior; such activities are best carried out at home, at work, and in other community settings. The Stanford Five-Cities study was a sophisticated program, making use of community organization principles and social marketing methods.

The Stanford study design included biennial assessments of cohorts followed over the 6 years and assessments of independent cross-sectional samples at 2-year intervals. Results at the end of the 6 years showed that the treatment cities exhibited greater improvements with regard to most of the risk factors being measured (cardiovascular disease knowledge, blood pressure, smoking behavior, resting pulse) than the controls.[22,29] Mixed results were found for body mass index,[86] which suggests less than fully effective results. What were not expected were the improvements in the control cities, presumably due to the widespread media publicity given to cardiovascular risk factors.[30] Although findings overall were positive, the beneficial trends in the control cities made the net changes attributable to the program rather small.

A major question after such large-scale projects is whether the good results achieved are maintained after the project's completion. To answer that question, participants in the Stanford project were followed up 4 years after the main project finished. Small net improvements in most risk factors measured were maintained in the treatment cities relative to the control cities, though trends in body mass index went the wrong way in both treatment and control cities.[97] This outcome was similar to the one found in the Minnesota Heart Health Program, in which strong efforts at obesity control ended in failure,[49] and in Pawtucket, where levels of physical exercise did not increase.[19] The conclusion of the Stanford researchers was that the modest net differences suggested that new designs and forms of intervention are needed to better reach those at highest risk. Later reflections on the Stanford study in health promotion included the rather humble admission that the researchers had learned little about the factors which determine population-level change, and the lowering of risk factors in the control cities was clearly unexpected.[27]

When the combined success of the interventions in all three of the cardiovascular health promotion projects was assessed, trends were in the favorable direction, although most differences between treatments and controls were not statistically significant.[64,96] There was agreement, however, that the success of community interventions of this type was linked to the community organization process.[68]

Cardiovascular disease is a life-and-death matter, and the modest impact of these extensive and expensive health promotional interventions on such a serious disease is sobering.

At the same time, most risk factors showed an overall secular decline in both treatment and control cities, which is good news. The conclusion that we really don't know much about how to effect community-wide behavioral change seems the correct one here. For dentistry, it is worth reflecting on the lessons from these cardiovascular studies, given that apart from oral cancer we do not deal with life-threatening diseases.

PROMOTION OF ORAL HEALTH

Health promotion requires active interventions at different levels and by different organizations, and the health professional organizations are certainly important components. Campaigns conducted by professional organizations themselves, however, are often a mix of health promotion and public relations. Public relations exercises may have their place, but they should not be confused with health promotion. The American Dental Association (ADA), for example, launched a television campaign in the mid-1980s to increase patient visits among adults over age 30 years, mostly by presenting the health benefits of regular dental care.[15] Although the ADA's House of Delegates voted not to finance this campaign nationally, several state associations picked it up for local use. The success of this campaign, in terms of improving oral health, is uncertain because of its narrow focus. The same could be said about an institution like National Children's Dental Health Month and special events in that month like Give Kids a Smile! Day. The activities aimed at getting dentists more involved in smoking cessation among their patients (see Chapter 30), although obviously focused on the individual patient, are also a contribution toward community health promotion.

Dentists and dental hygienists spend a lot of time in educating their patients, and the public, on the value of good oral health. Organized campaigns such as the ADA's Children's Dental Health Month have also been conducted fairly regularly. All this effort has probably had some impact, though we can't tell just how much. There is little question that over the last few decades the status of the public's oral health, and its standards of oral hygiene, have continued to improve. Once again, however, we do not know how much of this can be attributed directly to oral health education and how much to rising living standards and norms of personal cleanliness and grooming (i.e., the type of "external" influences that were noted earlier in the Stanford Five-City study: good things happening outside of our control). We can also accept that the rising utilization of dental services (see Chapter 2) is evidence of increasing public acceptance of the value of good oral health.

The mass media, especially television, are frequently used in promotional programs in oral health, but again the effects are hard to measure. For example, a national campaign in Finland in the early 1980s used the mass media to try to increase demand for dental services. Although the proportion of adults making an annual dental visit rose from 54% to 65%, the researchers concluded that the mass media were not effective in changing health behavior.[69] The value of the mass media in promoting dental visits and good oral health behavior was also questioned after a 1980s campaign in the Netherlands.[78] These findings were not really surprising, because researchers earlier had defined the limitations of mass media in changing health behavior.[9,32] The Stanford Five-City cardiovascular intervention program, described earlier, also reached ambivalent conclusions on intervention strategies that relied heavily on television and newspapers.

One problem in defining a role for mass media in oral health promotion is that evaluation carried out by market researchers, accustomed to dealing with commercial advertisements, is often "process" evaluation that stops short of detecting outcomes. An example is seen in the evaluation of a Michigan television campaign in the late 1980s. Correct description of the advertisements was given by 22% of a random sample of adults, up from 13% early in the campaign. Aided recall, meaning recall after some prompting, rose from 23% to 32%, and 12% of those interviewed said they were influenced by the commercials.[56] Recording whether the message was seen and understood is relatively cheap and easy to do by an experienced social research group, but measuring the actual impact of the campaign on oral health is more complicated.

An example of an oral health promotional campaign is a sealant program conducted by the Ohio Department of Health.[82] Results of an oral health survey of children in Columbus, which showed that caries experience was greatest among poorer children, were used as the rationale for grant support, which permitted continuation, and even expansion, of the sealant program in the city schools. But the data served wider purposes as well. They were invaluable in "marketing" the program among influential legislators, in developing a supportive constituency among parents and school personnel, and in educating the public. The end result was a preventive program that not only directly improved the oral health of the children concerned but that had the solid support of the community because its purposes were well understood and accepted.

Oral health promotion is more encompassing than dental health education and takes a broader approach to closing the oral health gap between the social strata. Oral health promotional efforts today should include the *common risk factor approach*, which brings oral health into the health mainstream by recognizing that much general health promotion (e.g., concerning tobacco use, diet, and hygiene) is also related to oral health.[81] The role of social capital in oral health promotion is still being worked out, though some role for it is generally accepted. The growth of interest in epidemiology across the life course, which addresses the question of how events and circumstances in childhood affect health in adulthood,[93] will also help give oral health promotion a stronger scientific basis.

GOALS FOR ORAL HEALTH

At the international level, global goals for oral health in the year 2000 were established by the Fédération Dentaire Internationale (FDI, now the World Dental Federation) in 1982 and are listed in Box 5-2. These goals were developed after a great deal of discussion and with the strong involvement of WHO. They have passed into history now but are shown because they pretty well did what they were supposed to do—that is, stimulate individual countries either to adopt them as they are for their own goals or to modify them to fit their own circumstances. The FDI followed up on these global goals with its guidelines for national dental associations to use in promoting the oral health of the public.[12] Unfortunately, new goals for the new century have not been established.

BOX 5-2   Global Goals for Oral Health in the Year 2000, Established by the World Dental Federation and the World Health Organization in 1982[24]

- 50% of 5- to 6-year-olds will be caries-free.
- The global average will be no more than three decayed, missing, and filled teeth at age 12.
- 85% of the population will retain all their permanent teeth at age 18.
- A 50% reduction from present levels of edentulousness at ages 35-40 years will be achieved.

- A 25% reduction from present levels of edentulousness at age 65 years and older will be achieved.
- A database will be established for monitoring changes in oral health.

The United States first adopted its own national goals for health in 1980[88] as part of a 10-year plan for improvement of national health status by 1990. A midcourse review[91] found that some of the oral health goals in this plan had already been achieved, others clearly would not be achieved, and still others could not be evaluated because of a lack of data. In the process, it became clearer than ever that goals were not going to be met without specific programs and that programs required funds and trained personnel if they were to have any impact. National goals for health for the year 2000 were announced in September 1990,[89] with generally favorable media publicity. Among them were 16 goals for oral health. Midcourse reviews found that, despite some progress, disparities were growing between some minority groups and the main population in some areas. As a result, new subobjectives were established for Native Americans for reduction of the number of edentulous persons and for African-Americans for the prevention of oropharyngeal cancer.[90]

The goals for the year 2010, known as *Healthy People 2010*,[87] included 467 health objectives altogether. One could argue whether a much smaller number of goals, perhaps a set that could be easily recalled, might be more effective—it is hard to remember 467 objectives, and it could be that the nation's resources are spread thin with that many. The purpose of the *Healthy People* objectives is to give guidance to public health departments in their choice of programs, to guide the nation's public health research agenda. The 17 oral health objectives from *Healthy People* are shown in Box 5-3. They are, of course, not everything that could be listed in the pursuit of oral health but are more of a consen-

sus priority listing. Some baseline data are presented for each objective (not shown in Box 5-3). These provide the point of reference against which progress will be measured.

As just mentioned, however, goals without a program to achieve them are little more than wishful thinking. Plans to reach the *Healthy People 2010* goals require a high level of agreement and coordination among federal, state, and local agencies, and between public and private sectors. Successful achievement of most goals is unlikely without the allocation of sufficient resources for the necessary programs.

KNOWLEDGE AND ATTITUDES ABOUT ORAL HEALTH

People demonstrate a wide variety of attitudes toward teeth, dental care, and dentists. These attitudes naturally reflect their own experiences, cultural perceptions, familial beliefs, and other life situations, and these attitudes strongly influence oral health behavior.[10,34,63,98,103]

Negative attitudes toward oral health are a strong factor in loss of teeth (see Chapter 19). For example, it was found in the Netherlands that the majority of decisions for full-mouth extractions are made by the patient rather than the dentist,[7] and a Scottish study related total tooth loss to negative attitudes about dental care and passivity about tooth loss.[70] It is possible that these negative attitudes might be unconsciously encouraged by dental professionals if the patient does not fit the "good patient" model. Not surprisingly, dentists' profile of a "good" patient was one who shared the dentist's values on oral health, complied with advice and accepted treatment plans, was

---

BOX 5-3 *Healthy People 2010* Objectives for Oral Health for the United States[87]

21-1. Reduce the proportion of children and adolescents who have dental caries experience in their primary or permanent teeth.

21-2. Reduce the proportion of children, adolescents, and adults with untreated dental decay.

21-3. Increase the proportion of adults who have never had a permanent tooth extracted because of dental caries or periodontal disease.

21-4. Reduce the proportion of older adults who have had all their natural teeth extracted.

21-5. Reduce periodontal disease.

21-6. Increase the proportion of oral and pharyngeal cancers detected at the earliest stage.

21-7. Increase the proportion of adults who, in the past 12 months, report having had an examination to detect oral and pharyngeal cancers.

21-8. Increase the proportion of children who have received dental sealants on their molar teeth.

21-9. Increase the proportion of the U.S. population served by community water systems with optimally fluoridated water.

21-10. Increase the proportion of children and adults who use the oral health care system each year.

21-11. Increase the proportion of long-term care residents who use the oral health care system each year.

21-12. Increase the proportion of low-income children and adolescents who received any preventive dental service during the past year.

21-13. Increase the proportion of school-based health centers with an oral health component.

21-14. Increase the proportion of local health departments and community-based health centers, including community, migrant, and homeless health centers, that have an oral health component.

21-15. Increase the number of states and the District of Columbia that have a system for recording and referring infants and children with cleft lips, cleft palates, and other craniofacial anomalies to craniofacial anomaly rehabilitative teams.

21-16. Increase the number of states and the District of Columbia that have an oral and craniofacial health surveillance system.

21-17. Increase the number of tribal, state (including the District of Columbia) and local health agencies that serve jurisdictions of 250,000 or more persons that have in place an effective public health dental program directed by a dental professional with public health training.

---

concerned about oral health, arrived on time, and paid the bills.[72] Because the same study found that "personal warmth" in a patient was valued by dentists, it is likely that many dentists have trouble in warming to patients who do not possess these attributes.

Knowledge gaps concerning a number of preventive procedures have been found between researchers, practitioners, and patients,[71] and lack of consensus between researchers and practitioners has been identified as a major barrier to more effective promotion of caries prevention. This unfortunate confusion can be alleviated by health promotional activities aimed at changing attitudes and practices. For example, dentists in one Indian Health Service region developed a significantly greater orientation toward preventive services after such a promotional campaign.[62] With the realization that positive attitudes toward health promotion need to be developed during student days rather than afterward, the FDI has recommended that substantial changes in the dental curriculum be implemented to give dentists the knowledge, skills, and attitudes they will need.[25] The behavioral sciences, and the control of fear and anxiety in patients, were listed among those areas needing more attention. Knowledge and attitudes on oral health among other influential professionals—schoolteachers, for example—also can be disappointingly poor,[37,58,61] which only underlines the responsibility of the dental professions to see that trainee teachers, nurses, and others who influence public attitudes receive correct information on oral health.

Even a relatively low level of serious oral disease in the community does not always reflect positive dental attitudes. In fluoridated Hong Kong, for example, where neither caries nor periodontitis were found to be major public health problems, ignorance and misconceptions about the most common oral conditions were widespread.[60] Poor knowledge of the oral diseases is common in many countries, including the United States and Canada, as shown by reports that many people do not associate existing symptoms, such as calculus deposits or bleeding gums, with periodontal diseases.[36,59] A more encouraging study in North Carolina found that patients of general practitioners were generally knowledgeable about the signs, causes, prevention, and treatment of periodontal conditions.[3] Few serious misconceptions were found in this study, though improvement was needed on the significance of bleeding gums. When incipient disease cannot be recognized, there will naturally be inadequate self-care, and promotion of self-care is one of the major goals of oral health education.

DENTAL HEALTH EDUCATION

In the past, unless health professionals were unusually sensitive to patients' reactions, health education often had a patronizing ring to it. When a health provider who believes she knows what is best for the patient "educates" a person who is tacitly assumed to know nothing, it is a safe bet that little of value eventuates. This has been called the "empty vessel" approach to health education: the patient is empty and waiting for the health professional to "pour in" the knowledge. This approach was enshrined in an early WHO report,[99] which saw the need to teach educational theory and methods to student dentists so that they could successfully "motivate" their patients and the public to behave as dentists would like them to. It also shows itself unconsciously in terminology such as *toothbrushing drills*, a so-called educational method in which children are taught to brush their teeth in a semimilitary manner. The empty vessel approach also dated from a time when the guild model of professionalism (see Chapter 1) was accepted, a model that saw the all-knowing professional as dominant in dentist-patient relations.

In more recent years, greater acceptance has been given to the idea that the recipients of all this attention might have some thoughts of their own. Item 4 in the Declaration of Alma-Ata, the outcome of a major international conference on primary health care, stated that "people have a right and duty to participate individually and collectively in the planning and implementation of their health care."[100] In

a subsequent WHO report, the evolution of professional attitudes was demonstrated when it was stated that (1) participant involvement was essential for success in health education, and (2) what is taught needed to be compatible with local customs and culture as well as with scientific knowledge.[102]

It is a basic precept that everyone has a right to the best available knowledge about caring for her own health. However, knowledge alone does not lead to action. Many health care workers can labor under the assumption that when people have knowledge about health care they will act upon that knowledge. It is a rational assumption, but human behavior is more complicated than that. Knowledge dissemination is a fundamental part of the mission of health professionals, but health care workers have to steel themselves to accept that much of their effort will go unheeded.

School-based oral health education programs, by definition, are aimed at more cohesive groups rather than at the public at large. Whatever approach is to be adopted, it will require a plan of action, with appropriate involvement of all parties concerned and clear delineation of responsibilities. Fundamental components of a school-based program for the promotion of oral health have been described as follows:

- Oral health services, meaning preventive procedures, health screening and treatment, referral, and follow-up.
- Health instruction, to include both personal and community health topics.
- A healthy environment, with attention to all aspects of the school environment that could affect the health of students or school personnel.[45]

Even though schoolchildren are more homogeneous than the public as a whole, any group of them still has a variety of beliefs and attitudes; in a multicultural society the differences can be profound.[18] Methods used in school programs should therefore be a mix of small group and mass approaches, and some are clearly more successful than others. The more successful approaches, as shown by evaluations of teachers and administrators, and by the oral health of participants, use a fair degree of active involvement.[13,14,26,43,73,80,84] This finding applies to all ages and social groups, for active involvement increased the effectiveness of programs conducted with employed adults[42,75] and with mothers of young children.[44] Nursing home residents who monitored their own progress toward oral hygiene goals showed improvements in psychological well-being and self-esteem as well as in oral hygiene.[54,55]

On the other hand, programs that involve less individual participation can increase knowledge of oral disease mechanisms and its prevention but have less impact on attitudes, beliefs, and behavior.[60,76,92] The mass media, which by definition do not develop personal involvement, are generally seen as effective in disseminating basic knowledge, but whether they do much to influence behavioral change is uncertain. We have learned from public oral health campaigns that personal involvement is needed to effect behavioral change. When the cultural competence needed to accommodate to the astonishing cultural variety in modern-day America is added in, designing programs for personal involvement becomes a challenge.

The most intensive form of oral health education is one-to-one instruction. Although oral health education is clearly an integral part of professional responsibility, simply passing across information does not by itself lead to desirable action; personal involvement (again) is necessary. A study of educational outcomes among "high-plaque" patients who received instruction in oral hygiene in dental practices in Washington found that only 28% substantially reduced their plaque scores over 6 weeks, and

in 13% scores actually got worse. The researchers concluded that the therapists often did not follow the principles of effective instruction, though outcomes were also related to patients' oral status and life situations.[94] The same study also found that educational effort was not being concentrated on those patients with greatest need but rather was more or less equally distributed.[67] A British project found that use of the Community Periodontal Index of Treatment Needs (as it was then named, see Chapter 16) was a useful way of improving patient awareness of periodontal conditions.[11]

Many health care professionals have enormous faith in the value of dental health education. Educational programs are rarely opposed on the grounds that the resources involved might better be placed elsewhere, and educational programs promote a general "feel-good" atmosphere among all concerned. There is no question that all people have a right to the best knowledge about how to care for their health, even though they will act on this knowledge in different ways. The conclusions from a searching review of dental health education outcomes should be borne in mind by all those planning educational programs: (1) educational programs work well in improving knowledge levels; (2) they have a positive but temporary effect on plaque levels; and (3) they have no discernible effect on caries experience.[53]

At a practical level, the principles of oral health education that emerge from the literature can be summarized as shown in Box 5-4.

BOX 5-4 Principles of Oral Health Education

- People interpret health messages through the filter of their own values, beliefs, and attitudes. These need to be understood as far as possible, if the educational process is to have any chance of success.
- The most successful education maximizes self-involvement of the participants.
- Mass media are effective in transmitting simple and consistent messages, although their value in influencing health behavior seems limited. They have been found effective in accomplishing some behavioral change related to cardiovascular disease,

but have been less effective in producing change in relation to oral conditions.
- Health professionals have to accept that not all people share their values about the importance of health. An acceptance of all components of wellness, not just physical health, will help in dealing with the infinite variety of human beliefs on health.
- Dental health education programs can improve knowledge and temporarily improve oral hygiene but have not demonstrated any direct effect on caries experience.

PROMOTION OF WATER FLUORIDATION

Water fluoridation is an issue that gives dental professionals the chance to promote oral health at the community level and to apply the experiences gained from other successful community-based campaigns. The ADA has a long-standing policy that dentists should work to promote fluoridation in their communities,[1] though it is recognized that the issue can provoke mixed feelings. Dentists and hygienists, accustomed to life outside the spotlight, are often far from comfortable in the public arena. For such individuals, there are still key roles for dental professionals as low-profile resource persons.

To begin with, dentists and hygienists should at least educate their patients about what fluoridation is and who benefits from it (see Chapter 25). They should actively persuade patients to vote for the measure if a referendum is coming. Patients, after all, are a more or less captive audience, and there is evidence that dentists could do better with this particular educational role.[48] Dental professionals should know the concentration of fluoride in their own community's drinking water, information that comes from the state or local health department. Cost estimates for fluoridating a community's water can be obtained from the state health department or water supply division, and from the fluoridation engineers at the Division of Oral Health of the Centers for Disease Control and Prevention (CDC) in Atlanta, Georgia. If there were previous attempts to fluoridate the community, it helps to have a history of which individuals were involved and what happened.

At the local community level, a decision by a city council to fluoridate has proven far more likely to result in a favorable outcome than a referendum. Lobbying of city councilors both answers questions and identifies the members who are for, against, and undecided, information that can then help shape the further promotional effort needed. When a city council decides to put fluoridation out for referendum, the role of dental professionals becomes more overtly political. Defining this role may not be easy. A thoughtful study in the 1960s, still relevant today, found that political efforts of dentists and other health professionals in a local fluoridation campaign got unfavorable reac-

tions for two different reasons.[77] First, the community expected partisans in a political campaign to be motivated by self-interest and to conduct a propaganda campaign to further those interests. Because the health professionals supporting fluoridation were seen as political partisans, their endorsements of fluoridation were not accepted as dispassionate expert testimony. Second, their efforts to maintain professional decorum and to avoid the hurly-burly of open controversy were interpreted as arrogance. This study suggests that, in a fluoridation referendum, the health professionals cannot expect to maintain a detached role, and referendum tactics must be structured accordingly.

Regardless of the nature of the political campaign, experience has shown that a successful outcome is more likely when the campaign is coordinated by a citizens' committee, often called Citizens for Healthy Teeth or some such name. The first task of the coordinating committee is to draw up a plan of action that will guide the promotional activities. Dental professionals can play the role of technical experts in this committee, though many have the qualities to take more prominent roles. If needed, the CDC and the ADA have materials to help. The composition of the citizens' committee should be as broadly based as possible, with attention to socioeconomic, age, and ethnic groupings, in order to accomplish the following:
- Represent the community and demonstrate that fluoridation has widespread political support.
- Increase the number of volunteer workers for telephoning potential voters, canvassing, and distributing materials.[65]
- Increase the base of financial support.[47]

Experience has also shown that a hired consultant in political organization can be very helpful.[21] A political expert can assist in these areas:
- Legal registration of the political action committee in those states in which it is required
- Outreach to the large segments of the population that ordinarily do not participate in organizations and are not much influenced by mass media
- Identification of the community power structure and the key individual leaders whose support will be needed.
- Campaign strategy and tactics

• Recruitment of "celebrities" and "outside experts," should it be decided to use them

The political tactics used vary with each community. There is no cookbook, although there are some standard issues. For example, should an invitation to publicly debate a fluoridation opponent be accepted? There is no easy answer. A refusal can be interpreted as professional arrogance, but at the same time a debate with a committed opponent cannot be "won." An opponent can imply, for example, that fluoridation is in the same category as toxic chemical waste or acid rain, and that proponents are trying to increase both unnecessary regulation and taxes. Despite the successful record of fluoridation in the courts (see Chapter 25), a good speaker can still score on the freedom-of-choice issue. Even the necessary dissemination of objective facts on fluoridation can be self-defeating, for the burden of proof always falls on those advocating change. Skilled opponents of fluoridation can quickly throw the proponents onto the defensive.

Successful referendum campaigns have been reported in the dental literature, and strategies for dealing with fluoridation in the political arena have now been well defined.[6,16,17,20,21,47,74,79] The common theme in these reports is that fluoridation is politics. It demands the use of the media, publicity, education, intensive door-to-door canvassing, telephone campaigns, and getting out the vote on polling day. Above all, it means consistent hard work over a long period and starting with a solid preparation.

REFERENCES

1. American Dental Association, Council on Dental Health. Statement of American Dental Association on role of dentists and dental societies in the promotion of fluoridation. Am Dent Assoc Trans 1962; 103:44.
2. Arnett DK, McGovern PG, Jacobs DR Jr, et al. Fifteen-year trends in cardiovascular risk factors (1980-1982 through 1995-1997): The Minnesota Heart Survey. Am J Epidemiol 2002;156:929-35.
3. Bader JD, Rozier RG, McFall WT, Ramsey DL. Dental patients' knowledge and beliefs about periodontal disease. Community Dent Oral Epidemiol 1989;17: 60-4.
4. Bandura A. A social learning theory. Englewood Cliffs NJ: Prentice Hall, 1977.
5. Birn H, Birn B. Education for wellness. Community Dent Health 1985;2:51-6.
6. Boriskin JM, Fine JI. Fluoridation election victory: A case study for dentistry in effective political action. J Am Dent Assoc 1981;102:486-91.
7. Bouma J, Westert G, Schaub RM, van de Poel F. Decision processes preceding full mouth extractions. Community Dent Oral Epidemiol 1987;15:268-72.
8. Carleton RA, Lasater TM, Assaf AR, et al. The Pawtucket Heart Health program: Community changes in cardiovascular risk factors and projected disease risk. Am J Public Health 1995;85:777-85.
9. Chambers DW. Susceptibility to preventive dental treatment. J Public Health Dent 1973;33:82-90.
10. Chen MS. Children's preventive dental behavior in relation to their mothers' socioeconomic status, health beliefs and dental behaviors. ASDC J Dent Child 1986;53:105-9.
11. Chesters RK, Dexter CH, Life JS, et al. Periodontal awareness project in the United Kingdom: CPITN and self-assessment. Int Dent J 1987;37:218-21.
12. Cohen LK. Promoting oral health: Guidelines for dental associations. Int Dent J 1990;40:79-102.
13. Craft M, Croucher R, Dickinson J. Preventive dental health in adolescents: Short and long term pupil response to trials of an integrated curriculum package. Community Dent Oral Epidemiol 1981;9:199-206.
14. Craft M, Croucher R, Dickinson J, et al. Natural Nashers: A programme of dental health education for adolescents in schools. Int Dent J 1984;34:204-13.
15. Decision 84: ADA's proposed paid public education program. J Am Dent Assoc 1984;108:740-8.
16. Dolinsky HB, McFadden RT, Kleinfeld L, Miller PT. A health systems agency and a fluoridation campaign. J Public Health Policy 1981;2:158-63.
17. Domoto PK, Faine RC, Rovin S. Seattle fluoridation 1973: Prescription for victory. J Am Dent Assoc 1975;91:583-8.
18. Durward CS, Wright FA. Dental knowledge, attitudes, and behaviors of Indochinese and Australian-born adolescents. Community Dent Oral Epidemiol 1989;17: 14-8.
19. Eaton CV, Lapane KL, Garber CE, et al. Effects of a community-based intervention on physical activity: The Pawtucket Heart Health Program. Am J Public Health 1999;89:1741-4.
20. Evans CA, Pickles T. Statewide antifluoridation initiatives: A new challenge to health workers. Am J Public Health 1978;68:59-62.
21. Faine RC, Collins JJ, Daniel J, et al. The 1980 fluoridation campaigns: A discussion of results. J Public Health Dent 1981;41:138-42.
22. Farquhar JW, Fortmann SP, Flora JA, et al. Effects of communitywide education on cardiovascular disease risk factors. JAMA 1990;264:359-65.
23. Farquhar JW, Maccoby N, Wood PD, et al. Community education for cardiovascular health. Lancet 1977; 1:1192-5.
24. Fédération Dentaire Internationale. Global goals for oral health in the year 2000. Int Dent J 1982;32:74-7.
25. Fédération Dentaire Internationale. The impact of changing disease trends on dental education and practice. FDI Technical Report No. 30. Int Dent J 1987; 37:127-30.

26. Flanders RA. Effectiveness of dental health educational programs in schools. J Am Dent Assoc 1987;114: 239-42.

27. Fortmann SP, Flora JA, Winkleby MA, et al. Community intervention trials: Reflections on the Stanford Five-City project experience. Am J Epidemiol 1995;142: 576-86.

28. Fortmann SP, Varady AN. Effects of a community-wide health education program on cardiovascular disease morbidity and mortality: The Stanford Five-City project. Am J Epidemiol 2000;152:316-23.

29. Fortmann SP, Winkleby MA, Flora JA, et al. Effect of long-term community health education on blood pressure and hypertension control. The Stanford Five-City project. Am J Epidemiol 1990;132: 629-46.

30. Frank E, Winkleby M, Fortmann SP, Farquhar JW. Cardiovascular disease risk factors: Improvements in knowledge and behavior in the 1980s. Am J Public Health 1993;83:590-3.

31. Frazier PJ, Horowitz AM. Oral health education and promotion in maternal and child health: A position paper. J Public Health Dent 1990;50:390-5.

32. Frazier PJ, Jenny J, Ostman R, Frenick C. Quality of information in mass media; a barrier to the dental health education of the public. J Public Health Dent 1974;34:244-57.

33. Freimuth VS, Mettger W. Is there a hard-to-reach audience? Public Health Rep 1990;105:232-8.

34. Friedman LA, Mackler IG, Hoggard GJ, French CI. A comparison of perceived and actual dental needs of a select group of children in Texas. Community Dent Oral Epidemiol 1976;4:89-93.

35. Gans KM, Assmann SF, Sallar A, Lasater TM. Knowledge of cardiovascular disease prevention: An analysis from two New England communities. Prev Med 1999;29: 229-37.

36. Gift HC. Awareness and assessment of periodontal problems among dentists and the public. Int Dent J 1988;38:147-53.

37. Glasrud PH, Frazier PJ. Future elementary schoolteachers' knowledge and opinions about oral health and community programs. J Public Health Dent 1988;48: 74-80.

38. Green LW. National policy in the promotion of health. Int J Health Educ 1979;22:161-8.

39. Green LW, Anderson CL. Community health. St. Louis: Mosby, 1986.

40. Green LW, Kreuter MW. Health promotion planning: An educational and environmental approach. 2nd ed. Mountain View CA: Mayfield, 1991.

41. Greenberg JS. Health education. Dubuque IA: Brown, 1989.

42. Hager B, Krasse B. Dental health education by "barefoot doctors." Community Dent Oral Epidemiol 1983;11: 333-6.

43. Hodge H, Buchanan M, O'Donnell P, et al. The evaluation of the junior dental health education programme developed in Sefton, England. Community Dent Health 1987;4:223-9.

44. Holt RD, Winter GB, Fox B, Askew R. Effects of dental health education for mothers with young children in

London. Community Dent Oral Epidemiol 1985;13: 148-51.

45. Horowitz AM, Frazier PJ. Effective oral health programs in school settings. In: Clark JW, ed: Clinical dentistry. Philadelphia PA: Harper and Row, 1986:1-15.

46. Irbarren C, Luepker RV, McGovern PG, et al. Twelve-year trends in cardiovascular disease risk factors in the Minnesota heart survey. Are socioeconomic differences widening? Arch Intern Med 1997;157:873-81.

47. Isman R. Fluoridation: Strategies for success. Am J Public Health 1981;71:717-21.

48. Isman R. Effects of the dentist as the primary information source about fluoridation. J Public Health Dent 1983;43:274-83.

49. Jeffery RW. Community programs for obesity prevention: The Minnesota Heart Health program. Obes Res 1995;3(Suppl 2):283s-288s.

50. Kaplan GA. People and places: Contrasting perspectives on the association between social class and health. Int J Health Serv 1996;26:507-19.

51. Kaplan GA, Lynch JW. Socioeconomic considerations in the primordial prevention of cardiovascular disease. Prev Med 1999;29:S30-5.

52. Kawachi I, Kennedy BP, Glass R. Social capital and self-rated health; a contextual analysis. Am J Public Health 1999;89:1187-93.

53. Kay EJ, Locker D. Is dental health education effective? A systematic review of current evidence. Community Dent Oral Epidemiol 1996;24:231-5.

54. Kiyak HA, Mulligan K. Studies of the relationship between oral health and psychological well-being. Gerodontics 1987;3:109-12.

55. Knazan YL. Application of PRECEDE to dental health promotion for a Canadian well-elderly population. Gerodontics 1986;2:180-5.

56. Kochheiser T. Latest consumer research reveals "Apple Lady" ads effective. J Mich Dent Assoc 1990;72: 227-9.

57. Lalonde M. A new perspective on the health of Canadians; a working document. Ottawa: Information Canada, 1974.

58. Lang WP, Woolfolk MW, Faja BW. Oral health knowledge and attitudes of elementary schoolteachers in Michigan. J Public Health Dent 1989;49:44-50.

59. Lie T, Mellingen JT. Periodontal awareness, health, and treatment need in dental school patients. I. Patient interviews. Acta Odontol Scand 1987;45:179-86.

60. Lind OP, Evans RW, Corbet EF, et al. Hong Kong survey of adult oral health. Part 2. Oral health related perceptions, knowledge and behaviour. Community Dent Health 1987;4:367-81.

61. Loupe MJ, Frazier PJ. Knowledge and attitudes of schoolteachers toward oral health programs and preventive dentistry. J Am Dent Assoc 1983;107:229-34.

62. Malvitz DM, Broderick EB. Assessment of a dental disease prevention program after three years. J Public Health Dent 1989;49:54-8.

63. McCaul KD, Glasgow RE, Gustafson C. Predicting levels of preventive dental behaviors. J Am Dent Assoc 1985;111:601-5.

64. McGovern PG, Jacobs DR Jr, Shahar E, et al. Trends in acute coronary heart disease mortality, morbidity, and

medical care from 1985 through 1997: The Minnesota heart survey. Circulation 2001;104;19-24.

65. McGuire KM. Strategies for a fluoridation campaign. J Mich Dent Assoc 1981;63:681-6.

66. McGuire MK, Sydney SB, Zink FJ, et al. Evaluation of an oral disease control program administered to a clinic population at a suburban dental school. J Periodontol 1980;51:607-13.

67. Milgrom P, Weinstein P, Melnick S, et al. Oral hygiene instruction and health risk assessment in dental practice. J Public Health Dent 1989;49:24-31.

68. Mittelmark MB, Hunt MK, Heath GW, Schmid TL. Realistic outcomes: Lessons from community-based research and demonstration programs for the prevention of cardiovascular diseases. J Public Health Policy 1993;14:437-62.

69. Murtomaa H, Masalin K. Effects of a national dental health campaign in Finland. Acta Odontol Scand 1984;42:297-303.

70. Nuttall NM. Characteristics of dentally successful and dentally unsuccessful adults. Community Dent Oral Epidemiol 1984;12:208-12.

71. O'Neill HW. Opinion study comparing attitudes about dental health. J Am Dent Assoc 1984;109:910-5.

72. O'Shea RM, Corah NL, Ayer WA. Dentists' perceptions of the "good" adult patient: An exploratory study. J Am Dent Assoc 1983;106:813-6.

73. Olsen CB, Brown DF, Wright FA. Dental health promotion in a group of children at high risk to dental disease. Community Dent Oral Epidemiol 1986;14:302-5.

74. Paul BD. Fluoridation and the social scientist: A review. J Soc Issues 1961;17:1-12.

75. Petersen PE. Evaluation of a dental preventive program for Danish chocolate workers. Community Dent Oral Epidemiol 1989;17:53-9.

76. Peterson FL Jr, Rubinson L. An evaluation of the effects of the American Dental Association's dental health education program on the knowledge, attitudes and health locus of control of high school students. J School Health 1982;52:63-9.

77. Raulet HM. The health professional and the fluoridation issue: A case of role conflict. J Soc Issues 1961;17:45-54.

78. Reelick NF, Verbeek MH. The Dutch dental campaign. J Am Dent Assoc 1986;113:803-4.

79. Rosenthal DB, Crain RL. Executive leadership and community innovation: The fluoridation experience. Urban Aff Q 1966;1:39-57.

80. Schou L. Active-involvement principle in dental health education. Community Dent Oral Epidemiol 1985; 13:128-32.

81. Sheiham A, Watt RG. The common risk factor approach: A rational basis for promoting oral health. Community Dent Oral Epidemiol 2000;28: 399-406.

82. Siegal MD, Martin B, Kuthy RA. Usefulness of a local oral health survey in program development. J Public Health Dent 1988;48:121-4.

83. Simons-Morton BG, Greene WH, Gottlieb NH. Introduction to health education and health promotion. 2nd ed. Prospect Heights IL: Waveland Press, 1995.

84. Sogaard AJ, Holst D. The effect of different school based dental health education programmes in Norway. Community Dent Health 1988;5: 169-84.

85. Sogaard AJ, Koch AL. Dental health education— a question of values. J Public Health Dent 1984;44: 169-71.

86. Taylor CB, Fortmann SP, Flora J, et al. Effect of long-term community health education on body mass index. The Stanford Five-City project. Am J Epidemiol 1991;134:235-49.

87. US Department of Health and Human Services. Healthy people 2010. 21: Oral health, website: http://www.healthypeople.gov/Document/pdf/Volume2/21Oral.pdf. Accessed October 31, 2003.

88. US Public Health Service. Promoting health: Objectives for the nation. Washington DC: Government Printing Office; 1980.

89. US Public Health Service. Healthy people 2000; national health promotion and disease prevention activities. Conference edition. Washington DC: Government Printing Office, 1990.

90. US Public Health Service, National Center for Health Statistics. Healthy people 2000 review 1997. DHHS Publication No. (PHS) 98-1256. Hyattsville MD: Public Health Service, 1997.

91. US Public Health Service, Office of Disease Prevention and Health Promotion. The 1990 health objectives for the nation: A midcourse review. Washington DC: Government Printing Office, 1986:147-61.

92. Walsh MM. Effects of school-based dental health education on knowledge, attitudes and behavior of adolescents in San Francisco. Community Dent Oral Epidemiol 1985;13:143-7.

93. Watt RG. Emerging theories into the social determinants of health: Implications for oral health promotion. Community Dent Oral Epidemiol 2002;30: 241-7.

94. Weinstein P, Milgrom P, Melnick S, et al. How effective is oral hygiene instruction? Results after 6 and 24 weeks. J Public Health Dent 1989;49:32-8.

95. White SL, Maloney SK. Promoting healthy diets and active lives to hard-to-reach groups: Market research study. Public Health Rep 1990;105:224-31.

96. Winkleby MA, Feldman HA, Murray DM. Joint analysis of three U.S. community intervention trials for reduction of cardiovascular disease risk. J Clin Epidemiol 1997;50:645-58.

97. Winkleby MA, Taylor CB, Jatulis D, Fortmann SP. The long-term effects of a cardiovascular disease prevention trial: The Stanford Five-City project. Am J Public Health 1996;86:1773-9.

98. Woolfolk MP, Sgan-Cohen HD, Bagramian RA, Gunn SM. Self-reported health behavior and dental knowledge of a migrant worker population. Community Dent Oral Epidemiol 1985;13:140-2.

99. World Health Organization. Dental health education. Technical Report Series No. 449. Geneva: WHO, 1970.

100. World Health Organization. Declaration of Alma-Ata. World Health, 1983 Sep 24-5.

101. World Health Organization. Ottawa Charter for Health Promotion, website: http://www.who.int/hpr/

NPH/docs/ottawa_charter_hp.pdf. Accessed December 17, 2003.

102. World Health Organization. Prevention methods and programmes for oral diseases. Technical Report Series No. 713. Geneva: WHO, 1984:24-32.

103. Wright FA. Children's perception of vulnerability to illness and dental disease. Community Dent Oral Epidemiol 1982;10:29-32.

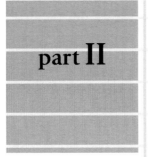

part **II** Dental Practice

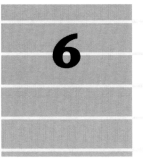

6   The Practice of Dentistry

Organized dentistry has two primary goals: to promote the oral health of the public and to preserve the autonomy and economic well-being of the profession. These goals can be in conflict, however, when dentistry's efforts to secure its own well-being are perceived as not being in harmony with the public interest, or when public efforts to improve oral health are seen by the professions as antagonistic to their self-interest. This type of conflict will continue, with just and acceptable outcomes more likely if the dental professions understand the pressures that produce them.

A *delivery system* is a collective health care expression that incorporates the various means by which care is provided to patients. The principal components are as follows:
  • The structure of the system, that is, the organizational arrangements by which patients meet up with providers.
  • The means by which the care is paid for.
  • The supply of various types of health care personnel.

Other elements of a delivery system can be identified, such as physical facilities and record keeping, but the three elements listed here are the most basic. They are interdependent; a change in any one affects the others, although this book divides the subject into three chapters to give these issues adequate consideration.

This chapter examines the structure of dental care provision systems in the United States, with some reference to methods used elsewhere.

PRIVATE DENTAL PRACTICE

Traditionally dental care in the United States has been delivered by independent private practitioners. The American Dental Association (ADA) estimated that approximately 93% of all active dentists were in private practice in 1998.[15] This proportion has remained remarkably stable over the years. Indeed, an essential feature of dental care delivery in the United States is the diversity of practice modes and their constant evolution within a private practice philosophy. Adaptability in a rapidly changing world is a major strength of private practice, an attribute that ensures that private practice will endure.

Private practice has a number of inherently desirable features. One advantage to both provider and patient is flexibility. Dental practitioners can provide care for as many hours per day and for as many days per year as they choose. When demand for care in a locality increases, private practitioners can respond if they wish by working longer hours, by increasing their productivity to meet it, by increasing their fees, or by all of these. There is a built-in economic incentive to be as efficient as possible in private practice, because it represents a big investment of private capital in facilities and equipment; the return on that investment is the practitioner's profit. Choice of equipment, materials, and employees therefore is made carefully, and all can be chosen to suit the tastes of the individual dentist.

Private practice has often been equated with free choice of a dentist by the prospective patient and, conversely, with freedom of the dentist to treat or not to treat anyone seeking care. Whether these concepts were ever fully true is arguable, but it is certain that current circumstances put some limits on these freedoms. In many inner city or small rural communities, for example, there is often little choice of dentist because dentists are less likely to establish practices there. Because dentists in private practice are self-employed business people, they tend to establish their practices in localities where they can be reasonably sure of adequate demand for their services; these localities are typically higher-income suburban areas. There is a clear association between the availability of dentists and the per capita income of an area.[7,8,14] Fig. 6-1 shows this association at the level of the states. Usually there are relatively more dentists in states with higher per capita incomes. This same phenomenon also is likely to apply to smaller geo-

graphic units such as counties, cities, and other natural market areas.

Even within communities that are well stocked with dentists, some groups are not readily treated in private practice (see Chapter 9). Treatment of the preschool child with behavioral difficulties, for example, requires a degree of time, patience, experience, and training that can make such treatment uneconomical for many general practitioners to provide, and pediatric dental specialists are not always available. Many elderly people cannot afford the care that they need, and many have difficulty traveling because of physical infirmities. In addition, there are people who are chronically ill, mentally retarded, or physically challenged, or who have illnesses that require them to receive dental treatment in a hospital. Private practices that are optimally designed for ambulatory, highly compliant patients are often not well suited to care for such persons.

Low-income individuals often have a double problem: care is less available near where they live, and when it can be found it is relatively expensive. It is hardly surprising that people in low socioeconomic areas are often thought "not to value dental care." That belief is not necessarily true; rather, the circumstances of their lives do not always permit the disadvantaged the luxury of "valuing dental care" the way that dentists would like.[30] Given this situation, "free

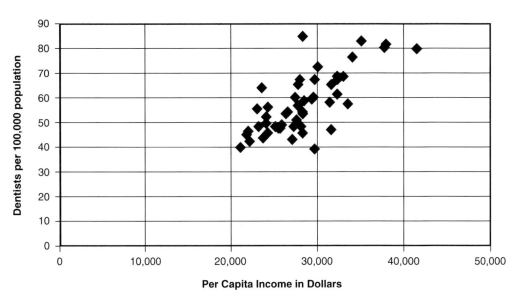

Fig. 6-1 The association between mean per capita income and the dentist/population ratio for individual states in the United States, 2000.[65,67]

choice" can be most accurately described as a middle-class value that may mean little in other socioeconomic contexts.

Free choice also cuts the other way: dentists have some freedom to reject patients (although not solely on the basis of race, ethnicity, or human immunodeficiency virus status; see Chapters 3 and 10). Some practitioners may believe that they are treating as many patients as they can manage and therefore will accept no new patients of any kind. Others may reject patients whose care is financed by public programs such as Medicaid (see Chapter 7). This rejection may be based on the dentist's view that such programs offer poor compensation and are bureaucratic nightmares, or the dentist may be unable to accept the attitudes and values of low-income individuals.

From the community viewpoint, the principal advantages and disadvantages of private practice as a delivery system relate to economics. Private funds are used to build the facilities, buy equipment, hire auxiliary staff, and pay for some of the expenses (although by no means all; see Chapter 8) of dental education. Dentists set their own fees. Dentists also have traditionally practiced *price discrimination*, meaning that they have charged wealthy patients higher fees than they have charged poorer ones. Wealthier patients in these practices therefore subsidized the poorer ones.

The business demands of running a dental practice can conflict with the need to provide for the dental treatment of all people. Dental fees simply are too high for some. The solo dental practitioner has certain overhead costs to meet: utilities, rent, equipment, supplies, staff payroll, and insurance. These expenses must be met regardless of whether or not patients come and whether or not fees are collected. In addition, the dentist is a highly trained and qualified professional and thus is deemed by American culture to be entitled to a good income. Many dentists graduate from dental school heavily in debt because of the high costs of their education and thus have a strong incentive to begin showing profits soon after they begin practice. The average debt among all dental graduates in 2003 was $118,750.[17] It is interesting to compare these facts of the dental practitioner's position with those of the position of the medical surgeon, who does not have to pay for hospital beds and hospital support staff out of the physician's fee.

Solo Practice

Within the overall realm of private practice, which is the principal form of dental practice in the United States, the solo practitioner is the most common form of practice. The ADA estimated that in 1998 almost two thirds (65%) of private practitioners worked in a practice with no other dentists, about 20.5% worked with one other dentist, and just over 14.5% worked with two or more other dentists.[16] This distribution is shown in Fig. 6-2.

Group Practice

The arrangements by which dentists can work together are so varied that the term *group practice* is difficult to define precisely. In fact, the ADA has adopted the term *nonsolo practice*. The ADA definition states the following:

A nonsolo dentist works in a practice with at least one other dentist. Some of these dentists may be employed by the owner dentist in the practice.[3]

As demonstrated in Fig. 6-2, solo practice remains the most common form of dental practice, and nonsolo practices generally are small, most of them consisting of two dentists. Although it is uncommon for newly graduating dentists to directly enter practice as a solo practitioner, the long-term pattern suggests that the dominance of solo and small group practices will continue, with a possible gradual shift toward small group practices.

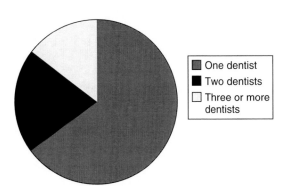

Fig. 6-2 Distribution of private practitioner dentists by type of practice in the United States, 1998.[16]

■ One dentist
■ Two dentists
□ Three or more dentists

Franchised Practices and Department Store Clinics

In the late 1970s, several major department store chains, including Sears and Montgomery Ward, opened dental clinics in some of their stores and announced their intention to open more. These clinics operated during usual store hours, and the stores' management viewed them as an extra service for their customers, no different from the pharmacies and optical departments. However, dental practices in department stores have not prospered and were few in number by the late 1990s.

The concept of franchises is common in the United States, encompassing such varied entities as motels, restaurants, automobile servicing, retail stores, and child care services. The franchisor, for some combination of initial fees and periodic payments, provides the name plus additional services such as advertising, training, coordinated purchasing, and management services. The franchisee runs the individual business location and, except for the agreed payments to the franchisor, retains the profits from the business.

By the early 1980s, there appeared to be the beginning of an explosive growth of franchised dental practices.[9,18,71] The idea as applied to dental practice varied in detail among franchises but tended to include such things as a franchise name; marketing and management services; bulk purchasing of supplies; and sometimes the design, construction, and equipping of the practice itself. The dental clinic space was usually leased by a dentist, because many state laws do not allow dental practices to be owned by a nondentist.

After a quick start in the early 1980s, most franchise dental organizations had fallen on difficult times by 1988;[73] all but a few were out of business or under bankruptcy protection. Reasons for this turn of events include undercapitalization, overexpansion, poor management control, unprofessional image, and high costs.[73] Fundamental conflicts between the traditional strengths of franchises and dental practice make it unlikely that franchised dental practice will ever be a major force. The standardization of process and procedures that leads to cost savings and uniform quality in many businesses is unlikely to produce cost savings in dental care.

In the mid-1990s, there were a few reports of dental insurers' buying individual dental offices. The reason for these purchases is usually to acquire the capacity to handle managed care offerings, particularly in areas where individual dental offices are reluctant to sign on. The impact of these arrangements will take some years to be properly evaluated.

HOSPITAL DENTISTRY

Although only a small fraction of dental care is provided in hospitals, dentists still have a substantial role in hospitals. In the mid-1980s, approximately 1000 hospitals in the United States had formally organized departments of dentistry, and about 40,000 dentists were members of the medical staff of at least one hospital.[10,33] In 1995, the number of dentists in the United States with hospital privileges was still about 40,000.[13]

The number of dental general practice residencies in hospitals grew rapidly through the 1970s, and as of 2003 there were 1423 first-year hospital-based residency positions.[17] The extended experience in the hospital environment that these residencies provide is likely to make it easier for these dentists to make use of hospital privileges later in their careers. Many dentists affiliated with these and other educational programs in hospitals have full-time or substantial part-time commitments to hospital-based care. Dentists in the military and with the Department of Veterans Affairs are also commonly in hospital-based practices. The majority of dentists who have hospital privileges, however, are in private practice and provide care only occasionally in the hospital.

Dental care provided in hospitals is for those situations in which general anesthesia and other resources of a hospital are required, such as for treatment of very young children with rampant caries, oral surgery to remove carcinomas, cleft palate repair, and maxillofacial prosthetic treatment for victims of burns or trauma. In addition, some routine dental care is provided in hospitals for patients who are suffering from serious systemic disease and for whom the risk of being treated in the private dental office would be unacceptably high. The inclusion of ADA representation on the board of the Joint Commission on Accreditation of Healthcare

Organizations since 1980 helps to ensure an appropriate role for dental consultation and services within hospitals.

Beyond the traditional role of educational programs and consultative services, a major challenge for hospital dental departments is economic justification. All departments within hospitals are increasingly being pressed to show that the income they produce is sufficient to justify their existence, and the traditional roles of teaching, consultation, and care for indigent patients do not provide high levels of revenue. On the other hand, moves by hospital-based programs to solicit insured patients through ambulatory care facilities are seen as unfair competition by some private practitioners.[35,57]

PUBLIC PROGRAMS

As stated earlier, private practice cannot meet the dental demands of all people. A number of public dental care programs therefore have been developed to meet the needs of specific groups. Some of these government-sponsored programs use a specific delivery system in addition to a funding mechanism. Many receive funding from the federal government, although most still remain under the control of state and local health departments. Many are under considerable strain because social services budgets, on which these programs heavily depend, have been severely cut over recent decades.

The oldest health care programs of the federal government are directed either at certain groups of its own employees or at other specific groups for whom it has an obligation or who would find it difficult to get care anywhere else. Each branch of the armed forces, for example, provides dental care for its own active-duty personnel. Care is provided for the most part by dentists who themselves are members of the armed services and is dispensed from clinical facilities wholly owned and maintained by the service concerned.

Many of the long-established clinical programs of the U.S. Public Health Service were described in Chapter 1. In addition, the Community and Migrant Health program of the U.S. Public Health Service provides grants to support public and nonprofit organizations to plan, develop, and operate health care facilities, known as community and migrant health centers, in rural and urban areas where existing health care resources are inadequate. These centers are primarily medical, but many provide dental services too. As of 2002 there were 1230 full-time-equivalent (FTE) dentists, 383 FTE dental hygienists, and 2291 FTE dental assistants, aides, and technicians employed at these health centers.[66] These centers are established in areas where access to private care is limited, and they employ salaried dental personnel.

Another program aimed at making care available in areas unattractive to private practice is the National Health Service Corps. This program, discussed more fully in Chapter 8, has provided incentives, including scholarships and loan repayment, to encourage dentists to practice in remote and underserved areas. Many National Health Service Corps dentists practice in community and migrant health centers.

Many states, counties, and cities have had their own dental care programs, with their own facilities and salaried personnel, operating for years. Most of these programs, which are often administered by an agency of the state or local government, have been aimed at providing care for people who are eligible to receive some form of public assistance. The services available through these programs vary widely. Many of these state and local dental treatment programs cover a portion of their costs of operation by billing Medicaid for eligible patients and by receiving Community and Migrant Health program grants from the Bureau of Primary Health Care.

Auxiliaries in Public Programs

Auxiliary-based programs have long been the backbone of public dental care in some countries, although not in the United States. The oldest and best known is the New Zealand school dental nurse plan, introduced in 1921. New Zealand is a nation of some 4 million people in the South Pacific, 1500 miles off the eastern coast of Australia. Living standards are high, and New Zealand has been a world leader in a number of social programs: old-age pensions, visiting maternal and child health nurses, and the secret ballot at political elections. A number of these programs began in the late nineteenth century, about the time that social security programs were initiated in Bismarck's Germany. Given these traditions, the introduction of the school dental nurse plan was not as radical an innovation as it might seem, although there was some concern among dentists at the time.[61] The stimuli for the program were the extensive dental disease found in army recruits during World War I (1914-18) and government intent to do something about this problem. Dentists were in short supply at the time, and treatment of young children was not as accepted in dental practice as it is now. Caries experience remained high for a long time in New Zealand[22,23] before that country joined in the worldwide decline in the late twentieth century (see Chapter 20).

When the service began, care was offered only to younger school-aged children, but eligibility was soon extended to all preschool-aged children and all children in primary and intermediate school. Although most care is provided by dental therapists (the current name for dental nurses), recent legislation will extend practice possibilities for dental therapists, including treating publicly funded clients in private practice and treating indigenous populations.[41] The traditional 2-year diploma program has also been supplemented with a 3-year degree program.[64]

The therapist's training concentrates on technical procedures, with considerable emphasis on learning to recognize conditions that are beyond the therapist's competence to treat. Individuals with these conditions are then referred to a private practitioner or to one of a small number of dentists employed by the School Dental Service. Therapists' clinical duties include performance of oral examinations, cavity preparation and placement of restorations, pulp capping, and extraction of primary teeth. Therapists also provide extensive dental health education, both in the classroom and to individual patients.

Dental therapists function with a high degree of independence. Many young children in New Zealand are examined and treated completely by dental nurses and never see a dentist until their teenage years. Although this fact has disturbed some American observers,[36,55] there is no evidence that the oral or general health of the children suffers as a result.

The decline in caries experience in New Zealand, as in most developed countries, has reduced the need for restorative treatment. In addition, women are staying in the workforce longer than they used to. As a result of these influences, the intake of new trainees had to be reduced. However, with many dental therapists approaching retirement age, there is concern that there may be a shortage in coming years.

The New Zealand school dental therapist plan has attracted the attention of dental organizations all over the world. Other countries and jurisdictions that have adopted similar programs, with modifications to suit the local environment, include Canada, Great Britain, Australia, Thailand, Malaysia, Singapore, Myanmar, Sri Lanka, Brunei, Hong Kong, and Indonesia. A small number of dental health aides are currently being trained in New Zealand to prepare for practice under Alaska's Community Health Aide Program that serves native populations in Alaska.[63]

The few attempts to introduce dental therapists in the United States have gone nowhere, at least partly because of the consistently strong opposition of the ADA.[11,12] An attempt to introduce an auxiliary-based school dental program in Massachusetts in the mid-1950s was defeated after political action by organized dentistry.[31] Despite this history, it is well established from research, much of it ironically conducted in the United States, that well-trained dental therapists are able to carry out many procedures as well as dentists can.[1,2,21,37,44-46,56,59] In most of the countries where these programs are established, children likely would be receiving no care at all were it not for the dental therapists.

Primary Health Care

Developing countries generally do not have the resources to train the number of dentists they need. Even if large numbers of dentists were available, the cost of care would still be beyond the reach of most. Recognition of this fact has led the World Health Organization to establish its principles of primary health care.[72] Under this concept, the focus of health care is to assist in maintaining health rather than to wait for problems to occur. In countries and localities where dentists are in short supply, much of the responsibility for first-level oral health care is assigned to a primary health care worker who resides in the community. In some places these individuals have been trained to provide dental examinations and to perform nonsurgical procedures such as calculus removal, application of topical fluorides, and the placement of sealants and glass ionomer restorations.[54] Under such a system, much of the preventive care is provided by people who are already part of the health care system in the community, and the more scarce and expensive personnel are used mainly as a second-level referral resource.

In circumstances of extreme shortage of trained oral health care professionals, the concept of primary health care tries to give to individuals as much practical information as possible for their own care and provides guidance for nondental health care workers when it is necessary for them to place temporary fillings or extract teeth.[27]

Dental care can be provided in ways that are markedly different from those in North America. If at first some of these alternative ways of meeting the needs of people seem unusual, it must be remembered that the system that seems right for any particular country is determined by a combination of its history, economics, cultural traditions, and prevailing philosophies on rights and responsibilities of health care.

QUALITY ASSURANCE

Regardless of the way that the care system is organized, every dental professional wants to provide the best possible care. However, defining what is meant by *quality*, and then reaching agreement on how to attain it, continue to be a major challenge. A typical dictionary definition of *quality* is "degree of excellence." Schoen[58] defined quality in dental care as "that characteristic that relates to the effective and efficient maintenance of optimum oral health when present, and improvement of oral health when needed." Although this definition gives us the general idea of quality in dental care, it leaves much room for disagreement about how quality is actually measured. Terms such as *effective and efficient maintenance* and *optimal oral health* do not have precise definitions. This ambiguity is behind the variety of approaches to quality assurance.

The term *quality assessment* is defined by the ADA as "the measure of the quality of care provided in a particular setting."[3] *Quality assurance*, in turn, is defined as:

. . . the assessment or measurement of the quality of care and the implementation of any necessary changes to either maintain or improve the quality of care rendered.[3]

The difference in these definitions is important: quality assessment is limited to the appraisal of whether or not standards of quality have been met, whereas quality assurance includes the additional dimension of action to take corrective steps if these are needed to improve the situation.

The most frequently used approach to quality assessment and quality assurance builds on the concepts of structure, process, and outcome, the classic evaluation model described by Donabedian.[28,29] The model is based on the idea that, although the outcome of treatment is important and should be evaluated, a desirable outcome is more likely if the structural arrangements meet adequate standards, such as with well-designed treatment facilities, proper equipment, and appropriate and properly trained staff. A good outcome is also more likely if the processes used, such as diagnostic methods, treatment planning, record keeping, and the treatment procedures themselves, follow recognized protocols. Perhaps even more important, Donabedian argues that if a less than satisfactory outcome is detected, the search for the cause is likely to be within the process of care and the structures that support it.

Numerous dental practice assessment procedures that follow the structure-process-outcome model have been developed.[50,58,69] Box 6-1 lists examples of some of the dimensions that can be assessed under this approach. These many dimensions of quality can present problems, because when people of good faith focus on different dimensions they can disagree as to whether quality has been attained. Furthermore, the same level of technical quality can be commendable in one setting and inappropriate in another. The picture can be even more confusing because much of the recent literature in this area uses different terms to describe some or all of the dimensions of quality assurance and quality assessment. Some examples of different terms in the literature are listed in Box 6-2.

Although the terms in Box 6-2 are not necessarily equivalent to quality assurance, they do fit easily within the broad concept. The purpose of quality assurance is to help provide the best possible health care. All of the items

BOX 6-1   Examples of Dental Practice Elements That Can Be Assessed Under the Structure, Process, and Outcome Approach

Structure	Process	Outcome
Facilities	**Management**	**Patient satisfaction**
Setting	Practice	
Physical structures	Personnel	**Oral health status**
Layout	Patient	Oral hygiene
Amenities		Tooth loss
Access	**Records**	Periodontitis
	Content	Caries
Equipment	Completeness	Function
Operatories	Availability	Comfort
Instruments	Legibility	Esthetics
Supplies		
Sterilization	**Diagnosis**	**Completion of treatment**
	Appropriateness	Timeliness and appropriateness
	Documentation	
Personnel	Thoroughness	**Recall pattern**
Types		Frequency
Training	**Treatment plan**	Needs at recall
Licensure	Written plan	
Certification	Sequencing	
Continuing education	Appropriateness	
Administration	**Treatment**	
Procedures	Appropriateness	
Record system	Timeliness	
Protocols		

BOX 6-2   Quality-Related Terms in the Literature

Quality improvement[60]
Continuous improvement[24]
Continuous quality improvement[42]
Quality ensurance[69]
Quality management[60]
Total quality management[35]
Outcomes management[70]
Clinical practice guidelines[68]
Practice parameters[4,5]
Standards of practice[43]
Evidence-based clinical guidelines[49]
Best practices[40]
Report cards[38]
Risk prevention[53]

are potential tools to accomplish this goal, and they all fit comfortably within the structure-process-outcome paradigm. In that sense, the proliferation of terms, rather than representing competing approaches to quality assurance, represents the development and refinement of the methods to implement quality assurance.

Evolution of Quality Assurance

We could begin with the work of Florence Nightingale, who gathered hospital statistics in an effort to improve clinical outcomes.[51] An important milestone in medicine was the Flexner report,[32] which led to a major overhaul in the education of physicians in North America that in turn affected medical practice. The publication of the Gies report on dental education[34] was a similar milestone for dentistry and dental education. One result of the Gies report was the eventual closure of proprietary dental schools in the United States and the development of a system of accreditation of dental schools that, with refinement, continues to this day (see Chapter 1). An example of these continuing refinements is that, since the late 1980s, the Accreditation Standards for Dental Education Programs of the ADA's Commission on Dental Accreditation have included an explicit requirement for a formal system of record review.

Activities that can legitimately be included as part of quality assurance in dentistry go back as far as the aptitude testing and scrutiny of the academic credentials of dental school applicants. The process of accreditation of the dental schools themselves is also part of quality assurance, as are the processes to acquire and periodically evaluate the faculty members who teach in these schools. The requirements for entering dental practice are also part of the quality assurance process. In most of the high-income countries there is a requirement for graduation from a properly accredited dental school, and virtually all states within the United States also require the passing of an independently administered set of examinations.

Furthermore, requirements for periodic continuing education for renewal of licensure, the establishment of peer bodies to review and adjudicate complaints against clinicians, and, when all else fails, the use of the legal system to resolve disputes between patients and providers of care can all be viewed as part of quality assurance. The development, testing, and certification of dental materials, devices, and equipment are also important quality-related functions.

Recent Emphasis in Quality Assurance

Although a broad spectrum of activities legitimately is part of quality assurance, most of the attention to quality assurance in dentistry in recent decades has focused much more narrowly on dental practice itself. This recent emphasis on formal quality assurance activities in the United States has been attributed to the following five influences.[26]

1. Rapid Growth of Dental Prepayment with Associated Cost and Quality Concerns
Before 1970, almost all payment for dental care in the United States was made by the individual patient. Government and third parties had little involvement. By about 1985, however, the proportion of the U.S. population with some form of prepayment for dental care approached 50%. This rapid change propelled third parties

into the dental care delivery system, and they brought collective interest in the overall cost of the insurance programs. Along with cost concerns came concerns about the quality of care.

2. Rapidly Rising Health Care Costs
Because both government and private purchasers were increasingly involved, there was great concern when it became evident that the costs of care were increasing faster than the overall rate of inflation in the economy. It was clear that if the costs of health care were not brought into line with overall cost increases, less and less money would be available for other desired purposes.

3. Professional Standards Review Legislation
Dentistry has also been influenced by the general climate of increasing demands for accountability that have been imposed on medical and hospital care through legislation. Especially since the advent of Medicare and Medicaid in 1965, government funds account for a large and growing part of medical care expenditures, and as a result requirements related to quality assurance have been imposed on medical and hospital-based care. Even though government involvement in the payment for dental care in the United States is small, dentistry has been affected both directly and indirectly by this increasing climate of accountability.

4. Growth of Consumer Involvement
Over the past several decades there has been an increase in the interest of consumers, as a group, in issues related to all sorts of services and products. Dentistry has been affected by this general movement, especially in the sense that it has created a climate in which providers of services are seen as being far more subject to scrutiny than had previously been the case.

5. Malpractice Litigation
Perhaps also related to the growth in consumerism, individual patients have become far more likely to seek relief through the legal system to redress perceived shortcomings in the care that they receive. One result has been the growth of quality-related activities such as risk prevention and development of standards of care, in an effort to reduce the likelihood that such lawsuits will need to be undertaken.

Examples of Quality Assurance Activities: The Dimensions of Quality

The types of activities that are part of quality assurance in dentistry illustrate the wide scope of the field. The following seven topics are representative of quality assurance approaches in dentistry.

1. On-Site Evaluation of Dental Practice

On-site evaluation of dental practice is perhaps the most widely used form of quality assurance, especially for programs directed by third-party payers. Various combinations of structure, process, and outcome are measured by trained auditors who visit the dental office. Although there are numerous examples of this approach in the dental literature,[50,58,69] it is the subject of many concerns. For one thing, the process is expensive. It is time consuming for a trained evaluator to visit each dental office and to conduct what is usually a highly detailed assessment. Marcus,[47] who has considerable experience with this approach to quality assurance, has stated the following:

I am not convinced that our quality assurance efforts have had a significant impact on improving the process of care, nor has it been effective in eliminating those providers who are unwilling to change their pattern of care delivery.[47]

The work of van der Wal and colleagues[69] also casts uncertainty on the validity of the process. This group was unable to find the expected associations between structural aspects and outcomes of dental care. Although there is much room to debate the validity and completeness of both the structure and outcome measures used in their study, it nevertheless does raise several important points. First, this study adds to the concern that the structure-process-outcome paradigm has not been empirically shown to represent accurately the "real world." It continues to be unsettling that we cannot produce good empirical evidence of the connection that is so widely believed to be present. Second, the authors suggest the possibility that the structural characteristics included in dental office evaluations are now so well known to dentists that virtually all are in compliance, so that structural indicators are no longer valid predictors of outcomes.

2. Audit of Dental Records

In addition to the assessment of technical quality of restorations, the record audit as a quality assurance mechanism is perhaps the most highly developed and widely used approach for institutions[20] such as dental schools and hospital dental departments.[6] In hospitals, record audits fit well with the approach that has been used for a long time in medicine for hospital accreditation. In dental schools, it fits well with the traditional teaching functions. Through the detailed review of dental records, not only can the dental care provided by the institution be assessed, but the student is also exposed to a review of the rationale and process of patient management and care.

As with several of the other approaches to quality assurance, the audit of dental records is a relatively expensive and time-consuming process. Apart from the institutional settings in which they are required by external auditors, record audits are not widely used.

3. Technical Quality

Assessment of the technical quality of restorative procedures has perhaps the most highly detailed criteria but is also one of the least-used forms of quality assurance in dentistry. First of all, measurement of technical quality is expensive. It is time consuming for examiners, and it is difficult to get cooperation from more than a small fraction of the patients who are selected for evaluation. Further, the results from random audits have not been encouraging, partly because of the low turnout of patients and also because unacceptable care is so infrequently found.[25] Because of the high costs and low yield, direct assessment of technical quality has not developed into a major area of quality assurance.

4. Oral Health Status

If there were a simple, valid, sensitive, and easily measured index of oral health status, the job of quality assurance would be much easier. After all, the ultimate objective of oral health care is to help patients attain and maintain the highest possible level of oral health.

Although there have been noteworthy efforts to develop such indexes of oral health,[48,52] their acceptance has been limited, and there has been little progress in this direction in the past decade. These indexes are discussed in Chapter 14.

5. Appropriateness of Care

Appropriateness of care is a dimension that has so far received little attention in dentistry. There is general agreement that the use of a technically superior restorative procedure when it is not needed is not acceptable quality. Standards for the appropriate use of dental care nevertheless continue to elude clear definition.

6. Consumer Satisfaction

Work in the area of consumer satisfaction is also in its infancy, but it is currently of considerable interest, especially to purchasers of group dental insurance. One of the primary reasons for employers to purchase dental insurance for their employees and their families is to make the employee happy and loyal to the employer. Although these purchasers are certainly interested in the oral health of their employees, of considerable importance is the satisfaction of these employees with the dental benefit. As a result, purchasers are increasingly pressing for measures of consumer satisfaction.

7. Profiling of Dental Providers

With the advent of computer-based records of dental treatment, especially in insurance companies, there have been attempts to make use of these kinds of data to evaluate the quality of dental care indirectly. If successful, this approach could be much less expensive than the direct methods already discussed. The idea is that by aggregating treatment records from large numbers of providers across many patients, inappropriate patterns of care can be detected and corrective actions taken.[39,62] At least in theory, this approach offers considerable promise. Not only can potentially inappropriate use of care be identified cross-sectionally, but patterns of care in individual patients over time also can be used to permit inferences about the effectiveness and appropriateness of the care provided.

Quality Assurance and Cost Control

In the often-heard accusations that quality assurance is being misused as a tool for cost control is the implication that quality and cost control are incompatible. However, an honest view of quality assurance must accept that quality assurance may result in higher costs. There is no doubt that quality assurance activities themselves are costly and that quite often they identify deficiencies that cost money to rectify. Quality assurance and cost control are not only compatible; they must be considered together for truly meaningful quality assurance.

Important to the issue of quality assurance is the fact that there is not, nor will there ever be, an unambiguous, universal, and stable formula for what constitutes quality dental care. The definition at any one time and place must be conditional on what is possible (the state of the science and art of dentistry) and what is affordable to the individual and to society. Even in the richest of societies, resources are finite. Therefore it follows that the definition of what constitutes quality dental care is a continuously variable one, and it will inevitably include consideration of cost.

Because cost considerations are fundamentally part of quality, it follows that if there are two or more equally effective and acceptable ways of reaching a desired outcome, the least expensive one (i.e., the most efficient one) is of higher quality. Simply put, if the desired outcome can be reached with fewer resources, the excess resources can be used by the individual and society to pursue additional desired goals, and the individual and society will be better off. This philosophy illustrates the fundamental role of cost in the quality equation.

Nevertheless, the tensions between quality assurance and cost containment are considerable. On the one hand, if cost containment reduces unnecessary care, quality should increase. On the other hand, substitution of lower-cost services might reduce the quality of care. Bailit[19] has pointed out that cost containment is not likely to be as simple as reducing so-called unnecessary services; the more expensive treatments usually do produce benefits for individual patients. Nevertheless, the same amount of money could often produce even more benefit for a large number of people if it were used for other, less expensive services.

Although it has been said that better-quality care is more expensive, the converse is not necessarily true: more expensive care is not necessarily of better quality. If too much of the available funds goes to a small number of the patient group, the overall oral health of the group may well suffer. This emphasizes a dilemma that is discussed further in Chapter 7, which is that there is no inherently "right" amount of health care. The amount of money that any individual, group, or society as a whole will want to spend for a particular health care procedure, or for health care in general, can be determined only by balancing it against other needs and desires. Implicit in this idea is that there is such a thing as too much health care, even if the use of a service can be shown to improve the medical or dental condition of a person. If the resources required to provide such a service are so large that other even more beneficial services cannot be provided, then it would be rational for individuals and society to conclude that such a procedure should not be used.

It has become more obvious with third-party payments that when there is a finite amount of money for care, priority decisions must be made as to who receives services, what services may be provided, or both. How these priorities will be set and how the inevitable trade-off between the benefit to the group versus the individual patient will be resolved will continue to be a topic of debate.

REFERENCES

1. Abramowitz J, Berg LE. A four-year study of the utilization of dental assistants with expanded functions. J Am Dent Assoc 1973;87:623-35.
2. Ambrose ER, Hord AB, Simpson WJ. A quality evaluation of specific dental services provided by the Saskatchewan Dental Plan: Final report. Regina: Government of Saskatchewan, 1976.
3. American Dental Association. CDT-4: Current dental terminology. Chicago: ADA, 2002.
4. American Dental Association. Dental practice parameters. Parameters for 12 oral health conditions. Adopted by the American Dental Association House of Delegates. October 1994. J Am Dent Assoc 1995;126(Suppl): 1-37.
5. American Dental Association. Dental practice parameters. Parameters for 12 oral health conditions. Adopted by the American Dental Association House of Delegates. October 1995. J Am Dent Assoc 1996;128(Suppl):iS–iiS, 1S-36S.
6. American Dental Association. Directory of dental quality assessment and quality assurance programs in the United States, 1989. Chicago: ADA, Office of Quality Assurance, 1990.
7. American Dental Association, Bureau of Economic Research and Statistics. Distribution of dentists in the United States by region and state; 1987. Chicago: ADA, 1987.
8. American Dental Association, Bureau of Economic Research and Statistics. Distribution of dentists in the United States by state, region, district, and county. Chicago: ADA, 1977.
9. American Dental Association, Council on Dental Practice. A brief overview of the franchise concept as applied to the practice of dentistry. J Am Dent Assoc 1983;106:518-9.
10. American Dental Association, Council on Hospital and Institutional Dental Services. Hospital dental statistics: An update. J Am Dent Assoc 1985;110:241-3.
11. American Dental Association, House of Delegates. Resolution 78-1972-H. Trans Am Dent Assoc 1973; 114:707-9.
12. American Dental Association, House of Delegates. Resolution 40-H-1976. Trans Am Dent Assoc 1977; 117:839.
13. American Dental Association, Survey Center. 1995 Survey of dental services in hospitals. Chicago: ADA, 1996.
14. American Dental Association, Survey Center. Distribution of dentists in the United States by region and state, 1995. Chicago: ADA, 1997.
15. American Dental Association, Survey Center. Distribution of dentists in the United States by region and state, 1998. Chicago: ADA, 2000.
16. American Dental Association, Survey Center. Key dental facts. Chicago: ADA, 2002.
17. American Dental Education Association, Institute for Public Policy and Advocacy. Dental education at-a-glance 2004, website: http://www.adea.org/CPPA_Materials/2004_Dental_Ed_At_A_Glance.pdf. Accessed May 5, 2004.
18. Anderson C. The arrival of franchise dentistry. J Mo Dent Assoc 1984;64:16-8.
19. Bailit HL. Is overutilization the major reason for increasing dental expenditures? Reflections on a complex issue. J Dent Pract Admin 1988;5:112-5.
20. Bailit HL, Gotowka T. Guidelines for the development of a quality assurance audit system for hospital dental programs. Chicago: American Dental Association, Office of Quality Assurance, 1983.
21. Baird KM, Purdy EC, Protheroe DH. Pilot study on advanced training and employment of auxiliary dental personnel in the Royal Canadian Dental Corps: Final report. J Can Dent Assoc 1963;29:778-87.
22. Barmes DE. Features of oral health care across cultures. Int Dent J 1976;26:253-66.
23. Beck DJ. Dental health status of the New Zealand population in late adolescence and young adulthood. National Health Statistics Centre Special Report No. 29. Wellington NZ: Government Printer, 1968.
24. Berwick DM. Continuous improvement as an ideal in health care. N Engl J Med 1989;320:53-6.
25. Boylan ME. Ongoing assessment of the quality of dental care. In: National Round Table on Quality Assurance. Summary of proceedings. Chicago: American Fund for Dental Health, 1983;121-4.
26. DeAngelis AJ. Quality assurance: Definition and direction for the 80s. J Dent Educ 1984;48:27-33.
27. Dickson M. Where there is no dentist. Palo Alto CA: Hesperian Foundation, 1987.

28. Donabedian A. Evaluating the quality of medical care. Milbank Q 1966;44:166-203.
29. Donabedian A. The definition of quality and approaches to its assessment. Vol I. Ann Arbor MI: Hospital Administration Press, 1980.
30. Dummett CO. Understanding the underprivileged patient. J Am Dent Assoc 1969;79:1363-7.
31. Dunning JM. Extending the field for dental auxiliary personnel in the United States. Am J Public Health 1958;48:1059-64.
32. Flexner A. Medical education in the United States and Canada: A report to the Carnegie Foundation for the Advancement of Teaching. New York: Carnegie Foundation, 1910.
33. Giangrego E. Dentistry in hospitals: Looking to the future. J Am Dent Assoc 1987;115:545-55.
34. Gies WJ. Dental education in the United States and Canada: A report to the Carnegie Foundation for the Advancement of Teaching. New York: Carnegie Foundation, 1926.
35. Goldfield N, Nash DB. Providing quality care: Future challenges. 2nd ed. Ann Arbor MI: Health Administration Press, 1995.
36. Gruebbel AO. A study of dental public health services in New Zealand. Chicago: American Dental Association, 1950.
37. Hammons PE, Jamison HC, Wilson LL. Quality of service provided by dental therapists in an experimental program at the University of Alabama. J Am Dent Assoc 1971;82:1060-6.
38. Harris N. Are health plans making the grade? Bus Health, 1994 Jun 22-8.
39. Hayden WJ, Marcus M, Lewis CE. Developing population profiles from dental claims data for conceptualizing effectiveness of care. J Dent Educ 1989;53:619-28.
40. Jensen UJ. From good medical practice to best medical practice. Int J Health Plann Manage 1989;4:167-80.
41. KiwiCareers. Dental therapist job market, website: http://www.careers.co.nz/jobs/3b_den/j35152e.htm. Accessed May 6, 2004.
42. Kritcheusky SB, Simmons BP. Continuous quality improvement: Concepts and applications for physician care. JAMA 1991;226:1817-23.
43. Leake JL, Woodward GL. Introduction to the quality assurance workshop in dentistry: Why dental educators need to learn how to develop practice guidelines. J Dent Educ 1994;58:610-2.
44. Lobene RR, Berman K, Chaisson LB, et al. The Forsyth experiment in training of advanced skills hygienists. Dent Hyg (Chic) 1974;48:204-13.
45. Lotzkar SJ, Johnson DW, Thompson MB. Experimental program in expanded functions for dental assistants. Phase I: Baseline, and Phase 2: Training. J Am Dent Assoc 1971;82:101-22.
46. Lotzkar SJ, Johnson DW, Thompson MB. Experimental program in expanded functions for dental assistants. Phase 3: Experiment with dental teams. J Am Dent Assoc 1971;82:1067-81.
47. Marcus M. Trends in quality assurance in the dental profession. J Dent Educ 1990;54:224-7.
48. Marcus M, Koch AL, Gershen JA. A population index of oral health status as derived from dentists' preferences. J Public Health Dent 1983;43:284-94.
49. McCulloch CAG. Can evidence-based dental health care assure quality? J Dent Educ 1994;58:654-6.
50. Morris AL, Bentley JM, Vito AA, Bomba MR. Assessment of private dental practice: Report of a study. J Am Dent Assoc 1988;117:153-62.
51. Nightingale F. Notes on hospitals. 3rd ed. London: Longman, Green, Longman, Roberts, and Green, 1863.
52. Nikias MK, Sollecito WA, Fink R. An oral health index based on ranking of oral status profiles by panels of dental professionals. J Public Health Dent 1979;39:16-26.
53. Owens JA, Tennenhouse DJ, Kasher MP. Dental risk prevention. San Rafael CA: Tennenhouse Professional Publications, 1990.
54. Phantumvanit P, Songpaisan Y, Pilot T, Frenken JE. Atraumatic restorative treatment (ART): A three-year community field trial in Thailand. Survival of one-surface restorations in the permanent dentition. J Public Health Dent 1996;56:141-5.
55. Redig DF, Dewhirst F, Nevitt G, Snyder M. Delivery of dental services in New Zealand and California. J South Calif Dent Assoc 1973;41:318-50.
56. Romcke RG, Lewis DW. Use of expanded function hygienists in the Prince Edward Island manpower study. J Can Dent Assoc 1973;39:247-62.
57. Rowe NH, Doelle PJ, Loos PJ, Herschfus L. Hospital dentistry—survival? J Mich Dent Assoc 1985;67:507-11.
58. Schoen MH. A quality assessment system: The search for validity. J Dent Educ 1989;53:658-61.
59. Smith QM, Pennell EH, Bothwell RD, Gailbreath MN. Dental care in a group purchase plan: A survey of attitudes and utilization at the St. Louis Labor Health Institute. PHS Publication No. 684. Washington DC: Government Printing Office, 1959.
60. Spath PL, ed. Quality management in ambulatory care. Chicago: American Hospital Publishing, 1992.
61. The state dental scheme and the New Zealand Dental Association [editorial]. N Z Dent J 1921;16:145-8.
62. Torchia M. Using data to improve quality. Bus Health, 1994, Mar 23-7.
63. University of Otago. 2003 Media release. Alaskans to begin dental studies at Otago, website: http://www.otago.ac.nz/news/news/2003/ 20-02-03_press_release.html. Accessed May 6, 2004.
64. University of Otago. 2003 Media release. NZ's first degree-qualified dental therapists to graduate, website: http://www.otago.ac.nz/news/news/2003/05b-12-03_press_release.html. Accessed May 6, 2004.
65. US Department of Commerce, Bureau of Economic Analysis. Regional accounts: State personal income, website:http://www.bea.gov/bea/regional/docs/Regional_SPI.pdf. Accessed May 6, 2004.
66. US Department of Health and Human Services, Health Resources and Services Administration, Bureau of Health Professions. The Uniform Data System (UDS)—data. Calendar year 2002 data (national rollup), website: http://bphc.hrsa.gov/uds/data.htm. Accessed May 6, 2004.

67. US Department of Health and Human Services, Health Resources and Services Administration, Bureau of Health Professions. US health workforce personnel factbook, website: http://bhpr.hrsa.gov/health-workforce/reports/factbook02/FB301.htm. Accessed February 16, 2004.

68. US Preventive Services Task Force. Guide to clinical preventive services: An assessment of the effectiveness of 169 interventions. Baltimore: Williams and Wilkins, 1989.

69. van der Wal CJP, Nakahata DT, Posl WM, et al. Dental office structure and treatment outcome—related or independent? J Calif Dent Assoc 1995;23(9):41-9.

70. Wojner AW. Outcomes management: An interdisciplinary search for the best practice. AACN Clin Issues 1996;7:133-45.

71. Wood WL, Scher AZ. Franchise dentistry. N Y State Dent J 1984;50:677-8.

72. World Health Organization. Report of the International Conference on Primary Health Care, Alma-Ata, USSR, 1978 Sept. Geneva: WHO, 1978.

73. Yavner SB, Yavner DL, Douglass CW. The failure of the dental franchise industry. J Dent Pract Admin 1988; 5(1):21-4.

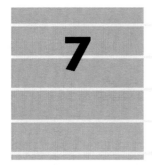

7 Financing Dental Care

Health care historically has been provided on a fee-for-service basis, in which the patient pays the provider directly for services. This two-party system is a private contract involving only the provider and the patient. Methods of financing health care in the United States, however, have progressed far beyond this traditional system since the mid-1930s and especially since 1965. A fundamental change has been the emergence of third parties, meaning that the financing of health services is no longer a matter of a purely private contract between provider and patient. In 2001, for example, 86% of the total outlays for health services and supplies involved a third party, and 46% of all health care services were paid for by government funds.[57] Dentistry's entry into the third-party system has been more recent, but third-party involvement in the payment for dental care is now a major and still-evolving part of dental practice.

This chapter reviews the various mechanisms used to finance dental care and the effects that these mechanisms have on care provision.

INSURANCE PRINCIPLES AND DENTAL CARE

To understand how dentistry fits into third-party payment, a review of insurance principles is helpful. During the years after World War II, when medical insurance was growing rapidly, dental care was one of the "fearful four" areas of health care (dental care, psychiatric care, prescription drugs, and long-term care) considered uninsurable by commercial insurers. This reasoning was based on the assumption that the nature of dental need violated the basic principles of insurance,[22] which state that to be insurable a risk must be the following:
- Precisely definable.
- Of sufficient magnitude that, if it occurs, it constitutes a major loss.
- Infrequent.

- Of an unwanted nature, such as destruction of a home through fire.
- Beyond the control of the individual.
- Without "moral hazard," which means that the presence of insurance itself should not lead to additional claims.

All health insurance violates some of these principles. For example, many of the benefits paid by health insurance represent relatively small amounts of money, and people with insurance are more likely to use care than those without it.[37,42] Insurance carriers found they could get around these problems in several ways, such as the following:

- Having patients pay a share of the costs.
- Limiting the range of services covered.
- Offering coverage only to groups.
- Including waiting periods after enrollment before benefits became payable.
- Using preauthorization and annual expenditure limits.

Requiring patients to pay part of the cost of some services is an economic disincentive to overutilization. The portion of the cost of the service that a patient pays is either a deductible or coinsurance (sometimes called *copayment*). A *deductible* is a set amount of money that the patient must pay toward the cost of treatment before benefits of the program go into effect.[4] A familiar example of a deductible is the "front-end" payment of a claim under automobile insurance. *Coinsurance* means that the patient pays a percentage of the total cost of treatment.[4] For example, if a patient is to pay 20% of the cost of an amalgam restoration, the amount the patient must pay varies depending on the approved fee for an amalgam but in any case will be 20% of that fee.

Insurance carriers also limit the range of health care services covered: some services are paid for and some are not, according to the plan. This is termed *coverage*, *covered charges*, or *schedule of benefits*. Examples of services that are not usually covered in dental policies are implants (although this is changing as implants become more common), cosmetic procedures, and extensive treatment for temporomandibular joint disorder. A common point of confusion is that, when a service is not covered by insurance, some patients take it to mean that they cannot have it, that the insurance company is somehow denying this service to the patient.

This is not the case; it is simply that the patient, rather than the insurer, is responsible for the payment.

An additional cost-control mechanism, preauthorization (sometimes called *predetermination*), means that treatment plans for more than a specified amount, or for especially costly services, must be reviewed by the carrier's dental consultants to ensure that the proposed treatment is reasonable and that the same quality of care could not be achieved at less expense.

Health insurance was at first offered only to groups, because illness experience is reasonably predictable for a group but much less so for an individual. The risk of *adverse selection*, which means the inclusion of too many high-risk beneficiaries, was reduced because insuring only large groups averaged out the risks. Although a large group would likely include people with high levels of need, there would also be many who had little need for care and who would still pay premiums. In fact, this is the essence of insurance. The fact that the cost of care required for a few people far exceeds the premiums paid for them is irrelevant as long as the average cost of care across the group is in balance with the premium.

The probability of adverse selection was further reduced by the use of waiting periods after enrollment. The waiting period ensured that people with existing disease were not simply going to use the plan to have that condition treated and then drop out. As experience with the administration of health insurance grew, carriers were able to offer individual policies. Today, many commercial and nonprofit insurance carriers make individual policies available for hospital and major medical coverage, although premiums are considerably higher and benefits are often more limited than for group policies.

After looking at the list of insurance principles, one can see why dental care was for a long time considered uninsurable. Nearly everyone has some dental treatment needs. They tend to be frequent rather than infrequent, and unlike the cost of hospital care the cost of dental treatment is rarely catastrophic. Nevertheless, evaluations of some of the earliest group prepayment plans indicated that dental care indeed was insurable because cost was found to be not the only barrier to dental care;[49-51] even when the cost barrier was removed, potential patients did not pour in as many had expected. Although utilization of dental service was increased, it stayed well short of 100%. In other words, although all members of the group may have needed dental care and all were paying a premium toward it, only some members were seeking treatment. Indeed, if 100% of the group seeks dental care on a regular basis, it might be less expensive for them to pay for their care individually rather than through prepayment.

EXPENDITURES FOR HEALTH CARE

Expenditures for health care have risen sharply in all industrialized countries over the last several decades, but nowhere has this pattern been as pronounced as in the United States. Fig. 7-1 shows that, in 1929, expenditures in the United States for health care (including dental care) accounted for 3.6% of the gross domestic product (GDP). Since 1929, the amount has gone steadily upward, reaching 14.9% of GDP in 2002.[26,57] Predictions suggest that spending for health care could rise to 20% of the GDP in the next few decades,[23,66] a level of national expenditure that is a cause for deep concern.

Fig. 7-2 shows how the per capita national health expenditures have risen since 1960. From an annual average of $141 in 1960, the average cost per person had risen to $5440 in 2002, a truly daunting figure.[36,57] For insurance to be able to cover these kinds of costs, it is easy to see why premiums must be high. Fig. 7-2 also shows that the portion of the cost of health care paid by public funds has grown since 1960. In 2002, 46% of total national health expenditures were paid by public (government) funds.[57] Some of the reasons given for this increase in the cost of health care in the United States include the following six factors:

Increasing Costs Incomes of health care workers have risen faster than the incomes for many other workers.

Difficult Economies of Scale It is harder to achieve economies of scale in health care than in many other sectors of the economy. In many manufacturing industries, for example, it does not require 10% more workers to produce an additional 10% of a product. In health care, by contrast, increasing the amount of care provided requires a nearly proportional increase in the workforce.

The Practice of "Defensive" Medicine Tests carried out to protect the provider against possible litigation, rather than to treat the patient, lead to a rise in costs.

The Aging Population An aging population causes an increase in per capita costs. Because older people use more health care services, the average cost of care will increase as the average age of the population increases. In addition, the

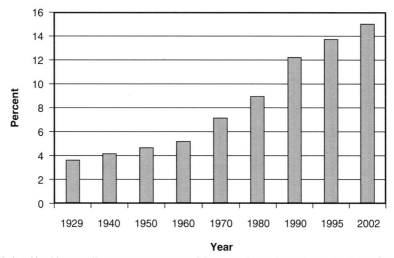

Fig. 7-1 National health expenditures as a percentage of the gross domestic product in the United States, selected years, 1929-2002.[26,36,57]

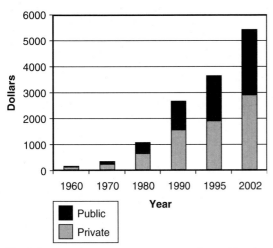

Fig. 7-2 Per capita national health expenditures, showing the proportionate expenditure of private and public funds in the United States, selected years, 1960-2002.[36,57]

expectation of longer life brings a greater willingness to provide heroic care for a person who in earlier days would not have been expected to live much longer even if healthy, but who today is thought to have a reasonable chance for more high-quality years of life.

Developments in Technology Some innovations reduce the costs of care because they are so much more effective than any available alternatives (antibiotics, for example, reduced the average length of a hospital stay when they were introduced in the 1940s and 1950s). Others, because they are providing care that was previously unavailable, can only add to aggregate costs. An example is treatment for end-stage renal disease for patients who in earlier days would have soon died. With dialysis they now live, but at a cost that was estimated to average $24,976 per patient per year as long ago as 1983.[48]

Third-Party Payment Insurance has provided large amounts of money for care that would otherwise have been unavailable. For example, many of the elderly and the poor who receive the benefits of Medicare and Medicaid would not otherwise have had the money to purchase this care. Without these programs, the total and per capita costs of care would undoubtedly be smaller. The same is true for private insurance, because many who otherwise

would have faced large bills for hospitalization and other services would have been forced to do without.

The spiraling costs of health care present American society with a classic trade-off dilemma. On the one hand, if people go without health care that can improve or prolong their lives, both the individual and society suffer. On the other hand, it should be evident that the proportion of the GDP going to health care cannot continue to climb indefinitely, because as more of our available resources go to health care there is less for housing, education, recreation, and other necessities that contribute to health, wealth, and happiness. Although there is ample reason to be concerned for people who receive too little health care, there is also the possibility that a point can be reached at which, at least in the aggregate, there is too much health care relative to life's other necessities. The dilemma is made even more difficult by the fact that, as of 2002, 43.6 million people in the United States had no health insurance.[56] Although there is a justifiable outcry that some form of coverage should be provided for these people, it is also obvious that to do so will further increase national expenditures.[30,42,78] Health care providers, in their honest desire to do the best for their patients, need to recognize that this tension between the individual and society will always exist.

Resolution of this dilemma is made even more complex by the inclusion of government and private third-party agencies in the equation. Because the total costs of care continue to climb and put more and more pressure on the economy, and because most health care costs are paid through third parties, the pressure for collective action to control these costs will continue. No one in health care should be surprised to see a continuing stream of proposals aimed at controlling or reforming the health care system.

EXPENDITURES FOR DENTAL CARE

Expenditures for dental care, although only a fraction of the total for health care, are nevertheless substantial. Fig. 7-3 illustrates that the total expenditures for dental care by Americans grew from less than $500 million in 1929 to an estimated $70.3 billion in 2002.[16,36,57] This latter

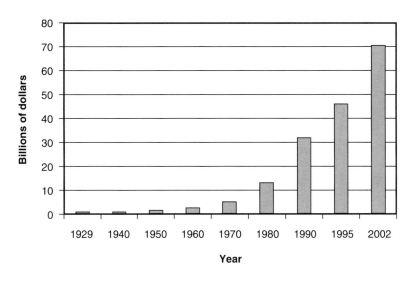

Fig. 7-3 Total expenditures for dental care in the United States, selected years, 1929–2002.[36,57]

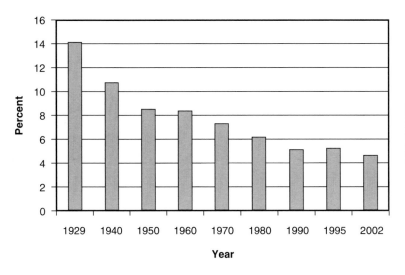

Fig. 7-4 Per capita expenditure for dental care as a percentage of total health expenditures in the United States, selected years, 1929–2002.[26,36,57]

figure represents an average per capita expenditure for dental care of $250 in 2002.

Figs. 7-4 and 7-5 present two additional views of the cost of dental care. Fig. 7-4 shows that, relative to the total cost of personal health care expenditures, dental expenditures have fallen steadily from the 14% reported in 1929 to 4.5% in 2002.[26,57] This pattern reflects the combination of the steep rise in the overall costs of medical care and the more modest rise in the costs of dental care. Fig. 7-5 presents the expenditures for dental care as a percentage of the GDP. The pattern here is especially interesting: the relative decline from 1929 to 1950 corresponds to the period of the Great Depression followed by World War II. Dental care is income and price

elastic, so that, as real income fell during the depression and as the cost of other goods and services rose during and after the war, there was simply less money available for dental care. The rise since 1970 coincides with a period of growth in real income and also in the extent of dental insurance. Economic theory suggests that both of these changes should result in a relative growth in dental expenditures, a phenomenon that has indeed occurred. The relative growth in dental expenditures has continued up to the present, to about 0.67% of the GDP in 2002, even though the percentage of the population covered by dental insurance has plateaued.[57] This is a sign that the dental sector continues to be a robust part of the national economy.

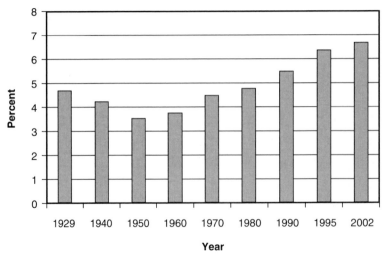

Fig. 7-5 National health expenditures for dental care as a percentage of the gross domestic product in the United States, selected years, 1929-2002.[26,36,57]

FEE-FOR-SERVICE DENTAL CARE

Private fee-for-service payment, the two-party arrangement, is the traditional form of reimbursement for dental services in the United States and elsewhere. Under this system, the patient decides when to visit a dentist, and the dentist suggests appropriate treatment and informs the patient of the fee for the service. If the patient chooses to follow the recommendations of the dentist and receives the services, the patient is then responsible for the fee. As shown in Fig. 7-6, as recently as 1970 almost all payments for dental services came directly from patients.[36] However, by 2002, because of the substantial growth in prepayment, direct consumer payment had dropped to about 44% of all payments, with nearly 50% being paid by private insurance.[57]

THIRD-PARTY PAYMENT IN DENTISTRY

In the language of contracts, the patient and dentist are the first and second parties, and the administrator of the finances is the third party, defined as the party to a dental prepayment contract that may collect premiums, assume financial risk, pay claims, and provide administrative services. Third-party payment for dental services therefore is payment for dental care that involves another party rather than payment directly by the patient. The third party is some-times called the *carrier, insurer, underwriter,* or *administrative agent.* The purchaser of the plan can be an organized private group such as a union, or it can be an employer, a union-employer welfare fund, a governmental agency, or an individual. Usually, however, the term *third party,* without further qualification, refers to an insurance company. When the government acts as the third party, the term more commonly used is *public financing of care.*

Growth of Third-Party Payment in Dentistry

In private third-party plans, periodic premiums are collected to meet the costs of providing care as well as the administrative costs of the third party. It has been argued that this arrangement should most properly be called *prepayment* rather than insurance, because it does not fulfill the classic definitions of insurance. Be that as it may, the term *dental insurance* has entered the language, and the terms *dental prepayment* and *dental insurance* as commonly used are virtually synonymous. The main difference between dental and some other forms of insurance is that traditional insurance involves a group of people making relatively small payments to cover the risk of a few suffering catastrophic loss, such as the loss of a home through fire. The expectation is that few of them will ever collect any insurance payments. Dental prepayment, on the other hand, is a mechanism to spread the financial load of dental care over a group and over time. Virtually all members of the group can

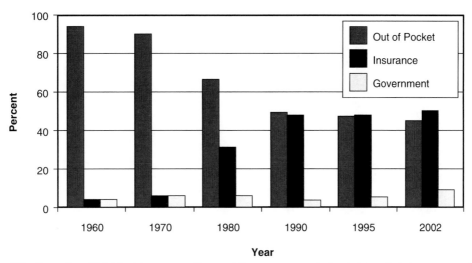

Fig. 7-6 Proportion of total dental care expenditures paid by consumers out of pocket, by private insurance, and by government funds in the United States, selected years, 1960-2002.[36,57]

reasonably expect to make regular and somewhat predictable use of the benefits.

For companies that administer these plans, the method for setting the premiums is essentially the same as it is for any other form of insurance. Based on the type of benefits involved and the characteristics and previous history of a group, the actuaries estimate how much dental care will be provided to the group in the coming period of time (usually at least 1 year). The expected reimbursable cost of that care plus the administrative expenses form the basis for premium calculations. Most private dental insurance in the United States is available only through group purchase; there are few individual policies. Individual policies that are available are characterized by high premiums or limited benefits. This is the carriers' method of countering the risk of high use and adverse selection.

Who actually pays for third-party care? A union that negotiates a dental plan as a fringe benefit is choosing to accept the plan rather than cash wages, so the union members pay for it in wages foregone. Ultimately, if the companies employing the union members increase the price of their products to finance the plan, the purchasers of those products pay for it. Reference to the third-party agency as the "payer for services," although common, is incorrect; nor are the union members getting "free" care, even if they do not pay directly out of pocket.

Passage of the Taft-Hartley Act in 1947 allowed labor unions to seek fringe benefits, in addition to wages, through collective bargaining. Since then, health care insurance has been a popular fringe benefit. One of the reasons for this popularity is that the premiums paid by the employer are not usually counted as taxable income for the employee. Each dollar of earnings taken in the form of health insurance therefore buys more health care than if it is taken as cash wages, because cash wages are taxed whereas the insurance benefits are not. (Health insurance as a fringe benefit, with protection from tax, is popular with the insurance and health care industries, too, because it actually is a subsidy for them.) There have been frequent unsuccessful attempts at the federal level to limit the amount of these health insurance premiums that are protected from taxes. It is reasonable to expect periodic attempts of this type in the future in times of budgetary difficulty. Such a "tax cap," if it were enacted, would reduce the popularity of dental insurance. It is assumed that if such a limit were to be placed on the tax deductibility of health insurance premiums, most people would apply the tax-deductible amount to their hospitalization and medical insurance. This would mean that the money paid by employers for dental insurance would be treated as taxable income, and additional wages would be deducted from each paycheck to pay this tax. Dental insurers fear that this change would cause some individuals and groups to drop their dental insurance.

By the late 1960s, with some 85% of the American population covered by hospital and surgical expense insurance,[33] coverage for dental expenses emerged as a popular area for negotiation by labor groups seeking additional fringe benefits. Growth of dental prepayment plans through the 1970s and 1980s therefore can be seen as an evolutionary step in the growth of employment fringe benefits.

The rapid growth of prepayment since 1970 has changed the nature of dental practice. The growth is illustrated in Fig. 7-6, which shows that the portion of dental care costs paid by prepayment plans increased more than tenfold between 1970 and 2002. The proportion of the U.S. population covered by some sort of dental insurance increased from less than 5% in 1970 to well over one half by the turn of the century. Today it is a rare dental practice indeed that sees no insured patients at all. In many parts of the country, the majority of the patients in most practices have dental insurance.

Although the growth in dental insurance has been spectacular since 1970, further rapid growth in the immediate future is not likely. This is because members of the large unions in the major U.S. industries are, for the most part, already covered. For dental insurance to grow, mechanisms will have to be developed to reach small businesses and individuals. A second reason why dental insurance will grow only slowly is the general climate of cost control in all aspects of business, which in turn comes from the fierce demands on the United States to be competitive in the global economy. Increased concern for worldwide competitiveness works against offering benefits to workers not already covered, and there are already some signs of cutbacks in some industries. A third factor that may work against further expansion of dental insurance is the improvement in oral health, which is especially evident in young adults and children (see Chapters 19-21). It may be that because people in these younger age cohorts have experienced little need for expensive and unexpected dental treatment, they will not push their employers as hard for dental insurance as did their elders, who had much higher levels of need for treatment.

Reimbursement of Dentists in Third-Party Plans

Control of the costs of third-party plans is essential to their success, for if the insurance plan is seen as a bottomless money pit, the plan will have to raise premiums to higher and higher levels, which makes it unlikely that anyone will be willing to buy the policy. Because the implications of "control" in this context are anathema to most practitioners, methods of reimbursing dentists under third-party plans have long preoccupied the American Dental Association (ADA). The ADA sees the need for controls but also tries to maximize the independence of the dental practitioner. Major forms of third-party reimbursement currently in use are:

- Usual, customary, and reasonable (UCR) fee
- Table of allowances
- Fee schedule
- Discounted fee (preferred provider organizations [PPOs])
- Capitation

In line with its philosophy of maximizing practitioner independence, the ADA has consistently supported the concept of the UCR fee as a reimbursement method for dentists in prepayment plans. However, ADA resolutions that UCR fees should be the preferred method of reimbursement were rescinded on legal grounds after the U.S. Supreme Court decision in June 1975 in *Goldfarb v. Virginia State Bar et al*. This decision ruled that learned professions were not exempt from antitrust laws.[5,7,8] In effect, the Court said that each practitioner should be free to choose how he or she wants to be reimbursed and that it was inappropriate for a professional association to suggest to its members which choice to make.

Usual, Customary, Reasonable Fee

The ADA definitions of usual, customary, and reasonable fees are as follows:

Usual fee: The fee that an individual dentist most frequently charges for a given dental service

Customary fee: The fee level determined by the administrator of a dental benefit plan from actual submitted fees for a specific dental procedure to establish the maximum benefit payable under a given plan for that specific procedure

Reasonable fee: The fee charged by a dentist for a specific dental procedure that has been modified by the nature and severity of the condition being treated and by any medical or dental complications or unusual circumstances, and that therefore may differ from the dentist's "usual" fee or the benefit administrator's "customary" fee[4]

When third-party dental programs first began, many dentists were opposed to them on the grounds that they would be forced to adopt lower fees than those that they usually charged. The evolution of the UCR fee concept as a mechanism acceptable both to dentists and carriers has allowed third-party dental care to be provided while still permitting individual dentists to charge what they believe their services are worth. It is reasonable to suggest that dental prepayment plans would not have been accepted by dentists to the extent they have been without the UCR fee concept.

Table of Allowances

A table of allowances (or schedule) is defined as a list of covered services with an assigned dollar amount that represents the total obligation of the plan with respect to payment for such service but that does not necessarily represent the dentist's full fee for that service.[4] For example, if a dentist's usual fee for a particular service is $20 and the plan lists a fee of $15 as payable for that service, the dentist will provide the service, collect $15 from the carrier, and may charge the patient $5 to make up the difference. Under the UCR fee method, on the other hand, the plan pays the dentist's usual fee in full (less any required patient copayment), in this case $20. Use of a table of allowances as a method of reimbursement requires that dentists carefully explain to patients the limited nature of the insurance payment, because some patients are unaware that their plan may not cover the costs in full.

Fee Schedule

A fee schedule is defined as a list of the charges established or agreed to by a dentist for specific dental services.[4] A fee schedule is usually taken to represent payment in full, whereas a table of allowances, as just explained, may not. With a fee schedule, the dentist must accept the listed amount as payment in full and not charge the patient at all. Fee schedules for dental care are sometimes established by public programs, such as Medicaid in many states. Dentistry's opposition to fee schedules is based on (1) the potential inflexibility of such sched-

ules, meaning that the fees listed can fall below customary fees, particularly in times of rapid inflation; (2) the implicit assumption that all dentists' treatment is of the same quality and therefore worth the same fee; and (3) the fear that autonomy is threatened, especially if the fee schedule is not controlled by the dentists. A potential risk with use of a fee schedule is that, if the fees paid are too far below the usual level, few dentists will be willing to treat the covered patients. This has been cited as one reason why many dentists either severely limit the number of their Medicaid patients or refuse to accept such patients altogether.[17,35,64]

Discounted fee

Discounted fees are usually the basis for PPO plans. Participating dentists have agreed to provide care for fees that are usually lower than those charged by many dentists in their area. Most preferred provider dental plans do provide partial payment for care received from a nonparticipating dentist, but in this case the patient is responsible for all of the difference between the dentist's fee and the amount paid by the plan.

Capitation

Reimbursement of the dentist by capitation, as in a medical health maintenance organization (HMO), became more common during the 1980s and 1990s but plays a much smaller role in dentistry than it has in medicine. The ADA defines capitation as a dental benefit program in which a dentist or dentists contract with the program's sponsor or administrator to provide all or most of the dental services covered under the program to subscribers in return for a payment on a per capita basis.[4] A capitation fee is usually a fixed monthly payment paid by a carrier to a dentist based on the number of patients assigned to the dentist for treatment. Capitation requires that patients be assigned to specific dentists or dental practices for care, so that the capitation payment can be paid to the appropriate dentist or practice. This assignment is important, because the dentist receives a fixed sum of money per enrolled person per month, regardless of whether the participants in the plan receive care during that particular month. The assumption is that, although some patients will need a lot of care, others will need little or none, and therefore the total amount of money paid to the dentist will be sufficient to cover the overall costs of care for the covered group.

Many dentists are resistant to capitation because of a fear that high utilization and demands for expensive forms of care could rapidly outrun the capitation fee and that dentists will thus be at an economic disadvantage. As a dissenting voice, Schoen[45-47] argued that capitation works every bit as well as fee for service and that with proper planning it is a highly efficient method of financing group dental care, especially for less affluent groups. Despite Schoen's claims of success with capitation in his own group practice, however, many dentists and the ADA remain cautious. The ADA is opposed to capitation and fee schedules as the sole forms of reimbursement in prepayment plans, arguing that where such mechanisms exist they should be on an equal footing with UCR fees so that prospective patients have a choice. In fact, by the 1990s there were very few "pure" capitation plans. Most capitation plans now include copayments, especially for more expensive services, and annual maximums, both of which limit the economic risks faced by the dentist.

NOT-FOR-PROFIT DENTAL PLANS
Delta Dental Plans

In June 1954, the Seattle District Dental Society in Washington State was approached by the International Longshoremen's and Warehousemen's Union-Pacific Maritime Association with a request that the society submit a proposal for a comprehensive dental care program for the children of the union's members up to 14 years of age. The proposal requested by the union required information on administration, fees, methods of operation, dental care provided, and control of quality. At that time there was almost no previous experience with plans of this type. The dental society nevertheless wished to discourage the union from setting up its own clinics, and it developed a plan whereby the children could be treated in the offices of private dentists. Shortly thereafter, the first dental service corporation was born.[72] Within a few years dental service corporations were also formed in Oregon and California, and in subsequent years the idea of the dental service corporation spread throughout the country from the West Coast.

A dental service corporation is a legally constituted not-for-profit organization, incorporated on a state-by-state basis, that negotiates and administers contracts for dental care. The original dental service corporations, now know as Delta Dental Plans in most states, were sponsored by the constituent dental societies in each state where they were initially formed. A service plan is a program in which the payment is meant to represent full payment, with no additional charge to the patient allowed beyond a preestablished copayment or deductible. Following the success of the early Delta plans, Blue Cross and Blue Shield organizations also began organizing dental plans in many states, which usually also were organized as not-for-profit service corporations.

As the number of state dental association–sponsored service corporations increased through the early 1960s and the size of the groups for which dental care benefits were negotiated grew, the need for a national organization of dental service organizations became apparent. Accordingly, the National Association of Dental Service Plans was formed in 1966, with staff and financial help from the ADA. The name became Delta Dental Plans Association (DDPA) in 1969,[28] and most of the member corporations became known as the Delta Dental Plan for the particular state.

DDPA has also become the vehicle through which the Delta plans in individual states compete with national for-profit insurance companies for contracts with companies with employees in more than one state. Through DDPA, an organization called DeltaUSA was formed to coordinate and administer these multistate contracts. In 2003 more than 108,000 participating dentists were available to DeltaUSA through the individual state Delta plans, accounting for at least 70% of all dentists in practice nationwide. Collectively, Delta plans cover approximately 42 million people in the United States.[18]

The underlying philosophy of the Delta Dental Plans was to permit dental practitioners to adapt their traditional patterns of practice to meet the demand for group purchase of dental care. In this sense, Delta plans have followed the lead of the professionally sponsored Blue Cross and Blue Shield hospital and medical plans. Most Delta plans were formed for the sole purpose of providing dental prepayment, and most have retained dental insurance as their sole or major business.

Delta also pioneered specific approaches to ensure the quality of care provided and to keep a program's costs under control, although other carriers now use many of these approaches as well. Quality of care is sometimes monitored by posttreatment examinations, in which a sample of individual patients who have received care through a plan are examined by a panel of independent consultant dentists to ensure (1) that the care claimed and paid for was in fact provided and (2) that it is of "acceptable" quality (see Chapter 7). When there are concerns about quality, referral can be made to the state's peer review mechanism if the matter cannot be resolved to the satisfaction of all involved.

Billing for services not actually provided and other instances of noncompliance with the contract such as waiving required copayments are taken seriously by insurers. Although the problem with billing for services not provided is obvious, that with waiving of copayment is perhaps less so. For insurers who base payments on the UCR method, the copayment is part of the "usual" fee and often an important part of the cost-control mechanism as well. If a dentist has claimed $40 as the usual fee for a service that has a 20% copayment, the insurer will pay the dentist $32 and expect the dentist to collect the remaining $8 from the patient. If the dentist chooses not to collect this $8, then the fee is in fact $32, not the $40 claimed, and the insurer should have paid 80% of $32 instead of 80% of $40. Further, if dentists were allowed to raise their submitted "usual" fees so that the fee minus the copayment equaled the fee that they really wanted, and then simply forgave the copayment, the cost-controlling effects of copayment would be lost. Concern over these billing practices has led to strict laws in many states, under which these practices are considered to be felonies. Any dentist dealing with third-party payment is well advised to read and understand the rules of participation and to make a good-faith effort to comply fully with the terms of the agreement.

Reimbursement of Dentists in Delta Plans

Because of Delta's initial close association with organized dentistry, Delta plans at first used the UCR fee-for-service concept almost exclusively, and this method of payment still dominates. Under the fee-for-service programs, the way in which a dentist is reimbursed depends on whether the dentist is participating or nonparticipating (often referred to as *par* and *nonpar* dentists) with Delta. A participating dentist is one who has entered into a contractual agreement to provide care to eligible persons.

Delta plans encourage all dentists to participate. Those who do generally agree to conditions similar to the following:

- Agreement to charge Delta-insured patients their usual and customary fees. The accumulated fees of all participating dentists form the basis of the UCR fee system. When a dentist decides to raise the fees charged to Delta patients, he or she must raise the fees to all fee-for-service patients. As long as the new fees are charged to all patients, they will become the fees that Delta uses for reimbursement purposes.
- Acceptance of payment for their services at an agreed-on percentile (to be described) as payment in full, which means the dentist will not assess the patient for any further charges, other than copayments as specified by a particular contract.
- Submission to fee audits by auditors from Delta, who may check the office records from time to time. The purpose of these audits is to ensure that the dentists are indeed charging their Delta patients the same fees as they charge their other patients and that copayments are being properly billed to the patient.

In the early days of dental insurance, participating dentists in many Delta plans also agreed to allow withholding of as much as 5% of the paid amount. This withheld amount was used by the new Delta plans to build up sufficient financial reserves to be able to take on more insurance risk and in turn to manage more business. As the corporations built up sufficient financial reserves, the withhold was reduced or eliminated in many states. Dentists who chose to become participating dentists agreed to the withhold because they supported the idea of developing a form of payment for dental care that they felt represented their interests and in which they had some voice. In addition, the prospect of direct, prompt payment from the insurer for their services, which greatly reduced bad debts and collection problems, was considered by many to be well worth the small amount withheld.

Nonparticipating dentists can also treat patients covered under Delta UCR plans and be reimbursed by Delta. Nonparticipating dentists are usually paid at the 50th percentile of fees, rather than the 80th or 90th percentile typically paid to participating dentists. A nonparticipating dentist also is free to charge the patient any difference between her fee and the amount paid by Delta. The incentive for a covered patient to go to a participating dentist is that the part of the fee that the patient must pay (i.e., the copayment) will usually be smaller than would be the case if the patient visited a nonparticipating dentist.

Percentile Fees

To illustrate how percentiles are applied to dental fees, suppose that in a given area there are 1000 participating dentists who have a range of fees for a particular service. The percentiles of a data set divide the total frequency into hundredths, so that the 90th percentile is that value below which 90% of the observations lie. In this example, let us assume that the range of fees charged for the service runs from $40 to $85. If each of these filed fees is spread out in a cumulative frequency distribution from the lowest to the highest, the result might be like that shown in Fig. 7-7. About 10% of dentists charge less than $60 for their service, 50% charge $65 or less, 80% charge $68 or less, and 90% charge $72 or less for this particular service. For this service, therefore, $72 is the 90th percentile fee. Ten percent of dentists charge more than $72.

When payment on UCR fees is made at the 90th percentile, 90% of the participating dentists receive their full fee for the service, and only 10% are paid less than their usual fee. Those dentists who normally charge $65 receive $65, those who normally charge $70 receive $70, and so on up to $72, the 90th percentile. Those who normally charge more than $72 are paid $72. If nonparticipating dentists are paid at the 50th percentile, which in this example is $65, they are paid whichever is lower, the fee that they actually charge or $65.

The rationale behind paying at the 80th or 90th percentile is to control payment at the top end of the scale while paying the vast majority of dentists (at least 80% or 90%) their full fee. This approach fits the definition of "customary." It is thus a cost-control mechanism usually written into Delta plan contracts with participating dentists.

Preauthorization

Another cost-control mechanism that is widely used by insurers is *preauthorization* (also called

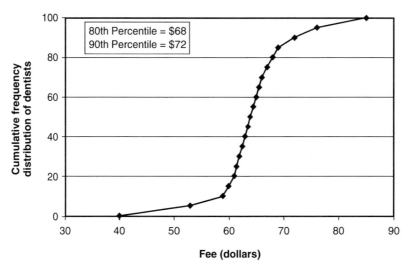

Fig. 7-7 Cumulative frequency distribution of hypothetical fees for a given dental service to illustrate the 80th and 90th percentiles.

predetermination, precertification, pretreatment review, or *prior authorization).*[4] With pre-authorization, when the costs of treatment are expected to exceed some limit (usually several hundred dollars), the dentist is required by some carriers, and advised by others, to submit the treatment plan to the insurer for review before the treatment begins. This review has several functions, including certification that the patient's insurance covers the planned treatment and at what level, and a review of the appropriateness of the care itself by a dental consultant who works for the insurer. These reviews reduce the cost of care directly, because some treatment plans are revised after discussion with a consultant. They also reduce it indirectly, because dentists soon learn that insurers are unlikely to allow expensive treatment when less expensive alternatives appear to be reasonable.

Procedure Codes

Dental procedure codes also were developed in the early days of dental prepayment. With the advent of third-party involvement, an unambiguous method had to be developed to define which procedures would be covered and which would not, as well as to facilitate the accurate reporting of which services were provided. There were various mechanisms for developing and maintaining these codes through the years, including the ADA's Code on Dental Procedures and Nomenclature. A single set of codes was mandated with the passage of the Health Insurance Portability and Accountability Act of 1996. The ADA is the designated agency for maintaining the dental codes and has established a Code Revision Committee for this purpose. Revised codes are issued every 2 years. Open meetings are held for input, and any interested party may submit requests for code revisions.[3] All dental insurers now use this standard set of procedure codes.

Blue Cross and Blue Shield Plans

Blue Cross and Blue Shield plans for many years offered only limited dental coverage as a part of their hospital-surgical-medical policies. Initially, this dental coverage was usually limited only to services provided in a hospital. The "Blues" showed little enthusiasm for going any further into dental prepayment on the grounds that it was a poor insurance risk, but their atti-

tude changed once dental prepayment was shown to be feasible.

Blue Cross and Blue Shield dental plans have adopted many of the cost-control features pioneered by Delta plans. Many now use UCR fees submitted by dentists, either to reimburse the dentists in the same way Delta does or to establish fee profiles or fee screens for different geographic areas as a basis for reimbursement. In some states, it is difficult to distinguish Blue Cross and Blue Shield dental plans from Delta plans in terms of benefits and administration.

As is now the case with Delta plans in some states, Blue Cross and Blue Shield plans are active in offering alternative reimbursement methods such as capitation, including independent practice associations (IPAs) and PPOs to meet the demands for cost reduction from purchasers. These alternative provider arrangements are described later in this chapter.

FOR-PROFIT DENTAL PLANS
Commercial Insurance Plans

Once it was clear that prepaid dental plans were viable and that they were likely to be a significant part of the health insurance market, commercial insurance companies began to view dental insurance as a potentially profitable area of business. The fundamental difference between commercial insurance companies and the dental service corporations is that the commercials operate for profit. Therefore, it might be expected that commercial insurance carriers would need to charge higher premiums than would the service corporations to allow for the profit margin. In practice, however, this is not necessarily true, for a number of reasons. Because there are so many different for-profit dental insurance carriers, collectively more people have dental insurance from commercial insurance carriers than from any other type of carrier.

Commercial insurance is often designed as an indemnity plan, meaning that cash payments are made to the providers, rather than as a service benefit plan. This allows the commercial carriers to organize reimbursement differently from the way that dental service corporations usually do. Dentists in most cases are not paid according to their UCR fees by a commercial insurance company; rather, the carrier develops fee profiles—that is, the carrier works out the "going rate" for services from the reported experience of fees in the area—and dentists are paid at that rate. The amounts paid can vary from one insurer to another.

MANAGED CARE

Managed care is a term that is in widespread use but for which there is no precise definition. The Health Insurance Association of America defined managed care as follows:

Systems that integrate the financing and delivery of appropriate health care services to covered individuals by means of arrangements with selected providers to furnish a comprehensive set of health-care services to members; explicit criteria for the selection of health-care providers; formal programs for ongoing quality assurance and utilization review; and significant financial incentives for members to use providers and procedures associated with the plan.[31]

This definition is a real mouthful, as complicated as managed care itself. Its key elements are the following:
- A comprehensive set of health care services
- Selected providers
- Financial incentives to use the selected providers

Simply stated, what has come to be called managed care is arrangements through which people receive all or most of their health care from providers (hospitals, physicians, and other personnel) who are formally linked to the organization. The patient's out-of-pocket cost is substantially lower than it would be if care were sought outside of the managed care organization.

The most common forms of these arrangements are HMOs and PPOs (described later in this chapter). There are also innumerable hybrids, with more coming every day. Although these types of arrangements are not new, the movement of the medically insured population to managed care in the 1990s has been on a massive scale. It was estimated that in 2001 about 93% of all insured individuals in the United States were enrolled in some type of managed care plan.[32] At the same time, there was a concerted effort under way by the federal Centers for Medicare and Medicaid Services to move Medicaid and Medicare enrollees from traditional fee-for-service to managed care. The effect of these trends on medicine has been pro-

found, for managed care has come to dominate the practicing life of many physicians.

The primary stimulus for the growth of managed care is concern over the seemingly endless increases in medical treatment costs, which were noted earlier in this chapter. The widespread hope is that managed care can somehow help control the costs of medical care. However, this hope begs the question as to what is the "correct" amount of care, and it assumes that there is some way that this can be determined for each patient. The hopes for cost control also depend on the assumption that the "correct" amount of care will be less expensive to provide than what people would buy outside of managed care.

No one system for organizing care, however, can be expected to solve all the underlying conflicts associated with health and health care. Although health care is sometimes judged only in terms of life and death, measuring the worth of a system is more complex. It is more sensible to look at how the system affects the quality of life, although the problem that immediately arises is that modern medicine's ability to add comfort and length to life usually comes at ever-increasing cost. Every dollar spent on health care is a dollar that is unavailable for some other purpose, which means that there is an implicit trade-off when an individual decides to spend money for more health care rather than for something else. The problem becomes especially difficult when small increases in comfort or longevity come at high dollar cost. These decisions are difficult enough when made by individuals with their own money; they are infinitely more difficult when made in a public forum with collective funds.

These tensions associated with deciding how much health care is appropriate, and for how much money, are driving the rapid evolution in the financing and delivery of medical care. That no single approach is going to be a panacea should be self-evident, because there is no single answer to the underlying question of how much health care is the right amount, and at what price. In fact, we see that, even as managed care is rapidly increasing market share, there is a growing backlash against it. It cannot satisfy everyone all of the time, and its promise of controlling costs is seen as the reason for its failures when inevitably some people experience unsatisfactory health care outcomes.

Dentistry in Managed Care

Dentistry is inevitably caught up to some extent in this financing maelstrom that affects medicine. Virtually all of the innovations that have been and are being tried in medicine are evident in dentistry. Some of this has occurred because purchasing groups have demanded the same kind of system from their dental coverage that they are using for their medical coverage. Some has come from entrepreneurs, both inside and outside dentistry, who see managed care as an opportunity to move dental practice into the future, or more crassly as a way to make quick money.

On the other hand, there are important differences between medicine and dentistry that make it unlikely that managed care will play as large a role in dentistry as it has in medicine. The most important difference is that, whereas about 85% of the population have medical insurance, only around 50% have coverage for dental care. Insured patients account for nearly all of the income of physicians and hospitals. If large purchasing groups want these providers to change their practices, physicians and hospitals are extremely vulnerable. With dentistry, on the other hand, there are still large numbers of patients who are not covered by dental insurance, so that dentists, individually and as a group, are far less susceptible to pressure from large purchasers.

The difference in governmental involvement in the payment for care is also important. For medical care in general, government funds account for almost one half of all expenditures, whereas government funds account for only about 6% of dental expenditures.[57] As government struggles to control expenditures, medical care costs cannot be ignored, but dental care costs are relatively unimportant. Because it controls such a large portion of medical reimbursement, government is in a position to exert an enormous influence over providers. In dental care, however, this is not the case. With Medicaid, for example, with reimbursement levels well below what many dentists deem reasonable, dentists can simply refuse to participate without affecting their economic well-being. This would not be possible for many practitioners in medicine.

Health Maintenance Organizations

Although the idea of HMOs is not new, its implementation was formally promoted with the passage of the Health Maintenance Organization Act of 1973 (Public Law 93-222). This act made federal funds for the development of HMOs available under certain conditions. It was intended to provide an acceptable alternative to the fee-for-service private practice system and help restrain the costs of care.

One of the principal advantages of HMOs, as a method of providing health care, lies in their claim to reduce the cost of care for those enrolled. These savings are purportedly due to the greater emphasis on ambulatory care and consequently on reduced hospital utilization as well as on close control of costly services. "Unnecessary" hospitalization, principally for routine diagnostic tests and minor surgery, is thereby curtailed. Dental care, however, is almost exclusively ambulatory care, because few dental procedures require inpatient hospitalization. The major advantage of the HMO concept in reducing hospitalization, therefore, has little application to dentistry, but the close monitoring of utilization emphasized in HMOs is relevant.

An HMO was defined in the 1973 act as "a legal entity which provides a prescribed range of health services . . . to each individual who has enrolled in the organization in return for a prepaid, fixed, and uniform payment."[55] Usually, but not always, an HMO looks like a large group practice with a number of services available under one roof. An HMO is described as having five essential elements: a managing organization, a delivery system, an enrolled population, a benefit package, and a system of financing and prepayment.[39] HMOs use a prepaid capitation system of financing medical services. Capitation means that the care provider is paid a fixed sum on a regular basis, usually monthly, for each enrolled person, whether or not the enrollee uses any care in that month.

Enrollment in HMOs grew rapidly, peaking at 80.8 million in 1999.[32] Since that time enrollment has begun to decline, likely due to consumer resistance to what was seen as restrictive access to some services. The decline in HMO enrollments have been more than balanced by rapid growth in PPOs and point-of-service arrangements (both to be described later).

Dental Personnel in Health Maintenance Organizations

Only a small proportion of HMOs offer dental services. When dental services are offered, they are financed through (1) the primary capitation premium, (2) a separate premium, or (3) a fee for service. When included, the dental care itself can be provided in an HMO according to one of four basic organizational models:

Staff model: Dentists, dental hygienists, and dental assistants are salaried employees of the HMO. The staff model is the only one of the four modes that affects auxiliary personnel directly, because in the other three, the terms of their employment in dental practices do not differ from those in traditional private practices.

Group model: The HMO contracts directly with a group practice, partnership, or corporation for the provision of dental services. The group receives a regular capitation premium from the HMO.

IPA: The IPA is an association of independent dentists (or physicians in medical practice) that develops its own management and fiscal structure for the treatment of patients enrolled in an HMO. An IPA is thus not a different form of practice but instead a legal arrangement through which individual dental offices can participate as providers to groups of patients who are enrolled in HMOs. Dentists continue to practice in their own offices. The IPA receives its capitation premium from the HMO (or other prepayment agency) and in turn reimburses the individual dentists on either a modified fee-for-service basis or a capitation basis.

Capitated network or direct contract model: The network is similar to the IPA, except that the HMO contracts directly with the individual provider for provision of services. This is the most common form of capitation arrangement in dentistry. Dental insurers who wish to offer a capitation product recruit and contract with dental offices that are willing to have patients assigned to them.

Assumption of Risk

The concept of assumption of (financial) risk is important in health care. In the case of patients who pay for their own care, the situation is uncomplicated: if the patient accepts the treatment proposed by the dentist, the patient is responsible for the necessary payment. With the advent of traditional fee-for-service insurance, the insurance companies typically agreed to assume the financial risk. In this arrangement, there are a set of covered services, usually subject to some copayments and an annual maximum, but the insurance company is responsible for paying for the care with the money it has collected from the premiums. The insurer carefully rates each group to estimate how much the group's care will cost, so that it can be sure to set the premiums at a level that is sufficient to cover the costs of care but not so high that a competitor will make a lower bid. In any case, with traditional insurance, the insurance company is "at risk" for most excess costs. Acceptance of this risk is part of what the insurer is selling.

In principle, one of the main features of the capitation method is that the risk, previously assumed by the insurer, is shifted to the provider. The essence of the capitation system of payment is that the provider receives a previously agreed-on sum per patient enrolled, regardless of whether or not the patient seeks care. In return, the provider agrees to provide specified services as necessary for a predetermined period.

Clearly, the concern of the provider is that the amount of money received (*known* before a contract is signed) be sufficient to cover the services needed (which are *unknown*, although they often can be reasonably estimated, especially for a large group of patients). If the cost of the services required exceeds the income received through the contract, the provider loses. Conversely, if the services required are less than the income provided by the contract, the provider gains. It follows that under some contracts there is the potential for undertreatment and discouragement of service utilization, which raises concerns about both ethics and the quality of care received.[38]

Therefore it is understandable that both the ADA and individual dentists are cautious about assumption of risk. Of course, risk is assumed by an HMO when it establishes its monthly premium for its enrollees, just as it is assumed by any insurer in a prepaid care plan. Capitation, however, brings the concept of assuming risk directly to the dentist. By the 1990s, features such as patient copayments and annual maximums had become common in capitation plans as ways to reduce the dentist's risk. These were and still are standard cost-control mechanisms in fee-for-service plans.

The pressure for innovative approaches to control the costs of medical care has in turn caused purchasers to demand, and insurers to provide, similar approaches for financing dental care. As a result, capitation plans are a part of many dental practices, especially when third-party payment involves a high proportion of patients. The basis of capitation, as previously described, is that the contracting provider, whether an HMO, group practice, IPA, or individual dentist, receives a fixed sum, usually on a monthly basis, for each eligible patient. The money is paid regardless of whether patients utilize care. In return, the patient is entitled to receive covered services that are needed. As of 2002, the National Association of Dental Plans estimated that about 23.5 million individuals were enrolled in dental HMOs (sometimes referred to as DHMOs).[41] Enrollment in DHMOs has actually declined over the past 10 years.

Preferred Provider Organizations

PPOs, along with HMOs, are one of the main managed care arrangements and the one that is growing most rapidly. PPOs typically involve contracts between insurers and a number of practitioners who agree to provide specific services for fees that are lower than the average for the area. Again following the pattern established in medicine, dental insurers have embraced the idea of selectively directing patients to specific providers (the preferred providers in a PPO) who have agreed to provide care to the insured group on a fee-for-service basis but at fees that are significantly lower than the usual fees for the area. The contracting dentists often agree to participate at the lower-than-usual fees to attract additional patients to their practices. Competition for patients is the driving force behind the willingness of some providers to discount their fees for PPO patients; clinicians who have ample demand for

their services at their usual fees, if these usual fees are higher than those required by the PPO, are not likely to be interested in a PPO agreement. PPOs differ from HMOs in that they are fee-for-service plans, so in PPOs a beneficiary can go to any participating provider for any covered service, because payment is made only when care is provided. By 2004, approximately 112 million Americans had medical coverage through PPOs.[1] Just as the popularity of medical PPOs has increased, PPO arrangements have grown rapidly in dentistry in the past decade. The National Association of Dental Plans estimated that dental PPO enrollment in 1999 was 65 million individuals nationwide.[41] Most PPOs (both medical and dental) allow patients to go to providers that are outside of the PPO panel. However, to encourage use of PPO providers, and thus to maintain the expected cost savings from the use of lower-fee providers, patients receiving care outside of the network are usually required to pay for a larger part of their care. With the continuing push to control the cost of health care, some PPOs have now come into being that pay nothing for out-of-network care (except for emergency care). This form of PPO is usually referred to as an *exclusive provider organization*.

Point-of-Service Plans

Point-of-service (POS) plans are managed care plans that allow enrollees to receive some of their care, if they wish, from providers who are outside of the managed care providers. For this feature, people who choose to receive care outside of the panel pay a larger part of the costs of their care. The recent increase in enrollment in POS plans indicates that many individuals are willing to pay extra for their health insurance to have the increased flexibility that these plans offer over more restrictive managed care arrangements.

Concerns Regarding Managed Care

For some, the primary concern with capitation is that it might encourage undertreatment. Under "pure" capitation, the dentist receives the same payment whether or not treatment is provided, which leads some to argue that this will encourage undertreatment and neglect. Others argue that this is a virtue of capitation, because the dentist is assured a predictable income and is thus able to make decisions about treatment without worrying about daily revenues if treatment need is low. Many think that the fee-for-service system, in which dentists are paid only if they find treatment to provide, has a high potential for producing overtreatment. They see this risk as even greater in the current era of lower disease levels. PPOs may also encourage overtreatment because the agreed-on fees are discounted, which thus provides incentive to provide multiple services per visit to make each patient visit more economically worthwhile for the practice. All of these concerns have led to increasing pressure on insurers to develop ways to monitor the quality and quantity of care. Purchasers and individual patients need to be assured that the care they pay for is appropriate and of acceptable quality, regardless of the way for which it is paid. To assure purchasers that the quality of care is high and the patterns of care provided are reasonable, some insurers are conducting increasingly sophisticated analyses of claims data to detect patterns that could be signs of substandard or fraudulent care. In this way, it is possible to focus most of the more expensive personal attention on the providers who are most likely to be providing care in ways that fall outside the patterns covered by insurance (also see Quality Assurance in Chapter 6).

DIRECT REIMBURSEMENT

Direct reimbursement is a form of payment for dental care that has existed informally for a long time. It continues to be promoted by the ADA as an alternative to the more common forms of dental insurance.[6] Direct reimbursement involves an agreement between an employer and its employees in which the employer agrees to reimburse the employees for some part of their expenses for dental care. Employees can go for care to any dentists they choose. The patient is responsible for paying the dentist, and the dentist has no responsibility to the insurer for such things as scope of covered services or limits on frequency of services. All treatment decisions are made by the patient and the dentist in a traditional two-party manner. After treatment has been provided and paid for, the patient takes the receipt to the employer and is reimbursed for these expenses according to the rules of the agreement. Reimbursement is usually on a percentage basis, and annual limits are common.

The ADA likes direct reimbursement because it keeps third parties out of the decisions on which services to provide, how frequently they can be provided, what the fee will be, and which dentists will provide them. It is also argued that direct reimbursement minimizes administrative costs, although the employer, or a hired administrator, still must process these reimbursements and keep track of annual limits.

Groups accustomed to the more conventional forms of third-party dental insurance have not readily embraced direct reimbursement because they have come to expect and value such things as direct payment from the insurer to the dentist, so that patients face fewer out-of-pocket expenses. They also expect the insurer to play an active role in ensuring that the type and quantity of services provided are reasonable and that the quality of care is acceptable. Direct reimbursement purposely attempts to keep third parties out of these areas, but for many purchasers the third-party involvement is an important part of what they expect from dental insurance. In any event, direct reimbursement has not become a major method of dental prepayment.

DISCOUNT DENTAL PLANS

In an attempt to find a way to capture markets beyond the traditional large groups, especially the individual market, a form of dental benefits that really is not properly called prepayment or insurance has arisen. These discount dental plans arise when carriers develop panels of dentists who agree to lower-than-average or discounted fees, similar to PPO panels, and agree to charge their low fees to patients who present a discount card. The carrier charges the patient a small monthly fee for the discount card. The major difference from other forms of coverage is that the patient is responsible for 100% of the discounted fee. What the monthly fee for the discount card is buying for the patient is access to a panel of dentists who have agreed to treat the patient at a discounted fee. This is a rapidly evolving product, and its long-term impact is difficult to predict.

ADMINISTRATIVE SERVICES ONLY

In addition to conventional insurance coverage, in which the insurer is at risk for the costs of care, insurers are increasingly providing for purchasers a service known as *administrative services only* (ASO). The distinguishing feature of an ASO contract is that the purchaser of the contract is at risk for the costs of care rather than the insurer. The purchaser pays a periodic fee that covers all of the normal administrative services associated with insurance, such as actuarial services, claims processing, preauthorization, posttreatment reviews, and processing of payments to providers. Virtually all of the types of payments to dentists that have been described, in which the insurer is usually at risk, can be managed on an ASO basis. Whether the insurance company or the purchaser is at risk does not affect the way the plan appears to the patient or the dentist. ASO contracts are popular with large groups, because the groups do not have to hand over the large sums of money needed for payment to the insurance company up front. Instead, the purchasers retain control over the funds until the time payment is actually made. The earnings on large amounts of cash, even if held for relatively short periods of time, can be considerable and therefore effectively reduce the cost of the insurance to the purchaser. Although insurance companies handle much of the ASO business, companies called third-party administrators have arisen that do no insuring at all. Third-party administrators handle only the administrative end of insurance, leaving responsibility for the funds to pay claims, and therefore the insurance risk, in the hands of the group.

MEDICAL SAVINGS ACCOUNTS, HEALTH SAVINGS ACCOUNTS, AND FLEXIBLE SAVINGS ACCOUNTS

Medical savings accounts and, more recently, health savings accounts are another attempt to control the continually rising expenditures for health care. Both of these allow a person to establish and add to a special savings account, protected from taxes, to be used as needed to cover medical expenses.[29,69] These accounts are meant to cover most small and often discretionary medical expenses and can be established

only in combination with a high-deductible insurance policy that covers the more expensive and infrequent expenses. The theory is that when individual patients are made responsible for and thus more aware of the actual cost of routine medical expenses, they will be more prudent users of care. Use of the high-deductible insurance policy would be reserved for those infrequent and high-cost needs that more ideally fit insurance principles. It is too early to say whether these types of accounts will be widely used or whether they will be effective in controlling the costs of care. Nevertheless, their recent development is further evidence of the high level of interest in finding a way to control the costs of health care. Flexible savings accounts are somewhat different, in that they allow employers to set up for their employees accounts into which employees make contributions that are not subject to income tax. These funds can then be used during the tax year for qualifying health care expenses that are not covered by insurance. They are different from medical savings accounts and health savings accounts in that they are not required to be created in conjunction with a high-deductible insurance policy, and any funds in the account not used for medical care in the year are forfeited by the employee, so the employee must carefully plan how much to have placed into such an account.[68] It is too early to know whether these mechanisms, in fact, will have a significant effect on use of medical or dental care.

FORCES AFFECTING THE DESIGN OF THIRD-PARTY DENTAL CARE PROGRAMS

Most mechanisms for controlling the costs of medical care also affect the way that dental care is provided and financed. Both HMOs and PPOs include substantial financial incentives to receive care from a participating provider. Both lower out-of-pocket payments and a wider range of covered services are common methods to encourage beneficiaries to choose managed care options. Even though the many forms of insurance options can seem bewilderingly complex, the underlying forces are straightforward and will always be present. Purchasing groups want to buy sufficiently easy and convenient access to care, at the lowest possible price. For some groups, the higher cost of wider access is worth higher premiums; for other groups it is not. In a growing number of cases, the cost of acceptable access is more than an employer can afford, and employees are increasingly being asked to pay a share of the premiums. In some cases, employees are required to pay the entire premium, and in these cases the coverage is voluntary. The only benefit to the employee in this case is the ability to buy insurance coverage through a group that might not otherwise be available as individual coverage. The continual pursuit by these groups of the best balance between access to care and cost will continue to put pressure on providers to keep costs unber control. To many dentists the expression *cost control* is synonymous with harassment, red tape, and poor quality of care. However, appropriate methods of cost control do not demand the use of inferior materials or techniques. Instead, cost control should be based on the concepts of evidence and cost effectiveness: that is, how can a purchasing group best spend the available money to gain maximum dental health benefits for its members?

Most dental practices have a vital stake in the continued economic health of the third-party payment system because it represents a substantial share of their income. At the same time, purchasers of care are taking increasing notice of the growing cost to them of providing dental insurance.[10,24,43] The dental insurance companies are then on notice that they must keep the costs of the plans that they offer under control, which in turn affects dentists' incomes. A number of such mechanisms have been described and are in common use; others are continually under development. If cost controls are not routinely and successfully incorporated, individual dental plans will simply not succeed in the marketplace. The challenge is to find ways of keeping the costs of dental care within the range that purchasers are willing to pay, while at the same time providing a level of care and access to providers that both dentists and patients find acceptable. Although dentists may have difficulty accepting the idea that not every patient should have all of the care that money can buy, purchasers of care for large groups are increasingly unwilling or unable to pay the insurance premiums needed to support open-ended benefits.

Although the cost of dental care is much smaller than the cost of medical care, dental care is nevertheless subject to the same kinds of pressure as is medical care. Although the mechanisms employed are numerous and are constantly evolving, and can thus be confusing and frustrating to providers and patients alike, the underlying principles are really quite simple. The challenge for those who design dental insurance products is to find the best balance between access and price. At one extreme, if insurance coverage will pay for whatever a patient and dentist decide is to be done, with few and small patient copayments, the premiums required will tend to be relatively high. Less expensive will be a plan that limits payments only to dentists who have agreed to provide services at low or discounted fees (i.e., a PPO) or one that requires substantial deductibles or patient copayments. Perhaps least expensive of all would be a plan that provides the beneficiary with a discount card which, when presented to a participating dentist, assures that the dentist will charge discounted fees, but these fees will be paid entirely by the patient. The number of variations is endless, and the resulting continuing dance of product designs is an attempt by the various insurance companies to match this balance between access and cost to create products that will be attractive to customers. This balance can be especially critical for dental insurance because, unlike with medical insurance, the risks of going without dental insurance are not large. Therefore the challenge for dental insurance companies is not only to meet the competition posed by other insurers but also to meet the challenge of the customer's deciding to go forward with no dental insurance at all. This concept is so important that it bears repeating. A prepayment system for dental care that cannot continue to provide to groups a level of coverage (access) that it wants at a cost that is acceptable is at risk of having the group decide that it can do without dental coverage altogether. Both patients and dentists would lose in such a situation. Without help to pay for the care, fewer patients would receive care, and dentists' incomes would decrease.

Third-party plans do not remove the cost barrier to dental care; they merely change its nature. The amount of care a plan can finance is still finite; the object of controls is to try to use the available financing to best advantage.[9] The more that dentists are able to accept this philosophy, the better they will be able to work with purchasers and administrators to devise mutually acceptable methods of cost control. The continual pushes and pulls of the prepayment marketplace are not there to harass dentists and patients, but instead are a manifestation of the unrelenting pressures of the marketplace to stay within the range of an acceptable access-price balance.

PUBLIC FINANCING OF HEALTH CARE

The federal government has been involved in the direct financing of health care almost from the founding of the United States. Congress in 1798 established the Marine Hospital Fund, the forerunner of the U.S. Public Health Service, to provide medical care for merchant seamen. The federal government gradually accepted responsibility for providing health care to other groups: the care received by military and Coast Guard personnel, American Indians, Alaska Natives, and inmates of federal penitentiaries is financed with federal funds and often provided at federal facilities. This limited and carefully defined role of the federal government was seen for a long time as its right and proper function in health care provision.

The relation between the various levels of government in the United States was permanently changed in 1935 with the passage of the first Social Security Act. This act was passed in the midst of the Great Depression, when unprecedented problems were caused by mass unemployment and widespread poverty. The act created a system financed from compulsory employee-employer contributions to provide income maintenance for the elderly. The Old Age Insurance (OAI) provisions of the original act of 1935 became extended to the Old Age and Survivors Insurance (OASI) in 1939 and then to the Old Age, Survivors, and Disability Insurance (OASDI) in 1960.[53] All provisions of the Social Security system until then were related to income security, rather than to the financing of health care. In addition, public welfare payments at that time were made directly to the recipients only. These payments were so low that most individuals could afford only limited emergency health care, and the choice was left to the recipient about whether to buy health care or something else. It is perhaps not surprising that recipients of public welfare tended to seek health care only when they perceived themselves or a member of their family to be seriously ill.

The Social Security Act of 1935 provided no funds expressly for the provision of health care. During the Great Depression, however, people's inability to purchase health care in the traditional way was recognized as a major social problem. A system of grants-in-aid was thus developed as a method of using federal finances for needed health care services without disturbing the traditional federal-state separation. Grants-in-aid were federal funds allocated to the states according to specified formulas. To receive these grants, the states had to expend their own funds for the same objectives as those supported by the grant-in-aid, often in the ratio of $1 from state or local sources to $2 from federal sources.[25] Grants-in-aid during this period were available only for support of specific categories of needy individuals, such as the blind, dependent children, permanently and totally disabled individuals, and the aged.

A significant change in methods of federal financing for health care came with the passage of the Kerr-Mills bill in 1960. This legislation, supported by both the ADA and the American Medical Association, linked health care needs to the general welfare of the aged indigent by a program known as Medical Assistance to the Aged. Although the effects of this program were relatively disappointing,[53] the Kerr-Mills bill introduced the use of vendor payments, meaning payments directly to those who provided service rather than to the recipients of care. This procedure ensured that allocated funds could be used only for health care.

Growing public awareness in the early 1960s of the problems of poverty and ill health set the stage for the 1965 amendments to the Social Security Act. These amendments were in their own way as landmark a piece of legislation as the original act 30 years earlier. Title XVIII, known as Medicare, provided for the receipt of health care services by all persons aged 65 and over, regardless of their ability to pay, and Title XIX, known as Medicaid, was intended to bring access to health care to the indigent and medically indigent segments of the population. The term *medically indigent* refers to those who are not dependent on public welfare to meet the basic necessities of life but who do not have sufficient income to purchase health care through the usual private practice channels. (This concept is meaningless, of course, because costly new developments in the diagnosis and treatment of previously untreatable diseases can make anyone but the super-rich medically indigent should they be unfortunate enough to get the wrong disease.)

In 1997 the Social Security Act was further amended through Title XXI, which created a State Children's Health Insurance Program (SCHIP). SCHIP provides federal funds to states and, like Medicaid, requires that the states also use some of their own funds to provide payment for health care for children in families whose income is too high to qualify for Medicaid but still too low to be able to afford health insurance.

Public Expenditures for Dental Care

By 2002 just over 6% of all dental expenditures were from public funds, compared with more than 46% of total health expenditures.[57] Fig. 7-8 shows the proportions of public and various types of private payments for different areas of health care in 2002. It can be seen that payment for dental care is close to evenly split between private insurance and out-of-pocket patient payments. Government, plus

other sources such as charity, account for the remaining 6% of dental payments.

The proportion of total public expenditures on health care services in 2002 that went to dental care was also very small, less than 0.7%. More than 40% of all public expenditures for health care went toward hospital care; the other major areas of public expenditure were physicians' services, nursing home care, public health activities, and research.[57]

North Carolina established the first state dental division in 1918, and many other state-level dental public health programs developed between 1935 and 1965. A great variety of dental care programs were instituted, financed, and administered by state and local communities during this period, frequently with the help of federal monies through grants-in-aid. Many state-level dental public health programs, focusing on maternal and child health populations, got their start via such grants-in-aid through what was then the Children's Bureau. These programs vary greatly from state to state. Although some are strong and active, in many states these programs are small and inadequately financed.

Medicare

Title XVIII of the Social Security amendments of 1965 is the program known as Medicare. As originally conceived, it removed financial barriers for hospital and physician services for persons age 65 and over, regardless of their financial means. Medicare also covers some people who are disabled as well as people with permanent kidney failure. Expenditures on the Medicare program in the first few years of operation were considerably higher than estimated, and it was not long before some financial constraints were introduced. By the mid-1970s, Medicare had two parts: Part A, hospital insurance, and Part B, voluntary supplemental medical insurance. Both parts contain a highly complex series of service benefits, and both parts also require some copayment by the individual. Apart from these copayments, Medicare is financed completely from Social Security funds.

Medicare was brought into being because the voluntary health insurance system was unable to provide adequately for people over age 65. The health insurance industry must collect premiums sufficient to cover what it must pay out, and the risk of adverse selection in those over

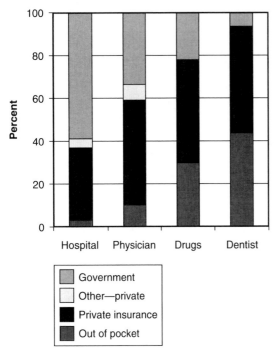

Fig. 7-8 Proportionate expenditures on various categories of health services by type of payment in the United States, 2002.[57]

age 65 is high. In addition, because the income of persons aged 65 and older is usually considerably less than that of those in the employed population, they have limited funds to spend on health care. Hence, there were twin problems of high health care needs and low income.

The uproar from the health professions that surrounded Medicare's birth in 1965 ("socialized medicine") subsided as the public realized that it filled a necessary gap in the financing of health care. Data from the website of the Centers for Medicare and Medicaid Services, the federal agency that administers Medicare and Medicaid, show that, in 2002, more than 40.5 million Americans, about 14.5% of the population, were enrolled in Medicare. Federal expenditures for the program were estimated to be approximately $236 billion in 2002, or $5800 per enrollee.[57] In late 2003 legislation was passed to add prescription drug benefits to Medicare by 2006. The dental segment of Medicare is limited to those services requiring hospitalization for treatment, usually surgical treatment for fractures and oral cancer, and hence constitutes a negligible part of the program.

Medicaid

Medicaid, Title XIX of the Social Security amendments of 1965, differs from Medicare in several important ways. Whereas Medicare is funded wholly from federal funds, Medicaid costs are shared jointly by the federal and state governments. In 2004 the federal government provided 53%–80% of the funds used by each state.[77] Federal allocations are made according to a formula based on the ratio of the state's per capita income to the national per capita income.[74] The original intent of Medicaid was to provide funds to meet the health care needs of all indigent and medically indigent persons. Eligibility standards vary widely from state to state, as do the expenditures on authorized services. For example, in 1998 the average Medicaid expenditure per recipient nationally was about $4300, but in some states it was almost $9000 and in others just over $2000.[60] Medicaid is a major source of health insurance for children. In 1998 almost 20% of children in the United States were insured by Medicaid.[58]

Expenditures for the overall Medicaid program have shown a steady growth through the decades, as indicated by Fig. 7-9. Even after adjustment for inflation, the pattern shows a steady increase over time. Medicaid expenditures for dental care, however, follow a quite different pattern, as shown in Fig. 7-10. Real (adjusted for inflation) dollar expenditures for dental care have changed relatively little since the early 1970s.[52,65,66]

A pattern of a relative decline in dental expenditures within Medicaid is demonstrated in Fig. 7-11, which shows that the proportion of the total Medicaid budget going to dental care has fallen steadily from nearly 3% in 1972 to well under 1% in the late 1990s. Small as this

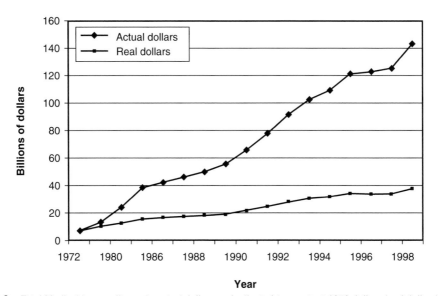

Fig. 7-9 Total Medicaid expenditures in actual dollars and adjusted to constant 1972 dollars (real dollars) in the United States, selected years, 1972–98.[52,65,66]

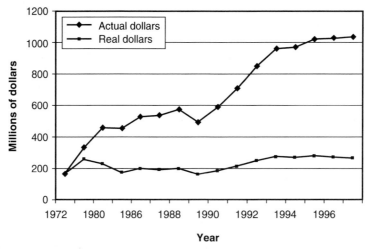

Fig. 7-10 Medicaid expenditures for dental care in actual dollars and adjusted to constant 1972 dollars (real dollars) in the United States, selected years, 1972-97.[52,65,66]

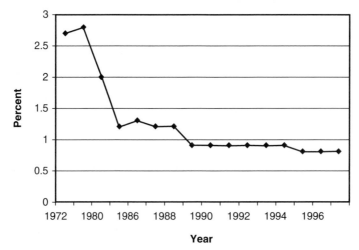

Fig. 7-11 Medicaid expenditures for dental care as a percentage of total Medicaid expenditures in the United States, selected years, 1972-97.[52,65,66]

fraction is, it still represents the bulk of public expenditures for dental care. This decline is made more severe by the rise in the number of recipients of dental services through this time from 2.4 million in 1972 to well over 5 million in 1998.[52,65,66] The result is that the expenditure for dental care per dental recipient fell throughout the period, as shown in Fig. 7-12. Expressed in constant 1972 dollars, payments dropped from nearly $71 per recipient in 1972 to $45 in 1997. In the mid and late 1990s, well under 20% of Medicaid recipients received dental care under the program.

To qualify for the federal government's share of Medicaid financing, every state Medicaid program is required to cover a set of basic services

for all children receiving federally supported financial assistance. In addition, amendments to the Medicaid program instituted in 1968 required that states offer early and periodic screening, diagnosis, and treatment (the EPSDT program) to needy children through age 20. Medical, dental, vision, and hearing services are mandatory under the EPSDT program.

Unfortunately, the EPSDT program continues to be a long way from fulfilling its promise. Of slightly more than 21 million children under the age of 21 who were eligible for EPSDT services in 1993, just over 4 million (under 20%) received preventive dental services.[64] With the exception of some relatively small demonstration projects to increase access, very little has

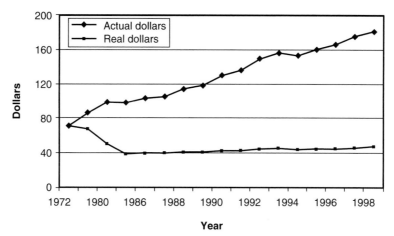

Fig. 7-12 Medicaid expenditures for dental care per dental recipient, in actual dollars and adjusted to constant 1972 dollars (real dollars) in the United States, selected years, 1972-98.[52,65,66]

improved over the past decade.[21] National statistics continue to show that only 20%-30% of Medicaid-enrolled children receive any dental care in a given year.[64,70,71]

Although Medicaid has reached a large number of people, there clearly are gaps. Despite the fact that well over 40 million people in the United States are without health insurance,[32] there have been and continue to be efforts to limit Medicaid expenditures.[14] The economic recessions of the early twenty-first century have sharply increased the number of people eligible for Medicaid, and because this happened during periods of rapidly increasing medical care costs, the higher costs of the Medicaid program were seen as excessive by many states. As a result, some states cut back on eligibility, reducing the availability of services and the levels of payment to providers. Unfortunately, dental services are often included among the first of these cutbacks, and Medicaid-funded services for adults have been especially hard hit. Many dentists, frustrated by rapidly changing eligibility standards for prospective patients, reductions in available services, changes in percentile fees paid, and delays in payment for services rendered, have refused to treat patients under Medicaid.

The future of Medicaid at the beginning of the twenty-first century remains clouded. For one thing, the pressure to reduce government spending at both the federal and state levels is relentless. Medicaid is a prime target for reduc-

tions, partly because it does not have a vocal constituency. Although the over-65 population is a powerful, articulate, and politically potent force in support of Medicare, the Medicaid-eligible population is not such an advocate. Although the federal government continues to push responsibility for Medicaid toward the states, the states already feel overburdened by Medicaid costs and are resisting. Whatever the outcome, the most likely losers are the Medicaid recipients, who are threatened with loss of access to health services provided by private practitioners.

The philosophy of shifting social welfare programs from the federal government to the states will cause continuing loss of needed services if funding is not also made available to already stretched state budgets. State governments, unlike the federal government, are unable to operate at a deficit. If tax revenues and other sources of funds are not sufficient to meet all of the budget needs, programs simply must be reduced or eliminated. The development of block grants, in which previously categorical federal funds (evolved from the grant-in-aid days) are lumped together to be allocated to specified programs at a state's discretion, is causing difficulties for dentistry. The total sum of federal funds received by the state is reduced, and there are heavy political pressures to use the funds for health-related purposes other than dental care. The immediate future for traditional public health programs does not look optimistic, although philosophies may change if large numbers of people are unable to get the care

*Reference 11–13,17,20,35,40,67,70,71,75,76.

they need. Although there have been innovative small-scale demonstration programs in some states that show promise for overcoming some of the access problems for the Medicaid population, the long-term success of these and other programs will ultimately depend on sufficient funding. There is simply no way to provide dental care, or anything else, without adequate funds.

On the positive side, the nearly $3.7 billion paid by Medicaid for dental services in 2002, although far short of what was needed, has still allowed dentists to treat many patients who would otherwise not have received care.[57] It should also be remembered that numerous public and philanthropic dental programs derive a substantial portion of their operating revenues by billing Medicaid for services that they provide to enrolled individuals, and in this way Medicaid plays a key part in sustaining and enlarging these safety net programs. Nevertheless, it is troubling that virtually all state Medicaid programs are out of compliance with the requirements for Medicaid and EPSDT, that this noncompliance is well known by all involved parties,[54] and that little enforcement is carried out. A vocal dental constituency is needed to force action.

In an effort to help control the costs of both Medicare and Medicaid, government has made a major effort to encourage enrollment in managed care plans. Although there has been some success in moving beneficiaries to managed care, especially in Medicaid, for which there is no other option in some states, it remains to be seen whether or not costs are actually controlled in the long run and whether access and other quality indicators will be at satisfactory levels.

State Children's Health Insurance Program

SCHIP, enacted in 1997 under Title XXI of the Social Security Act, is intended to encourage states to provide health coverage to many of the more than 10 million uninsured children in the United States. SCHIP is intended for children whose families have incomes that are above those for Medicaid but are too low to enable them to afford conventional health insurance. SCHIP covers children in families who have incomes up to at least 200% of the federal poverty level (a federally defined level of income that defines poverty for government purposes [see Chapter 2]), although states have some flexibility to set higher limits to

include more children. By 2003 about 5.8 million children in the United States were enrolled in SCHIP, a bit over 7% of the child population of the country and about one half of the uninsured children that SCHIP initially intended to reach.[59] Because the states have more flexibility in the design of their SCHIP programs than is the case for Medicaid, the programs can differ markedly from one state to another. They can vary from a simple expansion of the state's Medicaid program with no difference from the Medicaid program at all to a completely separate program with a different set of rules. These separate SCHIP programs may require patient copayments, monthly premiums, and annual payment limits, none of which is permitted under Medicaid.

Other Programs of Public Financing for Dental Care

The Indian Health Service (IHS) is responsible for medical and dental care for over 1.6 million American Indians and Alaska Natives who are members of federally recognized tribes.[2] The IHS provides care through over 230 hospitals and clinics in 35 states, and employs approximately 400 full-time dentists and 1400 hygienists and dental assistants.[63] The Division of Oral Health of the IHS is responsible for direct care through its own clinics and contract care through private dental offices for a large portion of this population. Federal funds also are provided for some tribes to run their own programs. Dentists who are commissioned officers in the U.S. Public Health Service are also assigned to provide dental care for U.S. Coast Guard personnel and inmates in federal prisons.

Community and migrant health centers are joint state-federal projects designed to bring primary and preventive health care to medically underserved areas throughout the United States and its territories.[61] Many of these centers provide dental services and preventive education. A substantial part of the federal Maternal and Child Health Services block grants (Title V funds) are also used by individual states for dental care, and funds are available for dental care through Head Start for prekindergarten and kindergarten children from deprived backgrounds who are otherwise not eligible for Medicaid. Other programs with federal involvement that have a dental care component are the Health Care for the Homeless program and the

National Hemophilia Program, which provides a wide range of services for hemophiliacs. There also are funds available for individuals with human immunodeficiency virus infection under the federal Ryan White CARE Act.[62]

Rehabilitative care for children born with cleft lips and palates has long been financed cooperatively by state funds and federal grants-in-aid because it was recognized that just about everybody is "medically indigent" when it comes to treatment of cleft lip and palate. All states have some resources available for team treatment of this condition. Dental personnel should be aware of resources available in or near their communities.

Unfortunately, public financing for the dental care of people with other handicapping conditions—for example, those with cerebral palsy, mental retardation, paraplegia, or quadriplegia—has never been as forthcoming. Although some states do have reasonable programs for the treatment of children with these conditions, few have any kind of financing available for their dental treatment when they become adults. The dental treatment of chronically ill and homebound adults has also been neglected almost completely, despite a successful demonstration program for providing dental care to the homebound.[73]

The program of the Department of Veterans Affairs (formerly the Veterans Administration, or VA) provides some dental care to eligible veterans through its inpatient and outpatient facilities nationwide. As previously noted, the various branches of the military also provide direct care for active duty personnel, and a voluntary dental insurance program, currently called TRICARE, which usually requires the participants to pay part of the cost, is available for dependents of military personnel. Similar voluntary insurance programs are available for military retirees and members of the reserve forces (National Guard). For all of these programs for other than active duty personnel, care is often provided through private dental offices, with payment partially paid according to the insurance coverage.[19]

National Health Insurance

Although the idea of national health insurance (NHI) in the United States is not new,[15] the fact that serious proposals for some form of it periodically resurface testifies to the persistence of the dual problems of (1) large numbers of people who have no insurance, and (2) the unrelenting increases in the costs of health care services.

If NHI is perceived as simply a financing mechanism without any restructuring of the care system, however, the rate of cost increases is not likely to diminish.[27,34] Indeed, the rate of increase in direct expenditures would far exceed present levels. The characteristics of the system that have fueled the continuing rise in the proportion of GDP that goes to health care would be magnified by an additional large infusion of funds. The trade-offs required to balance need against costs will present challenges for which American society seems unprepared.[44] This realization, added to concerns about a balanced federal budget and strong opposition from medicine, dentistry, and private health care and pharmaceutical interests, is responsible for the hesitancy in enacting NHI.

Although proposals for universal and comprehensive publicly financed health insurance have been consistently swept aside, the record clearly shows that government involvement in health care financing has been steadily increasing over the long term. Especially since 1965, when the federal government got involved in direct payment for care in a big way with Medicare and Medicaid, we have seen slow expansion in the groups covered. Given the relative success and popularity of these programs, and recent expansion to include prescription drugs in Medicare, which covers essentially all the over-65 population, and the expansion of the Social Security Act (Title XXI) in 1997 to include many uninsured children, there is some level of government-assisted health care coverage for virtually all but the working-aged population. There remain the dual concerns of, on the one hand, whether the funding for these programs is adequate, especially for Medicaid and the State Children's Health Insurance Program, and, on the other hand, whether taxpayers are willing to support what look to be ever-growing programs. Further, coverage for dental services continues to be a small part, at best, of these government health programs. For the foreseeable future, most Americans who receive regular dental care will continue to pay for it with private insurance or their own funds.

Those unable to pay will continue to be far less likely to receive regular care.

REFERENCES

1. American Association of Preferred Provider Organizations. Learn more about PPOs: PPO overview, website: http://www.aappo.org/ppo_about.html. Accessed May 11, 2004.
2. American Association of Public Health Dentistry. Dental public health residency, website: http://www.aaphd.org/print.asp?page-ihs.htm. Accessed Oct. 13, 2004.
3. American Dental Association, Council on Dental Benefit Programs. Code on dental procedures and nomenclature, website: http://www.ada.org/prof/resources/topics/cdt/index.asp. Accessed May 11, 2004.
4. American Dental Association, Council on Dental Benefit Programs. CDT 4: Current dental terminology. 4th ed. Chicago: ADA, 2002.
5. American Dental Association, Council on Dental Care Programs. Policies on dental care programs. Chicago: ADA, 1977.
6. American Dental Association, Council on Dental Care Programs. Policies on dental care programs. Chicago: ADA, 1991.
7. American Dental Association, House of Delegates. Resolution 9-1966-H. Trans Am Dent Assoc 1966; 107:311.
8. American Dental Association, House of Delegates. Resolution 30-1968-H. Trans Am Dent Assoc 1968; 109:305-6.
9. Bailit HL. Is overutilization the major reason for increasing dental expenditures? Reflections on a complex issue. J Dent Pract Admin 1988;5(3):112-5.
10. Bailit HL, Bailit JL. Corporate control of health care: Impact on medicine and dentistry. J Dent Educ 1988;52:108-13.
11. Brown LJ, Wall TP, Lazar V. Trends in untreated caries in permanent teeth of children 6 to 18 years old. J Am Dent Assoc 1999;130:1637-44.
12. Brown LJ, Wall TP, Lazar V. Trends in untreated caries in primary teeth of children 2 to 10 years old. J Am Dent Assoc 2000;131:93-100.
13. Brown LJ, Wall TP, Lazar V. Trends in total caries experience: Permanent and primary teeth. J Am Dent Assoc 2000;131:223-31.
14. Chang D, Holahan J. Medicaid spending in the 1980s: The access-cost containment trade-off revisited. Urban Institute Report 90-2. Washington DC: Urban Institute Press, 1990.
15. Chapman CB, Talmadge JM. The evolution of the right to health concept in the United States. Pharos 1971;34:30-51.
16. Cooper BS, Worthington NL. National health expenditures, 1929-72. Soc Secur Bull 1973;36(1):3-19, 40.
17. Damiano PC, Brown ER, Johnson JD, Scheetz JP. Factors affecting dentist participation in a state Medicaid program. J Dent Educ 1990;54:638-43.
18. Delta Dental Plans Association. Company information: Delta dental statistics, website: http://www.deltadental.com/servlets/Company/stats2.jsp?UserSection=employers. Accessed April 14, 2004.
19. Department of Defense, Office of the Assistant Secretary of Defense. What is TRICARE?, website: http://www.tricare.osd.mil/whatistricare.cfm. Accessed February 21, 2004.
20. Edelstein BL, Manski RJ, Moeller JF. Pediatric dental visits during 1996: An analysis of the federal Medical Expenditure Panel Survey. Pediatr Dent 2000;22:17-20.
21. Eklund SA, Pittman JL, Clark SJ. Michigan Medicaid's Healthy Kids Dental program. An assessment of the first 12 months. J Am Dent Assoc 2003;134:1509-15.
22. Faulkner EJ. The role of health insurance. In: Gregg DW, ed: Life and health insurance handbook. Homewood IL: Irwin, 1959:523-32.
23. Fuchs VR. The health sector's share of the gross national product. Science 1990;247:534-8.
24. Garrison J. Purchasers and payers: Who's driving the market? J Dent Educ 1996;60:356-9.
25. Gerrie NF. Grants-in-aid in federal-state dental public health program relationships. J Am Dent Assoc 1957; 54:182-8.
26. Gibson RM, Fisher CR. National health expenditures, fiscal year 1977. Soc Secur Bull 1978;41(7):3-20.
27. Gleicher N. Expansion of health care to the uninsured and underinsured has to be cost-neutral. JAMA 1991;265:2388-90.
28. Goetz J. The plan name and symbol. J Am Dent Assoc 1969;78:706-9.
29. Goodman JC, Musgrave GL. Patient power: Solving America's health care crisis. Washington DC: Cato Institute, 1992.
30. Hadley J, Steinberg EP, Feder J. Comparison of uninsured and privately insured hospital patients. Condition on admission, resource use, and outcome. JAMA 1991;265:374-9.
31. Health Insurance Association of America. Source book of health insurance data, 1995. Washington DC: HIAA, 1995.
32. Health Insurance Association of America. Source book of health insurance data, 2002. Washington DC: HIAA, 2002.
33. Health Insurance Institute. Source book of health insurance data, 1977-78. Washington DC: HII, 1978.
34. Jonas S. National health insurance. In: Jonas S, ed: Health care delivery in the United States. 1st ed. New York: Springer, 1977:434-66.
35. Lang WP, Weintraub JA. Comparison of Medicaid and non-Medicaid dental providers. J Public Health Dent 1986;46:207-11.
36. Levit KR, Lazenby HC, Braden BR, et al. National health expenditures, 1995. Health Care Financ Rev 1996; 18(1):175-202.
37. Manning WG, Bailit HL, Benjamin B, Newhouse JP. The demand for dental care: Evidence from a randomized clinical trial in health insurance. J Am Dent Assoc 1985;110:895-902.
38. Marcus M. Managed care and dentistry: Promise and problems. J Am Dent Assoc 1995;126:439-46.
39. Myers BA. Health maintenance organizations: Objectives and issues. HSMHA Health Rep 1971; 86:585-91.
40. Nainar SM, Tinanoff N. Effect of Medicaid reimbursement rates on children's access to dental care. Pediatr Dent 1997;19:315-6.

41. National Association of Dental Plans. 2000 Dental benefits enrollment data updated by joint study, website: http://www.nadp.org/resources/newsletters/2003_ Enrollment_Report_Release.pdf. Accessed February 16, 2004.

42. Oberg CN, Lia-Hoaberg B, Hodkinson E, et al. Prenatal care comparisons among privately insured, uninsured, and Medicaid-enrolled women. Public Health Rep 1990;105:533-5.

43. Olsen ED. Dental insurance: A successful model facing new challenges. J Dent Educ 1984;48:591-6.

44. Russell LB. Some of the tough decisions required by a national health plan. Science 1989;246:892-6.

45. Schoen MH. Group practice owned by a partnership using some salaried dentists and contracting directly with purchasers of group dental care. J Am Dent Assoc 1961;62:392-8.

46. Schoen MH. Group practice and poor communities: Dental care. Am J Public Health 1970;60:1125-32.

47. Schoen MH. Methodology of capitation payment to group dental practice and effects of such payment on care. Health Serv Rep 1974;89:16-24.

48. Smith DG, Harlan LC, Hawthorne VM. The charges for ESRD treatment of diabetics. J Clin Epidemiol 1989; 42:111-8.

49. Smith QE, Mitchell GE, Lucas GA. An experiment in dental prepayment: The Naismith Dental Plan. PHS Publication No. 970. Washington DC: Government Printing Office, 1962.

50. Smith QE, Pennell EH. Service requirements in dental prepayment: Predictability and adverse reaction. Public Health Rep 1961;76:11-8.

51. Smith QE, Pennell EH, Bothwell RD, Gailbreath MN. Dental care in a group purchase plan: A survey of attitudes and utilization at the St. Louis Labor Health Institute. PHS Publication No. 684. Washington DC: Government Printing Office, 1959.

52. Social Security Administration. Social Security Bulletin. Annual statistical supplement 2002, website: http://www.ssa.gov/policy/docs/statcomps/supplement/2002/8b.pdf. Accessed April 15, 2004.

53. Stevens R, Stevens R. Medicaid: Anatomy of a dilemma. Law Contemp Probl 1970;35:348-425.

54. US Congress, Office of Technology Assessment. Children's dental services under the Medicaid program: Background paper. OTA Publication No. OTA-BP-H-78. Washington DC: Government Printing Office, 1990.

55. US Congress, Senate. Health Maintenance Organization Act of 1973; Public Law 93-222. 93rd Congress, 2nd Session. Washington DC: Government Printing Office, 1974.

56. US Department of Commerce, Bureau of the Census. Number of Americans with and without health insurance rises, Census Bureau reports, website: http://www.census.gov/Press-Release/www/releases/archives/health_care_insurance/001372.html. Accessed February 19, 2004.

57. US Department of Health and Human Services, Centers for Medicare and Medicaid Services. Highlights—National health expenditures, 2002, website: http://www.cms.hhs.gov/statistics/nhe/historical/highlights.asp. Accessed November 13, 2003.

58. US Department of Health and Human Services, Centers for Medicare and Medicaid Services. State Children's Health Insurance Program (SCHIP): SCHIP summary, website: http://www.cms.hhs.gov/schip/. Accessed June 5, 2004.

59. US Department of Health and Human Services, Centers for Medicare and Medicaid Services. FY 2003 Number of Children Ever Enrolled in SCHIP by Program Type, website: http:// www.cms.hhs.gov/schip/enrollment/ schip03.pdf. Accessed 16 April, 2004.

60. US Department of Health and Human Services, Health Care Financing Administration. A profile of Medicaid. Chartbook 2000, website: http://www.cms.hhs.gov/ charts/medicaid/2Tchartbk.pdf. Accessed April 16, 2004.

61. US Department of Health and Human Services, Health Resources and Services Administration. Bureau of Primary Care [Community Health Center program], website: http://bphc.hrsa.gov/CHC/. Accessed April 16, 2004.

62. US Department of Health and Human Services, Health Resources and Services Administration, HIV/AIDS Bureau. 2004 Ryan White CARE act grantee conference information, 2004, website: http://hab.hrsa.gov. Accessed May 11, 2004.

63. US Department of Health and Human Services, Indian Health Service. Medical and professional programs: IHS Division of Oral Health, website: http://www.ihs. gov/MedicalPrograms/Dental/index.cfm. Accessed April 16, 2004.

64. US Department of Health and Human Services, Office of Inspector General. Children's dental services under Medicaid: Access and utilization. Publication No. OEI-09-93-00240. Washington DC: Government Printing Office, 1996.

65. US Department of Health and Human Services, Social Security Administration. Social Security Bulletin, annual statistical supplement, 1989. SSA Publication No. 13-11700. Washington DC: Government Printing Office, 1989.

66. US Department of Health and Human Services, Social Security Administration. Social Security Bulletin, annual statistical supplement, 1996. SSA Publication No. 13-11700. Washington DC: Government Printing Office, 1996.

67. US Department of Health and Human Services. Oral health in America: A report of the Surgeon General. NIH Publication No. 00-4713. Rockville MD: DHHS, National Institute of Dental and Craniofacial Research, National Institutes of Health, 2000.

68. US Department of Labor, Bureau of Labor Statistics. Health spending accounts, website: http://www.bls. gov/opub/cwc/cm20031022ar01p1.htm. Accessed April 16, 2004.

69. US Department of the Treasury. Treasury Secretary Snow Statement on health savings accounts, website: http://www.treas.gov/pressreleases/js1045.htm. Accessed February 22, 2004.

70. US General Accounting Office. Oral health: Dental disease is a chronic problem among low-income populations. GAO Publication No. HEHS-00-72. Washington DC: GAO, 2000.

71. US General Accounting Office. Oral health: Factors contributing to low use of dental services by low-income populations. GAO Publication No. HEHS-00-149. Washington DC: GAO, 2000.

72. US Public Health Service. The dental service corporation: A new approach to dental care. PHS Publication No. 570. Washington DC: Government Printing Office, 1961.

73. US Public Health Service, Division of Dental Public Health and Resources. Dental care for the chronically ill and aged: A community experiment. Washington DC: Government Printing Office, 1961.

74. US Public Health Service, Health Care Financing Administration. Medicare and Medicaid data book, 1988. HCFA Publication No. 03270. Washington DC: Government Printing Office, 1989.

75. Vargas CM, Crall JJ, Schneider DA. Sociodemographic distribution of pediatric dental caries: NHANES III, 1988–1994. J Am Dent Assoc 1998;129: 1229-38.

76. Venezie RD, Vann WF Jr. Pediatric dentists' participation in the North Carolina Medicaid program. Pediatr Dent 1993;15:175-81.

77. Wachino V, Schnider A, Rousseau D. Financing the Medicaid program: The many roles of federal and state matching funds. Washington DC: Kaiser Foundation, 2004.

78. Weissman J, Epstein AM. Case mix and resource utilization by uninsured hospital patients in the Boston metropolitan area. JAMA 1989;261:3572-6.

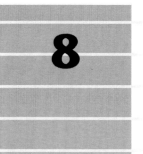

8   The Dental Workforce

The vision of the dental team is one of various people in dentistry with different roles, functions, and periods of training, all working together to treat patients.[106] *Dental team* is more a concept than a precise term, although the dental profession in the United States has long recognized that several different categories of personnel are fundamental to the efficient provision of care. Virtually all dentists employ at least one nondentist staff person, more than 94% of general practitioners employ at least one full- or part-time chairside assistant, and more than 63% employ at least one full- or part-time hygienist.[29]

This chapter defines the various types of personnel involved in the provision of dental services and assesses the factors that influence their supply and distribution.

TYPES OF DENTAL PERSONNEL

Dentists

A *dentist* is a person who is permitted to practice dentistry under the laws of the relevant state, province, territory, or nation. These laws are intended to ensure that a prospective dentist has satisfied certain requirements such as (1) completion of a specified period of profes-

sional education in an approved institution, (2) demonstration of competence, and (3) evidence of satisfactory personal qualities. Dentists are concerned with the prevention and control of the diseases of the oral cavity and the treatment of unfavorable conditions resulting from these diseases or from trauma or inherent malformations. A dentist is legally entitled to diagnose and treat patients independently, to prescribe certain drugs, and to employ and supervise auxiliary personnel. The mechanisms for fulfilling these requirements differ among nations. In the United States and Canada, for example, professional education is separate from the additional testing required for licensure. In many other countries, these two functions are combined under the authority of the educational institutions.

Dental Auxiliaries

Dental auxiliary is a generic term for all persons who assist the dentist in treating patients. It includes the categories of dental hygienist, dental assistant, hygienist or assistant with expanded functions, dental laboratory technician, receptionist, and secretary. Auxiliaries can be classified as operating and nonoperating,[107] depending on whether they carry out any intraoral procedures in the direct treatment of patients.

With rare exceptions, auxiliaries of all types operate under varying degrees of supervision by dentists. Even those auxiliaries who appear to operate more or less independently, such as the school dental therapist of New Zealand (see Chapter 6), work under some degree of supervision. Defining the extent of supervision required for various types of dental auxiliary can be confusing, because bodies concerned with supervision continue to modify their stance and definitions. As of 2002, the American Dental Association (ADA) acknowledged four levels of supervision of allied dental personnel as shown in Box 8-1.

The ADA policy statement on this issue declares: "General supervision is not acceptable to the American Dental Association because it fails to protect the health of the public."[8] This issue is important for public health programs because, without general supervision, it is far more expensive for dental hygienists to provide care in schools, nursing homes, and other institutional settings. Where general supervision is permitted, dentists in private practice can allow a hygienist to provide recall prophylactic services while the dentist is away from the office.

These policies of the ADA have no direct control on the practice of dentistry because the regulation of dental practice in the United States is determined by state licensing boards, not by the professional organization. Each state can have its own definition of supervision requirements and scope of practice, and indeed there is considerable diversity among states. The moves by the ADA to limit the scope of auxiliaries' practice are occurring as dental hygienists are working for a greater degree of autonomy, so conflicts are to be expected.

A *dental hygienist* is an operating auxiliary licensed to practice dental hygiene under the laws of the appropriate state, province, territory, or nation. In nearly all jurisdictions, to be licensed, hygienists, like dentists, must satisfy certain qualifications such as (1) completion of an approved period of education in an approved institution (only Alabama permits on-the-job training of hygienists),[81,99] (2) demonstration of competence, and (3) demonstration of satisfactory personal qualities. Hygienists are recognized auxiliaries in a number of countries, in which their duties and deployment are essentially similar.[62]

Dental hygienists have traditionally been concerned with prophylaxis, the health of the supporting structures of the teeth, and prevention of further diseases by direct clinical procedures and by the education of individual patients and groups. In most places, hygienists work under the supervision of dentists, either in private dental practice or in institutional settings such as health departments, nursing homes, or school dental programs.

BOX 8-1 Levels of Supervision of Allied Dental Personnel As Defined by the American Dental Association in 2002[8]

1. **Personal supervision:** The dentist is personally operating on a patient and authorizes the allied dental personnel to aid treatment by concurrently performing a supportive procedure.
2. **Direct supervision:** The dentist is in the dental office or treatment facility, personally diagnoses the condition to be treated, personally authorizes the procedures and remains in the dental office or treatment facility while procedures are being performed by the allied dental personnel and, before dismissal of the patient, evaluates the performance of the allied dental personnel.
3. **Indirect supervision:** The dentist is in the dental office or treatment facility, has personally diagnosed the condition to be treated, authorizes the procedures and remains in the dental office or treatment facility while the procedures are being performed by the allied dental personnel, and will evaluate the performance of the allied dental personnel.
4. **General supervision:** The dentist is not required to be in the dental office or treatment facility when the procedures are being performed by the allied dental personnel, but has personally diagnosed the condition to be treated, has personally authorized the procedures, and will evaluate the performance of the allied dental personnel.

The *expanded-function dental auxiliary* (EFDA) (sometimes called an expanded-duty dental auxiliary) is a more recent development among operating auxiliaries in the United States and Canada. An EFDA is usually a dental assistant, or a dental hygienist in some cases, who has received further training in duties related to the direct treatment of patients, although still working under the direct supervision of a dentist. Not all states in the United States recognize EFDAs, and the duties permitted in those that do vary considerably.

A *dental assistant* is a nonoperating auxiliary who assists the dentist or dental hygienist in treating patients but who is not legally permitted to treat patients independently. Traditionally the dental assistant's duties include immediate chairside assistance in the handling of dental equipment and materials used by the dentist or dental hygienist in treating patients.

Voluntary certification programs for dental assistants exist in many countries. *Certification* is the process by which a nongovernmental agency or association grants recognition to an individual who has met certain predetermined qualifications specified by that agency or association.[85] However, a dental assistant is not required to be legally certified or registered or to have completed any particular duration or amount of education. The vast majority of the world's dental assistants are trained on the job. However, to provide certain services, such as the exposure of radiographs, a growing number of American states require either some form of formal education or certification.

The *dental laboratory technician* is a nonoperating auxiliary who fills the prescriptions provided by dentists regarding the extraoral construction and repair of oral appliances. *Denturist* is a term applied to those dental laboratory technicians who are permitted in some American states, some provinces of Canada, and some other countries to fabricate dentures directly for patients without a dentist's prescription. These denturists must be licensed. Illegal denturists are also known to operate in other jurisdictions. The term can have strong political overtones in jurisdictions where denturists are trying to achieve legal recognition.

Dental nurse and *dental therapist* are more or less synonymous terms that describe an operating auxiliary who in some countries is legally permitted to treat special population groups, usually children, with little direct supervision from a dentist. The extent of their duties varies from one country to another, as does the degree of supervision required, but all dental nurses and therapists require specific training, licensure, and registration. Preventive dental nurses and therapists are trained in some countries to provide preventive services only, usually in a school dental service. Because their period of training is shorter than the training for dentists and their duties are limited, these auxiliaries can provide preventive services to specified groups at lower cost than can dentists or hygienists.

SUPPLY OF DENTISTS IN THE UNITED STATES

Table 8-1 shows the dentist/population ratios in several countries as of the late 1990s to give a perspective on the relative availability of dentists in the United States. The range is wide, with an especially large gap between developed and developing countries, and even within the more economically developed countries, the range is considerable. The numbers are given as the number of dentists per 100,000 population and as persons per dentist. The 55 dentists per

Table 8-1 Number of dentists per 100,000 population for 15 countries at various stages of economic development[108]

Country	Dentists per 100,000 Population	Population per Dentist
Sweden	143	700
Finland	98	1024
Denmark	92	1090
Norway	91	1100
Argentina	83	1200
France	72	1390
Switzerland	62	1613
United States	55	1810
Canada	54	1834
Spain	40	2525
Singapore	29	3500
Turkey	21	4668
Thailand	10	9800
India	3	36,538
Cameroon	1	119,200
Ethiopia	<1	1,200,000

Note: Rounded to the nearest whole number.

100,000 people in the United States in the mid-1990s are equivalent to 1810 persons per dentist.

Counting dentists and other dental personnel is not as straightforward as it might at first appear. Membership lists from professional associations and licensing lists are the most common source of counts, but these are seldom completely accurate. For example, some dentists maintain association membership even when they are retired or otherwise not actively engaged in professional practice; others are not members of a professional association. Dentists can hold a license in more than one jurisdiction, which leads to overcounting. As a result, one does well to realize that virtually all enumerations of dental personnel are estimates and that, in an attempt to be more precise, the counts are often qualified as all dentists, active dentists (those actually engaged in some activity related to dentistry), or practicing dentists (which often excludes dentists in full-time teaching, research, or administrative positions). Numbers obtained from different sources therefore can differ because they are based on different subgroups. This nomenclature is by no means standard and is often not clearly defined in source documents. Usually the differences are not of great consequence, but when interpretations are made within small geographic areas the differences can be important. For example, in a community where there is a dental school or a government agency that employs a number of dentists in nonclinical positions, a count of all dentists for that community could greatly overestimate the availability of dental care.

As of 2000, the ADA estimated that the number of professionally active dentists in the United States was about 168,000. Approximately 5000 of these were in the armed forces and other federal agencies.[21] About 155,200 dentists were in private practice in 2000, a more than 55% increase since 1975.[93]

From 1920 until the early 1980s, 1%–3% of dentists were women,[75,89] but since the early 1980s this percentage has increased. In 1998, over 13% of dentists were women, and almost one third of dentists who had graduated within the previous 10 years were women.[26] In 1969–70, women constituted only 1.3% of first-year enrollment in dental schools,[54] but by 1980–81 the first-year class was 19.8% female.[55] By the early years of the twenty-first century, dental school enrollments were over 40% women.[14]

Not all observers agree on the implications of the growing proportion of female dentists.[10,66,71,75,88,90,102,103] Although it is too early to be sure about trends, there are indications that women dentists are more likely to practice part time and to interrupt their practices for an extended period of time, thus spending fewer actual hours in practice during a career. Any differences between men and women in retirement patterns will also affect productivity, and it will be several decades yet before these can be observed. Further, it is likely that the practice patterns followed by those women in decades past, when women in the profession were rare, may be of little help in predicting the future practice patterns of the women now becoming dentists. Although any substantial shift in the average productivity of dentists would affect the adequacy of the dentist supply, it is at present not clear how the increasing proportion of female dentists is affecting productivity.

Not only are the numbers of women increasing, but dentistry is becoming more ethnically diverse. Although approximately 90% of dentists in practice as of 1995 reported themselves to be white non-Hispanic,[25] the picture for dental students indicates a decided shift. At the turn of the century, about 25% of dental school graduates listed themselves as other than white.[23]

Foreign-trained dentists, in contrast to foreign-trained medical graduates, have never been present in large numbers in the United States, in no small part due to difficulty in gaining licensure. Graduation from an accredited U.S. or Canadian dental school was for a long time a prerequisite for licensure in most states. However, rapid population growth, especially the growth of immigrant communities, is forcing some states to look at more radical ways of increasing dentist supply. California, for example, is considering accrediting certain foreign dental schools in a bid to attract dentists from other countries. The future of such policies remains uncertain, but their very existence certainly represents a major break with tradition. This is a rapidly changing area, and up-to-date information on the details for any particular state is usually available on the website of the ADA.[12,30]

Dental Specialists

The early development of dental specialists was informal, and such specialists did not require certification.[60] Varying patterns of formal training and certification developed as each specialty grew and matured relatively independently. Examining boards that certified specialty competence came into being, as did specialty societies, such as the American Academy of Pedodontics (now Pediatric Dentistry) and the American Association of Orthodontists, which maintained educational and experiential qualifications for membership. In addition, some states established specialty licensure following examination by the state board of dental examiners.

Under guidelines originally set by the ADA House of Delegates and the Council on Dental Education, and now maintained by the Commission on Dental Accreditation, examining boards have been established in nine areas of specialty practice: dental public health, endodontics, oral and maxillofacial pathology, oral and maxillofacial radiology, oral and maxillofacial surgery, orthodontics and dentofacial orthopedics, pediatric dentistry, periodontics, and prosthodontics. Minimum criteria for those entering a specialty are full-time limitation of practice, plus either the completion of at least 2 years of approved advanced study or specialty licensure by a state board. Certification as a diplomate by one of the specialty boards is not a prerequisite for limitation of practice. The stated purpose of specialty boards is to provide leadership in elevating standards for the practice of the specialty and, through examination and certification, to recognize those individuals who have demonstrated unusual competence. Numerous additional dental specialty groups are not officially recognized by the ADA, and the ADA actively discourages the announcement of practice limited to any area other than one of the nine recognized specialties.

Unlike the situation in medicine, in which by 1990 more than 60% of practitioners were practicing in a specialty outside of primary care, about 80% of dentists are general practitioners.[25,94] Since the early 1970s, the number of first-year positions in specialty training programs has remained stable at approximately 1200. More than 50% of all specialists work in orthodontics or oral surgery, the two longest-established specialties.

There has been strong sentiment in dentistry for some time that a further increase in the number of specialists would not benefit either the profession or the public.[59] This view was based on the contention that one of the chronic problems in the American health care system is fragmentation, the dispersal of many medical specialists and the frequent absence of coordination among them. The growth of General Practice Residency and Advanced Education in General Dentistry programs is a reflection of this emphasis on the general practice of dentistry. As of 2004 there were just over 1000 General Practice Residency and 650 Advanced Education in General Dentistry residency positions.[31]

Distribution of Dentists

In 2000 there were approximately 60.7 active dentists per 100,000 people in the United States.[93] These dentists, however, were not evenly distributed throughout the country, as seen in Chapter 6 (see Fig. 6-1). This situation is not unique to dentistry as a health profession nor to the United States, for it is found wherever there is relatively free choice of practice location. Table 8-2 provides data for the five most favorable and five least favorable states in terms of dentists relative to the population in 2000. The figures range from 84.7 dentists per 100,000 people in Hawaii to 39.2 per 100,000 in Nevada.[93]

Table 8-2 The five states with the highest number of dentists and the five states with the lowest number of dentists per 100,000 population in the United States, 2000[93]

State	Dentists per 100,000 Population
Hawaii	84.7
New York	83.1
Massachusetts	81.2
New Jersey	80.4
Connecticut	79.6
Alabama	43.5
North Carolina	43.1
Arkansas	42.2
Mississippi	39.7
Nevada	39.2

There are a number of reasons for this uneven distribution of dentists. The first and most fundamental is the relative freedom a dentist has in choosing a practice location. Dentists make this choice much as other people do, that is, because of personal preference: attachment to a home town, presence of good schools, or convenience to social, cultural, or recreational facilities.[6] Second, the location of dental schools also influences distribution, and the 56 American dental schools are located in only 34 states (plus the District of Columbia and Puerto Rico). Most dental schools are in state universities, at which tuition usually is less for state residents than for out-of-state residents. A third reason is market response, meaning that the availability of dentists reflects demand for services. Areas of high income and education where demand for services is highest, such as affluent suburbs, have more dentists than do poorer areas. The low number of dentists in Nevada is largely a reflection of the exceptionally rapid growth of the population of that state in the past decade. The dental school recently opened at the University of Nevada, Las Vegas, is expected eventually to help correct some of that imbalance.

Effect of Dental Education on the Supply of Dentists

Dentists were first enumerated separately in the 1850 census. It listed 2900 dentists serving a population of 23 million,[91] or 12.6 dentists per 100,000 population. With the growth of dental schools during the latter part of the nineteenth century, the supply of dentists in 1900 increased to 39 dentists per 100,000 population. By 1930, there were 57.7 dentists per 100,000 population.[98] This steady increase was caused principally by changes in dental education. Although in the second half of the nineteenth century many dentists were still being trained under an apprenticeship system, proprietary dental schools grew rapidly in response to demand (see Chapter 1). The number of dental graduates continued to grow until the closing of the last proprietary school in 1929.[70]

In the United States, the federal government has no direct jurisdiction over education, and there are considerable differences among states in the priority given to education. This is notably different from most other countries, where the national government directly determines how many practitioners, and of what type, will be produced. For these and related reasons, accreditation evolved as a voluntary, self-regulatory means of establishing and maintaining nationally acceptable standards of educational quality.[83] *Accreditation* is the process by which an agency or organization evaluates and recognizes a program of study or an institution as meeting certain predetermined qualifications or standards.[84,85] The Commission on Dental Accreditation of the ADA currently serves as the accrediting body for dental and auxiliary training schools and graduate programs in dentistry. The commission is a broad-based agency of the ADA; its membership includes auxiliaries, public members, and students in addition to dentists.

Enrollment in dental schools is obviously a prime influence on the future supply of dentists. During the 1960s and early 1970s, there was a widely held perception that more dentists were needed and that a critical shortage was inevitable if strong actions were not taken. Although the federal government in the United States has no direct control over dental education, it can provide incentives to increase supply. During the 1960s and 1970s, incentives were offered to dental schools to build new facilities and to increase the number of graduates at existing dental schools. The results were impressive, as shown in Fig. 8-1. The increased applications and enrollments through the 1970s also coincided with the time that the baby-boomer generation was deciding on careers. Applications to dental schools reached all-time highs during this period; the number of applicants per first-year position was 2.7:1 in 1974 and 1975. Applications began to decline in 1976; first-year enrollments began to decline in 1979. The federal incentives to dental education were reduced during this period, and the demographic bulge passed beyond college age.

The low point in applications and enrollments in the late 1980s coincided with a slow period in the U.S. economy and again with a public perception that there was an oversupply of dentists. During this period, dental schools made a remarkable adjustment in their capacity. Through a combination of the closing of six dental schools and the reduction of class size in most others, the first-year capacity declined

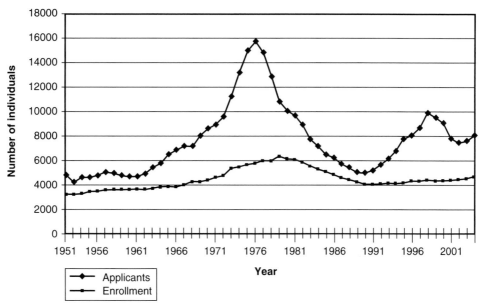

Fig. 8-1 Applicants and first-year enrollees in dental schools in the United States, 1951–2003.[2,22,31]

from its peak of 6301 in 1978 to approximately 4000 by 1990. Since 1990, applications and enrollments have recovered considerably, with first-year enrollments at 4618 in 2003, partly due to the opening of three new dental schools.

By the late 1990s, evidence suggested that the economic prospects for dentists, relative to those for physicians, were quite favorable. A 1994 report analyzing the return on educational investment among several professions projected that dentistry would provide a higher rate of return than primary care medicine and a virtually identical return to specialty medicine.[105] A more recent report suggests, perhaps because of the pressures on physicians from managed care, that in some parts of the country dentists average higher incomes than primary care physicians.[36] These favorable reports of dentists' economic prospects may have been a factor in the growing numbers of applicants to dental schools from the mid-1990s.

Fluctuations in dental school enrollments take considerable time to show their effect on the supply of dentists, and overall supply also is influenced by other factors. First, with approximately 160,000 dentists in practice in the United States, a change of a few hundred graduates in any one year does not make a large difference overall. Further, a major influence on the overall numbers is the number of dentists

retiring in any one year, which is itself a function of how many dentists graduated 40 or more years earlier. Choice of retirement age is highly variable. If demand for care is strong, a dentist may wait longer to retire than when there is an ample supply of younger dentists to take over. Finally, the population growth of the country is an additional variable. As population growth accelerates, more and more dentists are required to keep the supply constant.

The combination of these factors resulted in a gradual increase in the supply of dentists in the United States between 1970 and the mid-1990s, from 47 to 60 dentists per 100,000 population.[95,97] Much of this general increase in the relative number of dentists is the result of the large number of graduates through the 1970s and most of the 1980s. Virtually all projections at the end of the century suggested, however, that the relative supply of dentists was at its peak and was likely to decline for the next several decades. This projected decline will be the product of lower enrollment levels than in earlier decades, combined with continuing population growth and projected retirement levels of dentists. It is anticipated that the relative supply of dentists will decline especially sharply between 2010 and 2020, when many of the large cohort of dentists who graduated in the 1970s and 1980s are expected to retire. By 2020, it is expected that there will be about 55 dentists per 100,000 population, back to levels of the early 1980s. Whether this anticipated decline in the relative supply of dentists will be a problem or not is discussed further in Chapter 9.

State Practice Acts and Dentist Distribution

The requirement to hold a state license to practice inhibits the movement of dentists (and also licensed auxiliaries) from one state to another.[44,65] In addition, it has been suggested that certain states adopted deliberately restrictive policies in their licensing examinations in an effort to prevent what they saw as too many dentists, or dentists "of the wrong kind," from practicing in the state.[44,51,65,70] Results of state board examinations show a wide disparity among states in the proportion of applicants who fail.[5,44,56] Dentists in specialty practice also report difficulty in moving to states that do not have specialty licenses. In these instances, a specialist who may not have practiced general dentistry for many years may be required to take a clinical examination based on restorative procedures.

The ADA supports *licensure by credentials* to alleviate some of these problems. Under this concept, dentists who have passed a licensing examination in a state present their credentials to another state to which they want to move; if the credentials meet the criteria, the board grants a license. The actual process and requirements vary widely but generally include requirements for some minimum time in practice and no evidence of existing or pending disciplinary or legal actions. The ADA website shows that, in 2004, 43 states plus the District of Columbia and Puerto Rico allowed some form of licensure by credentials.[21] Encompassed within this concept is *reciprocity*, by which two or more states agree to honor each others' licenses.

Views differ on the value of licensure by credentials. Some say that the existence of individual state practice acts, and what is seen as parochial jealousies in their administration, is a major cause of maldistribution and that the problem would be greatly alleviated by licensure by credentials. Others argue that licensure by credentials could make maldistribution worse, because large numbers of dentists would then move to desirable locations.

Movement between states has been made somewhat easier, at least for the young dentist, by the development of regional examining boards. There are four regional boards (Northeast, Southern, Central, and Western), and a dentist passing the clinical licensing examination in any participating state can apply, usually within 5 years of the original examination, for license in any state in the same region without having to take another clinical examination. By 2001, 41 states and the District of Columbia were involved in one or more of these four regional examining boards.[12]

Whenever licensure and the assessment of dentists' competence are mentioned, the topic of mandatory continuing education as a requirement for license renewal also arises. If the competence of a dentist who moves from one state to another has to be tested, why should there not also be concern for those who stay in one place for many years? Although there is no clear evidence that mandatory continuing dental education improves dentists' competence, by the early part of the twenty-first century, continuing dental education requirements were virtually universal for both dentists and dental hygienists. As is the case with other regulatory matters, these requirements vary widely among states and can change rapidly.

ALLIED DENTAL PERSONNEL IN THE UNITED STATES
Dental Hygienists

In the early twenty-first century there were estimated to be approximately 120,000 registered dental hygienists in the United States, nearly an eightfold increase since 1970.[32,96] Table 8-3 shows the growth in the number of active hygienists and in particular the extremely rapid growth since the early 1970s (see Chapter 1). Even with this large increase in the number of hygienists, there are still some concerns about a shortage.[46,61,104] After declines in enrollment through the late 1980s, roughly parallel to the enrollment declines in dentistry, dental hygiene enrollments rebounded by the turn of the century to near-record levels. The majority of dental hygiene programs are in community colleges, and in 2004 there were a total of 266 programs in all 50 states, the District of Columbia, and Puerto Rico.[31]

Table 8-3   Dental hygienist statistics for the United States: selected years, 1950–2003[31]

Year	Number of Active Hygienists*	Active Hygienists per 100 Active Dentists	Training Programs in Dental Hygiene	First-Year Enrollment
1950	3190	4.0	26	862
1955	4160	4.9	33	1100
1960	8800	9.8	37	1440
1965	11,600	12.1	56	2070
1970	15,100	14.8	121	3265
1975	26,900	24.0	174	5337
1980	38,400	30.4	200	5619
1985	55,000	43.0	198	4866
1990	75,000	55.6	202	5419
1995	100,000	64.5	215	5669
2003	120,000	73.3	266	N/A

*Number of active hygienists is an estimate, because of the relative ease of movement into and out of active practice and the frequency of part-time practice for more than one employer.

The duties of a dental hygienist are similar in most countries where they are part of the dental team.[62] These duties, which are usually carried out under the supervision of a dentist, are associated with the preventive aspects of dental care: scaling and polishing teeth, applying fluorides and other preventive agents, and educating patients to practice sound dental habits. Expanded duties for hygienists have been developed in some states in the United States, where the training of hygienists is extended to teach them to carry out additional duties in the dental office. Since 1975, however, the ADA House of Delegates has repeatedly gone on record as being opposed to delegation of expanded functions to hygienists and other auxiliaries,[9,18-20] despite research evidence showing that trained hygienists can perform these duties competently. (There is a fuller discussion of expanded-function auxiliaries later in this chapter.)

Outside of the armed services, dental hygiene is an almost completely female profession. Even if this trend continues, the traditional passiveness of hygienists has changed. Hygienists, licensed and regulated by state boards of dentistry, have shown their dissatisfaction at not having a voice in their own licensing, and there continues to be considerable activity on the part of hygienists in many states to gain more control over their profession. Attempts continue, and some have succeeded, to develop separate licensing boards for dental hygiene, to increase the representation of hygienists on examining boards,

to relax supervision requirements, to allow direct third-party reimbursement to hygienists, to permit expanded functions, and to allow independent practice.[58] Not surprisingly, the ADA is firmly opposed to these moves, arguing that the only appropriate role for a hygienist is provision of care under the supervision of a dentist.[8,16,20]

Independent Practice

In 1986 Colorado became the first state in the United States to permit the *independent practice* of dental hygiene. In independent practice, the hygienist selects a site, rents or purchases space, secures equipment and supplies, and treats patients directly. The Colorado legislation, however, did not permit a full range of hygiene services; a dentist's supervision was required for a dental hygienist to take radiographs, remove live tissue, perform root planing, and inject local anesthetic.[101] As soon as the bill was signed into law, the ADA filed suit to block independent practice, but the court ruled that the ADA had no standing in the case. This ruling was upheld in appellate court.[81]

It is difficult to know how many dental hygienists have established independent practices in Colorado, because the law does not require them to register that fact. Nevertheless, as of 1998, the number was thought to be fewer than 20.[35] The costs of establishing and maintaining an office, the limited scope of services permitted, and the reluctance of insurers to reimburse hygienists for services appear to be major barriers to further development,[81] even though by 1997 insurers in Colorado were required to reimburse dental hygienists for covered services. The limited evidence from Colorado, and from an experiment in independent practice in California, indicates that independent dental hygiene practices compare favorably to dental offices on several measures of practice quality.[35,52,77]

The future of independent practice for hygienists remains uncertain, but the overall trend seems to be a slow expansion of the autonomy of dental hygiene practice, fought out on a state-by-state basis. Since the first law in Colorado permitting independent practice, California (1998) and New Mexico (1999) also have enacted laws that permit dental hygienists to own dental hygiene practices under some circumstances. Even more common is allowing dental hygienists to practice without direct supervision in public health settings, schools, health centers, nursing homes, and similar types of facilities. As of early 2004, 15 states had provision for allowing some forms of unsupervised practice in these types of facilities.[33] As of 2003, state Medicaid regulations in 10 states allowed dental hygienists to be paid directly for dental hygiene services provided by them.[34] Promoting expansion of dental hygienists' autonomy continues to be a major activity of the American Dental Hygienists' Association. At the same time, the ADA continues to watch and often resist these moves.

Dental Assistants

Dental assistants are the most numerous of all dental personnel groups in the United States and, along with dental laboratory technicians, are the longest-established auxiliaries. They began to be employed with regularity in dental practices toward the latter part of the nineteenth century. The first assistants were trained on the job by their dentist-employers to aid in receiving patients and performing "housekeeping" chores and office clerical procedures. Many assistants today still follow this same pattern, because formal training and licensure are not required for dental assistants who perform only the traditional extraoral functions .

In 2004 there were approximately 240,000 active dental assistants in the United States, or about 150 per 100 active dentists.[45] The ADA's *1998 Survey of Dental Practice* stated that 94.1% of dentists in practice employed at least one chairside assistant.[29] The number of assistants increased sharply during the 1970s and early 1980s, rising from an estimated 91 per 100 active dentists in 1965.[96] Some of the increase may be attributable to training programs in dental schools, originally encouraged by federal funds, in which dental students were taught how to use assistants effectively. Another measure of increased utilization of assistants can be seen in the same 1998 survey,[29] in which more than 60% of dentists reported employing two or more assistants.

During the 1980s there was a decline in training program enrollments that paralleled those in dentistry and dental hygiene. The peak first-year enrollment of 8386 in 1979 fell to 5388 in 1988,[2] but then rose to 5669 in 1995.[4] In 2004, approximately 250 institutions[11] offered accredited training programs, about double the number in 1968, although down from the peak of 296 in 1980.

In most states, dental assistants are now legally allowed to carry out more than their traditional duties. Many state laws and regulations have been changed to allow expanded functions of assistants. A bewildering and constantly changing variety of tasks is permitted from one state to another.[27,41,53,64] In some states, no certification or licensure is required; in others, certification is required; and in still others, testing and registration are required. Voluntary certification for dental assistants has been available since 1948 through the Certifying Board of the American Dental Assistants Association, now known as the Dental Assisting National Board (DANB), and this certification is accepted in some states as qualification to practice the expanded functions defined in its dental practice act. About 30,000 dental assistants are DANB certified.[45]

Expanded Function Dental Auxiliaries

Although dental assistants were used in the nineteenth century, it was not until the shortage of civilian dentists during World War II, owing to the enlistment of many dentists in the armed services, that serious consideration was given to their more efficient use.[63] The introduction of the air-turbine dental handpiece in the 1950s removed much of the drudgery from cavity and crown preparation and made greater productivity much more achievable. Development of "four-handed dentistry," with the dentist and assistant both seated, was a natural consequence. With it came sweeping changes in design of dental chairs, operating equipment, access to instruments, and layout of the dental office.

Continued developments in equipment, materials, and procedures are constantly making the role of the dental assistant more complex. The chairside assistant in a busy office must know instruments and understand procedures well for this type of practice to work. In the interest of greater operating efficiency, it was inevitable, therefore, that assistants began to do more and more intraoral procedures. Research has shown that both hygienists and assistants are capable of carrying out a wide range of extra duties at a high level of quality when adequately trained[1,37,41,57,67-69,87] and that the productivity and income of dentists can be greatly improved as a result.[39,73,74,76,82]

Moves toward utilization of EFDAs were given impetus during the 1960s, when a critical shortage of dental personnel was seen as imminent. If the country were to be short of dentists, the reasoning went, at least let those in practice be as productive as possible. Federal funds became available for dental schools to operate Dental Auxiliary Utilization programs, which trained dental students in four-handed dentistry, and later for Training in Expanded Auxiliary Management programs, which taught dental students to work with auxiliaries who carried out an even wider range of functions, including packing and carving amalgams in cavities prepared by the students.

The studies with EFDAs were carried out in a variety of special institutional settings, although considerable effort was made to simulate the characteristics of the private office. Limited studies in private offices also have been conducted,[47,73,74,79] and although they found some difficulties in adjustment of office routines, they confirmed that EFDAs can be successfully used there. EFDAs are also routinely used in the Indian Health Service and military and Department of Veterans Affairs facilities, and by some private practitioners in states where they are permitted.[53,64,73,74] Examples of the kinds of duties defined as expanded duties in various state dental practice acts are shown in Box 8-2.

The interest of government in promoting EFDAs is in increased productivity and in the subsequent presumed lower cost of care to the public. In fact, the U.S. General Accounting Office, in a 1980 report, urged states to develop practice acts that permitted expanded functions and recommended that all federal programs make wider use of EFDAs.[100]

Although the research literature makes it clear that auxiliaries can function as well as dentists in providing these expanded services, an appropriate cautionary note has been sounded.[41] A careful reading of the literature shows that even though the candidates for the demonstration projects were carefully selected and received rigorous training, not all candidates were able to perform successfully and some were dropped from the programs. These selective and rigorous training programs are quite different from the requirements for expanded functions in many states, some of which require no formal training or evaluation

---

BOX 8-2   Examples of Duties Permitted To Be Carried Out by Expanded-Duty Dental Auxiliaries in the United States[27,35,78]

- Applying topical fluorides
- Applying desensitizing agents
- Applying pit-and-fissure sealants
- Placing, carving, and polishing amalgam restorations
- Placing and finishing composite restorations
- Placing and removing matrix bands
- Placing and removing rubber dams
- Monitoring nitrous oxide use
- Taking impressions for study casts
- Exposing and developing radiographs
- Removing sutures
- Removing and replacing ligature wires on orthodontic appliances

at all. Caution is needed because the evidence that carefully trained auxiliaries can function at high levels when adequately trained does not necessarily mean that the same outcome can be assured in the absence of such training.

The American Dental Association and Expanded Function Dental Auxiliaries

A complicating factor in the legal status of EFDAs in the United States has been the position of the ADA, which, although it does not directly or legally control state boards, clearly has influence. During the mid-1960s, ADA policy encouraged experimental projects. By the early 1970s, however, when many became concerned about the possible oversupply of dentists, ADA policy reversed its stance and opposed such experimentation. As one health economist noted, an increase in EFDAs at the same time as an increase in dentists would clearly have a negative impact on dentists' willingness to employ them.[50]

Because most of the research studies on the use of EFDAs were based in dental schools, some dental educators became irritated at what they perceived as the ADA's efforts to interfere with academic freedom. The ADA's mood continued to become more opposed to experiments with EFDAs, however, and since 1975 the House of Delegates has passed a series of resolutions to that effect. These resolutions are opposed to (1) delegation of many of the procedures now permitted in some states, such as the taking of final impressions, placement or adjustment of appliances, performance of intraoral restorative procedures, and the use of local anesthetics; and (2) independent or unsupervised practice of any auxiliary personnel.[16,18,20]

Despite all of these activities with expanded functions over the last three decades, suggestions to develop operating auxiliaries like the New Zealand dental therapist (see Chapter 6) are rare. Part of the reason may be that, in the late 1940s, an attempt was made to establish such a plan in Massachusetts, but it was stopped by swift and effective political action by organized dentistry.[48] The recent initiation of a limited dental therapist program in Alaskan native communities (see Chapter 6) is a notable exception.

A possible additional reason for reduced enthusiasm about EFDAs is the change in the types and level of restorative need that has accompanied the decline in dental caries. The greatest benefits in increased productivity with EFDAs come with routine restorative care. Several decades ago it was quite common for children to require multiple restorations at each dental visit, and with the use of EFDAs, the process of quadrant and half-mouth restorative care was common. Today, however, the number of restorations placed per patient has declined substantially,[28,49] and therefore the potential efficiency of using EFDAs may also have declined.

Dental Laboratory Technicians

The dental laboratory technician, like the dental assistant, has been a part of dentistry for a long time. The technician's task is to fabricate crowns, bridges, dentures, and orthodontic and other appliances on the prescription of a dentist. Many of these tasks require high precision, and the technician's skill weighs heavily on the ultimate success of the treatment. Although many laboratory technicians are trained on the job, there are approximately 30 dental technology programs in the United States accredited by the ADA's Commission on Dental Accreditation.[13] Technicians also may become certified dental technicians in one or more of the areas of complete dentures, partial dentures, crowns and bridges, ceramics, and orthodontics.

Traditionally technicians were directly employed by dentists and worked in a laboratory in the same office as the dentist. Over time, however, this arrangement became uneconomical for most dentists. In addition, some technicians have become specialists, whose skills are properly at the disposal of many dentists. Most technicians now are employed by independent commercial laboratories, which provide their services to dentists. In the ADA's *1998 Survey of Dental Practice*, only 6.8% of responding dentists directly employed a laboratory technician either full or part time.[29]

The ADA estimated that in 1997 there were about 60,000 active technicians in the United States, or 40 per 100 active dentists. Enrollment in accredited training programs has declined from a peak of 1665 first-year enrollees in 1981 to 908 in 1990 and 487 in 1998.[2,24,61] These continuing declines in enrollments are causing some concern that it will become increasingly difficult for many dentists to find competent laboratory services.[15,86,104] Factors that affect the national staffing picture are relatively low hourly wages in the industry, growth in the use of dental laboratories overseas in low-wage countries, and a general decline in the need for some types of laboratory services because of changing patterns of disease in the population.

Denturists

During the 1970s and early 1980s, some dental laboratory technicians tried to change state dental practice acts to allow them to treat the public directly for the fabrication of dentures. These technicians call themselves denturists and their occupation denturism. This activity came at approximately the same time as similar movements in Canada. Denturists are now legally recognized in most Canadian provinces and six states (Arizona, Idaho, Maine, Montana, Oregon, and Washington). The requirements for licensing vary among the states but usually include some educational component.

The ADA has vigorously opposed the denturist movement. Its principal argument is that denturists are unqualified to treat patients and that poor-quality care and even actual harm could result to patients. In 1973 the ADA defined denturism as "the fitting and dispensing of dentures illegally to the public,"[17] a definition both clear and brief, even if no longer accurate for some states. Although the soundness of the ADA's argument may be evident in dental circles, it may be less so to the public and to legislators. This fact became painfully clear in the 1978 Oregon elections. Supporters of denturism had put the subject on the election ballot through the statewide initiative process, which meant that if it succeeded, the measure automatically became law. Not only was it successful, but the 3:1 margin of victory stunned organized dentistry. The conclusions of the ADA's postmortem analysis were as follows:

- The public viewed denturism as a consumer issue, not a health issue.
- The public believed that dentistry's campaign was spurred by economic self-interest.
- Some votes were based on sympathy for the elderly.
- Denturism provided consumers with freedom of choice.

- The media campaign organized by dentistry through a public relations firm was widely perceived as tasteless and unprofessional.[7]

The issue seems to have settled down from its peak in 1980, perhaps because in those states where denturists practice legally there appears to have been no major rush by patients to seek their care. With declining edentulism in the United States (see Chapter 19), the importance of the issue should continue to fade.

LEGISLATIVE INFLUENCE ON DENTIST SUPPLY AND DISTRIBUTION

Federal programs to provide financial aid to training institutions and to students between 1963 and 1980 were first intended to increase the *supply* of certain types of graduates. Legislation in the 1970s then attempted to alleviate the *maldistribution* of health personnel. However, what should be done about maldistribution continues to be a subject of debate. Some believe that a sufficient supply of dentists will permit free-market forces to sort out any problems. Some redistribution through the free movement of dentists undoubtedly does occur, but it also takes time and may be only partially effective. Others believe that only significant changes in the dental care system will solve the problem. If dentists are left as free as they now are to choose a practice location, so this argument goes, maldistribution will continue.

National Health Service Corps

One federally sponsored program aimed directly at easing maldistribution of health care providers is the National Health Service Corps (NHSC), the result of 1971 legislation.[80] The NHSC is designed mainly for physicians, but dentists and dental hygienists are also eligible. Although initially based on volunteers, the program has at various times provided scholarships and loan forgiveness to recent graduates to encourage them to practice in designated shortage areas.

After reaching a peak in 1980, when 6409 scholarships were awarded (both medical and dental), the program came under considerable strain. Severe budget cuts were enacted during the 1980s; by 1989 the scholarship program had ceased. Throughout the same period, a growing problem developed with defaults on student loans. The usual requirement was that each year of educational tuition and living expense support would be repaid by 1 year of practice in a shortage area, but by 1987 more than 1300 scholarship recipients were in default by having refused to serve in shortage areas.[43]

The phasing out of the scholarship program led to a rapid decline in the number of dentists going to shortage areas, which itself suggests that the scholarship program was achieving its goals. Community health centers (see Chapter 6) were particularly hard hit, because a high percentage of their staff had come from the scholarship programs. The program continues mainly through a loan repayment system, and as of 2004, a qualifying practitioner practicing in a federally designated health professional shortage area was potentially eligible for loan repayment of up to $25,000 per year for the first 2 years of service.[92]

Subsidies to Dental Schools and Dental Students

Before and since the NHSC, governmental programs to increase the supply of dental personnel existed in the form of financial incentives to dental schools and subsidies to dental students. Most dental schools are constructed and largely supported by state governments. Their object is to supply dentists for the state concerned, as indicated by the standard practice of charging higher rates of tuition for out-of-state residents.

Although some federal money has gone into dental schools for decades, the proportion of dental school budgets that come from federal funds rose dramatically in the years up to the early 1970s. The Health Professions Educational Assistance Act of 1963 was designed to alleviate the perceived shortage of health personnel, including dentists. This legislation subsidized existing schools, provided funds for new construction and renovation, and provided direct aid to students, all with few strings attached. An intended effect of this legislation was the sharp increase in the number of dental graduates (see Fig. 8-1).

The Comprehensive Health Manpower Act of 1971 continued financial aid to schools but with some stricter provisions for the use of the money attached. This act was followed by a period of financial recession, inflation, slower population growth, and growing belief in some dental circles that the perceived shortage of dentists had been alleviated and was tending toward an oversupply. The Health Professions Educational Assistance Act of 1976 was thus enacted in a different atmosphere from that of 1963. It concentrated on improving the distribution of primary care personnel rather than on simply increasing numbers. Part of the act's requirements were that dental schools could qualify for federal support funds only if they either (1) increased enrollment of first-year students by a specified proportion, or (2) provided "off-site" training for dental students. Some dental schools declined the federal aid rather than accept these conditions.

Between the mid-1970s and mid-1980s, there were substantial reductions in federal support to dental education. The institutional support grants that dental schools had come to rely on were eliminated. As a source of school operating revenue, federal funding fell from nearly 30% in 1973 to just over 10% by the early 1980s, where it has remained. The result has been intense financial pressure, reflected in higher tuition costs, because few states were able to fill the financial gap left by the loss of federal funds. To make matters more difficult, the reduced number of applicants put limits on how high tuition could go and therefore how much of the budget it could cover.

It is worth remembering that student tuition, high as it is and with an average indebtedness of $118,750 per graduate in 2003,[31] represents well under half of the cost of a dental student's education. At public dental schools in 1998, only about 15% of revenue came from tuition; in private schools it was just about 53%.[15] The combination of these pressures led to the decision during the late 1980s and early 1990s by six dental schools (all private) to close. Since 1997, however, three new dental schools (Nova Southeastern University College of Dental Medicine; University of Nevada, Las Vegas, School of Dental Medicine; and Arizona School of Dentistry and Oral Health) have opened, the first new dental schools in several decades. There may be more changes as dental education struggles to adjust to the new realities of extremely high costs of dental education, population shifts, generally stagnant levels of governmental support, and potential pressure on academic health centers, brought on by the demands of managed care, to reduce costs.[38] These negative forces may be balanced, however, by the generally favorable economic picture for dentists at the turn of the twenty-first century[36,42,72,105] and the apparent increase in the number of applicants to dental schools.

REFERENCES

1. Abramowitz J, Berg LE. A four-year study of the utilization of dental assistants with expanded functions. J Am Dent Assoc 1973;87:623–35.
2. American Association of Dental Schools. Deans' briefing book: Academic year 1988–89. Washington DC: AADS, 1989.
3. American Association of Dental Schools. Deans' briefing book; Academic year, 1994–95. Washington DC: AADS, 1995.
4. American Association of Dental Schools. Trends in dental education: 1997. Washington DC: AADS, 1997.
5. American Dental Association, Bureau of Economic and Behavioral Research. Facts about states for the dentist seeking a location. Chicago: ADA, 1979.
6. American Dental Association, Bureau of Economic Research and Statistics. Survey of recent graduates. II. Factors related to selection of a practice location. J Am Dent Assoc 1973;87:904–6.
7. American Dental Association, Bureau of Economic and Behavioral Research. The Oregon lesson: Results of postelection research. J Am Dent Assoc 1979;98: 749–54.
8. American Dental Association. Comprehensive policy statement on allied dental personnel, 2002, website: http://www.ada.org/members/advocacy/issues/auxiliary/policy.asp. Accessed May 11, 2004.
9. American Dental Association, Council on Dental Education. American Dental Association statement on expanded function dental auxiliary utilization and education. Trans Am Dent Assoc 1976;117:234.
10. American Dental Association, Council on Dental Practice. A comparative study of male and female dental practice patterns. Chicago: ADA, 1989.
11. American Dental Association. Dental assistant fact sheet. Chicago: ADA, 2004, website: http://www.ada.org/public/education/careers/assistant_fact.asp. Accessed May 11, 2004.
12. American Dental Association. Dental education and licensure in the United States and Canada: A comparison. Chicago: ADA, 2001, website: http://www.ada.org/prof/prac/licensure/factsheets_compare.pdf. Accessed June 4, 2004.
13. American Dental Association. Dental laboratory technician fact sheet. Chicago: ADA, 2004, website: http://www.ada.org/public/education/careers/technician_fact.asp. Accessed May 11, 2004.
14. American Dental Association. Dentistry as a career. Chicago: ADA, 2004, website: http://www.ada.org/includes/content/content_careers_dentistry_bro.asp. Accessed May 10, 2004.
15. American Dental Association, Health Policy Resources Center. Future of dentistry. Chicago: ADA, 2001.
16. American Dental Association, House of Delegates. Comprehensive policy statement on dental auxiliary personnel. Trans Am Dent Assoc 1996;739–42.
17. American Dental Association, House of Delegates. Resolution 97-1973-H. Trans Am Dent Assoc 1973;114: 743–4.
18. American Dental Association, House of Delegates. Resolution 50-1975-H. Trans Am Dent Assoc 1975;116: 701–2.
19. American Dental Association, House of Delegates. Resolution 33-1976-H. Trans Am Dent Assoc 1976;117: 836.
20. American Dental Association, House of Delegates. Resolution 10-H-1988. Trans Am Dent Assoc 1988;129: 464–8.
21. American Dental Association. ADA briefing. Chicago: ADA, 2004, website: http://www.ada.org/adaorganizations/ fds/fgmi_fdsppt.ppt. Accessed May 10, 2004.
22. American Dental Association, Survey Center. 1996/97 Survey of predoctoral dental educational institutions. Academic programs, enrollment, and graduates. Vol 1. Chicago: ADA, 1997.
23. American Dental Association, Survey Center. 1998 Survey of dental graduates. Chicago: ADA, 1999.
24. American Dental Association, Survey Center. 1998/99 survey of allied dental education. Chicago: ADA, 2000.
25. American Dental Association, Survey Center. Distribution of dentists in the United States by region and state, 1995. Chicago: ADA, 1997.
26. American Dental Association, Survey Center. Distribution of dentists in the United States by region and state, 1998. Chicago: ADA, 2000.
27. American Dental Association, Survey Center. Facts about states 1995. For the dentist seeking a location. Chicago: ADA, 1995.
28. American Dental Association, Survey Center. The 1990 survey of dental services rendered. Chicago: ADA, 1994.
29. American Dental Association, Survey Center. The 1998 survey of dental practice. Employment of dental practice personnel. Chicago: ADA, 2000.
30. American Dental Association. US licensure for international dentists. Chicago: ADA, 2004, website: http://www.ada.org/prof/prac/licensure/us.asp. Accessed May 10, 2004.
31. American Dental Education Association, Institute for Public Policy and Advocacy. Dental education at a glance 2004, website: http://www.adea.org/CPPA_Materials/ 2004_Dental_Ed_At_A_Glance.pdf. Accessed May 5, 2004.
32. American Dental Hygienists' Association. Profile of the ADHA, website: http://www.adha.org/aboutadha/profile.htm. Accessed May 5, 2004.
33. American Dental Hygienists' Association, Division of Governmental Affairs. States permitting unsupervised practice/less restrictive supervision, 2004, website: http//www.adha.org/governmental_affairs/downloads/unsupervisedchart.pdf. Accessed May 11, 2004.
34. American Dental Hygienists' Association, Division of Governmental Affairs. States which directly reimburse dental hygienists for services under the Medicaid

program, 2003, website: http//www.adha.org/govern-mental_affairs/downloads/medicaid2reimb.pdf. Accessed May 11, 2004.

35. Astroth DB, Cross-Poline GN. Pilot study of six Colorado dental hygiene independent practices. J Dent Hyg 1998;72:13–22.

36. Average dentist income nears or tops physician's. Manag Dent Care 1997;3(2):6–7.

37. Bader J, Mullins R, Lange K. Technical performance on amalgam restorations by dentists and auxiliaries in private practice. J Am Dent Assoc 1983;106:338–41.

38. Bailit H. Managed care and dental education and research: Should academicians be concerned? Crit Rev Oral Biol Med 1997;8:129–35.

39. Baird KM, Purdy EC, Protheroe DH. Pilot study on advanced training and employment of auxiliary dental personnel in the Royal Canadian Dental Corps: Final report. J Can Dent Assoc 1963;29:778–87.

40. Bergner M, Milgrom P, Chapko MK, et al. The Washington state dental auxiliary project: Quality of care in private practice. J Am Dent Assoc 1983;107: 781–6.

41. Boyer EM. A second look at expanded functions research: Unintended outcomes for the public's safety. J Dent Hyg 1996;70:35–42.

42. Brown LJ, Lazar V. Dentists and their practices. J Am Dent Assoc 1998;129:1692-9.

43. Can volunteers save the Health Service Corps? Med Health 1989;43(36):special insert.

44. Chambers DW. Who is qualified to practice dentistry? Contact Point 1987;65(3):8–15.

45. Dental Assisting National Board. DANB conducts salary survey of certified dental assistants, website: http://www.dentalassisting.com/. Accessed May 11, 2003.

46. Dental leaders discuss recruitment, retention of the dental team. J Mo Dent Assoc 1989;69(6):18–9, 21, 23–5, 27.

47. Douglass CW, Moore S, Lindahl RL, Gillings DB. Expanded duty dental assistants in solo private practice. J Am Coll Dent 1976;43:144–63.

48. Dunning JM. Extending the field for dental auxiliary personnel in the United States. Am J Public Health 1958;48:1059–64.

49. Eklund SA, Pittman JL, Smith RC. Trends in dental care in insured Americans: 1980 to 1995. J Am Dent Assoc 1997;128:171–8.

50. Fein R. Health manpower: Some economic considerations. J Dent Educ 1976;40:650–4.

51. Feldstein PJ. Financing dental care: An economic analysis. Lexington MA: Heath, 1973.

52. Freed JR, Perry DA, Kushman JE. Aspects of quality of dental hygiene care in supervised and unsupervised practice. J Public Health Dent 1997;57:68–75.

53. Govoni MM. Mandatory education and credentialing for dental assistants: Is it the answer to the manpower crisis? Dent Assist 1990;59(4):9–12.

54. Graham J. Dental education: Summary of the 1977–1978 annual report of the Council on Dental Education. J Am Dent Assoc 1978;96:767–71.

55. Graham J. Dental education 1980-1981. J Am Dent Assoc 1981;102:832–5.

56. Guarino RN. Licensure and certification of dentists and accreditation of dental schools. J Dent Educ 1995;59:205–33.

57. Hammons PE, Jamison HC, Wilson LL. Quality of service provided by dental therapists in an experimental program at the University of Alabama. J Am Dent Assoc 1971;82:1060–6.

58. Harrison B, West B. Rules & regs: Who needs them? J Am Dent Assoc 1991;122(1):155–7.

59. Hillenbrand H. The necessity for trained advanced dental professionals. J Dent Educ 1981;45:76–87.

60. Hollinshead BS. The survey of dentistry: The final report. Washington DC: American Council on Education, 1961.

61. Is shortage waning? ADA News 1991;22:1, 8.

62. Johnson PM. Dental hygiene practice: International profile and future directions. Int Dent J 1992;42:451–9.

63. Klein H. Civilian dentistry in war-time. J Am Dent Assoc 1944;31:648–61.

64. LeGallee-Byle BL. Trends in dental assistant utilization: A comparative study. Part I. Dent Assist 1989; 58(1):17–25.

65. Licensure by credentials: Is it working? J Am Dent Assoc 1985;111:18–32.

66. Linn EL. Professional activities of women dentists. J Am Dent Assoc 1970;81:1383–7.

67. Lobene RR, Berman K, Chaisson LB, et al. The Forsyth experiment in training of advanced skills hygienists. Dent Hyg 1974;48:204–13.

68. Lotzkar SJ, Johnson DW, Thompson MB. Experimental program in expanded functions for dental assistants. Phase 1: Baseline, and Phase 2: Training. J Am Dent Assoc 1971;82:101–22.

69. Lotzkar SJ, Johnson DW, Thompson MB. Experimental program in expanded functions for dental assistants. Phase 3: Experiment with dental teams. J Am Dent Assoc 1971;82:1067–81.

70. Mann WR. Dental education. In: Hollinshead BS: The survey of dentistry: The final report. Washington DC: American Council on Education, 1961:239–422.

71. Martens L, Glasrud PH, Burton KL. A profile of Minnesota's younger women dentists [abstract]. J Dent Res 1985;64:205.

72. Meskin LH. Healthier, wealthier and wiser. J Am Dent Assoc 1998;129:1660, 1662.

73. Milgrom P, Bergner M, Chapko MK, et al. The Washington state dental auxiliary project: Delegating expanded functions in general practice. J Am Dent Assoc 1983;107:776–80.

74. Mullins MR, Kaplan AL, Bader JD, et al. Summary results of the Kentucky dental practice demonstration: A cooperative project with practicing general dentists. J Am Dent Assoc 1983;106:817–25.

75. Niessen LC, Kleinman DV, Wilson AA. Practice characteristics of women dentists. J Am Dent Assoc 1986;113:883–8.

76. Pelton WJ, Overstreet GA, Embry OH, Dilworth JB. Economic implications of adding one therapist to a practice. J Am Dent Assoc 1973;86:1301–9.

77. Perry DA, Freed JR, Kushman JE. The California demonstration project in independent practice. J Dent Hyg 1994;68:137–42.

78. Pontecorvo DA. Expanded duties: Results of ADAA's nationwide survey. Dent Assist 1988;57(4):9–13.

79. Redig D, Snyder M, Nevitt G, Tocchini J. Expanded duty dental auxiliaries in four private dental offices: The first year's experience. J Am Dent Assoc 1974;88:969–84.

80. Redman E. The dance of legislation. New York: Simon and Schuster, 1973.

81. Reveal M. Dental hygiene regulation and practice. J Public Health Dent 1989;49:228–30.

82. Romcke RG, Lewis DW. Use of expanded function hygienists in the Prince Edward Island manpower study. J Can Dent Assoc 1973;39:247–62.

83. Santangelo MV. A review of dental school accreditation: Development and current philosophy. J Dent Educ 1977;41:233–8.

84. Santangelo MV. The dental accrediting process. J Dent Educ 1981;45:513–21.

85. Selden WK. Study of accreditation of selected health educational programs. Part one: Working papers. Washington DC: National Commission on Accrediting, 1971.

86. Shortage of qualified dental technicians. Gen Dent 1993;41:288, 290.

87. Soricelli DA. Implementation of the delivery of dental services by auxiliaries: The Philadelphia experience. Am J Public Health 1972;62:1077–87.

88. Talbot NS. Why not more women dentists? J Dent Educ 1960;60:114–22.

89. Tillman RS. Women in dentistry—a review of the literature. J Am Dent Assoc 1975;91:1214–20.

90. Tillman RS, Horowitz SL. Practice patterns of recent female dental graduates. J Am Dent Assoc 1983; 107:32–5.

91. US Department of Commerce, Bureau of the Census. Historical statistics of the United States: Colonial time to 1957. Washington DC: Government Printing Office, 1960.

92. US Department of Health and Human Services, Health Resources and Services Administration, Bureau of Health Professions. Fiscal year 2004 loan repayment program applicant information bulletin. E. Benefits.

93. US Department of Health and Human Services, Health Resources and Services Administration, Bureau of Health Professions. US health workforce personnel factbook, website: http://bhpr.hrsa.gov/healthworkforce/reports/factbook02/FB301.htm. Accessed February 16, 2004.

94. US Department of Health and Human Services, Public Health Service, Health Resources and Services Administration. Factbook—health personnel United States. Washington DC: Government Printing Office, 1993.

95. US Department of Health and Human Services, Public Health Service, Health Resources and Services Administration. Factbook—health personnel United States. Washington DC: Government Printing Office, 1997.

96. US Department of Health and Human Services, Public Health Service, Health Resources and Services Administration. Sixth report to the President and Congress on the status of health personnel in the United States. DHHS Publication No. HRS-P-OD-88-1. Washington DC: Government Printing Office, 1988.

97. US Department of Health, Education and Welfare, Public Health Service, Bureau of Health Manpower. Dental manpower fact book. DHEW Publication No. (HRA) 79-14. Washington DC: Government Printing Office, 1979.

98. US Department of Health, Education and Welfare, Public Health Service, Division of Dental Health. Manpower supply and educational statistics for dentists and dental auxiliaries. Bethesda MD: Division of Dental Health, 1972.

99. US Department of Labor, Bureau of Labor Statistics. Occupational outlook handbook 2004-05 edition. Bulletin 2540. Dental hygienists, website: http://www.bls.gov/oco/print/ocos097.htm. Accessed May 12, 2004.

100. US General Accounting Office. Increased use of expanded function dental auxiliaries would benefit consumers, dentists, and taxpayers. Publication No. HRD-80-51. Washington DC: Government Printing Office, 1980.

101. Vernon TM. The licensure of dental hygienists in Colorado: An update. J Public Health Dent 1989; 49:234.

102. Waldman HB. Female dentists: A factor in determining the available future dental work force. J Am Coll Dent 1985;52(4):22–7.

103. Waldman HB. Pediatric dentists: Evolving demography. ASDC J Dent Child 1990;57:111–3.

104. Waldman HB. Will there be enough trained dental auxiliaries? Ill Dent J 1992;61:253–6.

105. Weeks WB, Wallace AE, Wallace MM, Welch HG. A comparison of the educational costs and incomes of physicians and other professionals. N Engl J Med 1994;330:1280–6.

106. World Health Organization. Report of an expert committee on auxiliary dental personnel. Technical Report Series No. 163. Geneva: WHO, 1959.

107. World Health Organization. Inter-regional seminar on the training and utilization of dental personnel in developing countries, New Delhi, India, Dec 1967. WHO Document DH/68.2. Geneva: WHO, 1968.

108. Zillen PA, Mindak M. World dental demographics. Int Dent J 2000;50:194–7.

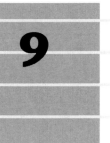

9   Access to Dental Care

In 2001, 65.6% of people ages 2 years and older in the United States reported that they had visited a dentist within the previous year.[30] According to a survey of American adults in 2003, slightly over 82% reported having a regular dentist.[7] These figures show that, for a large portion of the U.S. population, access to dental care is more routine than ever. But for a disturbingly large subset of the population regular access is not so simple. It is perhaps easy for many dentists in busy practices not to fully appreciate the difficulty experienced by many of those who do not get regular care, because their attention, understandably, is directed toward providing care to their established patients. Among those with lower levels of access are the poor, members of minority groups, the elderly, the very young, the institutionalized, and those with many types of disabilities. People living in sparsely populated rural areas or in run-down urban areas, where dentists are few, also have much reduced access to care. Often several of these characteristics apply simultaneously, which makes the situation especially difficult.

Access is a complex, multidimensional concept. It is also a continuum, not a matter of presence or absence. How much access is the right amount is probably undefinable in absolute terms, at least partly because how much is enough differs from one person to another and even for the same person over time. Defining adequate access also is complex because the ability to overcome impediments to access varies from person to person.

REASONS FOR ACCESS PROBLEMS

There are a multitude of reasons for access problems, and many of them are caused or made worse by lack of resources. Often this lack of resources is as simple as not having money to pay the usual fees for dental care. In other cases, it can be lack of program funds needed to meet the costs of providing care for the homebound, the very young, and people with disabilities. In still others, it can be lack of resources to ensure that health care personnel have developed competence beyond the norm required to deal with some of these special needs. Providing the means to overcome physical barriers also can be expensive, and cultural mismatches between providers and patients from ethnic minorities also can present a substantial barrier. People who are not in the mainstream of the population due to minority or immigrant status, inadequate financial resources, compromised mobility, or special needs simply do not have the ready access to dental care that is enjoyed by most of the population.

SCOPE OF THE ACCESS PROBLEM

The number of people enrolled in Medicaid in 2002 in the United States was estimated at

39.9 million, of whom 18.4 million were children.[26] By definition, all of these individuals need financial help to pay for dental care. Medicaid coverage for dental care is mandated for children (although it is chronically underfunded, see Chapter 7), but for adults any Medicaid dental care beyond the most rudimentary emergency services is now rare. In 2002 there were another 4.2 million children enrolled in the State Children's Health Insurance Program (see Chapter 7). In addition, of the 40.6 million individuals enrolled in Medicare in 2001, over 5.5 million were disabled (and under age 65) and approximately 4.5 million were 85 years or older, people who were likely to have mobility problems in accessing conventional dental practice. There is virtually no dental coverage in Medicare. These groups contain many of the people most likely to experience access problems, and they total nearly 50 million individuals (Medicaid, plus the disabled and those age 85 and older on Medicare), or more than 300 people per dentist, on average. Ensuring their dental care means that adequate means of financing must be forthcoming. Private dental practices, although they can and do provide some care of this type on a pro bono basis, require external help to provide care for this many individuals.

The largely government-subsidized safety net system, of which the migrant and community health centers are the major part, does play an important part in providing access where it might otherwise not be unavailable. Nevertheless, there needs to be more of these facilities and they need long-term support to be sustainable. In 2002 these health centers were able to provide dental care to 1.6 million people,[27] only a fraction of the nearly 45 million Medicaid and State Children's Health Insurance Program enrollees. It is evident that both the safety net system and private practices are required if the needs of these populations are to be met.

SUPPLY OF DENTISTS

It is tempting to blame lack of access on an insufficient number of dentists, but this is far too oversimplified. Of course, a sufficient supply of dental personnel is necessary for good access to dental care. The traditional way to estimate the adequacy of the supply of dentists has been the dentist/population ratio. Fig. 9-1 shows the historical pattern in the ratio of dentists to population in the United States, with projections through the year 2020. From a peak in the late 1990s, the supply of dentists is projected to decline because of (1) the growth in the U.S. population (see Chapter 2), and (2) the impending retirement of the large number of dentists who graduated in the 1970s and 1980s, combined with smaller dental school class sizes since then (see

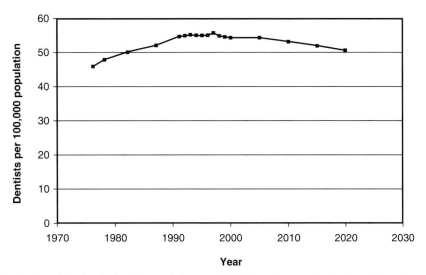

Fig. 9-1 Number of dentists in the U.S. population per 100,000 people, actual and projected, for selected years, 1967-2020.[3]

Chapter 8). Even if dental school classes were to be expanded to the peak seen in the late 1970s, it would take at least until the 2020s to restore the dentist/population ratios of the early 1990s.

In addition to measures of the dentist/population ratio, the two other most commonly used approaches to estimating personnel needs are demand-based and need-based models. The demand-based approach comes from economic theory and aims to make forecasts of the quantity of dental care that people will actually consume. The price and supply of services are key components of these models. Demand-based models have been used by the Health Resources and Services Administration of the U.S. Department of Health and Human Services and by the American Dental Association (ADA) for their workforce forecasts.[20,28,29] Through such models, it is possible to estimate how issues such as changes in insurance coverage, income levels, number of dentists, and population growth are likely to affect the use of dental care.

Need-based approaches to personnel requirements come from a philosophically different direction. Need-based models start from measurements of treatment need in a population, from which estimates are then derived of how much treatment would be required to meet those needs. The time required for treatment is added across the entire population, and from that an estimate of the number of required provider-hours of care can be determined.[31] A complication with the need-based approach is that both the accumulated backlog of need and estimates of future disease must be included. Other inherent difficulties are that dentists can treat the same condition in different ways and that demand is often poorly related to need. Demand for some types of care, cosmetic restorations, for example, is difficult to predict, which complicates the need-based approach even further.

Adequacy of the Supply of Dentists

Although the number of dentists relative to population clearly is an important consideration in estimating the adequacy of the supply of dental care, by itself it is not a sufficient indication of shortage or surplus. Careful examination of Fig. 9-1 demonstrates this fact. In the early 1980s, when there were about 50 dentists per 100,000 population, there was widely con-sidered to be "too many" dentists. Both the dental press and the popular media of the early 1980s contain a number of articles about the economic pinch that dentists were feeling because of what was perceived as a shortage of patients. Many dentists complained that they were not as busy as they wanted to be. By way of contrast, in the late 1990s, when there were nearly 55 dentists per 100,000 population (relatively about 10% more dentists), dentists reported being busier than ever, and their incomes had never been higher.[8,19] The fact that 2000 persons per dentist was "not enough" in 1982 whereas 1800 people per dentist was "plenty" in 2000 shows that additional factors must be important in determining the adequacy of the dentist supply.

Uncertainty over the supply of dentists is not new. The meaning of the relative increase in the number of dentists between 1970 and the mid-1990s, followed by the projected decline over the next several decades, has aroused considerable discussion.[6,14,16,17,21,23,29] For many years after World War II, both the dental profession and the public accepted that a shortage of dental personnel was imminent. It was expected that significant increases in demand, stemming from rising affluence, rapid increases in population (the postwar baby boom; see Chapter 2), and the high levels of caries at the time (see Chapter 20), would overwhelm the ability of the dental profession to provide all the care needed. The influential 1961 report *The Survey of Dentistry*[18] recommended marked increases in the number of dental graduates and auxiliaries and made projections of future personnel shortages. Indeed, the population figures from the 1960 U.S. census (Fig. 9-2) showed a continuing increase in the young population that, if continued, was expected to severely tax many of the nation's resources.

In 1963 the ADA referred to "the impending shortage of health personnel" as "probably the most critical problem in the health field today"[5] and again foresaw shortages in 1965.[1] These views were still in evidence in 1971, when the ADA's Task Force on National Health Programs stated the following as a basic assumption:

The United States faces a shortage of dental personnel in the next 20 years and the shortage will occur whether or not there is a national dental health program.[4]

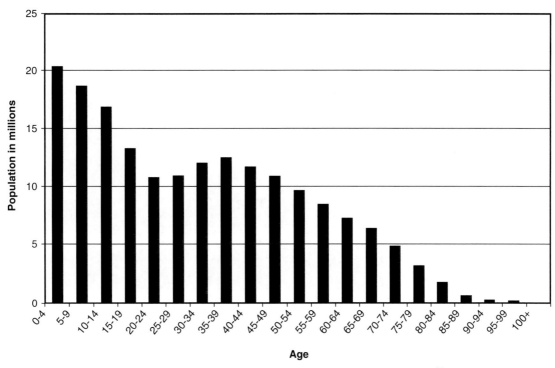

Fig. 9-2   Population of the United States by 5-year age increments, 1960.[24]

However, by the mid-1970s many in dentistry no longer accepted the existence of a personnel shortage.[9,17] The combined effect of a large increase in the numbers of graduates (see Chapter 8), chiefly as a result of increased federal support of dental schools, plus the large and unforeseen drop in the rate of population growth (Fig. 9-3), led to the increase in the relative supply of dentists. The ADA agreed in 1973 that the relative supply of dentists was going to increase considerably by 1985,[2] a notable reversal from its position of only 8 years before.[1]

No one in the early 1960s could foresee the dramatic drop in fertility rates with the consequent lowering of the rate of population increase, nor was the large decline in caries (see Chapter 20) anticipated. A further projection in 1977 indicated that the supply of dentists would slightly exceed demand by 1990.[25] Assumptions in this projection were that population growth would continue at the 1977 rate, that 43%-50% of the population would be covered by dental insurance, and that the number of dental graduates would peak at 5460 in 1982 and then remain stable through at least 1990. Of course, we now know that the number of

graduates fell as low as 3778 in 1993, substantially lower than any of these projections, and based on first-year enrollments, we can say that the number of dental graduates through the early twenty-first century will not be much more than 4500 per year. This whole matter is a further lesson that, although predictions are a necessary basis for rational policy decisions, predicting the future remains a hazardous business indeed.

It now seems likely that the dentist/population ratio will slowly decline for the foreseeable future, although the consequence of this trend on the practice of dentistry or the oral health of the public remains uncertain. It has become clear that there is no "correct" ratio of dentists to population; what may have been the "right" number of dentists in one decade is not necessarily "right" in the next. Although low levels of caries are already reducing the need for treatment in younger Americans,[13] substantial need will remain for maintenance and repair of the restorations placed in earlier generations.[6,10,22] This trend may be magnified by increasing tooth retention (see Chapter 19). More adults will have relatively complete dentitions that

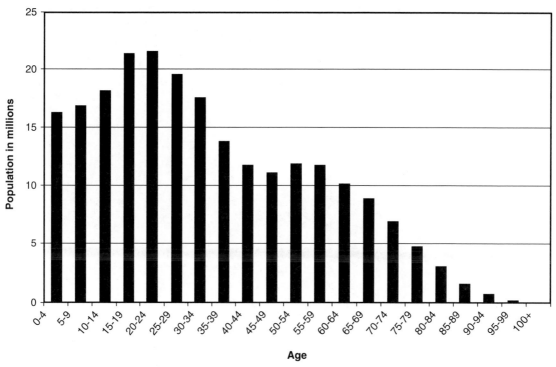

Fig. 9-3 Population of the United States by 5-year age increments, 1980.[24]

they expect to maintain throughout life and will thus require restorative and periodontal care. Although it now seems likely that the adult population will have substantially reduced need for care a few decades from now, the lessons from the recent past should be ample warning that speculations about the future should be treated as tentative at best. Even so, getting the personnel numbers "right" for the future demands policy now. The effects of policies like those embodied in the Health Professions Educational Assistance Act of 1963 are not seen for at least 10 years. Schools have to be built or expanded, faculty established, and the first new classes moved through to graduation and practice. Fig. 8-1 showed that the 1963 act first began to have real impact on the number of practicing dentists in the years 1970-75, and the effect of these graduates will be with us at least through 2020.

Factors Determining Adequacy

Skeptical about what they see as governmental ineptitude, many leaders in dentistry (and some in government) would prefer to leave the matter of workforce numbers to market forces. But

although market forces work well to regulate many aspects of the economy, health care presents a special challenge. Market forces attract or deter dental students based on conditions as they are now, and conditions can be very different in 20 years' time. In its comprehensive report on the future of dental education, the Institute of Medicine gave the issue of the dental workforce careful consideration.[15] In the face of the many uncertainties already cited, the Institute of Medicine recommended keeping the first-year enrollment levels at about 4000 for the foreseeable future, a level that has already been passed by about 10% (see Chapter 8).

Boxes 9-1 to 9-3 describe factors that are likely to play a role in determining the adequacy of the supply of dentists and dental care. As we have already seen, how these factors will balance out is exceedingly difficult to predict. Nevertheless, at least in terms of traditional disease-based dental care, it seems reasonable to expect that, with the ever-accumulating effect in the population of the declines in dental caries and related improvements in oral health, the average dental practice should in the future be able to manage the oral health of many

---

BOX 9-1 Factors Tending Toward a Shortage of Dentists

- **Good economic times.** As people have more disposable income, they are able to buy more dental care. Some dental care can be postponed, and with good economic times treatment for this postponed care may then be sought.
- **High expectations for oral health.** With the general improvement in oral health that has occurred over the past several decades, many people fully expect to maintain a healthy dentition throughout life and are willing to invest in dental care to that end.
- **Less edentulism.** As tooth loss diminishes in the population, there are more teeth to maintain throughout life.
- **Growing utilization.** Over the past several decades, a growing proportion of the population reports

receiving dental care on a regular basis. As this proportion continues to rise, more dental care will be consumed.
- **Effects of the baby boom group in the population.** The bulge in the population that resulted from the post–World War II baby boom (see Chapter 2) has affected many aspects of life in the United States and will continue to do so for several more decades. Because these birth cohorts were children when caries levels were high, they carried into adulthood many heavily restored teeth that continue to require increasingly expensive maintenance.
- **Decline in the dentist/population ratio.** All else being equal, fewer dentists means that less dental care will be available.

BOX 9-2 Factors Tending Toward a Surplus of Dentists

- **Falling disease levels.** Treatment of disease has historically been a major part of what motivates patients to visit dentists, and treatment of the consequences has been a major part of what dentists do. As succeeding birth cohorts benefit from lower disease levels, there will be less per patient for dentists to treat.
- **Changes in utilization.** As increasing numbers of individuals who experienced low levels of dental caries as children become young adults, they may not need nor seek dental care as frequently as their parents' generation did.
- **Effects of the "baby bust" generation.** In addition to having lower levels of past disease than their parents' generation, the birth cohorts since the early 1960 are much smaller than the generation that came before

them. Because middle-aged adults have traditionally been the group that provided large amounts of income to dental practices, the combination of much less need per capita and millions fewer of such patients could mean significantly less income to dental practices.
- **Economic downturns.** Just as improving economic conditions are associated with more demand for dental care, the inevitable periodic economic downturns will likely reduce demand for care, especially for cosmetic services.
- **Increasing role of auxiliary personnel.** With improving oral health, a larger proportion of the income to many dental practices comes from procedures associated with periodic recall visits. As more of these services are provided by auxiliary personnel, the need for dentists will decline.

---

more patients than in the past.[11] It is also the case that, because of improving oral health, the mix of dental services in most dental practices is shifting toward those that can be provided by allied dental personnel.[13] These facts alone should call into question concerns that a slowly declining dentist/population ratio over the next several decades is a sign of a looming shortage of dentists.

It also is evident, in some cases at least, that a shortage of dentists per se is not the problem in

lack of access for Medicaid enrollees. In a Medicaid demonstration program in Michigan, when fee levels were linked to those paid for privately insured patients and administration was managed by a commercial carrier in the same way as for private groups, access to care improved virtually immediately. Before this changeover, about 25% of dentists in the involved counties had treated Medicaid patients in the previous year. Within the first year of the demonstration program, over 85% of the

---

BOX 9-3 Factors Associated With Uncertainty Regarding the Adequacy of the Supply of Dentists

- **Possible changes in routine care.** The patterns of routine care, such as the 6-month recall visit, date to times when disease levels in the population were much higher than today and home care was less effective. As the oral health of the population continues to improve, the recommended time for recall visits for the healthiest patients could be significantly extended.
- **Demand for nondisease services.** Future levels of demand for services like cosmetic dentistry are difficult to predict and are especially likely to be subject to fluctuations associated with economic trends.
- **Demand from healthy people.** How the growing proportion of the population who have experienced little or no oral health problems will choose to use dental care is uncertain.
- **Patterns of dentists' retirements.** The group of dentists who graduated during the peak of dental school enrollments will likely be retiring over the next 20 years or so. Because this group is so large, how and when these dentists choose to retire will

significantly affect the supply of dentists. However, because dentists have so much flexibility in how they practice, for example, in how many days per week they practice and how many patients they see each day, it is extremely difficult to predict these retirement patterns.
- **Dental insurance trends.** The major growth in dental prepayment since the early 1970s has undoubtedly had an important role in the recent high levels of demand for dental care. However, that growth appears to have plateaued, and if the pressures to reduce the cost of health care (see Chapter 7) result in a significant drop in the proportion of the population with dental insurance, demand for dental care could also drop.
- **Government role in dental care.** Currently the role of government in paying for dental care is small (see Chapter 7). If dental coverage were to be added to Medicare, or the coverage under Medicaid were to be significantly improved, many people with high levels of need could suddenly be brought into the dental care system.

---

dentists in the affected counties treated Medicaid patients.[12] Many more children received dental care, and they received it without having to travel excessive distances to find an available provider. Although there clearly had been a shortage in dental care available at the conventional Medicaid fees, there appeared to be no shortage when dentists were reimbursed at their usual fee levels.

Access Problems for Certain Populations

Although there may be no across-the-board shortage of dentists, and thus no access problems for most people, it bears repeating that access will still be a problem for many. Those most likely to experience access problems are children, adults, and the elderly in families with low incomes, people of all ages with disabilities and special needs, and those living in areas where there are few dentists (these most often are low-income urban areas or low-population rural areas). However, assuring adequate access to dental care for these groups is not just a matter of training more dentists. Although dental

care for some of them, such as the disabled and institutionalized, requires special training, the major impediment to access is economic. It takes money to operate a dental practice, and if the patients don't have the money to purchase care, then access will continue to be a problem unless supplemental sources of funding are available. This will happen regardless of the number of dentists trained. The primary condition for solving the problem of access to dental care in the United States, in those places and for those individuals for whom access is a problem, is funding. Even the safety net providers of care such as the community and migrant health centers (see Chapter 6) cannot provide access over the long run without dependable long-term funding.

STRATEGIES TO SOLVE THE ACCESS PROBLEM

Because the reasons for access problems are many and varied, solutions will also require a multifaceted approach. The problem is too large and too diverse to think that a single approach will be adequate. Some of the approaches that are likely to be essential to a comprehensive solution are the following.

Strengthening of the Safety Net System

In many locations, both urban and rural, economic or other conditions are simply not adequate to support a sufficient number of conventional dental practices. Local, state, and federal support is necessary to build clinics and in many cases to subsidize the support of clinical staff. The current system of community and migrant health centers (see Chapter 6), which are usually jointly supported by local, state, and federal funds, is a prime example of this safety net system. Without continuing public support and additional support where new and expanded clinics are needed, many locations will remain areas of chronically low access.

Provision of Adequate Payment

For both the safety net providers and private practitioners, reimbursement levels must be adequate to cover the cost of providing care. It is simply a fact that no system can continue to exist in the long run if its costs are not met. Although all providers willingly provide some care without reimbursement, the size of the population in the United States is too large for such "free" care to be able to handle more than a small fraction of the need.

Optimal Use of Allied Dental Personnel

Because of the generally improving oral health of the U.S. population, a growing proportion of the care that is provided could be managed by auxiliary dental personnel. Dental practices could thus become more efficient, with the ability to reduce the per capita costs of providing dental care to many people. For this to happen, some states will need to modify their dental practice acts to permit practice by the types of personnel most suited to providing the necessary care under the most suitable practice arrangements. Although the best solution will vary from state to state, examples might include liberalized licensing of foreign-educated dentists as proposed in California, independent or unsupervised practice of dental hygienists, expansion of functions for auxiliary personnel, or use of dental therapists (see Chapters 6 and 8). If the cost of producing needed care can be

reduced, it will be economically feasible to provide care in places where otherwise it would not be possible.

Special Arrangements for Special Populations

In some circumstances, conventional dental practices are simply not suited to providing adequate access. For the elderly and disabled who are confined to extended care facilities, care often must be brought to them. Although some practices are able to manage some of this kind of care, many are not. Given the growing size of the elderly population, it is likely that more practices must be organized specifically for this purpose for such care to be most efficient. As with other forms of practice, sufficient treatment funds must be forthcoming to make these practices economically viable.

Development of Cultural Competency

Patient behaviors such as missing appointments and not following healthy lifestyles are sometimes cited as reasons for the frustrations that dental personnel experience in treating some patients from low-income and minority groups. Although it is appropriately a responsibility of health care providers to attempt to encourage optimum health-related behaviors, it is also a responsibility to do so in a manner that shows an understanding of the person's capabilities and circumstances. For example, for many individuals and families in these unusual circumstances, performing in ways that are typical of conventional patients can be exceedingly difficult, and this must be taken into account in working with them. The term *cultural competency* is often used to denote the knowledge and skills needed to be most effective in managing the dental care of these individuals.

Expansion of the Mindset of Dentistry

For any of the aforementioned solutions to be most effective they must have the strong support of the dental professions, both locally and nationally. Although the primary focus of most dental practitioners will necessarily be conventional dental patients in conventional dental practices, practitioners must also recognize that nonconventional patients are as much a part of their responsibility as are any other patients. The discharge of that responsibility can take many forms, from welcoming all patients that fit their practice arrangements to providing encouragement and political support for those practices that are organized to care for nonconventional patients.

Establishment of Responsibility for Providing Needed Resources

If the resources necessary to provide access are to be in place, someone must be willing to provide those resources. If that responsibility is not clearly defined and those resources are not made available on an ongoing and dependable basis, access will deteriorate. Discussions about improving access that do not include the identification of the resources to provide that access miss a necessary component for long-term success.

Most of the people who suffer from inadequate access to dental care do so because they simply do not have their own funds to pay for dental care. Those funds will become available only if society is willing to transfer funds from people who have money to pay for the care of those who do not. Until we as a society decide to put sufficient funds into paying for this care by adequately funding programs like Medicaid so that dental practices can afford to provide this care on a long-term basis, or by paying to build and staff community clinics to serve these populations, access is likely to remain a problem.

The resource demands to meet even the most modest definition of access in many groups within the population are far beyond those that dentistry alone can provide. The condition of current federal and state budgets is driving things in the wrong direction—with almost every state dropping all but emergency services for adults and looking for ways to further reduce benefits for children. There also is a serious proposal to reduce federal involvement in services to the low-income population, as evidenced by recent proposals to convert the federal Medicaid matching funds to a block grant. This projected move would include a cap on federal responsibility in return for liberalizing the states' requirements for comprehensive coverage of children. The irony of this approach is that it sets up a situation in which, just when people most need this kind of help because of temporary difficult economic times, the state will be least able to provide that help.

REFERENCES

1. American Dental Association, Bureau of Economic Research and Statistics. Number of dental graduates required annually to 1985. J Am Dent Assoc 1965; 71:697-8.
2. American Dental Association, Bureau of Economic Research and Statistics. Growth in population and numbers of dentists to 1985. J Am Dent Assoc 1973; 87:901-3.
3. American Dental Association, Health Policy Resources Center. Future of dentistry. Chicago: ADA, 2001.
4. American Dental Association, Task Force on National Health Programs. Dentistry in national health programs: A report with recommendations. J Am Dent Assoc 1971;83:569-600.
5. Association testifies in support of Educational Assistance Act. J Am Dent Assoc 1963;66:389-91.
6. Beazoglou TJ, Guay AH, Heffley DR. The economic health of dentistry: Past, present, and future. J Am Dent Assoc 1989;119:117-21.
7. Berry J. What do they think? ADA survey offers up the scoop on your patients. ADA News 2004;35(8):1.
8. Brown LJ, Lazar V. Dentists and their practices. J Am Dent Assoc 1998;129:1692-9.
9. Butts HC. Dental manpower shortage? [editorial]. J Am Dent Assoc 1976;93:507.
10. Douglass CW, Furino A. Balancing dental service requirements and supplies: Epidemiologic and demographic evidence. J Am Dent Assoc 1990;121:587-92.
11. Eklund SA. Dentistry 2000—clinical care: Changing treatment patterns. J Am Dent Assoc 1999;130: 1707-12.
12. Eklund SA, Pittman JL, Clark SJ. Michigan Medicaid's Healthy Kids Dental program. An assessment of the first 12 months. J Am Dent Assoc 2003;134:1509-15.
13. Eklund SA, Pittman JL, Smith RC. Trends in dental care among insured Americans: 1980 to 1995. J Am Dent Assoc 1997;128:171-8.
14. Feldstein PJ. Financing dental care: An economic analysis. Lexington MA: Heath, 1973.
15. Field MJ, ed. Dental education at the crossroads: Challenges and change. Washington DC: National Academy Press, 1995.
16. Furino A, Douglass CW. Balancing dental service requirements and supplies: The economic evidence. J Am Dent Assoc 1990;121:685-92.
17. Goodman SE. The dentist shortage that never was. Dent Manage 1976;July:33-8.
18. Hollinshead BS. The survey of dentistry: The final report. Washington DC: American Council on Education, 1961.
19. Meskin LH. Healthier, wealthier and wiser. J Am Dent Assoc 1998;129:1660, 1662.
20. Perich ML. American Dental Association manpower projections. J Dent Educ 1987;51:219-23.
21. Pew Health Professions Commission. Critical challenges: Revitalizing the health care professions for the twenty-first century. San Francisco: UCSF Center for the Health Professions, 1995.
22. Reinhardt JW, Douglass CW. The need for operative dentistry services: Projecting the effects of changing disease patterns. Oper Dent 1989;14:114-20.

23. Solomon ES. Errors in federal report on dental health personnel presents problems. J Dent Educ 1990; 54:499-501.

24. US Department of Commerce, Bureau of the Census. 1980 Census of the population. Vol 1, Characteristics of the population, Chapter A, Number of inhabitants, Part 1, United States summary. Table 45. Washington DC: Government Printing Office, 1983.

25. US Department of Health, Education and Welfare, Public Health Service, Division of Dentistry. Projections of national requirements for dentists 1980, 1985, and 1990. DHEW Publication No. (HRA) 77-48. Washington DC: Government Printing Office, 1977.

26. US Department of Health and Human Services, Center for Medicare and Medicaid Services, Office of Research, Development, and Information. 2003 CMS statistics. CMS Publication No. 03445, 2003, website: http://www.cms.hhs.gov/researchers/pubs/03cmsstats.pdf. Accessed May 13, 2004.

27. US Department of Health and Human Services, Health Resources and Services Administration, Bureau of Health Professions. Data from the Uniform Data System (UDS). Calendar year 2002 data (National rollup), website: http://bphc.hrsa.gov/uds/data.htm. Accessed May 6, 2004.

28. US Department of Health and Human Services, Public Health Service, Health Resources and Services Administration. Health personnel in the United States. Eighth report to Congress 1991. DHHS Publication No. HRS-P-OD-92-1. Washington DC: Government Printing Office, 1992.

29. US Department of Health and Human Services, Public Health Service, Health Resources and Services Administration. Seventh report to the President and Congress on the status of health personnel in the United States. DHHS Publication No. HRS-P-OD-90-1. Washington DC: Government Printing Office, 1990.

30. US Department of Health and Human Services, Public Health Service, National Center for Health Statistics. Health, United States. Dental visits in the past year according to selected characteristics: United States, selected years 1997-2001, web access: ftp://ftp.cdc.gov/pub/Health_Statistics/NCHS/Publications/Health_US/hus03/Table078.xls. Accessed April 27, 2004.

31. World Health Organization. Health through oral health. Guidelines for planning and monitoring for oral health care. London: Quintessence, 1989.

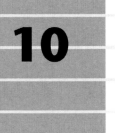

10 The Healthy Dental Practice: Infection Control and Mercury Safety

In dental practice not long ago, a blood-stained swab after a tooth extraction was simply thrown in the trash without further thought. Not any more. Today, dental offices must use *standard precautions*, a set of procedures based on the assumption that any patient, or any person working in the dental office, might carry a serious infection. All phases of dental treatment are then conducted so as to minimize the risk of cross-infection.

Some dentists look with nostalgia on the old days, a time when they did not have to work in gloves, mask, and eyewear; ensure that office waste went into the appropriate container; and worry about the latest regulations from the U.S. Occupational Safety and Health Administration (OSHA). This nostalgic view is misplaced. It is fair to say that dentistry should have been a lot more concerned about cross-infection in the old days than it was; it took a jolt from the human immunodeficiency virus (HIV) epidemic to force improvement. Although some dentists still see OSHA's regulations on waste disposal as just another bureaucratic burden, the management of the office environment has clearly become an integral part of running a modern dental practice. Given that many more people are infected with the HIV and hepatitis B and C viruses than demonstrate overt disease, the only defensible approach is to assume that any patient could be infected and to act accordingly. Dental practices today are far healthier

environments than they ever were, and both the public and the professions will continue to benefit as a result.

Our purpose in this chapter is to review the principal infection concerns in dental practice: HIV, hepatitis B virus (HBV), and hepatitis C virus (HCV). The chapter also reviews the issue of mercury safety as an example of an environmental concern.

INFECTION CONTROL

After the emergence of antibiotics during World War II (1939-45), the industrialized world lost much of its age-old concerns about infectious diseases. The major epidemics of the past were gone, and parents no longer feared the worst when they heard a child cough in the night. It was a short, complacent period during which some of the painful antisepsis lessons from the nineteenth century were neglected in our dependence on antibiotics. This period ended suddenly in the early 1980s with the harsh reminder that mortal infectious diseases were still with us. Not only is HIV infection a devastating disease that shredded the social fabric in a way not seen since tuberculosis in the nineteenth century, but the HIV epidemic is a humbling reminder that the path of biomedical advancement is not always smoothly upward.

Of course, HIV infection is not the only infectious disease to raise concerns about cross-infection during dental treatment. HBV infection is an ominous threat, and the risk of HBV infection is higher in the unprotected dental practice setting than in most other environments. Hepatitis B was around long before HIV infection, but it took the impact of HIV infection to force adoption of those old-fashioned barrier techniques of infection control that had never been a routine part of dental practice.

Guidelines for Infection Control

The American Dental Association (ADA) had a set of rather gentle infection-control guidelines in the pre-HIV era,[13] mostly concerned with hepatitis, but the advent of HIV in the early 1980s led to a more stringent approach. Detailed guidelines were then developed by the ADA,[16] and the American Association of Public Health Dentistry produced its guidelines in 1986.[4] The definitive guidelines for dental practice, however, are those issued by the U.S. Public Health Service's Centers for Disease Control and Prevention (CDC). These definitive guidelines were first issued in 1993,[103] and the updated and considerably extended version was released in late 2003 after extensive public comments.[104] The CDC has also developed infection control guidelines for field examinations for surveys or research studies.[98] The ADA has now merged its statement on infection control with the CDC guidelines.

All of these guidelines are based on the concept of *standard precautions* (previously called *universal precautions*). The underlying philosophy is that infected patients cannot be differentiated from uninfected ones, so the prudent thing to do is to assume that all patients may be infected. A parallel approach, first presented in 1987,[65] is referred to as *body substance isolation*, which focuses on reducing transmission of infectious material from any moist body substance of the patient to the health care worker. Both approaches emphasize that barrier procedures should be employed in treating all patients, which means that gloves, masks, and protective eyewear should be worn by dental personnel. They also focus on proper disposal of one-time-use materials, routine sterilization of other instruments and equipment, and proper handling of potentially infectious materials. The 2003 CDC guidelines moved toward combining the previous universal precautions regarding body substance isolation into a single set of recommendations known as *standard infection-control procedures.*[70] Each recommendation in these guidelines is graded according to the strength of the scientific evidence to support it.

The barrier principles that form the basis of the CDC guidelines hark back to the beginnings of antiseptic medical practice, and they are effective: HBV infection was found to be twice as high among dentists who never wore gloves as among dentists who wore gloves routinely.[48] With standard precautions, the risk of transmission of either HIV or HBV in the dental office is extremely low.[29]

OSHA and Dental Practice

OSHA was established by Congress as an agency in the U.S. Department of Labor in December 1970 (Public Law 91-596), and some amendments to the original act were passed in November 1990. The mission of this regulatory agency, as laid out in the introduction to the original act, is "to assure safe and healthful working conditions for working men and women." OSHA is responsible for establishing standards for safe and healthy working conditions for all employees and regulating maintenance of these standards. OSHA's standards cover just about all industries: mining, shipping, construction, logging, food service, health care, and many others. OSHA also has standards that are specific to workers handling hazardous or potentially hazardous substances and materials, so the reach of this federal agency is considerable. A number of states have set up their own OSHA-type agencies, and OSHA is required to work cooperatively with them.

Dentists, like all other employers, are subject to occupational health and safety laws and regulations that cover a variety of activities in the dental office. Although OSHA's interests include a wide range of issues like ergonomics, waterlines, and indoor air quality, the OSHA regulation that has most affected dental practitioners is the *bloodborne pathogen* (BP) standard. This standard came into effect in March 1992 after a period of intense public debate in which the ADA played a prominent role. The BP standard was revised in January 2001.[102] It applies to all activities in which health care workers come into contact with human blood or other bodily fluids, or are in a position where they may do so.

The BP standard applies to hospitals and other medical facilities, paramedical and ambulance services, blood banks, research facilities, and of course dental offices. The BP standard is comprehensive and highly detailed. It requires each dental office to prepare an exposure control plan, which is intended to minimize employee exposure to infection. The BP standard covers instrument sterilization and storage, handling of potentially contaminated equipment, disposal of medical waste, and many related topics. It specifies that dentists must offer HBV vaccination to staff and includes meticulous requirements for reporting "incidents," that is, accidents in which skin has been broken (e.g., a needlestick) and hence in which there is potential risk of infection. Details get down to the level of washing and storing laundry.

The ADA has not had a good relationship with OSHA in the development and application of these standards. The ADA has complained that it was not consulted adequately prior to the promulgation of the BP standard and that OSHA indiscriminately and inappropriately lumped dental practice in with hospitals and other facilities. The ADA considered that OSHA made no good attempt to understand dental practice, and its calls for industry-specific standards were not heeded. OSHA inspects health care facilities in response to complaints, and soon after the BP regulations went into effect the ADA began receiving complaints from dentists that some OSHA inspections of dental practices were heavy-handed and clumsy. OSHA admitted that there was some justification for these complaints, and with better communications the relations between the two organizations improved somewhat. A major step in improved relations came when OSHA permitted dentists to respond to complaints by phone or fax rather than be subjected to a site visit.

For dentists unaccustomed to reading the language of the federal government, the BP standard is a formidable document. To help practitioners meet the standards, the ADA has a set of manuals that outline the elements of an exposure control plan and put infection-control guidelines together with OSHA guidelines in standard operating routines for the dental office.[5]

Dentists have also complained about the high cost of compliance with OSHA standards,[32] sometimes implying that these are dollars not well spent. Some of the more trivial aspects of the BP standard have been refined over time, which should have the effect of reducing costs, but compliance will always carry some price. In the long run it is patients who foot the bill, and so far the public seems to view the cost of compliance as money well spent.

HIV INFECTION AND AIDS

AIDS is the acronym for *acquired immunodeficiency syndrome* and is the end point of HIV infection. With the dominant position this condition now occupies in the lives of all health professionals, it is sobering to recall that HIV was identified only in 1983.[76] The knowledge that has accumulated since then on the virology and epidemiology of the condition represents some impressive research, although the public hysteria that can surround AIDS is a reminder that humans have not fundamentally changed much since the Black Death in the fourteenth century.

The AIDS virus is human T-lymphotropic virus type 3 or lymphadenopathy-associated virus, a retrovirus usually called HIV. It attacks the CD4+ T lymphocytes in infected humans, which results in immunosuppression. As the number of CD4+ T lymphocytes is reduced, the affected patient becomes increasingly vulnerable to opportunistic infections, which can overwhelm the patient's compromised defense systems. *Pneumocystis carinii* pneumonia is the most common serious opportunistic infection, though there are many others, including pulmonary tuberculosis. AIDS was at first defined solely by clinical conditions, but a 1993 revision of the classification system by the CDC redefined the stages of HIV infection in terms of three ranges of CD4+ T-lymphocyte counts and three groups of clinical manifestations, set out in a nine-cell matrix.[25] These nine categories range from asymptomatic HIV infection or persistent generalized lymphadenopathy with a CD4+ T-cell count of 500/µl or more at the mild end of the scale, to the diagnosis of 1 of 25 AIDS-indicator clinical conditions plus a CD4+ T-cell count of 200/µl or less at the severe end. Dentally related conditions listed among the clinical diseases that are considered part of the AIDS diagnosis include oropharyngeal candidiasis, oral hairy leukoplakia, chronic herpes simplex, and Kaposi's sarcoma.

The disease we call AIDS is the "finale in a progressive process of immunologic deficit mediated by the virus."[76] The primary epidemiology of HIV infection has been well described in terms of risk factors and modes of transmission, although research is still needed on the dynamics of transmission and infection. The average time between infection with HIV virus and the onset of AIDS-like symptoms is estimated to be 10 years,[76] so that HIV disease is like a "time bomb." HIV infection is diagnosed when results of a serologic test are positive; the condition becomes AIDS when a low CD4+ count is found in combination with one of the AIDS-indicator clinical conditions.

The principal mode of transmission in North America is homosexual contact among men followed by intravenous drug injection with contaminated needles and heterosexual contact.[106] There are a small number of cases in which transmission has occurred perinatally (i.e., birth of an infant to an infected mother) and from transfusion with infected blood (e.g., as with the late tennis player Arthur Ashe in the early 1990s). The principal mode of transmission in poor countries is heterosexual contact. Despite the publicity given to the risk associated with certain sexual and drug-use activities, behavioral change among the highest-risk groups does not come easily. The epidemic is increasingly affecting women, minorities, the poor, and heterosexual persons.[55]

In the early days of the AIDS epidemic in North America, diagnosis with HIV infection meant virtually certain death within a few years.

Drug therapy developed quickly, and protease inhibitors showed some good effects. A few years later treatment evolved into the "cocktail" of antiretroviral drugs known as highly active antiretroviral therapy (HAART), which greatly extended life expectancy and has allowed many HIV-positive persons to live more or less normal lives. HAART has probably reduced much of the fear that surrounded HIV infection a generation ago, which may or may not be a good thing. In any event, the success of HAART should not blind us to the fact that AIDS is a pandemic, a global epidemic of massive proportions that is devastating a number of poor countries. HAART is far too expensive to be used widely in these poor countries at market prices. Box 10-1, which shows some of the global data for 2002, indicates the enormity of the HIV pandemic.

Figures for the United States are not as mind boggling as the global data but still tell us that AIDS is a major epidemic.[106] At the end of 2002, there had been 501,669 deaths from AIDS in the United States, including 5315 children under age 15. The death count had increased 39% over 6 years. The cumulative number of cases reported since the beginning of the epidemic in the United States was 886,575. The number of adults and adolescents living with AIDS was 384,906, an increase of 73% over a 6-year period. No one knows how many people are infected with HIV who have not yet been diagnosed, but it is likely to be over a million. It is because of this large number of undiagnosed HIV carriers that the estimates of the growth of the epidemic are ominous. Development of successful vaccines is not

---

BOX 10-1 Global Extent of AIDS/HIV Infection in December 2002[118]

- Globally, 42 million people, 38.6 million adults and 3.2 million children, are estimated to be living with AIDS/HIV.
- In 2002, 70% of these cases were in sub-Saharan Africa and another 14% in South and Southeast Asia.
- In 2002, HIV-associated illnesses caused the death of 3.1 million people, including 610,000 children under age 15.
- Women are becoming increasingly affected. Women accounted for half of the HIV-infected adults and half of the HIV-related deaths in 2002.

- Newly infected persons during 2002 included 5 million adults and 800,000 children under age 15.
- The main mode of transmission in North America and Europe is sexual contact between men, intravenous drug use is second, and sexual relations between heterosexual individuals is third. In sub-Saharan Africa, transmission is almost entirely from heterosexual contact.

considered likely, and HAART treatment is expensive, so control of the epidemic falls back on the toughest measure of all: education to control risky human behavior.

AIDS presents some paradoxes. For example, despite the "time-bomb" implications of the extent of current infection and thus the near certainty of the continued growth of the epidemic, the responsible virus is really quite delicate and hard to transmit. Although dental professionals are at relatively greater risk than average members of the public because of their close contact with saliva and blood, they still have an extremely low risk of occupational exposure.[56] A small number of health care workers have become HIV infected through occupational exposure, but the risk of seroconversion even after needlestick exposure to HIV-infected blood is still only about 1 in 200.[111]

A possible case of HIV transmission from an infected dentist in Florida to a patient was reported in 1990; the dentist died soon after the patient was diagnosed. In this case the patient had two maxillary third molars removed by the dentist. She reported pharyngitis 4 months later and had oral candidiasis 17 months later. Two years after the extractions, she was seropositive for HIV antibody and was diagnosed with *P. carinii* pneumonia. The dentist was reported to have worn gloves and mask throughout the procedure, and from the patient's statement there was no evidence of exposure to the dentist's blood. There were similar DNA sequences in peripheral blood mononuclear cells of both dentist and patient, like those found in many cases that have been epidemiologically linked. Soon afterward, evidence emerged that eight other patients treated in this practice were HIV infected, and there were strong indications that the dentist was the source of infection for at least five of them.[26] The ADA responded quickly to this disclosure in early 1991 with an interim policy that HIV-infected dentists should not perform invasive procedures or should disclose their seropositive status to their patients.[69] The CDC closed the case in 1992 without being able to reach firm conclusions about whether the dentist infected his patients.

Since then, the CDC has issued guidelines that place some limitations on HIV-infected practitioners, mostly restricting the performance of major invasive procedures. Some states

have a legal requirement that an HIV-infected practitioner disclose this status to the patient, although usually this does not mean that the practitioner is not permitted to perform a given procedure.[11] Again, it can be seen that the basis for these requirements is the effectiveness of the standard precautions.

Oral Manifestations of HIV Infection

All dental professionals should be thoroughly familiar with the oral manifestations of HIV infection. The principal signs are oral candidiasis, oral hairy leukoplakia, and Kaposi's sarcoma, although periodontal conditions are frequently bad in persons with advanced immunosuppression[117] and a number of less common disease entities are also found.[89] The details of these conditions are covered thoroughly in oral pathology texts[50] and workshop proceedings.[81] The three principal signs are described only briefly here.

1. *Oral candidiasis:* A fungal infection, candidiasis (called candidosis in Britain) usually presents as a semi-adherent white plaque on the palate, although glossitis and angular stomatitis forms are not uncommon. The plaques can be sore, and they are very common among HIV-positive individuals. An excellent presentation by Pindborg on the diagnosis and treatment of oral candidiasis is available.[77]

2. *Oral hairy leukoplakia:* In a study of 375 homosexual males who either had AIDS or were considered at risk for the disease, 28% presented with oral hairy leukoplakia. The lesions appeared most commonly on the lateral surface of the tongue, with wide variation in the size, severity, and surface characteristics.[88] The condition is highly predictive of the future development of AIDS. In a longitudinal study of a group with oral hairy leukoplakia, survival analysis showed that the probability of AIDS' developing in the patients was 48% after 16 months and 83% after 31 months.[49]

3. *Kaposi's sarcoma:* Kaposi's sarcoma is diagnostic for AIDS and is found in some 20%-34% of AIDS patients.[42] The oral cavity may be the first or only site of the lesion. The most common intraoral site is the palate. The pathogenesis of the disorder

is still not well understood, nor is its inter-action with HIV infection. Treatment is required because of functional impairment, pain, or bleeding, or for cosmetic reasons.

The particularly distressing condition of pediatric AIDS, in which HIV is transmitted from an infected mother, appears to be on the increase. Recognition can be difficult because of the varied presentation of the condition, but the most common oral findings include candidiasis, parotid salivary gland enlargement, and herpetic infections.[94]

HEPATITIS B AND C

Hepatitis is a far more prevalent disease than HIV, both worldwide and in the United States. The CDC estimates that 45% of the world's population live in areas of high prevalence, 43% in areas of moderate prevalence, and only 12% in areas of low prevalence.[107] Globally, the World Health Organization estimates that 2 billion people have been infected with HBV and that currently some 350 million people have chronic infection.[119] In poor countries, 8%-10% of the total population is chronically infected, and in these regions liver cancer, a result of chronic HBV infection, is among the top three causes of death in men.[119] By contrast, fewer than 1% of the population in high-income countries is chronically infected.

The United States and other high-income nations are areas of low prevalence, although there are still around 80,000 new infections per year in the United States.[108] Hepatitis B is primarily a disease of young adults in the United States (peak age for new infections is 20-29 years), whereas in poor countries it is a childhood disease. Both HBV and HCV are transmitted by contact with infected blood, so the primary transmission routes are:

- Sexual contact, both homosexual and heterosexual, especially unprotected sex
- Sharing of infected needles
- Perinatal transmission to an infant born to an infected mother

Although the case fatality rate from HBV infection is low (0.5%-1%) and most infected people recover completely in due course, a significant number of people develop chronic infection. It is in these chronically infected peo-

ple that the most serious sequelae are found. HBV carriers are at risk of long-term sequelae such as chronic liver disease, cirrhosis, and liver cancer, though a more common outcome than death is severe and usually lifelong debilitation. The risk of becoming a chronic carrier of HBV varies with age at first infection. Among those first infected as young children, 30%-90% develop chronic infection, whereas among those who were adults when first infected only 2%-10% do. Chronic infection can be asymptomatic, but 15%-25% of this group can die prematurely from cirrhosis or liver cancer. The CDC estimates that there are some 150 deaths per year from acute hepatitis, although there are around 5000 deaths each year from chronic liver disease. Although the good news is that the number of new infections has been dropping in recent years (Fig. 10-1), the bad news is that there are still 1.25 million persons chronically infected with HBV and 2.7 million HCV-infected persons in the United States.[108]

Signs and symptoms of hepatitis B and C are very general (fatigue, abdominal pain, loss of appetite, intermittent nausea and vomiting, jaundice), and hence the condition can easily be misdiagnosed. Health care workers are at higher risk than the general population because of their likely contact with chronic carriers. The CDC has estimated that there are some 18,000 infections each year among health care workers in the United States, the majority through exposure to infected blood. Blood and serous fluids have the highest concentration of HBV in infected persons; the concentration in saliva is a little lower. However one looks at it, hepatitis B is a disease to be taken seriously.

Fig. 10-1 shows the annual incidence of HBV and HCV infection in the United States from 1980 to 2001. The prevalence of tuberculosis, another infectious disease that has caused concern in dental practices, has been included in this graphic. The drop in incidence of HBV infection through the 1990s is thought to be due partly to the effectiveness of the HBV vaccine but mostly to behavioral change among risk groups (injection drug users, the indiscriminately sexually active, and immigrants from high-prevalence areas) because of their fear of AIDS.

The most insidious aspect of HBV infection is the relative ease with which carriers can

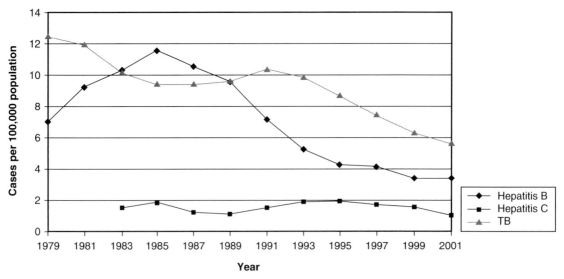

Fig. 10-1 Incidence of hepatitis B (HBV) and hepatitis C (HCV), and prevalence of tuberculosis in the United States, 1980-2001.[107,108]

inadvertently transmit the disease to anyone with whom they come in contact in day-to-day life. The worst reported instance of an infected dentist's inadvertently transmitting HBV to his patients was in Indiana in 1984-85. Nine patients of a dentist in a rural county came down with HBV infection within 2-5 months after being treated by the dentist, a vastly higher incidence than had previously been reported in the area. Two of the patients died. Although the dentist had never had hepatitis symptoms, serum tests showed that he was probably a carrier.[92]

In contrast to the AIDS virus, HBV is hardy and capable of being transmitted much more readily via percutaneous and nonpercutaneous routes.[33] To heighten the contrast, it was reported in 1989 that whereas 15 health care workers had become seropositive for HIV over the previous 7 years in the absence of outside risk factors, a total of between 1750 and 2100 health care providers had died from complications associated with HBV infection over the same period.[64] Because carrier states of HBV are not uncommon, with only 20% of infections being recognized, the patient history can be of little value for dental practitioners.[33] The risk of contracting HBV infection has been estimated to be 3-10 times greater for dentists than for the general population,[3,116] although those estimates came from the days before standard pre-

cautions were widely used. The greatest risk of infection in the dental office clearly comes from the undiagnosed carrier, whether it be a patient, the dentist, or one of the office staff.[34]

Hepatitis viruses A, B, C, D, and E have been identified. Some 90% of non-A, non-B viruses are now recognized as HCV. The designation *non-A, non-B* came after more stringent screening of blood donors in the 1970s resulted in a sharp decrease in the incidence of hepatitis B due to blood transfusion; the non-A, non-B designation was given to the type of hepatitis that continued to occur after blood transfusion despite the new screening program. HCV was identified as the causative agent in 1989.[119] HCV infection has an insidious onset, and like HBV infection it can be easily missed in its early stages. Only some patients become symptomatic (symptoms are similar to those for HBV infection); the majority of infected persons show no symptoms. It is estimated that 2.7 million Americans are infected with HCV, with infection more common in minority populations.[110] Some 85% of infected persons develop chronic infection. As with HBV, transmission of HCV is by infected blood, so the main routes are sexual contact, both heterosexual and homosexual; use of infected needles; and perinatal infection. Also as with HBV infection, health care workers are considered to be at higher risk than the general population. Unlike for HBV, however, no vaccine has yet been developed for HCV. Hepatitis C is responsible for 8,000-10,000 deaths from chronic liver disease annually in the United States (i.e., more than from HBV infection), and without effective intervention that number is expected to grow over the next 10-20 years.

The barrier precautions (gloves, masks, and eyewear) and sterilization procedures for preventing HCV transmission are the same as those for preventing HBV transmission. However, unlike with AIDS, there has been an effective vaccine against HBV since 1982.[119] Since that time, both the CDC and the ADA have strongly recommended immunization against HBV for all dental office staff who contact patients, and as described earlier, OSHA regulations now require that dentists provide HBV vaccination for their office staff. Immunity status is readily tested. For most, immunization through a series of three injections over 6 months will be required. Vaccination is specific to HBV and does not protect against HCV or other non-A, non-B forms of hepatitis.[79]

Dentists have responded well to the need to ensure their immune status to HBV. Among dentist participants in the ADA's health screening at the annual meeting, those reporting vaccination increased from 22% in 1983 to 84% in 1992, and the number whose blood tests showed current infection (i.e., presence of the HBV surface antigen) dropped from 14% to 9% over the same period. Chronic carrier status (i.e., positive result for both the HBV surface antigen and core antigen) dropped among dentists from 0.95% in 1983 to 0.25% in 1992.[30] Even higher rates of immunization were reported by a national survey of dental personnel in Britain.[90] Vaccination is more common among younger than among older dentists, so in time virtually all dental personnel should be immune to HBV.

PUBLIC AND PROFESSIONAL PERCEPTIONS OF INFECTIOUS DISEASES

As the public has come to accept the existence of an HIV epidemic, attitudes of dentists toward treating infected people have also matured. Not surprisingly, dentists in a number of countries demonstrated ambivalent attitudes toward treating infected patients, especially in the early days of the epidemic.[44,83,87,101] Treating infected patients was seen as a professional responsibility fulfilled reluctantly, and many clearly would have preferred not to treat infected patients.[20,57,84] With the adoption of standard precautions and the realization that adherence to them greatly reduces the risk of transmission of HIV, HBV, and HCV, rational fears on the part of dentists seem to be allayed. However, there are still a lot of dark, irrational fears and anxieties,[20,68,86] especially of HIV infection, that do not abate with continuing education and evidence of extremely low risk of transmission. A general willingness to treat HIV-positive patients was expressed by two-thirds of dentists in a New York City study in the early 1990s, but this proportion dropped when the patients concerned were not patients of record in the practice.[85] HIV-infected patients, who used to be referred to clinics dedicated to treating them, are increasingly feeling comfortable in general dentists' offices.[19] As noted earlier in this chapter, dentists do not have the legal right to turn away prospective patients who are, or may be, HIV or HBV infected. By the same token, with standard precautions there is no need for anxiety when treating such patients.

Surveys in the mid-1980s found variable adherence to infection-control procedures in the dental office[44]; some dentists were apparently slow to accept that they were at risk without them. Dental professionals who accepted that some of their patients were probably infected were more likely to adhere to the recommendations,[46] and educational programs for dental personnel were effective in improving adherence to these procedures.[39,45] Attitudes and infection-control practices appeared to move forward considerably in the late 1980s, however, because a national survey of general dentists in 1990 found virtually universal acceptance of the need for infection-control procedures in the dental office.[84] These advances in attitudes and practice continued for dentists through the 1990s,[31,47] although it has been pointed out that, while use of standard precautions has become common, the poor communication between dentists and HIV-infected patients has changed little.[51] A study of hygienists in Mississippi also disclosed that their attitudes and beliefs had not kept pace with modern knowledge, so there is still apparently a need for continuing education on infection control.[37]

HIV ISSUES IN DENTAL PRACTICE AND DENTAL EDUCATION

The legal implications of cross-infection continue to evolve, and all dental practitioners need to be constantly aware of them. HIV-infected dentists are in a particularly difficult position. A number of states have responded to public clamor with laws restricting the rights of infected dentists to practice. Many interpret these laws as overreaction, although in states without them the dentist's legal obligation to tell patients and staff that he or she or a staff member is HIV- or HBV-infected is not clear. If the dentist does so, then the ensuing hysteria would probably force the practice to close; if the dentist does not, he or she is probably liable should a patient become infected.[61]

On the other hand, dentists have a clear legal obligation, under the Americans with Disabilities Act of 1990, not to deny treatment to a patient solely on the grounds of the patient's infection. This became clear in a 1997 U.S. District Court judgment against a dentist who, it was alleged, denied treatment to a patient solely on the grounds of the patient's HIV status.[36] The dentist appealed, but the U.S. Court of Appeals reaffirmed the District Court's decision. The ruling was based on the evidence that standard precautions reduce the risk of transmission to extremely low levels.

Willingness to treat HIV-infected patients is an issue that organized dentistry, and the dental schools in their curricula, should deal with vigorously. The ADA has included in its code of ethics (see Chapter 3) the statement that refusal to treat an HIV-infected patient, solely on those grounds, is unethical. As just discussed, it is also illegal. It is a position that also makes little sense because (1) the risk of transmission of HIV from patient to dentist, as already discussed, is extremely low when the dentist is using standard precautions, and (2) many dentists already have treated HIV-infected persons without knowing it.

The fact remains that a level of anxiety persists about treating infected patients, especially HIV-infected patients. Some dentists are adamant that they do not have an ethical responsibility to treat HIV-positive patients.[86] These dentists cite a lack of confidence in standard precautions and concerns about what will happen to their practices if it becomes known that HIV-positive patients are treated there. The majority of dentists accept their ethical responsibility to treat infected patients, though most would rather not do so if they had the choice.[20] In a 1991 national survey of senior dental students, 76% agreed that an ethical responsibility existed to treat infected patients, although 54% admitted to having some fear about treating infected patients and 53% would prefer not to do so if given the choice.[96] AIDS clinics appeared in a number of major cities, manned by dental practitioners whose commitment to equality of care for all represented the highest degree of professionalism. However, by the end of the twentieth century the trend was toward "mainstreaming" (i.e., treatment in private dental offices rather than in segregated facilities).

The issues raised in dental education by the AIDS epidemic are many and will take years to become resolved. Two questions that readily arise are the following:

1. Should an HIV-positive student applicant be admitted to dental school?
2. What is the dental school's obligation if a student becomes HIV positive in the course of clinical duties?

Some experience in these matters has accumulated. There are several documented cases of students who were identified as HIV positive during their studies and after they had begun treating patients,[35,52,100] and at least one documented case of a faculty member who died of AIDS.[23] In each instance the experience was disruptive for all concerned. In the cases of the students, what followed was similar in each school. The student was immediately removed from patient contact, patients treated by the student were offered free testing and counseling, and confidentiality of the student's identity was maintained in the face of intense media pressure. Reviews were made of the student's compliance with infection-control procedures and of the school's procedures for sterilizing instruments. Extensive meetings of school administration with faculty and students were held to explain the actions taken and the reason for them. (None of the patients tested was seropositive.) At least one of the students concerned completed his dental degree, carrying out his remaining required clinical procedures on patients known to be HIV infected.[52]

Dental schools should have clear policies on these issues and an established plan of action to be followed when an incident arises. There are many implications to whatever policies are adopted, but experience has shown that the worst thing to do is to stick our collective heads in the sand and hope that nothing unpleasant will happen with respect to HIV in dental educational settings. Almost certainly the situations described earlier will occur at other schools, and the schools should be ready to handle the situation.

The AIDS epidemic has already had a dramatic effect on the practice of dentistry, and it will continue to affect it in complex ways for the foreseeable future. As was said the day after the first nuclear bomb was dropped on Hiroshima in 1945, nothing will ever be the same again.

DENTAL UNIT WATERLINES

There is evidence that the water used in the dental operatory for cooling, irrigation, and flushing can be infected, sometimes quite heavily infected.[38] Certain microbial species can form biofilms in the waterlines, and small bits of biofilm can break off and infect the water going into the patient's mouth. Human pathogens have been isolated from this water, including *Legionella pneumophila*, the causative organism for Legionnaires' disease. Although outbreaks of Legionnaires' disease occur periodically, none has been associated with dental procedures, and there are no specific recommendations for preventing *L. pneumophila* infection in dental practice. However, given the increasing number of immunologically compromised patients now being seen in dental practices, the possibility of infection is clear.

There is no good research base from which to provide recommendations on how to deal with the problem. The CDC's recommendations include the use of sterile water for invasive procedures and regular flushing of the waterlines.[105] The CDC also states, however, that although these procedures help to reduce the numbers of microorganisms in the water they do not reduce biofilm formation.

In 1995 the ADA set a goal of having equipment available by the year 2000 that would provide unfiltered water with no more than 200 colony-forming units/ml.[10] This is the same standard that applies to kidney dialysis machines. Although some advances have been made, progress toward this goal is slow.

An issue related to waterline infection is backflow. Cross-connection is the name given to the link by which contaminated materials may enter a public water supply when the pressure from the polluted source exceeds the pressure of the water supply. The risk of such an occurrence, already extremely low, is reduced even further when backflow prevention devices, or antiretraction valves, are used to prevent back-siphonage of contaminated fluids. Although a cross-connection is also theoretically possible through the high-speed handpiece and the air and water syringe, this risk, too, is extremely low and has not yet been documented.[10]

Much of the concern expressed about backflow relates to the chance of HIV, HBV, or HCV infection through this route, but this possibility is close enough to zero, because none of these viruses is transmitted through contaminated water. The use of self-contained water systems in the dental office—that is, water systems not connected to the public water supply—is a recommended measure to reduce any possible risk even further.

DENTAL AMALGAM: SAFETY AND ENVIRONMENTAL ISSUES

Amalgam restorations have been used in dental practice since the mid-nineteenth century, and it would be impossible to calculate how many have been placed since then. Today, millions of people around the world are carrying amalgam restorations around in their mouths without apparent ill effects. Amalgam use has lasted so long because amalgam is stable in the complicated oral environment, it is easy to handle, and it is relatively cheap. Even with new composite and bonding materials now in use, amalgam remains a basic restorative material. However, the toxic properties of mercury have been known for years, and with current environmental sensitivities some observers have charged that it is no longer conscionable to use a mercury compound in the human mouth.

Mercury vapor is released from amalgams, and average daily intake of mercury from amalgam restorations is estimated to be 1.2-1.3 mcg when tested subjects have seven or eight restorations.[66,97] This amount constitutes 6%-12% of total mercury intake from all sources.[67] Earlier estimates of up to 20 mcg/day from amalgams[112] have been criticized as being some 16 times too high because of the failure to account for the difference between the flow rate of the mercury vapor detector and that of human respiration.[67] However, opponents of amalgam use still insist that exposure to mercury from dental amalgams exceeds the sum of exposures from all other sources.[62]

The evidence against the use of amalgam restorations on health grounds is largely circumstantial. Among patients, intraoral measurements of mercury vapor show higher readings in adults with amalgam restorations than in those without, and the differential is higher after chewing.[99,112,113] Computer simulations based on these data have led to the estimate that long-term inhalation of mercury vapor from restorations results in an increasing mercury burden in the tissues.[114] In animal studies deleterious effects on brain tissue and intestinal microbial flora have been reported from amalgams.[63] In humans blood mercury levels have been correlated with the number and surface area of amalgam restorations, and have been measured as significantly lower in people without amalgam restorations.[1,59,97] However, raised levels of mercury in urine could not be demonstrated in child patients after a single session of restorative dentistry,[75] although this finding could have resulted from the relatively small amounts of amalgam used.

Dentists generally have levels of urinary mercury that are higher than those found in the general population but are still well below safety limits. Mercury levels among dentists attending the ADA annual session show wide variability but generally are higher in dentists who have greater exposure to mercury. Thus higher levels are seen in older dentists and in generalists rather than specialists and are related to the number of amalgams placed, form of amalgam preparation, and type of heating and cooling system in the office. Dentists in the New England and mid-Atlantic regions, on average, had twice the urinary mercury levels found in West Coast dentists.[71] Swedish studies have shown higher urinary mercury levels in dental personnel than in nondental controls, although all values were well below those set in occupational health standards.[73,74]

Because one of the outcomes of mercury toxicity is neurologic damage, some studies had looked specifically for neurologic syndromes related to amalgam restorations. The evidence here is weak. One researcher concluded that the prevalence of multiple sclerosis was related to the use of amalgam restorations,[54] although the evidence presented was so broad that this conclusion was hard to accept. (The evidence presented was ecologic: there are more amalgams placed in the northern United States than in the south, and there is also more multiple sclerosis in the north. The prime weakness in this argument is that the people with the disease are not necessarily the people with the restorations.) Evidence of neurologic damage has been reported in some dentists with exceptionally high mercury tissue levels,[91] and there are a few reports of mental distress in dentists and patients supposedly resulting from exposure to mercury.[93,95] Other reports have concluded that the symptoms reported by patients who believed that amalgams were making them sick were of psychosomatic origin.[60]

Widespread media publicity has been given to the results of animal studies with amalgam. Reports on studies of sheep, for example, have concluded that mercury inhaled from amalgams placed in pregnant ewes appears in the fetal circulation within 2 days.[115] Critics contend that the sheep, a ruminant, is a poor model in which to study mercury inhalation.

The validity of a number of these studies, involving both humans and animals, remains a subject of debate; firm conclusions are hard to reach from them. Critical reviews of the literature have concluded that mercury from amalgam restorations does find its way into human tissues,[27,41,58,89] although these same reviewers all consider there to be no evidence for ill effects in humans from the amounts in question. For example, no difference in lymphocyte levels could be found in comparisons between persons with amalgam restorations and those without.[67] Subsequent studies examining the potential effects of amalgam on human health have all concluded that amalgam use has no adverse consequences.[2,21,22] But in a debate that sometimes has overtones of that surrounding water fluoridation (see Chapter 25), not every single health hypothesis can be tested, and the question of whether subtle side effects exist would require a lot of additional research to be fully answered. Literature reviews have also concluded that bad health effects result from amalgams,[63,78] but others have concluded that mercury from amalgams had no effect on Alzheimer's disease.[28] The issue has even provoked a spirited response from the antiquackery watchdog group the National Council Against Health Fraud,[72] which came out firmly in favor of amalgam restorations.

By the early 1990s the issue had become an emotional debate that spilled over from scientific discussions into the public arena, with numerous lawsuits filed by antiamalgam activists. The ADA has consistently maintained its support for the use of amalgams on the grounds that there are no substantiated reports of ill health to humans resulting from their use. The courts have agreed. Over 2 years beginning in June 2001, 32 very similar amalgam-related complaints were filed in different parts of the United States. All were dismissed.[24] Bills to ban amalgams have also been introduced in Congress and some state legislatures. All have alleged environmental pollution from amalgam waste and adverse health effects among people with amalgams. The ADA has vigorously and successfully campaigned against these bills.

The amalgam health issue is not new in ADA circles; a 1971 review concluded that normal handling of mercury in practice does not present a threat to patients, although it can present a threat to dental personnel if precautions are not taken.[82] This review led to formulation of the ADA's first set of 15 recommendations on mercury hygiene in 1974.[12] In its own review of the literature, the ADA concluded that there was no need to remove amalgams from patients except in the rare cases of mercury allergy.[14] A second set of recommendations on mercury hygiene was issued in 1984, rather more stringent than the first edition, which included reference to OSHA requirements for disposal of scrap amalgam.[15] Further updates of these recommendations followed in 1999[8] and 2003,[9] and the ADA will no doubt continue to give this issue close attention.

The ADA derided the claims that removal of amalgams could improve the condition of multiple sclerosis sufferers as "a cruel hoax"[17] and

made a strong statement with an advisory opinion in the code of ethics, which states the following:

The removal of amalgam restorations from the non-allergenic patient for the alleged purpose of removing toxic substances from the body, when such treatment is performed solely at the recommendation or suggestion of the dentist, is improper and unethical.[7]

It is clear that research and public inquiry on this issue should continue, though as with many environmental questions the determination of cause and effect is extraordinarily difficult. Symptoms of mercury toxicity are general in nature, similar to those of dozens of other medical conditions. Threshold limits in occupational medicine are at best broad estimates, and extrapolation from animal studies to human conditions is always difficult. Humans are also exposed to environmental mercury from other sources, such as organic mercury from seafood. As was mentioned earlier, mercury from amalgams constitutes only some 6%-12% of daily intake for adults with amalgam restorations. Improvements in alternative restorative materials are nevertheless to be encouraged, and the sealants and minimum-preparation restoration procedures that are evolving (see Chapter 27) are increasingly appropriate for restorations in children.[43] The mercury issue can be expected to diminish over time as composites and sealants replace amalgams in children and complex restorations in young people become increasingly uncommon.[40]

The U.S. Public Health Service conducted an exhaustive review of amalgam safety in 1993.[109] The review concluded that amalgam use was declining as caries experience diminished and other materials were used more often. However, there was an appropriate note of caution. The committee (which could hardly be accused of bias because it did not contain a dentist) concluded that, although there was no clear evidence that amalgam caused harm in humans apart from rare allergic reactions, the very paucity of reliable studies required that further investigation of the issue should continue. As with all issues in infection control and environmental safety, however, the dental profession cannot determine policy by itself. Although the dental profession should act as a leader, both these subjects are public health issues and must be handled as such.

REFERENCES

1. Abraham JE, Svare CW, Frank CW. The effect of dental amalgam restorations on blood mercury levels. J Dent Res 1984;63:71-3.
2. Ahlqwist M, Bengtsson C, Lapidus L, et al. Concentrations of blood, serum and urine components in relation to number of amalgam tooth fillings in Swedish women. Community Dent Oral Epidemiol 1995;23:217-21.
3. AIDS less prevalent than hepatitis B virus. J Am Dent Assoc 1986;112:464-5.
4. American Association of Public Health Dentistry. The control of transmissible diseases in dental practice: A position paper of the American Association of Public Health Dentistry. J Public Health Dent 1986;46:13-22.
5. American Dental Association. ADA infopaks: OSHA, website: http://www.ada.org/prof/ed/careers/infopaks/osha.asp. Accessed November 6, 2003.
6. American Dental Association. ADA positions and statements: ADA statement on backflow prevention and the dental office, website: http://www.ada.org/prof/resources/positions/statements/backflow.asp. Accessed November 14, 2003.
7. American Dental Association, Council on Ethics, Bylaws, and Judicial Affairs. ADA principles of ethics and code of professional conduct, website: http://www.ada.org/prof/prac/law/code/index.asp. Accessed September 26, 2003.
8. American Dental Association, Council on Scientific Affairs. Dental mercury hygiene recommendations. J Am Dent Assoc 1999;130:1125-6.
9. American Dental Association, Council on Scientific Affairs. Dental mercury hygiene recommendations. J Am Dent Assoc 2003;134:1498-9.
10. American Dental Association. Dental unit waterlines (biofilms), website: http://www.ada.org/public/topics/waterlines_faq.asp. Accessed November 14, 2003.
11. American Dental Association. Human immunodeficiency virus (HIV): Resource manual for support of dentists with HIV, HBV, TB and other infectious diseases, website: http://www.ada.org/prof/resources/topics/hiv/legal.asp#state. Accessed November 6, 2003.
12. American Dental Association, Council on Dental Materials and Devices. Recommendations in mercury hygiene, February 1974. J Am Dent Assoc 1974;88:391-2.
13. American Dental Association, Council on Dental Materials and Devices and Council on Dental Therapeutics. Infection control in the dental office. J Am Dent Assoc 1978;97:673-7.
14. American Dental Association, Council on Dental Materials, Instruments, and Equipment and Council on Dental Therapeutics. Safety of dental amalgam. J Am Dent Assoc 1983;106:519-20.
15. American Dental Association, Council on Dental Materials, Instruments, and Equipment. Recommendations in dental mercury hygiene, 1984. J Am Dent Assoc 1984;109:617-9.
16. American Dental Association, Council on Dental Therapeutics and Council on Prosthetic Services and Dental Laboratory Relations. Guidelines for infection control in the dental office and the commercial dental laboratory. J Am Dent Assoc 1985;110:969-72.
17. American Dental Association, Council on Ethics, Bylaws, and Judicial Affairs. American Dental Association principles of ethics and code of professional conduct. J Am Dent Assoc 1990;120:585-92.
18. American Dental Association, Council on Scientific Affairs and Council on Dental Practice. Infection control recommendations for the dental practice and the dental laboratory, website: http://www.ada.org/prof/resources/positions/statements/infectioncontrol.asp. Accessed November 1, 2004.
19. Barnes DB, Gerbert B, McMaster JR, Greenblatt RM. Self-disclosure experience of people with HIV infection in dedicated and mainstreamed dental facilities. J Public Health Dent 1996;56:223-5.
20. Bennett EM, Weyant RJ, Wallisch JM, Green G. A national survey: Dentists' attitudes toward the treatment of HIV-positive patients. J Am Dent Assoc 1995;126:509-14.
21. Bergdahl BJ, Anneroth G, Anneroth I. Clinical study of patients with burning mouth. Scand J Dent Res 1994;102:299-305.
22. Berglund A, Molin M. Mercury vapor release from dental amalgam in patients with symptoms allegedly caused by amalgam fillings. Eur J Oral Sci 1996;104:56-63.
23. Butters JM, Hutchinson RA, Koebl JJ, Williams JN. A dental school's experience with the death of an HIV-positive faculty member. J Dent Educ 1994;58:19-25.
24. Case dismissals nationwide. ADA News, 2003 Aug 18.
25. Castro KG, Ward JW, Slutsker L, et al. 1993 Revised classification system for HIV infection and expanded surveillance case definition for AIDS among adolescents and adults. MMWR Recomm Rep 1992;41(RR-17);1-19.
26. Ciesielski C, Marianos D, Ou CY, et al. Transmission of human immunodeficiency virus in a dental practice. Ann Intern Med 1992;116:798-805.
27. Clarkson TH, Hursh JB, Sager PR, Syversen TLM. Mercury. In: Clarkson TH, Friberg L, Nordberg GF, Sager PR, eds: Biological monitoring of toxic metals. New York: Plenum Press, 1988:199-246.
28. Clarkson TW, Magos L, Myers GJ. The toxicology of mercury—current exposures and clinical manifestations. N Engl J Med 2003;349:1731-7.
29. Cleveland JL, Barker L, Gooch BF, et al. Use of HIV postexposure prophylaxis by dental health care personnel: An overview and updated recommendations. J Am Dent Assoc 2002;133:1619-26.
30. Cleveland JL, Siew C, Lockwood SA, et al. Hepatitis B vaccination and infection among U.S. dentists, 1983-1992. J Am Dent Assoc 1996;127:1385-90.
31. Cohen AS, Jacobsen EL, BeGole EA. National survey of endodontists and selected patient samples: Infectious diseases and attitudes toward infection control. Oral Surg Oral Med Oral Pathol Oral Radiol Endod 1997;83:696-702.
32. Cost of OSHA compliance gets mixed response. ADA News, 1994 Oct 3.
33. Cottone JA. Hepatitis B virus infection in the dental profession. J Am Dent Assoc 1985;110:617-21.
34. Cottone JA, Goebel WM. Hepatitis B: The clinical detection of the chronic carrier dental patient and the effects

of immunization via vaccine. Oral Surg Oral Med Oral Pathol 1983;56:449-54.

35. Cottone JA, Kalkwarf KL, Kuebker WA. The assessment of an HIV seropositive student at the University of Texas Health Science Center at San Antonio Dental School. J Dent Educ 1992;56:536-9.

36. Court says dentist cannot deny care to HIV-positive patient. Nations Health, 1997 Apr.

37. Daniel SJ, Silberman SL, Bryant EM, Meydrech EF. Infection control knowledge, practice, and attitudes of Mississippi dental hygienists. J Dent Hyg 1996;70: 22-34.

38. DePaola LG, Mangan D, Mills SE, et al. A review of the science regarding dental unit waterlines. J Am Dent Assoc 2002;133:1199-1206.

39. DiAngelis AJ, Martens LV, Little JW, Hastreiter RJ. Infection control practices of Minnesota dentists: Changes during 1 year. J Am Dent Assoc 1989;118: 299-303.

40. Eklund SA. Changing treatment patterns. J Am Dent Assoc 1999;130:1707-12.

41. Enwonwu CO. Potential health hazard of use of mercury in dentistry: Critical review of the literature. Environ Res 1987;42:257-74.

42. Ficarra G, Berson AM, Silverman S Jr, et al. Kaposi's sarcoma of the oral cavity: A study of 134 patients with a review of the pathogenesis, epidemiology, clinical aspects, and treatment. Oral Surg Oral Med Oral Pathol 1988;66:543-50.

43. Fuks AB. The use of amalgam in pediatric dentistry. Pediatr Dent 2002;24:448-55.

44. Gerbert B. AIDS and infection control in dental practice: Dentists' attitudes, knowledge, and behavior. J Am Dent Assoc 1987;114:311-4.

45. Gerbert B, Badner V, Maguire B. AIDS and dental practice. J Public Health Dent 1988;48:68-73.

46. Gerbert B, Maguire B, Badner V, et al. Changing dentists' knowledge, attitudes, and behaviors relating to AIDS: A controlled educational intervention. J Am Dent Assoc 1988;116:851-4.

47. Gibson GB, Mathias RG, Epstein JB. Compliance to recommended infection control procedures: Changes over six years among British Columbia dentists. J Can Dent Assoc 1995;61:526-32.

48. Gonzalez E, Naleway C. Assessment of the effectiveness of glove use as a barrier technique in the dental operatory. J Am Dent Assoc 1988;117:467-9.

49. Greenspan D, Greenspan JS, Hearst NG, et al. Relation of oral hairy leukoplakia to infection with the human immunodeficiency virus and the risk of developing AIDS. J Infect Dis 1987;155:475-81.

50. Greenspan D, Greenspan JS, Schiodt M, Pindborg JJ. AIDS and the mouth. Copenhagen: Munksgaard, 1990.

51. Hazelkorn HM, Bloom BE, Jovanovic BD. Infection control in the dental office: Has anything changed? J Am Dent Assoc 1996;127:786-90.

52. Heuer MA. Recent dental school experiences concerning HIV positive students: Northwestern, 1991-92. J Dent Educ 1992;56:528-35.

53. HIV discrimination ruled; judge says Maine dentist violated disabilities law. ADA News 1996;27:1, 6, 23.

54. Ingalls TH. Epidemiology, etiology, and prevention of multiple sclerosis. Hypothesis and fact. Am J Forensic Med Pathol 1983;4:55-61.

55. Karon JM, Fleming PL, Steketee RW, De Cock KM. HIV in the United States at the turn of the century: An epidemic in transition. Am J Public Health 2001; 91:1060-8.

56. Klein RS, Phelan JA, Freeman K, et al. Low occupational risk of human immunodeficiency virus infection among dental professionals. N Engl J Med 1988; 318:86-90.

57. Kunzel C, Sadowsky D. Comparing dentists' attitudes and knowledge concerning AIDS: Differences and similarities by locale. J Am Dent Assoc 1991;122(3):55-61.

58. Langan DC, Fan PL, Hoos AA. The use of mercury in dentistry: A critical review. J Am Dent Assoc 1987; 115:867-80.

59. Langworth S, Elinder C-G, Akesson A. Mercury exposure from dental fillings. I. Mercury concentrations in blood and urine. Swed Dent J 1988;12:69-70.

60. Lindberg NE, Lindberg E, Larsson G. Psychologic factors in the etiology of amalgam illness. Acta Odont Scand 1994;52:219-28.

61. Logan MK. Legal implications of infectious disease in the dental office. J Am Dent Assoc 1987;115:850-4.

62. Lorscheider FL, Vimy MJ, Summers AO. Mercury exposure from "silver" tooth fillings: Emerging evidence questions a traditional dental paradigm. FASEB J 1995;9:504-8.

63. Lorscheider FL, Vimy MJ, Summers AO, Zweirs H. The dental amalgam mercury controversy—inorganic mercury and the CNS; genetic linkage of mercury and antibiotic resistances in intestinal bacteria. Toxicology 1995;97:19-22.

64. Lundberg JF. Legal and ethical aspects of the AIDS crisis. J Dent Educ 1989;53:515-7.

65. Lynch P, Jackson M, Cummings M, Stamm W. Rethinking the role of isolation precautions in the prevention of nosocomial infections. Ann Intern Med 1987;107:243-6.

66. Mackert JR Jr. Factors affecting estimation of dental amalgam mercury exposure from measurements of mercury vapor levels in intra-oral and expired air. J Dent Res 1987;66:1775-80.

67. Mackert JR Jr, Leffell MS, Wagner DA, Powell BJ. Lymphocyte levels in subjects with and without amalgam restorations. J Am Dent Assoc 1991;122(3):49-53.

68. Manz MC, Weyant RJ, Adelson R, et al. Impact of HIV on VA dental services: Report of a survey. J Public Health Dent 1994;54:197-204.

69. Meskin LH. A letter of importance [editorial]. J Am Dent Assoc 1991;122:8-10.

70. Molinari JA. Infection control; its evolution to the current standard precautions. J Am Dent Assoc 2003; 134:569-74.

71. Naleway C, Sakaguchi R, Mitchell E, et al. Urinary mercury levels in US dentists, 1975-1983: Review of Health Assessment Program. J Am Dent Assoc 1985;111:37-42.

72. National Council Against Health Fraud. NCAHF position paper on amalgam fillings (2002), website: http://www.ncahf.org/pp/amalgampp.html. Accessed November 14, 2003.

73. Nilsson B, Gerhardsson L, Nordberg GF. Urine mercury levels and associated symptoms in dental personnel. Sci Total Envir 1990;94:179-85.

74. Nilsson B, Nilsson B. Mercury in dental practice. II. Urinary mercury excretion in dental personnel. Swed Dent J 1986;10:221-32.

75. Olstad ML, Holland RI, Pettersen AH. Effect of placement of amalgam restorations on urinary mercury concentrations. J Dent Res 1990;69:1607-9.

76. Osborn JE. Dispelling myths about the AIDS epidemic. In: Fransen VE, ed: Proceedings of the AIDS prevention and services workshop. Princeton NJ: Robert Wood Johnson Foundation, 1990:15-21.

77. Pindborg JJ. Oral candidiasis in HIV infection. In: Robertson PB, Greenspan JS, eds: Perspectives on oral manifestations of AIDS. Littleton MA: PSG Publishing, 1988:28-37.

78. Pleva J. Dental mercury—a public health hazard. Rev Environ Health 1994;10:1-27.

79. Porter SR, Scully C. Non-A, non-B hepatitis and dentistry. Br Dent J 1990;168:257-61.

80. Reinhardt JW. Risk assessment of mercury exposure from dental amalgams. J Public Health Dent 1988;48:172-7.

81. Robertson PB, Greenspan JS, eds. Perspectives on oral manifestations of AIDS. Littleton MA: PSG Publishing, 1988.

82. Rupp NW, Paffenbarger GC. Significance to health of mercury used in dental practice: A review. J Am Dent Assoc 1971;82:1401-7.

83. Rydman RJ, Yale SH, Mullner RM, et al. Preventive control of AIDS by the dental profession: A survey of practices in a large urban area. J Public Health Dent 1990;50:7-12.

84. Sadowsky D, Kunzel C. Are you willing to treat AIDS patients? J Am Dent Assoc 1991;122(2):29-32.

85. Sadowsky D, Kunzel C. Measuring dentists' willingness to treat HIV-positive patients. J Am Dent Assoc 1994;125:705-10.

86. Sadowsky D, Kunzel C. Dentists' HIV-related ethicality: An empirical test. J Am Coll Dent 1997;64(1):27-9.

87. Scheutz F. Dental care of HIV-infected patients: Attitudes and behavior among Danish dentists. Community Dent Oral Epidemiol 1989;17:117-9.

88. Schiodt M, Greenspan D, Daniels TE, Greenspan JS. Clinical and histologic spectrum of oral hairy leukoplakia. Oral Surg Oral Med Oral Pathol 1987;64:716-20.

89. Scully C, Epstein JB, Porter S, Luker J. Recognition of oral lesions of HIV infection. 1. Candidosis. Br Dent J 1990;169:295-6.

90. Scully C, Griffiths M, Levers H, et al. The control of cross-infection in UK clinical dentistry in the 1990s: Immunisation against hepatitis B. Br Dent J 1993;174:29-31.

91. Shapiro IM, Cornblath DR, Sumner AJ, et al. Neurophysiological and neuropsychological function in mercury-exposed dentists. Lancet 1982;1:1147-50.

92. Shaw FE Jr, Barrett CL, Hamm R, et al. Lethal outbreak of hepatitis B in a dental practice. JAMA 1986;255:3260-4.

93. Siblerud RL. The relationship between mercury from dental amalgam and mental health. Am J Psychother 1989;43:575-87.

94. Silverman S Jr, Wara D. Oral manifestations of pediatric AIDS. Pediatrician 1989;16:185-7.

95. Smith DL Jr. Mental effects of mercury poisoning. South Med J 1978;71:904-5.

96. Solomon ES, Gray CF, Gerbert B. Issues in the dental care management of patients with bloodborne infectious diseases: An opinion survey of dental school seniors. J Dent Educ 1991;54:594-7.

97. Snapp KR, Boyer DB, Peterson LC, Svare CW. The contribution of dental amalgam to mercury in blood. J Dent Res 1989;68:780-5.

98. Summers CJ, Gooch BF, Marianos DW, et al. Practical infection control in oral health surveys and screenings. J Am Dent Assoc 1994;125:1213-7.

99. Svare CW, Peterson LC, Reinhardt JW, et al. The effect of dental amalgams on mercury levels in expired air. J Dent Res 1981;60:1668-71.

100. Taylor M. Recent dental school experiences concerning HIV-positive students: Creighton University. J Dent Educ 1992;56:540-7.

101. ter Horst G, Hammann-Konings GM, van Hegten MJ, et al. AIDS and infection control: Amsterdam dentists surveyed. J Public Health Dent 1989;49:201-5.

102. US Department of Labor, Occupational Safety and Health Administration. Bloodborne pathogens—1910.1030, website: http://www.osha-slc.gov/pls/oshaweb/owadisp.show_document?p_table=STANDARDS&p_id=10051. Accessed November 6, 2003.

103. US Public Health Service, Centers for Disease Control and Prevention. Recommended infection-control practices for dentistry. MMWR Recomm Rep 1993;42(RR-8):1-12.

104. US Public Health Service, Centers for Disease Control and Prevention. Guidelines for infection control in dental health-care settings. MMWR Recomm Rep 2003;52(RR-17):1-66.

105. US Public Health Service, Centers for Disease Control and Prevention. Statement from CDC regarding biofilm and dental unit water quality, website: http://www.cdc.gov/oralhealth/infectioncontrol/fact_sheet/biofilm.htm. Accessed November 14, 2003.

106. US Public Health Service, Centers for Disease Control and Prevention, Divisions of HIV/AIDS Prevention. Basic statistics, website: http://www.cdc.gov/hiv/stats.htm#cumaids. Accessed November 6, 2003.

107. From U.S. Public Health Service, Centers for Disease Control, National Center for Infectious Diseases. Hepatitis Surveillance Report no. 59. website: http:/www.cdc.gov/neidod/diseases/hepatitis/resource/PDFs/hep_surveillance_59.pdf. Accessed November 1, 2004.

108. U.S. Public Health Service, Centers for Disease Control and Prevention. Division of Tuberculosis Elimination; Surveilance Reports, website: http://www.cdc.gov/nihstp/tb/surv/surv.htm. Accessed November 1, 2004.

109. US Public Health Service, Committee to Coordinate Environmental Health and Related Programs. Dental amalgam: A scientific review and recommended

Public Health Service strategy for research, education, and regulation. Washington DC: Government Printing Office, 1993.

110. US Public Health Service, National Institutes of Health. Management of hepatitis C. NIH Consens Statement Online 1997 Mar 24-26;15(3):1-41.

111. Verrusio AC. Risk of transmission of the human immunodeficiency virus to health care workers exposed to HIV-infected patients: A review. J Am Dent Assoc 1989;118:339-42.

112. Vimy MJ, Lorscheider FL. Intra-oral air mercury released from dental amalgam. J Dent Res 1985;64: 1069-71.

113. Vimy MJ, Lorscheider FL. Serial measurements of intra-oral air mercury: Estimation of daily dose from dental amalgam. J Dent Res 1985;64:1072-5.

114. Vimy MJ, Luft AJ, Lorscheider FL. Estimation of mercury body burden from dental amalgam: Computer stimulation of a metabolic compartmental model. J Dent Res 1986;65:1415-9.

115. Vimy MJ, Takahashi Y, Lorscheider FL. Maternal-fetal distribution of mercury (^{203}Hg) released from dental amalgam fillings. Am J Physiol 1990;258:R939-45.

116. West DJ. The risk of hepatitis B infection among health professionals in the United States: A review. Am J Med Sci 1984;287:26-33.

117. Winkler JR, Robertson PB. Periodontal disease associated with HIV infection. Oral Surg Oral Med Oral Pathol 1992;73:145-50.

118. World Health Organization. AIDS epidemic update: December 2002, website: http://www.who.int/hiv/pub/epidemiology/epi2002/en/. Accessed November 6, 2003.

119. World Health Organization. Hepatitis B, website: http://www.who.int/mediacentre/factsheets/fs204/en. Accessed November 1, 2004.

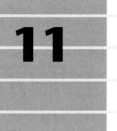

11 Reading the Dental Literature

The literature is the generic name given to the body of writing in books, journals, reports, and other sources that makes up the sum of knowledge in a branch of science. In the case of dentistry we refer to the *dental literature*. However, the literature is more than just our compendium of knowledge and our scientific base; it is our very identity. It defines who we are and what we do; it charts the progress of dentistry to its present status and provides guidelines for future directions.

Technologic and social developments, in dentistry as elsewhere, are proceeding at a speed that can be both bewildering and overwhelming. Although dental and dental hygiene graduates learn enough in professional school to begin practice, "keeping up" is absolutely essential for professional growth. Attendance at continuing education courses is one way to do so (such attendance is required in most states), but the literature is the primary source of new knowledge. Therefore it follows that dentists and hygienists must keep familiar with those sections of the literature that most concern them if they are to function properly. To do this, they need to be able to locate the literature they need and read it critically; they need to distinguish front-line from mediocre journals and be aware of how to distinguish good from poor research. Acquiring these skills requires some time and practice, but confidence with them will pay off in helping practitioners use their time efficiently while they grow professionally. Professional training, unfortunately, does not usually include critical reading. The usual progression begins with accepting the veracity of reports unquestioningly and without conscious thought, because "if it weren't true, it wouldn't be printed." After being misled a few times, readers can become increasingly skeptical. In the extreme, they can move full circle from believing everything they read to believing nothing. The ideal course is between the two extremes, somewhere between blind acceptance and blanket mistrust.

This is the first of two chapters on how to efficiently locate and interpret information that is needed for effective clinical practice. This chapter deals with assessing the quality of an individual report in the literature, whereas Chapter 12 is devoted to evidence-based dentistry and assessment of a body of literature to determine best clinical practices.

TEXTBOOKS AND PEER-REVIEWED JOURNALS

Textbooks are the most familiar source of information for students. Although good books may be the first source to be consulted on a subject, books can soon become dated. The copy a student buys from the bookshop may be new, but if it was published 10 years ago then at least parts of it risk being obsolete. That proviso accepted, the best textbooks present the state of the science, at least at the date of publication, as well as a sound foundation on which to build further information.

Journals are the basic source of current information in any science-based field, dentistry included. The number of journals in dentistry, as in most other disciplines, has proliferated in recent years. It is virtually impossible for anyone to keep up with all journals, so selectivity is needed. There are good journals and not-so-good ones, and there are some clues to picking which is which. The most basic is that good journals are all peer reviewed.

Peer Review

Peer review means that manuscripts, when first received by the journal editor, are sent out to be reviewed by several experts in the subject area of the manuscript. Usually two reviewers are selected, sometimes more, and the identity of the reviewers is concealed from the authors to promote candid reviews. Some journals, though not all, also mask the identity of the authors from the reviewers in an effort to remove any bias from the reviewers' judgment. The reviewers' task is to assess the manuscript critically for the quality of its science, its logic, its manner of presentation, and any other feature that might reflect on its value in the literature. Poor-quality manuscripts can be rejected outright at this stage or returned to the authors for revision if the papers are basically sound but have room for improvement. Most articles published in journals have been returned to the authors for revisions at least once prior to acceptance. Many prestigious journals, such as the *New England Journal of Medicine*, reject far more manuscripts than they publish; their reviewing standards are extremely rigorous. The top dental journals publish well under half of the manuscripts they receive.

Peer review is a system that has evolved through the years, and there is no question that it has served to greatly elevate the standards of published material. However, it does have some limitations. For example, the process can suffer when the reviewers chosen are inappropriate, either because they are not sufficiently expert in the field of study or because their own prejudices get in the way of an objective review. More common are reviewers who simply do not give a manuscript the attention it deserves. An inherent problem is the tendency of the peer-review process to inhibit original research or creativity and to push imaginative thoughts into a safe middle ground. On balance, however, peer review has served to greatly elevate the quality of the literature.

Judging the Quality of a Journal

The first step in judging a journal's quality is to find out whether it is peer reviewed or not. Some provide this information in their instructions to contributors, which journals publish regularly and which can usually be found on the journal's website. The second thing to find out is the journal's sponsorship: who puts it out? Here are four broad categories of sponsorship:

A Learned Society Learned societies frequently present the best and most important research papers—their reason for existing, after all, is to promote and disseminate research findings. Some, like the International Association for Dental Research, which publishes the *Journal of Dental Research, Critical Reviews in Oral Biology and Medicine,* and *Advances in Dental Research,* promote dental research in all fields; others advance research in specialized or semispecialized areas. Journals published by learned societies are invariably peer reviewed and have a strong emphasis on scientific rigor. These journals are characterized by a straightforward format with a relative absence of advertising, a strong editorial board, and explicit instructions to contributors. On the down side, a relatively small circulation to a specialized group often makes them expensive.

A Professional Organization A professional organization is a dental or dental hygiene association, a specialty society, or any other professional group. The best journals in this category, such as the *New England Journal of Medicine, British Medical Journal,* and *Journal of the American Medical Association,* rank among the most prestigious in biomedicine. The majority of journals in this group are peer reviewed. In contrast to the journals published by learned societies, these can show some bias in choice of material: there can be a tendency to publish papers favorable to the organization's views and not to publish papers with contrary views, regardless of their quality. These journals can carry a fair amount of advertising, which together with wide distribution to the association's membership keeps the price moderate. In the better journals, advertising material must pass editorial scrutiny for factual content and taste.

A Reputable Scientific Publisher Some journals are produced by publishers of medical and dental texts to fill a need: *Community Dentistry and Oral Epidemiology* and *Journal of Periodontal Research*, published by Blackwell Scietific Publishers, are examples. The best journals in this group are rigorously peer reviewed and generally are the equal of those issued by learned societies in terms of quality.

A Commercial Publisher Journals issued by commercial publishers comprise a category often referred to as "throwaways," and some can be more accurately described as magazines rather than journals. They carry a lot of advertising, which often permits them to be distributed free of charge, and their articles are often written by professional in-house staff. Some do accept contributed papers, but peer review is unusual. The scientific quality of these journals is usually not high, for that is not their function. These journals fill a niche, as long as readers recognize them for what they are.

The third step in quality determination is to look for a listing of an editorial board, advisory board, or consultants. These terms can be used loosely and interchangeably, and the functions of these groups can vary widely, from taking an active role in journal policies to being little more than window dressing. The presence of such a list, however, suggests that the journal is at least trying to keep up standards.

As the fourth step, a reader should be able to judge the nature of the papers from a quick perusal: research reports, case reports, opinion pieces, reviews, political commentary. First and most important, the reader should be able to tell which is which. Looking over the editorials, in those journals that carry them, can give a feeling for any particular political stance the journal may take.

The fifth step can be to scan the advertising for the products and services presented, and the advertising style. Better-quality journals either have no advertising or a reasonably restrained advertising style. Look for some statement of advertising policy, such as is found in the advertising index of each issue of the *Journal of the American Dental Association*.

Finally, the production standards should be checked. Typographical errors, lack of consistency, and inadequate citations in references can make a reader wonder what else is wrong that is less readily apparent.

A professional's ability to understand scientific reports in the literature demands some grasp of research design. Although the principles of research apply to all kinds of scientific inquiry, the details described in the following paragraphs relate specifically to epidemiologic studies and to clinical trials.

CRITICAL READING—EVALUATING THE QUALITY OF A PUBLISHED PAPER

Hierarchy of the Quality of Information

As far as possible, knowledge upon which treatment procedures and other actions are based should come from the results of carefully structured research designs, free of bias, minimizing random error, and carried out with human subjects. This is inherently impossible in some instances and simply lacking in others, so a reader needs to judge the source of information carefully when assessing the state of knowledge on any subject. It was this need, often frustratingly unresolved, that spawned the move toward evidence-based medicine (see Chapter 12).

The best-developed measuring scales for assessing the quality of information in a published report are for studies of therapeutic and preventive products and interventions. A number of such scales have been suggested. The first of these was developed by a Canadian panel that had the task of appraising the value of the routine physical examination in preventing morbidity.[2] The scale the panel constructed was used, more or less unchanged, by the U.S. Preventive Services Task Force a few years later and with some modification is still being used by that group.[3] These pioneering scales can be seen in retrospect as early steps in the growth of evidence-based medicine. The scale in Box 11-1 gives a hierarchy for judging the quality of an individual study that tests the value of a therapeutic or preventive product or intervention. This is a broad guide, with many overlaps, but provides a framework for judging the *internal validity* of a paper, that is, the extent to which its conclusions are supported by its methods and results. (Note that this scale is not applicable to judging papers on diagnosis, prognosis, appropriateness of policy, or economic analysis.)

Many questions regarding treatment or prevention in dentistry are simply not amenable to testing in randomized trials, either for ethical reasons (Are amalgams harmful to human health?) or because of inherent difficulties (Is group practice more efficient than solo practice?). In such instances, evidence from less rigorous study designs must do. Case studies can be helpful in guiding appropriate treatment, but individual patients may be atypical, and the treatment outcome therefore not generalizable; that is, case studies lack *external validity*—they cannot be generalized to the base population. The opinion of an acknowledged expert is always worth listening to, but experts are human too and subject to bias.

In many areas of basic science, animal studies and other laboratory experiments are a major source of information that can be applied to humans. The fundamentals of trials involving rats, hamsters, guinea pigs, dogs, monkeys, and other animals used in studies are the same as those for trials with humans. The reader should look for the special complications of animal studies: Was the strain of rat used susceptible to the disease? Were the results potentially biased by an undue number of deaths in one group? An ever-present difficulty with animal studies is the extent to which results should be applied to humans. The same concern applies to all laboratory procedures: Does the dental enamel in the test tube react the same way as it does in the mouth? Are the bacteria produced from pure culture the same as those found in the oral environment? The ideal occurrence for reaching conclusions is when the results of laboratory studies are confirmed in humans, but again this happy circumstance often is not possible.

Criteria for Judging the Quality of an Individual Paper

There are essentially four kinds of papers published in journals. These can be categorized as follows:

Research Reports, which describe original clinical, basic, or epidemiologic research. A question is identified, a study is designed to test the question, the results are discussed, and some conclusions are reached.

Case Reports, which are accounts by clinicians of unusual manifestations of disease conditions, treatment outcomes, or disease progression. In many areas of surgery, randomized trials will never be carried out because of the inherent difficulties, so case reports form the body of literature on many surgical procedures.

Reviews of the literature, which summarize knowledge in a particular area (the narrative review is referred to here; systematic reviews are discussed in Chapter 12). A *narrative review* is a

---

BOX 11-1 Scale for Judging the Quality of Information in Reports on Therapeutic and Preventive Interventions in Human Studies, Ordered From Best Quality (1) to Weakest (8)[2,5]

1. Randomized clinical trials in humans, in which all criteria described in Experimental Study Designs in Chapter 13 are met.
2. Clinical trials in humans that employ concurrent randomized controls but in which one or more elements described in Experimental Study Designs in Chapter 13 are missing. The more that these elements are missing or the criteria inadequately satisfied, the greater the threat to internal validity.
3. Well-controlled cohort and case-control studies, or clinical trials without random allocation, or field trials (in which the community, rather than the individual, is the unit of study).
4. Clinical trials without concurrent control groups, such as those using historical controls, and retrospective cohort studies. The better examples here can be considered equal to those in item 3.
5. Cross-sectional studies without controls, in which a group's oral health status is matched against some past exposure to suspected disease-causing or disease-preventing agents.
6. Descriptive surveys, in which present oral health is surveyed and there is informed speculation as to the influences that led to the observed status.
7. Case reports.
8. Personal opinion, subjective impressions, and anecdotal accounts.

traditional approach in which a knowledgeable person or persons collects the published information on a subject and reaches conclusions on what the literature collectively says about the issue in question. The best narrative reviews are superb additions to the literature; the poorest ones, narrow and biased. This type of review is frequently presented at a conference or symposium, and when such reviews are done well they can be among the most influential and valuable works in the literature.

Commentaries, in which some documented facts are used as a basis for urging program development, health policy, or some other kind of action. Commentaries can vary greatly in quality, ranging from beautiful insights to hopelessly biased diatribes.

The essential features to look for when reading a paper in the literature can be presented in semichecklist form, and this is done for three types of reports in Boxes 11-2 to 11-4 (case reports do not fit this model). The list may seem rather long at first, but with practice readers will soon be able to apply these criteria quickly and in due course almost unconsciously. The goal, in fact, is that their application become an automatic feature of reading reports in journals.

As evidence-based medicine developed, it quickly became apparent that a major stumbling block to synthesizing clinical trial reports from the literature was their lack of homogeneity. Vital information (e.g., method of subject allocation, control of exposure, data reliability) was often presented in vague terms or, worse, not mentioned at all. The response to this problem was the development of a protocol known as the CONSORT Statement (CONSORT is an acronym for Consolidated Standards of Reporting Trials), which journals are urged to adopt as a means of ensuring that all published clinical trials contain adequate detail on the methods used. The goal is to achieve homogeneity in reporting, which in turn permits meta-analysis (see Chapter 12) and improves the quality of systematic reviews.[4] When authors adhere to CONSORT standards their papers are easier to read, and it is also easier for readers to judge the quality of the papers. Protocols for reporting other kinds of scientific study have been developed in the wake of CONSORT; these are discussed in Chapter 12.

There are a few other aspects common to all reports in the literature. Reports should have a concise yet informative title that allows the reader to recognize the content and assists in electronic retrieval. A good abstract permits readers to identify quickly the basic contents of the paper. An abstract for a research paper should (1) state the objectives and scope of the investigation, (2) describe briefly the methods used, (3) summarize the findings, and (4) state the main conclusions. Some journals require that an abstract be written strictly to that format. The wise author chooses words for the abstract that are similar to the MeSH (Medical Subject Headings) terms under which the paper will be indexed. Headings specific to dentistry are especially helpful because these are underrepresented in MEDLINE (Medical Literature, Analysis, and Retrieval System Online, described in the next section). Abstracts should never contain information or conclusions not stated in the body of the report. Brevity (no more than 250 words helps electronic storage and retrieval) requires that abstracts be objective, straightforward, and free of opinion or speculation.

FINDING THE REPORTS YOU NEED IN THE LITERATURE

Practitioners often need to find information about a given subject: What is this material that a supply house salesman is pushing? Do sealants work on primary teeth? Has this new cavity liner been adequately tested? The list is endless. Dental professionals need to know how to search the vast literature efficiently to find the information they need to reach a conclusion. Fortunately, the rapidly developing electronic methods for searching the literature make this task much less arduous than it once was.

A useful start is the reference lists at the ends of textbook chapters, although the earlier caveats on obsolete material in textbooks pertains to the references too. Not only do they risk being dated, but such reference lists often are not complete, or they can reflect an author's bias or incomplete grasp of a subject. These reference lists can be a good starting place, although usually more is needed. Good reviews of the literature on a related topic can be useful. Although the conclusions of the review may be

---

BOX 11-2 Quality Issues in Judging Research Reports

General Issues
- Nature of the journal in which the report appeared (see discussion on journals in the text).
- Qualifications of the authors. Is at least one a well-known researcher? Is there evidence of research training among the authors? Are they affiliated with a reputable institution?
- Research funding. If the work was commercially funded, is there any reason to believe that the sponsors might have influenced the results?
- Date of publication. Knowledge is moving rapidly in some fields, less so in others. Is the report likely to have been superseded by more recent work?

Research Specifics
- Is the research question, purpose of the paper, and a hypothesis clear and succinctly stated? If not, is a hypothesis at least implied?
- Although the review of current knowledge must often be brief in a research report, is it a balanced summary of previous work? (The "selective" review to support a particular point of view is unfortunately not unknown.)
- Are the measurement variables and other terms specifically defined? If standard terms and measures are being used, are references given for their definition? If new measures are being introduced, are they clearly defined and is it made clear why existing ones cannot be used? (These questions are all aimed at checking internal validity.)
- If the study involves humans, is the population studied appropriate in view of the stated purposes? Does the report give details on participants in the study: the numbers of people approached, those who agreed to begin the study, and those who remained at the end?

- Is the research design appropriate to test the hypothesis and thus answer the underlying question?
- Are the materials and methods clearly detailed? Are measurements applied as described? Have the researchers taken steps to ensure that the measures are being recorded as reliably as possible? With regard to this latter point, if there are several examiners in an epidemiologic study, are they experienced in such research or have they been trained and their evaluations calibrated for this project? Are any checks made to ensure examiner reliability?
- Is the statistical analysis appropriate for the types of data collected? Have the authors presented sufficient data in the way of tables or graphics to permit the reader to check this question? Are the statistical tests used appropriate for testing the stated hypothesis?
- Does the discussion look critically at any limitations of the methods used? Are appropriate comparisons made with previous work and reasons discerned for similarities or differences? Is a fair assessment of the relevance of the work made, with some specifics given for the next steps?
- Are the conclusions clear and warranted by the results of the research? Have the authors made suitable distinction between statistical significance and clinical importance?
- Is the paper clearly and concisely written? Does the abstract give a clear profile of the study?
- Have the issues of informed consent and ethical research been dealt with adequately and clearly stated?
- If the report is a clinical trial, have the reporting requirements listed in the CONSORT (Consolidated Standards of Reporting Trials) Statement been met?

---

enough for some purposes, the reader will often want to follow up on some of the papers cited in the review.

The main repository of bibliographic information on the biomedical literature is the *Index Medicus*, a vast compendium managed by the National Library of Medicine (NLM), located on the campus of the National Institutes of Health in Bethesda, Maryland. A bibliographic guide to the dental literature for years was to be found in the bound copies of the *Index to Dental Literature*, although NLM stopped production of

the printed Index in the late 1990s. Searching the biomedical literature today is a computerized operation, involving a search of electronic databases and the World Wide Web. All biomedical literature since 1966 indexed by the NLM is now searchable on-line through MEDLINE, biomedicine's primary database, though by no means the only one in which dental practitioners will be interested. MEDLINE indexes most, but not all, of the world's biomedical research literature, although EMBASE, another biomedical database, is stronger in non-English

---

BOX 11-3 Quality Issues in Judging Narrative Reviews of the Literature

- Is the subject of the review clearly stated and are its boundaries delineated?
- As far as you can determine, is all appropriate work included in the review?
- Is there a fair but critical analysis of the reports reviewed, or does the author(s) seem to be emphasizing only one side of an issue?

- Does the review critically assess the value of different research reports, or are they all taken at face value and given equal merit? Lack of critical assessment weakens a review.

BOX 11-4 Quality Issues in Judging Commentaries

- Has the author used whatever factual basis is available to develop the case? (Hard data should always be used as much as possible, even though some conclusions must be reached with less information than is desirable.)

- Is there respect for various points of view?
- Are conclusions warranted by the argument made, or is there a sense of preconceived conclusions?

---

publications and the drug literature. The most popular version of MEDLINE is PubMed, designed for quick and easy use by the busy practitioner. The Clinical Queries option in PubMed allows the clinician to quickly focus a large search on the question of interest. Practitioners anywhere in the world need only a personal computer, appropriate web browser software, and a connection (preferably high-speed) to the World Wide Web (of course, this service also needs to be paid for). A number of commercial services carry MEDLINE and related databases, and the search process is becoming more and more user friendly.

When one first begins to use MEDLINE, the effect can be overwhelming: a tidal wave of information gushes over the user, often far more than can be readily digested. Sometimes this reflects reality; there is just so much more published on an issue than the user may have imagined. At other times it means that the search is too broad and that a lot of inappropriate material is included. Practice in the use of keywords and increasing familiarity with the MeSH terminology make searching much more efficient. It does not take long for even a technophobe to conduct an efficient search. A dental practitioner with a computer in the back room of the practice can easily search an issue over a lunchtime sandwich and refine the search to a usable number of relevant references. Abstracts now accompany the reference citation for most journals, which makes the search even more efficient, and full-text paging is becoming more common. This means that the full article is available from the web for an increasing number of biomedical journals. On-line subscriptions can be purchased in the same way as are regular subscriptions; indeed, many see on-line subscriptions as the future of the scientific literature.

The result of a search is a stream of references, most with abstracts, that flow across the screen; unless they are captured and stored, the search is a transitory thing. Therefore, to go along with the electronic searching procedures, bibliographic database software permits downloading of the search results into the storage database. The search is performed, the desired references are selected from among those perused, and these are downloaded into the database; then they are on hand permanently. Once we get accustomed to this way of searching the literature, it is difficult to know how we ever got along without it.

The amount of useful information on the World Wide Web is growing at a staggering rate. It is assumed that readers are familiar with the web to some extent. For those who are not, the World Wide Web is a means of storing text, graphics, and audio material in a computer server in such a way that anyone in the world with web-browsing software can retrieve it. Although the web generally remains a delightfully anarchic affair, a lot of useful information can be found there. An example was given in Chapter 3, which noted that the ADA's Principles of Ethics are now accessed through the ADA home page on the web rather than published in print. A vast amount of health-related information can be found on the websites for the ADA, National Institutes of Health, Centers for Disease Control and Prevention, and World Health Organization. Also available now is an encyclopedic guide to searching and finding information on the web, available both as a traditional book (three volumes) and on CD-ROM.[1]

The only snag in these developments is that information located in the search still has to be read! Photocopying is getting easier and cheaper, and dental school librarians will obtain a needed journal from interlibrary loan if necessary. Whether or not they have access to a dental school library, health practitioners can submit on-line requests for interlibrary loans from anywhere in the country using PubMed's *Loansome Doc* system. Even photocopying from a journal may become largely obsolete as full-text electronic storage grows. When full-text storage develops completely, practitioners in the most remote geographic locations will need only a computer and an Internet connection to have the entire dental literature at their fingertips, literally! The technology for all this is in existence now, and future developments will depend on sorting out the legal and economic ramifications. We can be virtually certain that progress in the area of keeping up with the literature will continue to be rapid and that scientific knowledge will continue to become more readily available all the time.

REFERENCES

1. Anderson PL, Allee NJ. Medical Library Association encyclopedic guide to searching and finding health information on the web. New York: Medical Library Association and Neal-Schuman Publishers, 2004, website: http://www-personal.umich.edu/~pfa/mlaguide/indextest.html. Accessed April 3, 2004.
2. Canadian Task Force on the Periodic Health Examination. The periodic health examination. J Can Med Assoc 1979;121:1193–1254.
3. Harris RP, Helfand M, Woolf SH, et al. Current methods of the US Preventive Services Task Force; a review of the process. Am J Prev Med 2002;20(3 Suppl):21–35.
4. Moher D, Schultz KF, Altman DG, for the CONSORT group. Revised recommendations for improving the quality of reports of parallel group randomized trials 2001, website: http://www.consort-statement.org/revisedstatement.htm#app. Accessed November 28, 2003.
5. US Preventive Services Task Force. Guide to clinical preventive services. 2nd ed. Washington DC: US Department of Health and Human Services, 1996.

12 Evidence-Based Dentistry

What do you do when a periodontal patient says, "I read in a magazine that gum disease can cause a heart attack but that there is a drug available to prevent this. Should I be taking this drug?" Chances are that you don't know how to respond. You may have studied the relationship between periodontitis and cardiovascular disease (see Chapters 21 and 29), but you have never heard of the drug the patient describes. Your first instinct is probably to dismiss the whole thing, but you have a nagging feeling that perhaps there is something in it. So what do you do? That is the theme of this chapter: to look at the emerging field of evidence-based dentistry (EBD) and to see how you can use it in practice. This chapter describes what EBD is, why increased attention is being given to EBD, how this emphasis will affect oral health professionals in the future, and what responsibilities come with adherence to evidence-based practice.

WHAT IS EVIDENCE-BASED DENTISTRY?

EBD is sometimes described as doing the right thing, for the right patient, at the right time. This definition is succinct and hard to dispute, but it still leaves the practitioner with little concrete direction in the day-to-day, patient-by-patient decisions that must be made in practice. What, in fact, is the right thing to do in each sit-

uation that presents itself, who is the right patient to treat with which procedure, and when is the time right? These are complex questions and usually do not have clear-cut answers.

A more detailed definition of evidence-based medicine (EBM), from which EBD is derived, is the following:

The conscientious, explicit and judicious use of current best evidence in making decisions about the care of individual patients. The practice of evidence-based medicine means integrating individual clinical expertise with the best available external clinical evidence from systematic research.[21]

There are three essential components of EBM: the scientific base for any treatment decision a practitioner makes, the clinical expertise of the practitioner, and the patient's values. Dentistry has come to this field later than medicine and has for the most part adopted the same language and conventions. So the definition just given for EBM is applied to EBD, as are the three components, although this more detailed definition also requires interpretation before the clinician can be confident about how it applies in the day-to-day clinical practice of dentistry. Both EBM and EBD relate to patient care (rather than research or administration) and are invoked when the practitioner is seeking to make the best treatment decision for a particular patient.

But hasn't dentistry always based treatment decisions on scientific evidence? Well, yes and no, as we'll discuss further. The landmark Gies report of 1926 noted "the growth of quackery" during the nineteenth century,[9] and even the 1995 Institute of Medicine report on the future of dental education recommended greater development of the scientific base in dental practice.[11] The modern evidence-based approach in medicine, which got underway during the 1970s, is now well established, one could almost say institutionalized. The years between the 1970s and the present day saw an evolution of the methods for the systematic collection of information in EBM and its application to clinical practice, so that today, as we develop EBD, we can benefit from the experience of our medical colleagues. What is now emerging in dentistry is the formal recognition that clinical decision making requires the application of the rigorous rules of evidence. One sign of this increased attention is the establishment of two journals on the topic: *Evidence-Based Dentistry* first appeared as a supplement to the *British Dental Journal* in 1998 and became a stand-alone journal in 2000. The *Journal of Evidence-Based Dental Practice* began publication in the United States in 2001.

THE ART AND SCIENCE OF DENTISTRY

The phrase *the art and science of dentistry* means that when we care for our patients we combine our clinical acumen, experience, and human sensitivity with procedures that are based on the most up-to-date science. Essentially, the "art" of dentistry is the acceptance of the individuality of each patient. We recognize that a treatment we think appropriate for one person will not necessarily be appropriate for another with the same condition. We use the art side of our practice to assess the patient's interest in his or her oral health when formulating a treatment plan. We also factor into the treatment plan the patient's age, existing state of oral and general health, and ability and willingness to pay for treatment. The art of dentistry also includes the clinician's individual ability in using certain materials or techniques. Sometimes a clinician will have a special knack for working with a material or procedure and so can make a given

treatment perform better than the average clinician would.

This art aspect of clinical dentistry should remain. It is only out of place when the opinions, beliefs, and attitudes of the dentist, no matter how well intentioned, are allowed to override facts that are clearly demonstrated through science. There should be a mix of art and science in each treatment plan, but the procedures that we consider as treatment options should, as far as possible, be justified by science. There will be occasions in which a scientific base for a treatment option is nonexistent, and in these cases the practitioner has to determine what the best practices are. In such cases it is up to the dental research community to see that resources are directed into these areas to ensure that the necessary scientific base is developed.

It is useful to distinguish between the principles of EBD and the methods that have been proposed for implementing it. Regarding the principles there is little dispute, for no one can argue against using evidence as the basis for care. This philosophical stance, however, is immediately followed by the practical issues of (1) what qualifies as evidence, and (2) how we evaluate that evidence. With EBD, the traditional ad hoc and subjective approach to these issues is replaced by explicit and objective methods to evaluate the available evidence. We recognize that today it is more difficult than ever for clinicians to assess all of the rapidly expanding treatment options before deciding on their value to their patients. Although the methods of EBD are not a panacea for the challenge of increased options, they do provide a framework for a systematic and unbiased approach to evaluating those options. Rather than requiring an ad hoc assessment by each individual clinician to determine the strength of the scientific evidence on each aspect of dental care, EBD uses a systematic process to assemble, evaluate, and summarize the evidence on particular treatment questions.

RATING THE QUALITY OF THE LITERATURE

If the quality of the scientific evidence is to form an important part of our clinical decision making, then how do we judge the quality of that evidence? In Chapter 11, we looked at how to

Table 12-1 Scale for categorizing the strength of evidence for a program or procedure[4]

Code	Criteria
I	Evidence obtained from one or more properly conducted randomized clinical trials (i.e., one using concurrent controls, double-blind design, placebo, valid and reliable measurements, and well-controlled study protocols).
II-1	Evidence obtained from one or more controlled clinical trials without randomization (i.e., one using systematic subject selection, some type of concurrent controls, valid and reliable measurements, and well-controlled study protocols).
II-2	Evidence obtained from one or more well-designed cohort or case-control analytic studies, preferably from more than one center or research group.
II-3	Evidence obtained from cross-sectional comparisons involving subjects at different times and places, or studies with historical controls. Dramatic results in uncontrolled experiments (such as the results of the introduction of penicillin treatment in the 1940s) could also be regarded as this type of evidence.
III	Opinions of respected authorities, based on clinical experience; descriptive studies or case reports; or reports of expert committees.

evaluate the quality of an individual paper. In terms of assembling components of the scientific base to support a treatment procedure, EBM and EBD extend that analysis by objectively measuring the quantity and quality of the *body of evidence* on a subject. The traditional process is by means of the *narrative review* (see Chapter 11) in which an expert, or experts, assesses the literature on the subject and then reaches conclusions. Again as noted in Chapter 11, the quality of such reviews varies from brilliant to mediocre or even misleading. This range results from differences in the research attention the subject has received, the thoroughness of the literature search, and the ability and objectivity of the reviewer.

An inherent problem in any literature review is the variation in quality of research reports on the subject. As stated in Chapter 11, to be of value any review must be a critical review; that is, the variation in quality of the various research reports must be explicitly recognized. Recognition is a good first step, but the reviewer still has to deal with the issue. This variation in the quality of the literature was a problem facing a Canadian expert panel in the 1970s whose task was to assess the value of the annual physical examination in preventing mortality and morbidity.[4] To deal with the range in quality of the papers on the subject, the Canadian group developed a hierarchical scale to give a quality score to each paper the members were reading. This scale is shown in Table 12-1. These quality scores were the basis for the recommendations issued on the use or rejection of the procedure

(Table 12-2). This methodologic approach had sufficient appeal to be adopted a few years later by the U.S. Preventive Services Task Force[25] and, in slightly modified form, by the Centers for Disease Control and Prevention for a major report on fluoride (see Chapter 26) a few years later.[26] This approach does require some summary judgments by the review panel when the research reports on testing of a procedure are of mixed quality. Scaling the quality of a whole body of evidence as a unit still has some application, although the principal method now used for assessing the quality of a body of evidence is the *systematic review*, which is based on grading each of the individual reports selected and then reaching an overall conclusion.

THE SYSTEMATIC REVIEW

For most of us, the most convenient way to catch up on a subject is to read reviews of the literature. The traditional format is the narrative review, which often takes the form of a paper given at a conference or symposium, in which the authors assess the information from published reports on a topic and then reach a conclusion based on the weight of evidence. Narrative reviews have been around for ages and generally have served a valuable purpose, but they can have limitations because of their subjective nature.[18] The first problem with any type of review is that not all research gets published. A significant number of clinical trials, in particular, do not find their way into our journals.[5] Corporate sponsors are generally reluctant to

Table 12-2   Scale for strength of recommendation on the use or rejection of a procedure.[4]

Grade	Criterion
A	There is good evidence to support the use of the procedure.
B	There is fair evidence to support the use of the procedure.
C	There is a lack of evidence to enable a specific recommendation to be made; i.e., the subject has not been adequately tested. This grade will also apply to mixed evidence; i.e., some studies support the use of the procedure and some oppose it.
D	There is fair evidence to reject the use of the procedure.
E	There is good evidence to reject the use of the procedure.

publish clinical trials with so-called negative results,[6] meaning that a benefit from the tested product or procedure could not be demonstrated, and accordingly researchers tend not to submit reports with negative results.[19] This particular problem is called *publication bias*. Another aspect of publication bias is the fact that only two thirds of published abstracts, which cannot provide methodologic detail, get into print as full publications within a 2-year period.[22]

So, what can be done about this? The response to these problems of bias and incomplete information in narrative reviews is the *systematic review*, which reduces the potential for bias at all levels. A systematic review is defined as one in which there is a comprehensive search for all relevant studies on a specific topic and those identified are then appraised and synthesized according to predetermined and explicit criteria.[13]

There is a philosophical link between a systematic review and a scientific study. Just as a good report of an experiment carried out in the laboratory gives sufficient methodologic detail to let the reader know just how the results were achieved, the existence of written protocols in a systematic review lets the reader know just how the authors came to the conclusions they did. The word is *transparency*. Systematic reviews are transparent in that the reader is given all the details of the search strategy, inclusion and exclusion criteria, quality ratings, and the way final conclusions were reached. This is rarely the case with a narrative review, for which the reader usually must just trust the authors. In a systematic review, the reader knows exactly how the authors arrived at their conclusions.

The systematic review was developed for judging the efficacy of preventive or therapeutic procedures and hence is best geared to assess the quality of randomized clinical trials (RCTs). It

quickly became evident that judging the quality of an RCT could be frustrated when the original report was deficient in some essential details (e.g., group allocation procedures, control of the procedure, statistical methods). This issue is separate from the quality of the study itself—the study may or may not be of top quality, but the report is deficient. This problem led a group of concerned researchers and editors to develop criteria for what should be included in the report of an RCT so that the quality of the study could be determined. The result was a checklist known as the CONSORT Statement.[15] CONSORT is an acronym for Consolidated Standards of Reporting Trials. The more journals that subscribe to CONSORT principles, the more readily comparable RCT reports will become, and the more precise systematic reviews will become.

The idea of standards to promote more uniform reporting has now spread to encompass other types of research manuscripts. For meta-analyses, in which a number of RCTs are combined to increase statistical power, there is QUORUM (Quality of Reporting Meta-Analyses)[15] and for papers studying diagnostic accuracy there is STARD (Standards for Reporting of Diagnostic Accuracy).[3] The other member of this menagerie is MOOSE (Meta-Analyses of Observational Studies in Epidemiology), which specifies reporting standards for observational studies, the designs of which cover a broader spectrum than do those of RCTs.[23]

Conducting A Systematic Review

Because the systematic review is the cornerstone of EBD, some detail are given on how a systematic review is put together. Just as with a research proposal, all the protocols are written down before the search begins: making up the rules or acting on whims as one goes along is not allowed.

Question to Be Examined

The purpose of a narrative review is usually rather general, for example, to assess the effect of oral hygiene on the prevention of gingivitis. In a systematic review, the question is sharpened, just as in a research proposal a broad research question is honed into a hypothesis that can be tested experimentally. The oral hygiene and gingivitis question for systematic review would then become, for example, "Does toothbrushing once every 48 hours prevent gingivitis?" Or the time interval selected might be 24 hours, which could result in the inclusion of some different studies in the review and might lead to a different conclusion. Or the question could substitute dental flossing for toothbrushing, which again would change the direction of the search. The question to be examined in a systematic review *must* be stated precisely and explicitly.

Inclusion and Exclusion Criteria

The inclusion and exclusion criteria follow from the question, and the criteria must be stated so the reader can be satisfied that there is little chance of inclusion bias, that is, that not all publications were considered or that inappropriate ones were included. To illustrate, one such criterion is language of publication. Americans tend to read only the English-language literature, but in some fields this can be a clear source of inclusion bias.[16] Another criterion is the range of the outcome. If the subject is the effect of fluoride varnish in preventing caries, for example, the reviewers must specify whether they intend to include root caries as well as coronal caries, caries in the primary as well as the permanent dentition, noncavitated lesions as well as cavities, secondary caries, and so on. Age of people studied must also be considered.

Search Strategy

Electronic searching is the logical starting point, and the reader needs to know which databases were searched. MEDLINE (Medical Literature, Analysis, and Retrieval System Online) is the principal database for reports in dentistry, but only about half the papers on most topics can be found readily in MEDLINE, mainly because of inappropriate indexing.[7] It may also take up to a year for recent papers to be indexed in MEDLINE. This is not a criticism of MEDLINE, for relevant reports are usually in the MEDLINE database somewhere, but if they are inappropriately indexed they will not be found with the usual keywords. Other databases can profitably be added to the search for many fields of study. The reviewers also must state the keywords used in the search,[12] again to make the search method as transparent as possible.

Electronic searching usually needs to be augmented by hand searching, largely because of the chances of missing improperly indexed reports in MEDLINE and other databases, as mentioned earlier. Hand searching is what we used to do all the time before there were electronic databases. It consists of going through the references listed at the ends of some publications and going through back copies of specific journals in which publications on the topic are most likely to have appeared. Hand searching is tedious and time consuming, but it is absolutely necessary if inclusion bias is to be avoided.

Criteria for Study Quality

The step of developing criteria for study quality sets the attributes that a report must possess to be included in the final analysis. For example, with RCTs the reviewer wants a description of how subjects were allocated to groups. If the use of random allocation as an inclusion criterion results in the discarding of virtually all the studies because no trials used random allocation, then a less rigorous criterion would probably have to be written. Because one of the results of systematic reviews is identification of further research needs, in this instance a recommendation for true RCTs might be a logical conclusion.

Development of Conclusions

Assessment of the final group of reports can be qualitative or quantitative. *Qualitative* means that no further statistical analysis is done by the reviewer; instead, the studies are grouped as being on one side of the question or another, and a final conclusion is then reached, based on where most results lie. Further *quantitative* analysis can in some circumstances be carried out by combining the data from a number of studies to produce a single estimate of effect, a process called *meta-analysis*.[13] The rationale for meta-analysis is that the statistical power of the estimate can be increased by enlarging the sample size. The limitation to this procedure is that there must be design homogeneity among the studies to be combined; otherwise, the exercise loses validity.

EXAMPLES OF EVIDENCE-BASED DENTISTRY

Now that formal EBD approaches to evaluating the research literature have been developed, there is a rapidly growing body of such reviews. Many can be found in the Cochrane Library (http://www.update-software.com/cochrane/abstract.htm), an on-line catalog of systematic reviews to augment the published journals (Box 12-1). Two such reviews are outlined here as examples of how these reviews can help the clinician provide authoritative scientifically based information and treatment choices to patients.

EBD Example: Are Powered Toothbrushes Superior to Manual Cleaning for Oral Health?

With the proliferation of powered toothbrushes that are marketed directly to the consumer, dentists are asked about them by patients. The analysis[27] of a Cochrane review[10] compares plaque removal and gingivitis in people using manual toothbrushes and in those using one of six different types of powered toothbrushes. An early problem was that most of the studies in the literature were excluded from the review because of various shortcomings in their design, execution, or reporting. This immediately points up to the reader the importance of not being unduly influenced by individual literature reports that do not meet contemporary standards for quality research and reporting.

BOX 12-1   The Cochrane Collaboration

The Cochrane Collaboration, launched in 1993 and named after the late British epidemiologist Archie Cochrane, is an international nonprofit organization whose mission is to make up-to-date information about the effects of health care readily available to clinicians. It was born from Cochrane's frequent observations that, although many clinical trials had been carried out in medicine, there was no systematic collection of these trials that a busy practitioner could consult. The main product of the Cochrane Collaboration is the Cochrane Database of Systematic Reviews, which forms part of the Cochrane Library.[24] The Cochrane Library is an electronic resource that by 2004 contained some 2000 regularly updated systematic reviews and other sources of information. There are 51 Cochrane review groups around the world, each focusing on a specific disease or group of problems, including an oral health group (http://www.cochrane-oral.man.ac.uk/) through which a number of systematic reviews have already been archived. There are a number of funding sources for the Cochrane Collaboration, but its acceptance around the world in such a short time is largely due to volunteer effort.

Much of this success is a result of the rigorous standards that the Collaboration maintains at all levels (http://www.cochrane.dk/cochrane/handbook/hbook. htm). Anyone wishing to carry out a systematic review for the Cochrane Library must first register a title with a Cochrane review group, have the title accepted, and then submit a protocol for the systematic review. The

protocol is then sent out for internal and external peer review. Protocols, like papers submitted to a journal, can at this stage be accepted, rejected, or revised. Protocols for which the final review has not been completed are listed, so readers can see what reviews are coming up. The same rigorous refereeing process is carried out when the systematic review is completed. A particular feature of the Cochrane system is that reviews are not intended to be carved in stone and left there. Quite the opposite in fact, for it is intended that reviews be updated periodically as new information comes out. Because the protocols and procedural methods are published as an integral part of the review, updating can be carried out by the original author(s) or by someone else. Readers can then be assured that what they read in a Cochrane review represents the most up-to-date summation there is.

There is already an impressive list of completed Cochrane reviews. Although access to the full reviews in the Cochrane Library usually requires a subscription, detailed abstracts of the Cochrane reviews are available on-line without charge (http://www.cochrane.org/cochrane/revabstr/ORALAbstractIndex.htm) and are beginning to appear in other publications.

Access to the Cochrane Library is free of charge in many countries. Further details can be found at http://www.update-software.com/cochrane/provisions.htm.

After carefully proceeding through the statement of the question, inclusion and exclusion criteria, the search strategy, and the criteria for judging quality, this systematic review reported the following primary findings:

- For powered toothbrushes with oscillation-rotation action, plaque and gingivitis scores were 7%-17% lower than for manual toothbrushes.
- The studies were of insufficient duration to determine whether these reductions are relevant to the development of destructive periodontal disease.
- An insufficient number of high-quality studies were available to judge whether other types of powered toothbrushes were superior to manual toothbrushes.
- There was no evidence that powered toothbrushes were more likely to cause injury than manual toothbrushes.
- No information on durability, reliability, and cost of powered toothbrushes was provided by the available studies.

With this kind of information, the clinician is able to provide authoritative information to patients and can be confident that the information provided is realistic and does not promise more than can be supported by the best-quality research available.

EBD Example: What Are the Success Rates of Different Implant Systems?

Estimates were that in the year 2000 there were nearly 1300 different implant configurations available, and manufacturers are rapidly placing new systems on the market while just as rapidly removing older ones.[2] The clinician is thus swamped with a bewildering array of choices when trying to make the best selection to recommend to a patient. The systematic review on implant success rates provides the clinician with some assurance in selecting from this otherwise very confusing morass.[8,28] Within the limitations imposed by the rapid turnover of available implant types and by the fact that only five high-quality RCTs were identified, the primary conclusions reached by the reviewers were the following:

- There was no difference in apparent success, up to 3 years after placement, among the implant systems of the six manufacturers whose systems were studied.

- During the follow-up periods of 1-3 years, only 25 of 957 implants were judged to have failed. This indicates a high success rate, at least in the short term.

The reviewers noted that, in the case of implants, the results of RCTs may provide only part of the story about the level of success that a clinician might expect. The level of care given to patient selection in an RCT, and the level of experience of the clinicians involved, may differ from that in the average clinical practice, and these factors probably contributed to the likelihood of success.

RESPONSIBILITIES OF PRACTITIONERS

Individual dental practitioners are not expected to conduct systematic reviews on their own for each clinical question that they encounter. Conducting systematic reviews efficiently and effectively requires extensive training and practice, well beyond what can be reasonably expected from all clinicians. The responsibility for most clinicians is thus to be aware of, and to use wherever applicable, the findings from systemic reviews carried out by others. If the process were to stop when a review was completed, and the review were simply to gather dust on the library shelf, it would provide little benefit in improving oral health care. What obviously must follow the systematic review is a process to put the results into practice. Indeed, EBD explicitly incorporates both a research component (along with the systematic review) and the translation of that research into practice.[1]

Dental and dental hygiene education has at least two primary tasks. The first is to teach students what are the best available procedures and how to perform them competently, a process demanding an emphasis on manual skills. The second is to instill in students the recognition, indeed the certainty, that much of what they are learning will become obsolete during their lives in practice. The challenge for the busy clinician is to recognize when this has occurred, yet neither to replace the outmoded treatment with the latest inadequately tested fad nor to wait too long so that patients are receiving outdated care.

At the very least, the concept of EBD should make it routine for the clinician to consider all options when treating each patient, rather than relying on comfortable habits and familiar procedures. The clinician must routinely ask, "Could I have misdiagnosed this condition?" and "What are the possible alternative diagnoses?" When preventive and restorative choices are made, the clinician must ask, "What is the state of knowledge concerning this procedure or material?" and "What is the likelihood that this patient will benefit from this procedure?" Also, "What are the possible risks associated with this procedure and is the probability of success sufficient to tolerate those risks?" Furthermore, "How does the balance among these considerations fit with the preferences of the patient and the costs involved?" Although the process may at first seem cumbersome and involved, with routine use it will become second nature. Moreover, it is part of the fundamental responsibility of a health care professional to assure that the best possible care is being provided to each patient. At the very least, EBD has made us aware of the continuing responsibility of every practitioner to be as up to date as possible in knowledge of the scientific literature. It further has shown us that simply providing the same service or set of services to virtually every patient is unlikely to be consistent with providing the best possible care.

The concepts of EBD also make it clear that the challenge for the clinician is never ending. The right thing, the right patient, and the right time will constantly evolve as change inexorably takes place in disease patterns, our understanding of oral diseases and conditions, the available therapies and materials, and patient preferences.

CURRENT STATE OF THE SCIENCE

It will be a long and slow process to conduct the necessary RCTs and then to mount the systematic reviews to cover even a small proportion of all of the necessary details of modern dental practice. Even in some of the most widely researched areas, the available systematic reviews do not always provide clear direction for the clinician in choosing which patients to treat in which way. An example is found in a systematic review of professionally applied fluorides in which virtually all of the vehicles tested were shown to be effective, but the clinician was still left with no clear direction as to which patients should receive fluorides, what fluoride product to use, and how long they need to be provided to each patient.[14] The clinician must still rely on professional judgment in areas such as the trade-off between the cost of treatment, on the one hand, and the likelihood that the patient will develop caries in its absence. It is also possible that the experimental subjects in the studies on which the systematic reviews are based are fundamentally different from the patients in a particular dentist's practice. Some patients may be at very low risk for certain conditions, so the appropriateness of using some preventive methods on a frequent basis may be questionable. Other patients may be at higher than average risk and may need more aggressive treatment. Evaluation of these types of subtle distinctions is not common in the current scientific literature, and thus recommendations by systematic reviews on these dimensions are rarely available. Nevertheless, the shortcomings of the literature that are identified in scientific reviews can help to define the future research agenda and to address the current gaps in knowledge, so that the level of specificity possible in future systematic reviews will make them even more valuable to clinicians in the future.

LIMITATIONS OF EVIDENCE-BASED DENTISTRY

EBD is an important evolution in the continuing drive to provide the right care, to the right patient, at the right time. It is not an infallible prescription for what to do in all clinical situations, and in many areas the underlying clinical research has simply not been done. Nevertheless, the research base will continue to develop, and the approach provides a workable method to give the busy clinician a rigorous review and balanced summary of the evidence available up to the present, in a form that is readily accessible and digestible. This body of underlying evidence and systematic summaries will grow rapidly and should be an ever-increasing part of both clinical teaching and everyday clinical practice.

Systematic reviews are not always unambiguous, and they are always open to reinterpretation and revision.[20] As with all of science, new evidence or reinterpretation of current evidence may in the future change the conclusions of a review. It must further be remembered that there is not a single truth that, once discovered, will remain so forever. By its very nature, science is always open to revision and reevaluation. Therefore, EBD, based as it is firmly on science, is always open to revision. These facts place significant demands on the clinician. On the one hand, it is imperative that the current best practices, as supported by rigorous science and systematic reviews when available, be carefully considered when making treatment decisions. On the other hand, such practices emphatically must not be taken as immutable fact and used without further thought throughout a career. The competent clinician must constantly look for systematic reviews to find new evidence as it becomes available and watch for signs of changes in what had previously been considered the best evidence.

REFERENCES

1. Bader J, Ismail A, Clarkson J. Evidence-based dentistry and the dental research community. J Dent Res 1999;78:1480-3.
2. Binon PP. Implants and components: Entering the new millennium. Int J Oral Maxillofac Surg 2000;232-6.
3. Bossuyt PM, Reitsma JB, Bruns DE, et al. Towards complete and accurate reporting of studies of diagnostic accuracy: The STARD initiative. Clin Radiol 2003; 58:575-80.
4. Canadian Task Force on the Periodic Health Examination. The periodic health examination. Can Med Assoc J 1979;121:1193-1254.
5. Dickersin K. How important is publication bias? A synthesis of available data. AIDS Educ Prev 1997;9(1 Suppl):15-21.
6. Dickersin K, Min YI. Publication bias: The problem that won't go away. Ann N Y Acad Sci 1993;703:135-46.
7. Dickersin K, Scherer R, Lefebvre C. Identifying relevant studies for systematic reviews. Br Med J 1994;309 (6964):1286-91.
8. Esposito M, Coulthard P, Worthington HV, et al. Interventions for replacing missing teeth: Different types of dental implants (Cochrane Review). In: *The Cochrane Library*, Issue I, 2003. Chichester, UK: John Wiley and Sons.
9. Gies WJ. Dental education in the United States and Canada. New York: Carnegie Foundation, 1926.
10. Heanue M, Deacon SA, Deery C, et al. Manual versus powered toothbrushing for oral health (Cochrane Review). In: *The Cochrane Library*, Issue I, 2003. Chichester, UK: John Wiley and Sons.
11. Institute of Medicine, Committee on the Future of Dental Education. Dental education at the crossroads: Challenges and change. Washington DC: National Academy Press, 1995.
12. Jadad AR, Rennie D. The randomized controlled trial gets a middle-aged checkup [editorial]. JAMA 1998; 279:319-20.
13. Klassen TP, Jadad AR, Moher D. Guides for reading and interpreting systematic reviews: I. Getting started. Arch Pediatr Adolesc Med 1998;152:700-4.
14. Marinho VCC, Higgins JPT, Sheiham A, Logan S. Combinations of topical fluoride (toothpastes, mouthrinses, gels, varnishes) versus single topical fluoride for preventing dental caries in children and adolescents (Cochrane Review). In: *The Cochrane Library*, Issue 3, 2004. Chichester, UK: John Wiley and Sons, website: http://www.cochrane.org/cochrane/revabstr/ORALAbstractIndex.htm. Accessed March 15, 2004.
15. Moher D, Cook DJ, Eastwood S, et al. Improving the quality of reports of meta-analyses of randomised controlled trials: The QUOROM statement. Lancet 1999;354:1896-1900.
16. Moher D, Fortin P, Jadad AR, et al. Completeness of reporting of trials published in languages other than English: Implications for conduct and reporting of systematic reviews. Lancet 1996;347(8998):363-6.
17. Moher D, Schultz KF, Altman DG, for the CONSORT group. Revised recommendations for improving the quality of reports of parallel group randomized trials 2001, website: http://www.consort-statement.org/revisedstatement.htm#a. Accessed November 20, 2003.
18. Mulrow CD. The medical review article: State of the science. Ann Intern Med 1987;106:485-8.
19. Olson CM, Rennie D, Cook D, et al. Publication bias in editorial decision making. JAMA 2002;287:2825-8.
20. Sackett DL, Rosenberg WM, Gray JA, et al. Evidence-based medicine; what it is and what it isn't [editorial]. Br Med J 1996;312:71-2.
21. Sackett DL, Straus SE, Richardson WS, et al. Evidence-based medicine: How to practice and teach EBM. 2nd ed. New York: Churchill Livingstone, 2000.
22. Scherer RW, Dickersin K, Langenberg P. Full publication of results initially presented in abstracts. A meta-analysis. JAMA 1994;272:158-62.
23. Stroup DF, Berlin JA, Morton SC, et al. Meta-analysis of observational studies in epidemiology: A proposal for reporting. Meta-analysis of Observational Studies in Epidemiology (MOOSE) group. JAMA 2000;283: 2008-12.
24. The Cochrane Collaboration: A brief introduction, website: http://www.cochrane.org/resources/leaflet.pdf. Accessed March 15, 2004.
25. US Preventive Services Task Force. Guide to clinical preventive services. 2nd ed. Washington DC: Department of Health and Human Services, 1996.
26. US Public Health Service, Centers for Disease Control and Prevention. Recommendations for using fluoride to prevent and control dental caries in the United States. MMWR Recomm Rep 2001;50(RR-14):1-42.
27. Weyant RJ. Powered toothbrushes with a rotation action remove plaque and reduce gingivitis more effectively than manual toothbrushes. J Evid Based Dent Pract 2003;3:72-6.
28. Weyant RJ. Short-term clinical success of root-form titanium implant systems. J Evid Based Dent Pract 2003; 3:127-30.

part **III**

The Methods of Oral Epidemiology

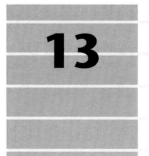

13

Research Designs in Oral Epidemiology

Numerous books have been written about research design and the characteristics of good research. This is not one of them, but we do set out in this chapter to give a bare-bones presentation of the essentials of valid research reports. This coverage is intended to permit the reader to make good sense of epidemiologic studies, especially clinical trials, and of other studies involving human beings.

Epidemiology is the study of health and disease in populations, and of how these states are influenced by heredity, biology, physical environment, social environment, and ways of living. Some definitions extend the meaning to include the application of this study to control health problems.[14] Epidemiologic studies can first be classified either as *descriptive*, meaning that the data only describe the distribution of a condition in a population and no specific hypothesis is tested, or as *analytic*, meaning that the data collection and analysis are designed to answer a particular question. Descriptive and most analytic studies are *observational*; that is, they observe outcomes without intervening to affect them. Analytic studies in epidemiology look at people with and without the disease in question (the *effect* or *outcome*) and with and without exposure to the putative influences that may increase the risk of disease (the *exposure*).

The clinical trial, an experimental design to test the efficacy of a preventive-control agent or treatment procedure in humans, is an aspect of analytic epidemiology sometimes classified separately as *experimental* epidemiology. The clinical trial is also an *interventional* design; that is, something is intervening in the natural history of a condition in an effort to give a beneficial outcome.

Good research demands careful, sometimes exhaustive planning. Every study, no matter how modest, needs a protocol, which is a written plan encompassing the purpose and the detailed operation of the study. The essential elements of a protocol are listed in Box 13-1. A protocol demands careful thinking through of a project, a process that aids its design and also helps the researchers to anticipate potential problems. It also simplifies the writing of a final report, because the protocol forms the basis of the report.

CAUSALITY AND RISK

Causality, meaning that a certain exposure results in a particular outcome, can only be demonstrated unequivocally within the experimental study design of a clinical trial (discussed in a later section). Because clinical trials cannot be conducted on many topics for both practical and ethical reasons, causality in the study of disease usually must be imputed from studies with nonexperimental designs. Criteria by which a conclusion of causality can be reached from nonexperimental epidemiologic analyses,

173

BOX 13-1   Essential Features of a Protocol for Research With Humans

- A precise definition of the research problem, the reasons for undertaking the research, and a review of pertinent literature.
- Objectives of the study or hypotheses to be tested. A hypothesis is a conjecture cast in a form (the null hypothesis) that will allow it to be tested and refuted if it is false.
- Population to be studied, including its selection, source, size, method of sampling, and method of allocation to groups (if a clinical trial).
- Data to be collected, including a description of each item needed to accomplish the objectives or to test the hypotheses.
- Procedures to be carried out, with details of exactly how the needed data will be obtained from the participants in the study and by whom.

- Data collection methods, with examples of all data collection forms or computer methods of data collection and a list of all necessary supplies, equipment, and instruments.
- Plans for data processing and analysis, including how the data get from field collection to computer, computer file organization, and statistical distributions to be examined.
- Time schedule for planning, procurement of informed consent from study subjects, data collection and analysis, and report writing.
- An assessment of any ethical issues involved in the study and certification that the necessary institutional human subjects clearance has been obtained.

BOX 13-2   Criteria for Inferring Causality From Observational Studies (the Bradford Hill Criteria)[3]

The following conditions must he satisfied before a particular exposure can be accepted as the cause of a disease:

- **Time sequence of events:** To be causal, an exposure must precede the occurrence of the disease. Demonstration of this temporal sequence requires longitudinal study. This is the only condition in this list that is absolute, a *sine qua non*.
- **Consistency of association:** If there are a good number of studies on whether a particular exposure is a cause of a disease, and if all of them produce fairly similar positive results, it is more likely that the factor is causal.
- **Strength of association:** In valid studies, the stronger the association between exposure and outcome, the more likely it is that the association is causal.

- **Specificity of association:** If a given exposure is related to other diseases as well as the disease in question, it is less likely to be seen as causal. However, lack of specificity by itself does not justify rejecting causality (e.g., tobacco is nonspecific in its effects but is clearly a causal factor in many of them).
- **Degree of exposure (dose response):** If an exposure is causal, then the risk of disease should be related to the degree of exposure. An exception could be exposure to a toxin with a threshold effect.
- **Biologic plausibility:** The association must make biologic sense from our knowledge of the disease. It follows that the better understood a disease is, the more stringent this criterion can become.

---

known as the Bradford Hill Criteria after the British statistician who developed them, were suggested in 1965[3] and have become well accepted over the years. The original Bradford Hill criteria have evolved over the years and are summarized in Box 13-2 as they are usually understood today.

Analytic studies, in contrast to descriptive studies, have the general aim of seeking out cause-and-effect associations. Because analytic observational studies cannot directly address cause and effect, however, they seek to quantify the degree of disease risk in specified circumstances. *Risk* is the probability that a specified event will occur, for example, that an individual will exhibit a disease or die within a stated period of time or by a particular age.[14]

The criteria listed in Box 13-2 are not all imperative; in fact the only absolute among them is the time sequence—exposure must precede outcome. In many exposure-outcome relationships there are factors that both researchers and clinicians think play a role in causing a disease but which do not satisfy all these criteria. If researchers had to proceed with just the dichotomous judgment of whether a factor is or is not involved in causing a disease, our knowledge of disease causation and development would be seriously hindered. The concept of a risk factor permits quantification of the degree of importance of a particular factor in the development of a disease; some causal factors are more important than others.

A *risk factor* is broadly defined as an attribute or exposure that is known, from epidemiologic evidence, to be associated with a health condition considered important to prevent.[14] Although the term *risk factor* is applied loosely in the literature, modern usage ascribes a strong causal role to a risk factor: it is either part of the causal chain or is something that brings a person into contact with the causal chain. (An example of the latter situation is an occupation that requires handling toxic materials. The occupation itself is not a risk factor for toxicity, but because it brings a person into contact with toxic materials, which are the risk factors, it does increase the chance of disease.) We prefer the following more complete definition of risk factor:

An environmental, behavioral, or biologic factor confirmed by temporal sequence, usually in longitudinal studies, which if present directly increases the probability of a disease occurring, and if absent or removed reduces the probability. Risk factors are part of the causal chain, or expose the host to the causal chain. Once disease occurs, removal of the risk factor may not result in a cure.[2]

Part of the concept of a risk factor is that it can be modified: people can stop smoking, lose weight, change to a healthier diet, improve their oral hygiene. The identification of risk factors for a disease then allows the potential for prevention by removing or modifying the risk factors. As examples, smoking is a risk factor for lung cancer; poor oral hygiene is a risk factor for gingivitis. In both instances, removing or modifying the risk factor reduces the risk of disease, although neither exposure is a sole cause of the disease.

As stated in this definition, a risk factor for a disease must be demonstrated as such longitudinally. This is because confirming the necessary time sequence—that is, ensuring that exposure to the risk factor occurs before the disease outcome—can nearly always be demonstrated only longitudinally. This time sequence

---

> **BOX 13-3** Criteria to be Met to Accept a Given Exposure as a Risk Factor for a Particular Disease[13]
>
> - **Time sequence:** The exposure must precede the occurrence of the disease.
> - **Statistical association:** The exposure must covary with the disease; that is, that the frequency of the disease must be observed to differ by category or value of the exposure.
> - **Absence of error:** The observed association must not be the result of error, whether that be bias, sampling error, analytic errors, or the intrusion of other extraneous factors.

---

is one of three criteria that must be met before we can suggest that a particular exposure is a risk factor for a particular disease (Box 13-3 lists the criteria for identifying a risk factor. Box 13-2 gives the criteria for imputing a cause.) The ultimate test of a risk factor is that, if exposure to it is reduced, the risk of subsequent disease diminishes. As an example, quitting smoking reduces the risk of a heart attack.

What if a suspected risk factor cannot be confirmed as such because the necessary longitudinal studies are impractical or unethical? The factor may be classed as a *risk indicator*, defined as a factor shown to be associated with a disease in cross-sectional data and assumed, on theoretical grounds, to play some causal role.[15] Research experience has shown that risk indicators which emerge from cross-sectional studies can disappear in a more rigorous longitudinal analysis, so without longitudinal assessment it cannot be known whether a risk indicator is or is not a true risk factor. As would be expected, many more risk indicators for oral diseases than true risk factors have been identified.

A *risk marker* is an attribute or exposure that is associated with the increased probability of disease although it is not considered part of the causal chain. A risk marker can also be called a *risk predictor* when included in predictive statistical models. Some immutable characteristics of a person or group—namely, age, gender, and race or ethnicity—can influence disease occurrence, progression, or outcome. These attributes do not fit the concept of a risk factor because they are not modifiable. Although they can be useful in statistical models whose purpose is to predict disease occurrence, they clearly are of no use when considering disease prevention based on control of risk factors. The literature is unfortunately muddled about what to call these attributes. We suggest the term *demographic risk factors* to refer to these immutable influences. In addition to age, gender, and race or ethnicity, socioeconomic status is usually considered a demographic risk factor. Theoretically it can be modified, but in practice this is hard to do.

NONEXPERIMENTAL STUDY DESIGNS

The collection of data to be used for descriptive purposes is commonly called a *survey* (see Chapter 4). Surveys record the *prevalence* of various conditions, meaning the number or proportion of persons in the population who exhibit a condition at any given time. (Data from national surveys in the United States are reported in Chapters 19-22.) Although surveys are important in assessing trends in health and disease, the field of oral epidemiology encompasses much more than surveys.

At the most basic level, epidemiologic study designs are *cross-sectional* or *longitudinal*. A cross-sectional study is one in which both exposure to risk factors and the health outcomes in a group of people who are, or are assumed to be, a sample of a particular population (a "cross section") are assessed at the same time. A *longitudinal* study is one in which the same group of people is studied on two or more occasions so that *incidence*, the change in a condition over time, can be assessed. A survey collects cross-sectional data. Comparison of trends by examining the results of a sequence of surveys, even if the same study protocols are used in all of them, is still a cross-sectional comparison because different people are examined in the different surveys.

Longitudinal studies require at least two series of measurements among the same people at different times to determine the progress of the condition over the specified time period. Such a study is also an *incidence* study. Sometimes an analytic study can be cross-sectional, such as when several cross-sectional studies are performed over a period of time for analytic purposes. An examination of mortality trends, for example, must be cross-sectional (obviously it cannot be the same people who

die on different occasions!). A comparison of the prevalence of dental caries in today's sixth-graders with that of sixth-graders 10 years ago must be a cross-sectional study, although it could also be an analytic one; again it is obvious that different persons are studied each time. But if all the children originally in first grade in a school system are studied periodically until they finish sixth grade some years later, the study is longitudinal because the same children are seen on several occasions.

Analytic studies are either *prospective* (looking forward) or *retrospective* (looking backward). Prospective studies collect information on an exposure of interest and compare eventual outcomes, whereas retrospective studies begin with the outcome of interest and probe back for exposure information. A *cohort* study is a prospective design: a cohort is a group of people from whom data are collected longitudinally. Members of a cohort often have some particular characteristic in common, frequently age; thus, the expression "the 1955 birth cohort" means all persons born in 1955. In cohort studies, some individuals will have the exposure of interest and some will not, and some will have the outcome of interest and some will not. This permits the computation of *relative risk*, the chance that the outcome will occur in an exposed person compared to the risk among the unexposed.[14]

Science has long viewed retrospective studies as being inherently of poorer quality than prospective studies. This view is unjustified, however, because many unusual conditions or conditions that develop over a long period of time can only be studied realistically through retrospective designs. Indeed, the noted epidemiologist Rothman considers the development of the retrospective study design to be one of the major advances in epidemiologic methods in recent years.[20] The principal retrospective design is the *case-control* study, in which people who have a given condition ("cases") are compared to, and sometimes matched with, people who do not have the condition ("controls") but who may be similar with regard to some other characteristics. The exposures of interest are then sought in the past of the participants. This design permits the derivation of an *odds ratio*, a numerical statement of probability very similar to relative risk.

Case-control studies must be planned thoughtfully, because the characteristics on which the groups are matched (e.g., ethnic group) cannot be analyzed further as possible etiologic factors. Case-control studies can demonstrate risk indicators for a disease, but the retrospective design means that risk factors cannot be identified in this way. Risk factors for a disease can be confirmed only through cohort or experimental study designs.

An *ecologic* study is an analytic study in which data for both exposures and outcomes come from the population rather than from individuals. For example, studies addressing the question of whether water fluoridation is related to hip fracture experience (i.e., suggesting that fluoridation is a risk factor for hip fracture) have used community data for both water fluoridation (the exposure) and for hip fractures (the outcome) to derive a relationship.[11,21] Such studies are relatively quick and inexpensive because they avoid sampling, interviewing, clinical examinations, or access to individual medical records. Their weakness, however, is that they cannot be certain that the people with the outcome condition (in this case, the hip fracture) are the same ones who had the exposure (drank fluoridated water). This weakness is often called the *ecologic fallacy*. Ecologic studies can be useful, though usually they are not definitive. They have a clearer role when a variable under consideration, for example, community income level, is by definition a group measure rather than an individual one.

All of these study designs are nonexperimental and noninterventional, meaning that they study conditions as they occur rather than manipulate conditions in the manner of a classical laboratory experiment. However, there are experimental designs in epidemiology that are used to test the efficacy or effectiveness of a therapeutic drug, a preventive material, or a treatment regimen.

EXPERIMENTAL STUDY DESIGNS

In medical terminology, *clinical trials* are carried out among patients, frequently hospital inpatients, and *field trials* are carried out among people in the community who may not necessarily be patients. This medical model does not transfer well to dentistry, where the definition of a patient is less clear-cut and only a small part of dental care is provided in hospitals. The term *clinical trial* tends to be loosely applied in dentistry to both types of study, so we will use it in this chapter when describing research principles common to both clinical trials and field trials. We will use the term *field trial* (sometimes called a *community trial*, or an *effectiveness study*) only when specific reference to a field trial is needed.

A clinical trial is a controlled experimental study or group comparison, based on epidemiologic principles and designed to test the hypothesis that a particular agent or procedure favorably alters the natural history of a disease. The group receiving the agent or regimen under study is the *test group*, sometimes called the *experimental* or *study group*, whereas a comparable group not subject to the agent or regimen is the *control group*. Clinical trials compare results in two or more samples of a single population, divided into groups that are essentially similar (in distribution of age, sex, race, socioeconomic status, and previous disease experience). The aim is to ensure that the only difference between the groups is the fact that the test group receives the treatment under study whereas the control group does not.

Much of the basis for preventive procedures in dentistry has come from the results of clinical trials, although the quality of trials described in the dental literature varies from excellent to poor. The reader can judge the validity of a trial by determining how closely the report adheres to certain principles in its conduct. These principles are described in brief in the following sections.

Choice of Population in Which the Trial Will Be Conducted

Choice of population should be determined by the purpose of the trial. If the prime purpose of a clinical trial is to test the *efficacy* of a particular agent, that is, whether it works or not, then the most favorable conditions should be created to show that it does work. For that reason, the project should be conducted with subjects who are selected for their susceptibility to the disease or condition. This means that a population of a specific age range is usually chosen deliberately, because many oral diseases are age specific (see Chapters 19-23). Sex, race, socioeconomic status, and geographic location are other factors considered in the choice of a study population for efficacy trials. If, however, the purpose is to assess the *effectiveness* of an agent under everyday conditions, then broad community populations, those with varying degrees of the disease or condition under study, should be chosen.[16] Confusing the purposes of trials can lead to the error of generalizing the results of efficacy trials conducted in special populations with unusual disease distributions, such as institutionalized people, to the general population.

Adequacy of the Numbers of Subjects

Loss of subjects during a prospective clinical trial is a fact of life and must be planned for. If the numbers of subjects in the groups are not large enough to begin with, at the end of the trial the researcher will be left with too few subjects to be able to show by statistical logic whether it is likely that an observed difference between the groups is real or a chance result. The result may then be that a real difference cannot be detected, and an agent that in fact is effective will not seem to be so. This issue relates to data analysis and the conclusions from the trial, and is discussed more fully later in this chapter.

Comparability of Study and Control Groups

The randomized trial, always the most elegant design for efficacy studies[4] and a cornerstone of evidence-based dentistry (see Chapter 12), is one in which group similarity is achieved by *random allocation* of subjects to the study and control groups. Random allocation means that each participant has an equal chance of being assigned to either the study or the control group. Statistical probability is such that the assumption can then be made that bias is not intruding and that at the end of the trial any differences between the groups can be attributed only to the agent under study. Any uncontrolled variables influencing the outcome, which are usually undetected by the researchers, are likely to affect subjects in both groups equally and therefore not to affect the relative differences between the groups.

The principle of random allocation is simple, although it is a carefully planned and controlled procedure. Random allocation is not haphazard assignment or one based on volunteering or self-selection. A statistician can further improve the probability of establishing comparable groups by *stratification*, which means that before allocation the base population is separated by those factors known or thought to influence disease occurrence (usually age, sex, race, socioeconomic status, and previous disease experience). Subjects from each stratum are then randomly allocated to study and control groups.

Nonrandomized trial designs are not uncommon in the dental literature.[18,19] Although they are weaker than randomized designs, sometimes practical considerations dictate their use. For example, the landmark Vipehölm study on diet and caries (see Chapter 28) was a prospective study, but participants were assigned to groups on a convenience basis rather than by randomization. This could have influenced the results to some extent. Some studies dispense with a control group altogether and determine efficacy by comparison with historical controls; that is, they use a before-and-after design in which disease levels at the end of the project are compared with those at the beginning.[10] The weakness in this design is that uncontrolled change could take place during the trial to invalidate results. For example, in a trial of a fluoride mouthrinse, children in sixth grade at the completion of a 3-year trial may have brushed with fluoride toothpaste more often than did the sixth-graders examined at the beginning of the trial. Without use of a concurrent control group it is impossible to tell if beneficial outcomes were due entirely to the mouthrinse or were due at least in part to the additional toothpaste use.

Before-and-after trials are often called *demonstrations*, intended to "demonstrate" the value of accepted preventive measures.[12] Presenting a case for the scientific validity of demonstrations can get complicated,[9,10] although it is worth noting that the pioneering Grand Rapids fluoridation trial used this design (see Chapter 25). A major threat to the validity of a before-and-after design comes from undetected sociodemographic change in the population under study during the period of the trial.

Some studies have used a *comparison group*, defined as any group to which the study group is compared and a term that too often is used synonymously with *control group*.[14] It is less confusing, however, if the term *control group* is reserved for randomized controls and the term *comparison group* is used for nonrandomized comparisons. Examples of comparison groups are the control communities used in fluoridation field trials (see Chapter 25). Some comparison groups can be similar to study groups and thus permit fairly valid comparisons, but others are so far removed from the study group that they serve little purpose.

Certain types of trial use a *crossover* design, in which subjects serve as their own controls. Each subject receives an active treatment for a specific time and a placebo (or no treatment) during a control period. Crossover designs are useful in short-term trials (weeks or months, rather than years) for preventing reversible conditions like gingivitis or calculus accumulation but are unsuitable for caries prevention trials because the time needed for new lesions to develop is too long. They are also not appropriate for testing of regimens that have a carryover effect, because the effects of the treatment phase could influence responses during the nontreatment phase. Crossover designs are also inappropriate when the tested regimen may produce a permanent effect, when test agents may be retained at the site of action for prolonged periods, or when conditions may naturally undergo a rapid change in prevalence, incidence, or morbidity. The principal advantage of a crossover design is that results are not affected by variations in response among participating subjects.

In studying efficacy trials, readers should take care not to confuse the need to carefully select the study population with the necessity to randomly allocate the individuals in that population to the study and control groups.

Use of a Placebo in the Control Group

A *placebo* is a material or formulation like the test product but without the active ingredient, such as a toothpaste that feels and tastes like a fluoride toothpaste but contains no fluoride. The purpose of using a placebo in a trial is to keep subjects unaware of whether they are in the test or control group (a *blind* study), so that their health behavior will not be consciously or unconsciously affected by group allocation. *Bias*, which is systematic though usually unconscious error, can affect examiners as well: an examiner who expects a product to be effective may unconsciously apply stricter criteria for caries in a control group if he or she knows which children are in which group. Examiners

therefore also should not know the group allocation of subjects. When neither participants nor examiners know the group allocations, the trial is termed *double-blind*.

Use of a placebo is inherently impossible in some instances, such as in trials of water fluoridation (where the fluoridating community is a matter of public record), fissure sealant (where sealant visibility determines the outcome), or dental health education (where the control at best is a comparable group that receives no program, a *passive control*). Placebos raise ethical issues, because it is usually considered unethical to deny established beneficial products to trial participants. If a manufacturer wants to test fluoride toothpaste with a stronger formulation than is standard, for example, the control group does not use a nonfluoride toothpaste but rather a standard-strength product. This is called a *positive control*; the results then compare the effects of the new product with the effects of the old one. Because the difference between these two groups would be expected to be less than if a placebo were used, the trial needs larger numbers of participants to permit any true difference to be shown.

The ethical issue is recognized, but the weakness of efficacy trials without controls is that we never know if using a tested product in a public health program is any better than having no program. In an age of low caries experience and extensive fluoride exposure (apart from any that may be associated with the test product), that can be a fair question.

Control of Operational Procedure

An efficacy study, designed to answer the question of whether a particular agent or regimen works or not, must give the test agent every chance to succeed. Susceptible populations are chosen for the trial, participants are randomly allocated to test and control groups, and double-blind conditions prevail. But in addition the researchers need to be sure that the agent is used as intended. If it is a professionally applied agent or a treatment regimen, the protocol must specify precisely how the agent will be used, for how long, how often, at what concentration, and by whom. A placebo, or positive control, would be applied the same way. If a self-applied agent is being tested, such as a mouthrinse, the protocol should call for the agent to be used under professional supervision. It is the researchers' task to ensure that the protocol is adhered to throughout the course of the study.

In an effectiveness trial, the agent or treatment can be used as it normally would. That means that professionals are given instructions in the use of a procedure or participants are given the rinse to take home and use as instructed. Therefore there is less certainty in an effectiveness trial that the material has been used as intended, but part of the aims of an effectiveness trial is to evaluate how the material works under everyday conditions. In operational control, as in other aspects of a trial, the purpose of the study must be kept in mind.

Examiner Reliability

Examiners in clinical trials must record disease that has developed over a relatively short period of time. This requirement forces the examiner to diagnose disease at an early stage of its development, which increases the risk of error. In caries trials, the most troublesome form of error is that an early lesion classed as carious at the first round of examinations may be classified as sound in subsequent examinations, a *negative reversal*, more commonly referred to just as a *reversal*. Reversals are virtually unavoidable in any form of sequential diagnosis,[17] although they should remain a fairly small proportion of all diagnoses. The ways of dealing with reversals in data analysis are discussed in Chapter 15, and further discussion of examiner reliability is found in Chapter 14.

The validity of clinical trial results depends heavily on the reliability of the examiner(s). This factor is usually referred to as *intraexaminer reliability* (i.e., within-examiner consistency) or the ability of an examiner to record the same conditions the same way over time. Most examiners with training and experience can develop an acceptable degree of intraexaminer consistency. Consistency between different examiners, *interexaminer reliability*, is more difficult to achieve, even when the examiners train together from the same written criteria. It is best to use one well-qualified examiner, but large-scale studies usually require more than one examiner, and multicenter trials certainly do. In such cases the examiners should undergo a period of training to bring their diagnostic standards as close together as can possibly be managed. This train-

ing procedure is referred to as *standardization*. When one of the group serves as the "gold standard" examiner and the training is to enable other examiners to record similarly, the term *calibration* can be applied.

Radiographs can be helpful in a trial, but the same issues of examiner consistency are present. Diagnostic criteria must be established, and intraexaminer and interexaminer consistency maintained with radiographic interpretation just as with clinical examinations. Given the logistic and ethical issues that also arise, use of radiographs is usually not recommended in field trials.[8] That is not necessarily the case in clinical trials in a dental school setting, where patients may undergo radiography anyway in the course of treatment.

Duration of the Trial

Clinical trials must be continued long enough to permit detection of new disease or extension of lesions already present. For caries trials, the minimum duration is usually 2-3 years, although precise timing depends on the purposes of the trial.[7] The longer the trial, the more expensive it is, so trade-offs are again required. The FDI World Dental Federation suggested in 1977 that trials of plaque-inhibiting agents could be as short as 8-21 days,[6] but that guideline was for plaque measurements only. The FDI also recommended that studies of calculus-preventing agents should last at least 90 days for supragingival calculus and longer for subgingival calculus. The American Dental Association requires that plaque-inhibiting agents for which the association's seal of approval is sought (see Chapter 29) demonstrate gingivitis reduction as well as plaque reduction; it requires such trials to be at least 6 months long.[1]

Statistical Analysis

It is not our purpose to cover the methods of statistical analysis in this text, because numerous excellent biostatistics textbooks are available. One particular analytic issue that can bother readers of the literature, however, is that of the relationship between *statistical significance* and *clinical importance*. This issue is worth some discussion here.

A clinical trial to test a preventive agent or treatment regimen begins with a null hypothesis (i.e., the proposition that there is no difference in disease experience between the test and control groups). When large differences between test and control groups are expected, the groups can be smaller than when small differences are expected. In either case, groups must be large enough (i.e., the trial must have sufficient *statistical power*) to permit the observed differences in disease increment between test and control groups to be reasonably tested for *statistical significance*, which is the probability that the observed results are due to chance rather than to the efficacy of the tested product or regimen. *Chance* in this context means that even with random allocation one group had more disease-susceptible or disease-resistant individuals. (It does not mean the probability of a chance result because of poor design or sloppy conduct of the study!) Such differences are not always apparent when the groups are compared following allocation, but if it is apparent immediately after allocation that the groups differ in some important respect, the groups can be disbanded and the allocation procedure repeated.

When comparing the observed results in a clinical trial, it has been traditional to accept 5% (sometimes stated as 0.05) as the outer limit of acceptable statistical significance. The statement $p = 0.05$ thus means that the risk of accepting the observed difference between the groups as real when actually it is due to chance is 5 in 100. In this case, the 5% chance of falsely accepting that a regimen is effective is termed type I error and the Greek letter α (alpha) is the probability of making a type I error. To offer greater assurance that an observed difference is real, investigators may set α at 1% ($p = 0.01$), although the trade-off here is that larger group sizes are necessary.

However, the selection of a small α level does not protect investigators from the possibility of failing to identify an effective agent or regimen. If the group size is too small, it is possible to conclude mistakenly that a treatment has no effect when in fact it really does. This latter mistake is known as type II error, and the probability of making a type II error is signified by the Greek letter β (beta).

The chance of detecting a true effect, if it exists, is denoted as the *power* of the test and is defined as $1 - \beta$. Power is dependent on (1) the magnitude of the difference observed between the two treatments, (2) the number of subjects in each group, (3) the population variance, and (4) the α level chosen. If the findings of a study are negative (meaning that the null hypothesis cannot be rejected), the power of the test indicates how confident one can be that the findings are truly negative. The goal in considering power when calculating group sizes is to enhance the chances of finding effects if they really do exist.

The power of a test is critically important in trials using a positive control, for example, those testing a higher-concentration fluoride toothpaste against the positive control of a standard fluoride product. Differences in caries increments between the groups are likely to be small. If the investigators judge that differences as small as 15% between groups are clinically meaningful, they will need to be able to demonstrate that differences this small are statistically significant. The group sizes then have to be extremely large.[5] Otherwise, with smaller groups, the researchers may falsely conclude that the regimens were equivalent because they failed to demonstrate statistical significance, when in fact the chance of demonstrating such significance, or the power of the test, was small to begin with.

In a well-conducted study, type I errors usually arise from the fact that sometimes the random allocation process results in bias in the composition of the groups. In a less well-conducted study, it can come from an absence of random allocation and from lack of blindness in either examiners or participants. In an otherwise well-conducted study, type II errors typically come from group sizes that are too small to permit demonstrating statistical significance when clinical differences are apparent (i.e., the trial is *underpowered*). Imprecise diagnosis by examiners, in which a lot of random error will result in high error variance, can also lead to type II error. In a trial in which there has been no random allocation, the assumptions underlying the statistical probability tests have been violated, so the p values presented in such reports have little value.

Overcoming problems of sample size requires more care than simply making study groups as large as possible. The reason is that, when groups are large, the most trivial difference in disease increment between them will reach statistical significance. This can be misleading if there is no clinical importance to the difference observed; therapeutic importance cannot be concluded simply because statistical significance has been determined. Using sample sizes larger than necessary is also inefficient; each additional subject in a study adds extra expense, consuming funds that could be used to conduct other important studies.

Ethical Considerations

Group sizes in a clinical trial should not be unduly large, because it is unethical to involve participants in research when their involvement is scientifically unnecessary and needlessly exposes them to the inconvenience and possible risks of participation. Humans taking part in clinical trials must give informed consent, which means providing a written acceptance that the participant understands the conduct of the trial and the nature of any risks involved. Researchers must certify in the report of the trial that the study protocol has been accepted by their institution's review board, which any institution conducting research is required to maintain. If the study raises special issues (e.g., if it includes illiterate or mentally retarded people), extra explanations are usually required in the report. Additional explanation of how the rights of participants have been safeguarded may also be needed if the study is conducted in a developing country that does not have the same rigorous standards for human subject protection as do the developed nations.

REFERENCES

1. American Dental Association, Council on Dental Therapeutics. Guidelines for acceptance of chemotherapeutic products for the control of supragingival plaque and gingivitis. J Am Dent Assoc 1986;112:529-32.
2. Beck JD. Risk revisited. Community Dent Oral Epidemiol 1998;26:220-5.
3. Bradford Hill A. The environment and disease: Association or causation? Proc R Soc Med 1965;58:295-300.
4. Cochrane AL. Effectiveness and efficiency: Random reflections on health services. London: Nuffield Provincial Hospitals Trust, 1971:20-5.
5. Conti AJ, Lotzkar S, Daly R, et al. A 3-year clinical trial to compare efficacy of dentifrices containing 1.14% and 0.76% sodium monofluorophosphate. Community Dent Oral Epidemiol 1988;16:135-8.
6. Fédération Dentaire Internationale, Commission on Classification and Statistics for Oral Conditions. Principal requirements for controlled clinical trials in periodontal diseases. Int Dent J 1977;27:62-76.
7. Fédération Dentaire Internationale, Commission on Oral Health, Research and Epidemiology. Principal requirements for controlled clinical trials of caries preventive agents and procedures. Int Dent J 1982;32:292-310.
8. Horowitz HS. Ethical considerations of study participants in dental caries clinical trials. Community Dent Oral Epidemiol 1976;4:43-50.
9. Horowitz HS, Meyers RJ, Heifetz SB, Driscoll WS. Eight-year evaluation of a combined fluoride program in a nonfluoride area. J Am Dent Assoc 1984;109:575-8.
10. Horowitz HS, Meyers RJ, Heifetz SB, et al. Combined fluoride, school-based program in a fluoride-deficient area: Results of an 11-year study. J Am Dent Assoc 1986;112:621-5.
11. Jacobsen SJ, Goldberg J, Cooper C, Lockwood SA. The association between water fluoridation and hip fracture among white women and men aged 65 years and older. A national ecologic study. Ann Epidemiol 1992;2:617-26.
12. Klein SP, Bohannan HM. The first year of field activities in the National Preventive Dentistry Demonstration Program. Rand Report No. R-2536/1-RWJ. Santa Monica CA: Rand Corporation, 1979.
13. Kleinbaum DG, Kupper LL, Morgenstern H. Epidemiologic research: Principles and quantitative methods. Belmont CA: Lifetime Learning Publications, 1982:25-34.
14. Last JM, ed. A dictionary of epidemiology. 4th ed. New York: Oxford University Press, 2001.
15. Locker D, Leake JL. Risk indicators and risk markers for periodontal disease experience in older adults living independently in Ontario, Canada. J Dent Res 1993;72:9-17.
16. O'Mullane DM. Efficiency in clinical trials of caries preventive agents and methods. Community Dent Oral Epidemiol 1976;4:190-4.
17. Radike AW. Examiner error and reversals in diagnosis. In: Proceedings of the conference on the clinical testing of cariostatic agents. Chicago: American Dental Association, 1972:92-5.
18. Ringleberg ML, Conti AJ, Webster DB. An evaluation of single and combined self-applied fluoride programs in schools. J Public Health Dent 1976;36:229-36.
19. Ripa LW, Leske GS, Levinson A. Supervised weekly rinsing with a 0.2% neutral NaF solution: Results from a demonstration program after two school years. J Am Dent Assoc 1978;97:793-8.
20. Rothman KJ. Modern epidemiology. Boston: Little Brown, 1986:3.
21. Suarez-Almazor ME, Flowerdew G, Saunders LD, et al. The fluoridation of drinking water and hip fracture hospitalization rates in two Canadian communities. Am J Public Health 1993;83:689-93.

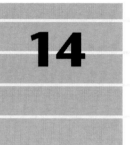

14   The Measurement of Oral Disease

Why do some patients have serious periodontitis whereas apparently similar patients do not? Why does a child who seems to eat candies all day not get caries? Frequently there is no obvious answer. That branch of scientific inquiry which seeks to find order among these apparently haphazard patterns of disease is *epidemiology*. Epidemiology is defined as the study of health and disease in populations, and of how these states are influenced by heredity, biology, physical environment, social environment, and ways of living.

Epidemiologic study requires that disease be measured quantitatively. This chapter describes the philosophies that underlie disease measurement and some of the procedures used. These methods are fundamental to the conduct of research, and they can also be of value to practitioners in monitoring their patients.

EPIDEMIOLOGY: AN INTRODUCTION

Although there are commonalities in the philosophies of all scientific research, biologic laws tend to be less universally true than are physical laws. The set of circumstances that leads to a heart attack in one person will not necessarily do so in another person of the same age, gender, and race. Biologic variation, meaning the different disease susceptibility among individuals, leads the epidemiologist to seek patterns among people who can be grouped by particular characteristics. Using the characteristics listed in the definition of epidemiology given earlier, one may relate these patterns to the following:

- *Heredity:* a person's genetic endowment
- *Biology:* age, gender, race
- *Physical environment:* sanitation levels, food and water supply, air quality, occupational hazards, housing quality, neighborhood characteristics
- *Social environment:* educational attainment, cultural beliefs and practices, neighborhood quality
- *Lifestyle:* smoking, exercise, dietary patterns, dental attendance, toothbrushing habits

Heredity has received a lot of recent attention with the rapid growth of molecular epidemiology, that is, the application of the techniques of molecular biology to epidemiology. DNA typing has been used to identify the genotype of pathogenic microorganisms, and viral DNA can be measured in host cells and their genomes.[13] DNA typing can also identify the genotypes of people who are especially susceptible to certain diseases. Molecular epidemiology holds enormous potential for disease control during the twenty-first century.

We should remember, however, that this is not the first time in history that there has been great optimism about prospects for disease control. In the late nineteenth century, when the bacterial agents in many infectious diseases were being identified, the "end of disease" was confidently being predicted. The concept of disease at that time was dominated by acute, mortal infections with a single bacterial agent, and little thought was given to chronic conditions. Today we are more aware that disease is multifactorial, meaning that multiple causative circumstances can be defined for just about any disease. Heart disease, the leading cause of death in the United States, is associated with genetics, stress, diet, exercise, smoking, blood pressure, and blood cholesterol levels. So what is the "cause" of heart disease? Dental caries is of bacterial origin but is also associated with sugar consumption, fluoride exposure, saliva quality and quantity (which are likely to be genetically controlled), family education and income, and other factors in the physical and social environment. So what is the "cause" of dental caries? Within the multifactorial tangle, epidemiology attempts to identify the risk factors (see Chapter 13) associated with a disease and to determine which of them are the most important for prevention and control.

Early Studies

Epidemiology was learned and practiced empirically long before it was named. For example, people have known for ages that malaria is a disease of wet lowlands, so they have avoided living in such places. But there was little true understanding about conditions that led to disease. The periodic epidemics that swept Europe from the Middle Ages until fairly recent times, for example, were often seen as religious signs rather than as a result of squalid living conditions. It was from the more rational study of these epidemics that epidemiology evolved to its present form. Samuel Pepys, who wrote vivid chronicles of life in seventeenth-century London, used the Bills of Mortality, the forerunner of modern death certificates, to measure the onset and decline of a plague epidemic in London in 1665. Percivall Pott's *Treatise of the Chimney Sweep's Cancer*, in 1775, described the unusually high occurrence of scrotal cancer among chimney sweeps and is thus an early scientific description of an occupational hazard.

In 1854 John Snow, a medical practitioner in the Soho area of London, went so far as to control an outbreak of cholera by the application of

his epidemiologic conclusions. His investigation took place some years before the germ theory of disease was understood, so Snow began by trying to identify the features common to those who died from the disease. After he mapped out the residences of those who had died (Fig. 14-1), his subsequent inquiries disclosed that all of the victims had used water from the same source. That source, in the days before indoor plumbing, was a pump on Broad Street (now Broadwick Street, where the site of the pump is currently occupied by a public toilet). Snow reached the rational conclusion that something in the water was responsible for the spread of the disease. Snow's method of controlling the epidemic, still without knowing its cause, was to persuade the authorities to remove the pump handle. The epidemic soon subsided.

Snow's subsequent investigations on the relation between cholera and the source of water supply are epidemiologic classics. The results of the patiently executed research of nineteenth-century workers such as Snow still benefit present-day society. Their investigations led to gradual but profound improvements in sanitation and personal hygiene, and the development of the public health codes for housing, water supply, and food processing that are now taken for granted. The fact that infectious diseases such as cholera, typhoid, yellow fever, plague, scarlet fever, and relapsing fever are now rare in high-income countries is not simply chance but is due largely to the pioneering work of these early epidemiologists. Their work continues today: our understanding of the mode of transmission of the human immunodeficiency virus and its translation into public health education to prevent acquired immunodeficiency syndrome followed remarkably quickly on the first identification of the virus in 1983.[21,30] That, too, is epidemiology.

The types of study design used in epidemiology were described in Chapter 13 and the various uses of the epidemiologic method in research are shown in Box 14-1.

The Concept of Measuring Disease

The good clinician thinks in qualitative terms. During a diagnostic examination the dental practitioner not only looks for existing disease but also tries to look ahead to the possibility of future disease. Measuring the oral health of a

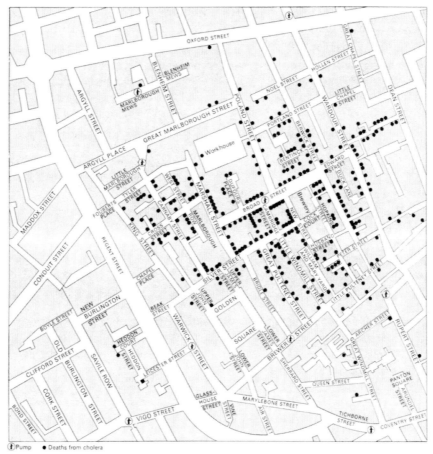

Fig. 14-1 John Snow's map of the Soho area of London, showing deaths from cholera during the epidemic of 1854.[18] (From Longmate, N. Alive and well: Medicine and public health, 1830 to the present day. Hammondsworth, Penguin, 1970.)

population, however, requires a more standardized and objective approach. Specific *diagnostic criteria*, written explicitly for clinical, radiographic, microbiologic, or pathologic examination, provide an objective framework for the practitioner's judgment. These criteria are applied to judge the condition of the oral tissues as they are at examination time, not as they might be in the future. This objective application of diagnostic criteria is the most important philosophical difference between the epidemiologic examination and the examination carried out for treatment planning.

Measurement, the quantification of observations, is the crux of science. Measurement variability is inherent in all fields of science; it is one reason why laboratory experiments are repeated before their findings can be accepted. In studies of oral disease, a count of carious lesions in a population is almost never duplicated; a repeat

examination of the same group of patients frequently results in a different count of carious lesions. Any one count of disease in a group is therefore an estimate of conditions, rather than absolute truth. As long as criteria are applied consistently, however, valid estimates will still result, because diagnostic drifts in one direction will be balanced by drifts the other way.

Acute diseases, such as measles, are characterized by a sudden onset of symptoms, so that the patient progresses rapidly from a state in which the disease is clearly absent to one in which the disease is clearly present. Remission of the acute phase of the disease is equally rapid, so little time is spent in the "gray areas." Chronic diseases, however, are usually characterized by a much slower onset. It is difficult to establish exactly when arthritis, alcoholism, mental illness, dental caries, and periodontitis become definitely established; there is a considerable

- **Describing normal biologic processes.** Examples are height at various stages of growth, blood groups, and times and order of tooth eruption.
- **Understanding the natural history of diseases.** Observations of disease progression and outcome in populations have enabled investigators to distinguish those diseases that are fatal or disabling from those that will resolve uneventfully.
- **Revealing the distribution of disease.** Indicating how disease occurs in the population by age, gender, race, geographic region, and socioeconomic status. Comparisons of cross-sectional surveys conducted at different times demonstrate trends in disease prevalence and distribution. It was the comparison of survey results in the early 1980s which first clearly showed that caries experience had declined among children in the United States (see Chapter 20).
- **Identifying the determinants of disease.** Within the multifactorial causes of disease referred to earlier, specific study designs (see Chapter 13) can identify the risk factors and risk indicators associated with a disease. Even if the causal pathway of a disease is not fully understood, knowledge of risk factors can lead to intervention strategies for prevention and control.
- **Testing hypotheses for disease prevention and control.** Agents, regimens, or procedures for the prevention and control of disease can be experimentally tested in clinical trials (see Chapter 13). As a dental example, the various uses of fluorides to reduce caries incidence have been subjected to numerous field trials in human populations (see Chapters 25 and 26).
- **Planning and evaluating health care services.** Data that describe (1) the distribution of disease, both treated and untreated, in the population under study; (2) the population's utilization of health care services; and (3) the availability and productivity of health care services can be employed to assist planning decisions on services and types of personnel required. Related applications are validation of the effectiveness of treatment techniques, both new and traditional, and determination of the quality of treatment provided.

gray area. In dentistry this problem is handled by counting as lesions only those that meet specific criteria.

SAMPLING FROM HUMAN POPULATIONS

Because the intent of a survey is to project results from a sample back to the base population from which the sample was drawn, clearly the sample should closely represent the population.

Examples of representative sampling are found in the national surveys of the health status of the United States population carried out continuously by the National Center for Health Statistics (http://www.cdc.gov/nchs). Obviously no one project can physically examine or ask questions of all 280 million or so Americans, so sampling is required. The process itself is complicated and requires specialized training, but sampling precision is such that the 100,618 persons interviewed in the 2000 National Health Interview Survey[28] could represent the whole country with a low degree of sampling error. *Sampling error* is the discrepancy between the sample and the base population in one or more important characteristics, and with modern statistical methods it can be remarkably small. The type of sample used in the National Health Interview Survey is a *probability sample*, which means that the chance of each person's being selected in the sample is known, though not necessarily equal. A greater proportion of older people than younger people, for example, may be deliberately sampled to compensate for the poorer response that is characteristic of older people. What is important is that the sampling probability be *known*, because then the degree of sampling error can be calculated.

When a nonprobability sample is used for a survey, however, interpretive problems arise because sampling error cannot be calculated from nonprobability samples. As an example, the National Survey of Oral Health in U.S. Employed Adults and Seniors in 1985-86[29] sought to obtain a profile of oral health in

American adults by examining employed adults and seniors who visited senior centers. This was a practical and budget-conscious way of obtaining a reasonable profile, but the restricted sampling most likely introduced bias into the results. For example, the survey found that only 4.2% of persons under age 65 were edentulous, but this is almost certainly an underestimate because various groups (e.g., the unemployed and self-employed) were excluded from the sampling frame, which means that they had no chance of selection in the sample.

Note that analytic studies in epidemiology usually do not use probability samples. In fact, case-control and cohort studies, as well as clinical trials (see Chapter 13), are usually conducted with groups carefully chosen for required attributes such as age, accessibility, presence of both the disease and the exposures under study, and willingness to participate. In analytic study designs, a prime critical issue is the selection and categorization of participants as cases or controls, or exposed and unexposed. In clinical trials, the prime critical issue is the allocation of participants to test or control group.

More than one analytic study is usually required before the identification of a risk factor can be confirmed or the results of a clinical trial can be generalized. If weekly use of a fluoride mouthrinse is found to reduce caries incidence by 22% over 30 months among 12-year-old children in fluoridated Des Moines,[6] what does that mean for the children of the United States as a whole? Even assuming experimental conditions could be identical (which they never are), results need not necessarily be the same for children of different ethnic backgrounds, living in different climatic zones, and with differing dietary practices and exposure to fluoridated water. When additional studies are carried out by different researchers in different places with fairly similar results, however, then the weight of evidence increases the likelihood that the observed effect is real and generalizable to the population at large.

METHODS OF MEASURING ORAL DISEASES
Counts

The simplest way of measuring any disease is by counting the number of cases of its occurrence.

Simple counts of cases are most useful for unusual conditions of low prevalence (e.g., the 130 or so incident cases of Ewing's tumor in children under 15 years of age in the United States each year). Simple counts become less useful as prevalence increases.

Proportions

A count becomes a proportion when a denominator is added, and prevalence is thus determined. The count of cancers in males ages 55-64 years can be divided by the population of that group to give prevalence: 22 cases in a population of 845 men ages 55-64 years yields a prevalence of 0.026, or 2.6%. Proportions do not include a time dimension; the figure just given would include newly diagnosed cases as well as longstanding ones. Proportions can also be useful in expressing the prevalence of caries among schoolchildren, the prevalence of total tooth loss in adults, or the prevalence of other conditions whose occurrence is somewhere between common and rare.

Rates

A rate is a proportion that uses a standardized denominator and includes a time dimension. Infant mortality rate, for example, is the number of deaths of newborn infants within the first year of life per 1000 live births, usually stated for particular calendar years to illustrate trends. In the United States the infant mortality rate for white children dropped from 6.3 per 1000 live births in 1995 to 5.7 in 2001; for African-American children the same measures were 14.6 and 13.3.[28]

Rates have not been used much in oral disease measurement, except to describe caries incidence over a period of time in clinical trials[6] and annual rate of loss of periodontal attachment in longitudinal studies.[17] Proportions or index values are often mistakenly referred to as rates in the literature.

Indexes

The individual who suffers from caries in only 2 of 32 teeth clearly has a much lower intensity of disease than does the person who has carious lesions in 16 of 26 teeth. Simple prevalence does not discriminate between these degrees of intensity, which is usually determined in oral epidemiology by use of an index (the plural

BOX 14-2 Properties of an Ideal Index

- **Validity.** The index must measure what it is intended to measure, so it should correspond with the clinical stages of the disease under study at each point.
- **Reliability.** The index should be able to measure consistently at different times and under a variety of conditions. The term *reliability* is virtually synonymous with *reproducibility, repeatability,* and *consistency,* meaning the ability of the same or different examiners to interpret and use the index in the same way.
- **Clarity, simplicity, and objectivity.** The criteria should be clear and unambiguous, with mutually

exclusive categories. Ideally, they should be able to be readily memorized by an examiner after some practice.
- **Quantifiability.** The index must be amenable to statistical analysis, so that the status of a group can be expressed by a distribution, mean, median, or other statistical measure.
- **Sensitivity.** The index should be able to detect reasonably small shifts, in either direction, in the condition.
- **Acceptability.** The use of the index should not be painful or demeaning to the subject.

form we will use is *indexes*, although *indices* is also used).

An *index* is a numerical scale with upper and lower limits, with scores on the scale corresponding to specific criteria. Index scores can be expressed for an individual; populations can be characterized by distributions or mean scores. The properties of an ideal index are listed in Box 14-2. Index scores frequently are clinical abstractions (e.g., a Plaque Index score of 1.2), which only make sense when used for comparisons between individuals or groups measured in a similar way. In the literature, the word *index* is often used broadly to mean any form of disease quantification, including proportions and rates. We encourage confining its use to scales meeting the aforementioned definition. The criteria for assigning a particular score to a condition are an integral part of the description of any index.

The different types of scales used in disease measurement are shown in Box 14-3. The majority of indexes used in oral epidemiology are ordinal scales, although some are treated statistically as though they were interval or ratio scales. This statistical impropriety can be a bit academic, however, because such deviations usually do not give seriously misleading results.

There are other terms used in the literature to describe indexes, such as *reversible* and *irreversible*. An irreversible index is one that measures cumulative conditions that cannot be reversed: dental caries (e.g., caries that has resulted in tissue loss, either restored or unre-

BOX 14-3 Types of Scale Used in Disease Measurement

- **Nominal.** A scale that simply gives names to different conditions and therefore is not strictly a scale at all, e.g., Angle's classification of malocclusions.[3]
- **Ordinal.** A scale that lists conditions in some order of severity without attempting to define any mathematical relation between the categories, e.g., the Gingival Index of Löe and Silness.[17]
- **Interval.** A scale in which the numbers used in the scale purport to have a mathematical relation to each other, although the scale does not have a true zero point. Examples are the Fahrenheit and Celsius temperature scales; none known in dentistry.
- **Ratio.** A scale in which the numbers used in the scale purport to have a mathematical relation to each other, and the scale has a true zero point. An example is the Kelvin temperature scale, which goes to absolute zero. A dental example, though one no longer in use (see Chapter 16) is the Russell Periodontal Index.[27]

stored, or tooth loss itself). However, gingivitis is a reversible inflammatory condition, so an index of gingivitis is considered reversible.

A final general point about disease measurement is that, just as there is no perfect method, there are also no generic, all-purpose scales that meet every need. Choice of measurement scale in any situation, whether it be for a practitioner monitoring a patient's progress or for a researcher conducting a highly sophisticated clinical trial, is dictated by the needs. The first response to the often-asked question of "What index should I use?" is "What is the question you want to answer?" The process a practitioner goes through to select a measure by which to monitor the oral hygiene progress of a middle-aged periodontal patient is little different from that followed by the researcher in a complex study. Both have to determine why they are using that particular measure, how to handle it reliably, and what it is they want to demonstrate.

EXAMINER RELIABILITY

When any measurements of disease are made over a period of time, conclusions reached are based on the comparison between two sets of results. It follows that the diagnostic criteria must be applied the same way at different times, because if they are not, the comparisons have little value. This is the issue of examiner *reliability*, which was introduced in Chapter 13. Assuming that the index is inherently reproducible, the ability of an examiner to record the same conditions the same way over time is termed *intraexaminer reliability*. This quality can be developed by most examiners with some training and experience, but it needs to be demonstrated in research studies. Intraexaminer reliability can be assessed by having an examiner record conditions in a group of 10-20 persons and then repeat the process a few hours to a few days later. The time between the first and second examinations should be long enough for memory to fade but short enough so that real change in the condition itself will not be noticeable. Reaching agreement between two or more examiners, *interexaminer reliability*, is usually more tedious. It requires initial agreement on interpretation of diagnostic criteria, then a period of training with repeated patient examinations to ensure that examiners' judgments are comparable. Interexaminer reliability is rarely perfect, but when examination findings from two or more examiners are being pooled, a measure of interexaminer reliability training should be recorded. This conforms with the CONSORT (Consolidated Standards of Reporting Trials) Statement, a set of criteria for explicit reporting of

clinical trials (see Chapter 12), which lists "any methods used to enhance quality of measurements" as one of the elements to be reported.[19]

The issue of examiner reliability can make people uncomfortable, because to have one's inconsistencies exposed for the world to see can be humbling. (We stress that examiner reliability is totally unrelated to clinical skills or ability to care for patients.) In the literature, examiner reliability is sometimes vaguely dismissed with a statement like "the examiners achieved 96% agreement," which by itself is of little value because of its uncertain meaning (it usually seems to mean that one examiner's group mean score was 96% of the mean score of the other examiner's group). In addition, such a comparison does not account for decisions requiring little diagnostic judgment (e.g., inclusion of many obviously sound lower incisors in the denominator), nor does it account for agreement that would be expected by chance alone.[10] The measure most frequently used for expressing interexaminer reliability is the *kappa* statistic, a value between 0 and 1.0 that expresses the degree of agreement beyond that expected by chance alone.[10,12] Correlation statistics and specified percent agreement, along with kappa, give a good picture of interexaminer reliability in a cross-sectional study.

Reversals can be exasperating in longitudinal studies, notably in clinical trials. A *reversal*, more properly called a *negative reversal*, is a change of diagnosis in an illogical direction over a period of time long enough for real change to have taken place. For example, when a surface scored as caries into dentin at the first examination is scored as sound 1 year later, this is an illogical change. In a clinical trial, the examiner has to record disease that developed over a relatively short time; hence, much of it is at incipient stages. Diagnosis of borderline lesions as caries inevitably results in some degree of negative reversals, so reversals are an inherent part of any clinical trial.[25] What must be remembered about reversals, however, is that if the examiner is consistent then negative reversals will be balanced by *positive reversals*, which are changes in a logical direction made in error. In a caries trial this means that a lesion diagnosed as sound at the first examination is marked as carious a year later, when the diagnosis really should have been sound-sound or carious-carious. The snag, of course, is that at data analysis the positive reversals cannot be separated from normal disease progression. That is where a demonstration of reliability is important: even if the examinations are all of incipient lesions in first molars, where many reversals would be expected, a consistent examiner will have negative reversals balanced by positive reversals. Net results should therefore be analyzed without subtracting out the negative reversals.

Reversals are illustrated in Fig. 14-2, which uses 10 tooth surfaces being measured for caries to illustrate the point. Surfaces A to C have progressed from sound to decayed, but D and E (shaded) show negative reversals. The remaining teeth have not changed in diagnosis between examinations. The net result is that the four D lesions at baseline have become five lesions a year later. But how is this analysis affected by the negative reversals in D and E? Reversals at best can be disturbing (indeed, if the reliability examinations cast doubt on the examiner's reliability, then the entire set of data is suspect). If, however, the examiner is acceptably consistent, then it can be assumed that the two negative reversals in D and E are random errors and will be balanced by two positive reversals in A, B, or C. There could also have been random error in the diagnoses for surfaces F to J, but because all these diagnoses are in a logical direction, such error cannot be detected. The net result of four decayed lesions progressing to five therefore is retained and referred to as the *net caries increment.*

Reversals in longitudinal studies of periodontitis are especially troublesome because reattachment has been demonstrated by experienced examiners.[15] A loss of periodontal attachment of 6 mm at initial examination that is then recorded as 5 mm a year later could represent examiner error or it could be true reattachment. A demonstration of examiner reliability in diagnosis is especially important in these circumstances. Reliability in periodontal examinations has been improved with the advent of pressure-sensitive and computerized probes,[11,24] although the use of these instruments is largely restricted to clinical research studies.

Note the difference between an examination to check reliability and the occurrence of reversals. A reliability check consists of repeat examinations only hours apart, too close together for real change to have occurred. Differences in diagnosis are therefore all examiner variation. Reversals occur over a period of time long enough for real change to have occurred, so examiner variation can be mixed in with real change. In a reliability check, the duplicate examinations do not form a part of the data set, whereas reversals are detected from the study data.

Fig. 14-2 Representation of positive and negative diagnostic reversals in a longitudinal study.

Surface	Baseline	1 Year
A	S	→ D
B	S	→ D
C	S	→ D
D	D	→ S
E	D	→ S
F	S	→ S
G	S	→ S
H	S	→ S
I	D	→ D
J	D	→ D

MEASURING THE VALUE OF A DIAGNOSTIC TEST

We discussed in Chapters 12 and 13 that the ultimate test for the efficacy of a preventive agent or procedure was the randomized clinical trial, but this design does not fit when the purpose is evaluation of a diagnostic test.

Diagnostic tests in medicine are numerous and well established. The criteria for an ideal test are that it should be simple, inexpensive (relative to the direct or social cost of the disease), acceptable to the patient, valid, and reliable. A test should also be *sensitive*, which in this context means that it yields a positive result in those with the disease, and *specific*, meaning that it gives a negative result in those who do not have the disease. There are only a few tests that rate highly in both sensitivity and specificity, so the choice may be whether to use a test that is highly sensitive but not very specific (which would capture a lot of false positives—people who test positive but really don't have the disease), specific but not sensitive (which would lead to a lot of false negatives—people who test negative but really do have the disease), or not to test at all. Fig. 14-3 summarizes how sensitivity, specificity, and related predictive values can be derived from the results of tests and subsequent disease outcome.

In dentistry a considerable number of predictive tests intended to identify caries-susceptible individuals have been explored down the years without much success. A 1977 conference at Niagara Falls concluded that there was little at that time in the way of bacteriologic, enzymatic, or other biologic tests that could predict caries with sufficient sensitivity and specificity. The best predictor of future caries was past caries experience,[5] a result that is consistently found in more recent studies as well.[9,14,26] This finding is not much help to a practitioner trying to control caries in a susceptible patient.

Research aimed at finding tests for susceptibility to severe periodontitis still has some way to go.[1,22] The only true risk factors established are tobacco use and diabetes,[1] although inflammatory mediators identified in gingival crevicular fluid may in time form the basis of practical tests of susceptibility.[2] Clinical signs such as gingivitis, plaque deposits, suppuration, and bleeding on probing have demonstrated poor sensitivity, and even a pocket depth of 4 mm or more is only weakly predictive at best for severe periodontitis.[8,20] There has been some modest progress in exploring risk factors in the physical and social environment such as stress and anxiety, income level, and poor ability to cope with life's pressures.[4,7] Although many of these factors, apart from smoking and diabetes, have not yet been unequivocally related to periodontitis, some have been put together into a "risk calculator" that is reasonably valid.[23] Further refinements in this area can be expected.

EPIDEMIOLOGY AND THE PRACTITIONER

Epidemiology joins the basic sciences and clinical studies to increase our understanding of diseases. The practitioner can factor knowledge of risk factors into diagnosis and treatment

Test result	Disease	No disease	Total
Positive	TP	FP	TP + FP
Negative	FN	TN	TN + FN
Total	TP + FN	FP + TN	ALL

Sensitivity: Proportion of people with disease who test positive: **TP/(TP + FN)**

Specificity: Proportion of people without disease who test negative: **TN/(FP + TN)**

Positive predictive value: Probability that a person who tests positive will have disease: **TP/(TP + FP)**

Negative predictive value: Probability that a person who tests negative will not have disease: **TN/(FN + TN)**

False-positive rate: Proportion of people with positive tests who do not have disease: **FP/(FP + TN)**

False-negative rate: Proportion of people with negative tests who have disease: **FN/(TP + FN)**

Fig. 14-3 Information that can be derived from the results of a predictive test related to disease outcome. *TP,* True positive; *TN,* true negative; *FP,* false positive; *FN,* false negative.

planning decisions; that is, a patient is more likely to develop a particular disease if he or she exhibits certain characteristics. For example, a man who smokes may or may not get lung cancer, but he certainly runs more risk of developing lung cancer than if he did not smoke. Similarly, an elderly man who both smokes and drinks heavily is more at risk of oral cancer than one who does not.

Another immediate use of epidemiology to the practitioner is application of the results from clinical trials, preferably from systematic reviews, which form the cornerstone of evidence-based dentistry (see Chapter 12). Although not every member of a test group in a clinical trial necessarily benefits from the tested procedure, the probabilities are high that a given patient will benefit from a procedure that has been successfully tested.

Biologic variation also applies the other way: a practitioner cannot generalize from the results of an individual patient's treatment to the population at large. Successful treatment can result from a practitioner's personality, from serendipitous characteristics of the particular patient, or from outside influences, as well as from the treatment itself. Clinical experience is important, but only with controls and the appropriate design can effective prevention and treatment methods be clearly identified.

REFERENCES

1. Albandar JM. Global risk factors and risks indicators for periodontal disease. Periodontol 2000; 2002;29: 177-206.
2. Alpagot T, Bell C, Lundergan W, et al. Longitudinal evaluation of GCF MMP-3 and TIMP-1 levels as prognostic factors for progression of periodontitis. J Clin Periodontol 2001;28:353-9.
3. Angle EH. Classification of malocclusion. Dent Cosmos 1899;41:248-64.
4. Beck JD, Koch GG, Offenbacher S. Incidence of attachment loss over 3 years in older adults—new and progressing lesions. Community Dent Oral Epidemiol 1995;23:291-6.
5. Bibby BG, Shern RJ, eds. Methods of caries prediction; proceedings of a workshop conference. Washington DC: Information Retrieval, 1978.
6. Driscoll WS, Swango PA, Horowitz AM, Kingman A. Caries-preventive effects of daily and weekly fluoride mouthrinsing in a fluoridated community: Final results after 30 months. J Am Dent Assoc 1982;105:1010-3.
7. Genco RJ, Ho AW, Grossi SG, et al. Relationship of stress, distress, and inadequate coping behaviors to periodontal disease. J Periodontol 1999;70:711-23.
8. Haffajee AD, Socransky SS, Goodson JM. Clinical parameters as predictors of destructive disease activity. J Clin Periodontol 1983;10:257-65.
9. Hausen H, Seppä L, Fejerskov O. Can caries be predicted? In: Thylstrup A, Fejerskov O, eds: Textbook of clinical cariology. 2nd ed. Copenhagen: Munksgaard, 1994:393-411.
10. Hunt RJ. Percent agreement, Pearson's correlation, and kappa as measures of inter-examiner reliability. J Dent Res 1986;65:128-30.
11. Jeffcoat MK, Jeffcoat RL, Jens SC, Captain K. A new periodontal probe with automated cemento-enamel junction detection. J Clin Periodontol 1986;13:276-80.
12. Landis JR, Koch GG. The measurement of observer agreement for categorical data. Biometrics 1977;33: 159-74.
13. Last JM. A dictionary of epidemiology. 3rd ed. New York: OUP, 1995.
14. Leverett DH, Proskin HM, Featherstone JD, et al. Caries risk assessment in a longitudinal discrimination study. J Dent Res 1993;72:538-43.
15. Lindhe J, Haffajee AD, Socransky SS. Progression of periodontal disease in adult subjects in the absence of periodontal therapy. J Clin Periodontol 1983;10:433-42.
16. Löe H, Ånerud A, Boysen H, Morrison E. Natural history of periodontal disease in man. Rapid, moderate and no loss of attachment in Sri Lankan laborers 14 to 46 years of age. J Clin Periodontol 1986;13:431-40.
17. Löe H, Silness J. Periodontal disease in pregnancy. I. Prevalence and severity. Acta Odontol Scand 1963;21: 533-51.
18. Longmate N. Alive and well: Medicine and public health from 1830 to the present day. Harmondsworth UK: Penguin, 1970.
19. Moher D, Schultz KF, Altman DG, for the CONSORT group. Revised recommendations for improving the quality of reports of parallel group randomized trials 2001, website: http://www.consort-statement.org/. Accessed November 20, 2003.
20. Norderyd O, Hugoson A, Grusovin G. Risk of severe periodontal disease in a Swedish adult population. A longitudinal study. J Clin Periodontol 1999;26: 608-15.
21. Osborn JE. Dispelling myths about the AIDS epidemic. In: Fransen VE, ed: Proceedings of the AIDS prevention and services workshop. Princeton NJ: Robert Wood Johnson Foundation, 1990:15-21.
22. Page RC, Beck JD. Risk assessment for periodontal diseases. Int Dent J 1997;47:61-87.
23. Page RC, Krall EA, Martin J, et al. Validity and accuracy of a risk calculator in predicting periodontal disease. J Am Dent Assoc 2002;133:569-76.
24. Polson AM, Goodson JM. Periodontal diagnosis; current status and future needs. J Periodontol 1985;56:25-34.
25. Radike AW. Examiner error and reversals in diagnosis. In: Proceedings of the conference on the clinical testing of cariostatic agents. Chicago: American Dental Association, 1972:92-5.
26. Reich E, Lussi A, Newbrun E. Caries risk assessment. Int Dent J 1999;49:15-26.
27. Russell AL. A system of scoring for prevalence surveys of periodontal disease. J Dent Res 1956;35:350-9.

28. US Public Health Service, National Center for Health Statistics. Summary health statistics for US children: National Health Interview Survey 2000. DHHS Publication No. (PHS) 2003-1541, Series 10 No. 213. Washington DC: Government Printing Office, 2003.

29. US Public Health Service, National Institute of Dental Research. Oral health of United States adults; national findings. NIH Publication No. 87-2868. Washington DC: Government Printing Office, 1987.

30. Yankauer A. AIDS and public health [editorial]. Am J Public Health 1988;78:364-6.

15 Measuring Dental Caries

DMF INDEX
CRITERIA FOR DIAGNOSING CORONAL
  CARIES

ROOT CARIES
EARLY CHILDHOOD CARIES
CARIES TREATMENT NEEDS

This chapter describes the methods for measuring dental caries in human populations. Some historical measures from the early twentieth century include the proportion of first molars lost through caries[21,22] and the percentage of erupted permanent teeth affected by caries.[1] Both of these measures were useful when there was little information of any kind about the disease, though they lacked sensitivity. At the other extreme, the Bodeckers' index of surfaces affected by caries, described in 1931,[10] was sensitive but complicated. Dean and his colleagues,[14] in their pioneering studies of the caries-fluoride relationship, counted the number of teeth in the mouth visibly affected by caries, which was a forerunner of the DMF count. The first description of what is now known as the DMF index is attributed to Klein, Palmer, and Knutson in their studies of dental caries in Hagerstown, Maryland, in the 1930s.[32] Since then, the DMF index has received practically universal acceptance and is the best known and most widely used of all dental indexes.

DMF INDEX

The DMF index, an irreversible index, is applied only to permanent teeth. As originally described, it defined three categories of teeth that were counted to calculate the index:

  D for decayed teeth

  M for teeth missing due to caries

  F for teeth that had been previously filled

  Filled teeth were assumed to have been unequivocally decayed prior to restoration. The DMF score for any one individual can range from 0 to 32, in whole numbers. A mean DMF score for a group, which is the total of individual values divided by the number of subjects examined, can have a decimal value. The DMF index can be applied to whole teeth (designated as DMFT) or to surfaces (DMFS). Modifications can be made to the index for factors such as filled teeth that have redecayed, crowned teeth, bridge pontics, and any other particular attribute required for a given study. To save time in a large survey, the DMF index can be used half-mouth; that is, it can be applied to opposite diagonal quadrants and the score doubled, an approach which assumes that the carious attack is bilateral. The DMF index can be applied to all 32 teeth, although because of the widespread removal of third molars in young adults some prefer to record a score for 28 teeth. Either approach is acceptable as long as the method is clearly stated.

Although the DMF index has been used universally since its introduction in 1938, its limitations need to be recognized. The main ones are shown in Box 15-1.

The DMF index for permanent teeth is always signified by uppercase letters; the equivalent index for the primary dentition is the *def* index and its modifications.[19] The teeth counted to derive this index were originally defined as follows:

  d for decayed teeth

  e for teeth indicated for extraction

  f for filled teeth.

Teeth missing because of caries are not recorded because of the complications of exfoliation and lack of knowledge as to whether missing teeth were carious prior to exfoliation.

BOX 15-1 Limitations of the DMF Index

The DMF index has received remarkably little challenge over some 70 years of life, probably because it is simple and versatile. It was developed for use in children a long time ago, however, and accordingly it shows its age in a few areas. The principal limitations are the following:

- DMF values are not related to the number of teeth at risk. A DMF score for an individual is a simple count of those teeth that in the examiner's judgment have been affected by caries; it has no denominator. A DMF score thus does not directly give an indication of the intensity of the attack in any one individual. A 7-year-old child with a DMF score of 3.0 may have only 9 permanent teeth in the mouth; thus one third of these teeth have already been attacked by caries in a short space of time. An adult may have a DMF score of 8.0 with a full complement of 32 teeth; thus over a longer period of time only one quarter of the teeth have been affected. DMF scores therefore have little meaning unless age is also stated.
- The DMF index gives equal weight to missing, untreated decayed, and well-restored teeth. Common sense suggests that this philosophical basis is faulty for many purposes.

- The DMF index is invalid when teeth have been lost for reasons other than caries. Teeth can be lost for periodontal reasons in older adults and for orthodontic reasons in teenagers. Decision rules, which go along with criteria, are required to determine how to deal with these instances.
- The DMF index can overestimate caries experience in teeth with "preventive restorations." In an epidemiologic survey, such teeth must be included in the F component of DMF, although had they not been filled in the first place they might have been diagnosed as sound teeth. DMF scores will thus be inflated.[5] Composite restorations judged to have been placed only for cosmetic reasons likewise should not be included in DMF counts.
- DMF data are of little use for estimating treatment needs (see Caries Treatment Needs).
- The DMF index cannot account for sealed teeth. Sealants did not exist in 1938 and thus are obviously not included in the description of the index. Here is where the DMF index shows its age; sealants and other composite restorations for cosmetic purposes have to be dealt with separately.

Modifications of this index are (1) the dmf index for use in children before the age of exfoliation, (2) the dmf index applied only to the primary molar teeth, and (3) the df index. Values for df and def should be numerically the same; def allows for two grades of caries, and neither index counts missing teeth. Both the def and df indexes may therefore understate the true extent of the carious attack; the trade-off is presumably greater reliability from ignoring missing teeth.

Because of the present-day skewed distribution of caries prevalence in the population, the Significant Caries Index (SiC Index) was developed.[11] The SiC Index is not a new index, because it is based on the distribution of DMF values in a population, but is a way of expressing caries distribution that goes beyond mean DMF. It is actually the mean DMF score for the third of the distribution most affected by caries and is intended to be used alongside the mean DMF value to give a more complete summary of caries in the whole population. The more

skewed the distribution, the greater the gap between the mean DMF score and the SiC value. A new global goal of an SiC score of 3.0 or less for 2015 has been suggested[57] and, if adopted and used, would provide some further information on caries distribution.[38]

Other methods of measuring dental caries with a different philosophical base have been suggested. One is Grainger's hierarchy, an ordinal scale designed to simplify the recording of the caries status of a population, which uses five zones of severity of the carious attack.[18] This scale appears to be valid[29,31,45] but has received little further use, probably because of low sensitivity. More recently, "composite" indicators have been suggested that attempt to measure health rather than disease by weighting healthy restored teeth differently from missing or decayed teeth.[46] The first of these is the FS-T, which sums the sound and healthy restored teeth. The second is T-Health, which seeks to measure the amount of healthy dental tissue and assigns descending numerical weights for a sound healthy tooth, a filled tooth, and a decayed tooth. These are conceptually sound approaches to measuring dental health and function (rather than disease), and they deserve more attention than they have received.

Sealants had not arrived when the DMF index first appeared, but there are two reasonable approaches for dealing with sealants in the DMF system. One view holds that the sealed tooth is not restored in the classic sense and should therefore be considered sound. The other contends that it has required hands-on, one-to-one dental attention and so should be considered a filled tooth. Probably the best way to deal with sealed teeth is to put them into a category by themselves, S for sealed. The DMFS index would then become DMFSS. Depending on the purpose of a given study, the S teeth can be left separate, included with the F teeth, or regarded as sound.

With modern preventive and restorative technology, the DMF index is really outdated as a measure of caries attack; the index may be more valid as a measure of treatment received. It is philosophically questionable to use a disease index that is so dependent on the treatment judgments of many practitioners, and combining previous treatment (i.e., the M and F components) with current treatment need (the D component) is unsuitable for surveillance purposes (see Chapter 4). A measure of caries activity would be preferable for many purposes, but approaches to scoring caries activity are still based on clinical acumen.[41] Until a more objective measure is developed and accepted, the DMF index will continue to be used. The results of its use, however, should always be interpreted with care.

CRITERIA FOR DIAGNOSING CORONAL CARIES

There is no global consensus on the criteria for diagnosing dental caries, despite a vast quantity of words on the subject. Different traditions about defining a lesion in the gray area, where it is difficult to tell whether the disease is irreversibly established or not, have grown up and are still adhered to. Apart from the inherent problem of diagnosing a borderline lesion, the major philosophical issue is how to score an early carious lesion that has not yet become cav-itated, whether diagnosed clinically or radiographically. Such a lesion appears as a discolored fissure without loss of substance, as a "white spot" on visible smooth surfaces, or radiographically as an early interproximal shadow. The issue is that not all noncavitated lesions progress to become dentinal lesions requiring restorative treatment; a good proportion of them remain static or even remineralize, especially smooth surface lesions.[43] These lesions are thus reversible, as opposed to a dentinal lesion, which is generally considered irreversible. Because there are usually more noncavitated than cavitated lesions at any one time in both high-caries and low-caries populations,[9,23,44] the decision as to whether to include or exclude them, and how to express them if included, can make a substantial difference in the oral health profiles obtained.

Examples of these two different approaches to diagnostic criteria for dental caries are shown in Box 15-2. Traditionally, European investigators have recorded caries on a scale that extends through the full range of disease from the earliest detectable noncavitated lesion through to pulpal involvement.[3] The criteria in Box 15-2 are based on those first published by the World Health Organization (WHO) in 1979[54] and now usually referred to as the *D1-D3 scale*. Clinical researchers in Europe have expanded on this concept to produce a scale with up to 10 points, combining increasing depths of lesion development with clinical signs of activity or inactivity.[37] On the other hand, investigators in North America, Britain, and the other English-speaking countries have traditionally recorded caries as a dichotomous condition, meaning that caries is diagnosed only as present or absent. (We refer to this as the *dichotomous scale*.) In dichotomous recording, caries is only noted when it has reached the level of dentinal involvement,[20] that is, the D3 level. Use of the D1-D3 scale requires that the teeth be dried and be given a longer, more meticulous survey examination. Although there are more diagnostic decisions to make when the D1-D3 scale is used, adequate examiner reliability can be maintained when examiners have been trained in this system.[43]

The D1-D3 scale is extremely valuable in research studies on dental caries, because it permits identification of lesion progression as well

---

BOX 15-2 Criteria for Diagnosis of Caries Through the Full Range of Lesion Development (D1-D3 Scale) Compared With Criteria for Diagnosis at the Dentinal Lesion Stage Only (Dichotomous Scale)[20,44,55]

Diagnosis through the Full Range of Caries: the D1-D3 scale

0. Surface sound. No evidence of treated or untreated clinical caries (slight staining allowed in an otherwise sound fissure).

D1. Initial caries. No clinically detectable loss of substance. For pits and fissures, there may be significant staining, discoloration, or rough spots in the enamel that do not catch the explorer, but loss of substance cannot be positively diagnosed. For smooth surfaces, these may be white, opaque areas with loss of luster.

D2. Enamel caries. Demonstrable loss of tooth substance in pits, fissures, or on smooth surfaces, but no softened floor or wall or undermined enamel. The texture of the material within the cavity may be chalky or crumbly, but there is no evidence that cavitation has penetrated the dentin.

D3. Caries of dentin. Detectably softened floor, undermined enamel, or a softened wall, or the tooth has a temporary filling. On approximal surfaces, the explorer point must enter a lesion with certainty.

D4. Pulpal involvement. Deep cavity with probable pulpal involvement. Pulp should not be probed. (Usually included with D3 in data analysis.)

Diagnosis at the Dentinal Lesion Stage Only: the Dichotomous Scale

Pits and fissures on the occlusal, vestibular, and lingual surfaces are carious when the explorer "catches" after insertion with moderate to firm pressure and when the "catch" is accompanied by one or more of the following signs of decay:

1. Softness at the base of the area.
2. Opacity adjacent to the area* providing evidence of undermining or demineralization.
3. Softened enamel adjacent to the area that may be scraped away by the explorer.

*The area should be diagnosed as sound when there is apparent evidence of demineralization but no evidence of softness.

---

as initiation. Research questions on the conditions under which early lesions progress, regress, or remain static can thus be answered only with the use of such a measurement scale. Its application demands meticulous examiner training because D1 lesions are capable of remineralizing back to sound enamel, and it thus becomes difficult to differentiate examiner error from natural phenomena. There is less consensus on whether the D1-D3 scale should be used in large-scale surveys, and there are no examples of this having been done. Arguments can be made both ways, but on balance we believe that more benefit is to be gained if surveys continue to diagnose caries at the D3 level only, that is, using the dichotomous scale.[12]

Caries diagnosis by clinical means, irrespective of the criteria adopted, has traditionally used visual-tactile methods; that is, it has used the explorer as well as vision. Indeed, the criteria listed in the dichotomous scale in Box 15-2 explicitly require use of the explorer. Our current understanding of caries, however, indicates that

routine use of the explorer in this way is likely to damage the enamel matrix of noncavitated lesions where remineralization is taking place. As a result, European criteria for diagnosing caries in the 1990s have moved toward exclusively visual criteria.[42] Initial studies with a group of dentists using extracted teeth that later were sectioned and histologically examined found that use of the explorer did not add to the value of visual diagnosis.[34,35] The series of surveys for monitoring caries in British children that is carried out by the British Association for the Study of Community Dentistry, really a surveillance system, uses the exclusively visual approach in its protocol. Caries is recorded at the D3 level, and the criterion for caries is the following: "if, in the opinion of a trained examiner, after visual inspection there is a carious lesion into dentine," then caries is recorded.[43] Use of this criterion requires extensive examiner training and meticulous drying of the teeth. The third National Health and Nutrition Examination Survey (NHANES III) in the United States, 1988-94, retained the traditional dichotomous criteria shown in Box 15-2.[25]

Caries diagnosis is also complicated by *hidden caries*, the name given to dentinal caries found radiographically beneath an apparently sound occlusal surface.[30,43,52] This condition is poorly understood, although it is hardly rare; studies found hidden caries in 7.5% of a group of Dutch children[53] and 2%-5% of Lithuanian children.[37] Some see it as a by-product of the fluoride age, in which the original break in the enamel remineralizes before the dentinal lesion has reached the pulp, but its natural history is really unknown. Additional research on this condition is clearly needed. The possibility of hidden caries has led to a further look at the use of radiographs for caries diagnosis at a time when they generally are not employed in caries epidemiologic studies and clinical trials for ethical reasons (unnecessary radiation exposure when not used in the course of treatment), costs, and the risk of bias that comes from the refusal of some study participants to undergo radiography.

Newer methods of caries diagnosis, such as fiberoptic transillumination, electrical conductance, and laser fluorescence, have shown promise[2,30,36] and may find a role in epidemiologic study as well as in patient care. These diagnostic aids do not change the philosophical approach to measuring caries, although if reliable they will permit noncavitated lesions to be detected at earlier stages of development. Whether this is always necessary or not depends on the aims of the given study and the purposes for which the resulting data will be used.

ROOT CARIES

The criteria most frequently used to diagnose root caries were first described in 1980.[7] The clinical examination was carried out after a thorough prophylaxis, after which root caries was diagnosed according to the criteria shown in Box 15-3. Although these criteria have proved to be versatile, there are several diagnostic issues in root caries that have not yet been fully settled. These problems include the lack of a universally accepted case definition,[8] difficulty in differentiating active from nonactive lesions,[27] and uncertainties in diagnostic reliability.[6]

Root lesions are frequently difficult to detect because many appear as small, discrete lesions

---

BOX 15-3 Criteria For Diagnosing Root Surface Caries[6]

- A discrete, well-defined, and discolored soft area is present.
- The explorer enters easily and displays some resistance to withdrawal.
- The lesion is located either at the cemento-enamel junction or wholly on the root surface.
- Restored root lesions are counted only if it was obvious that the lesion originated at the cemento-enamel junction or is confined to the root surface completely.

---

on a single root surface rather than circumscribing a root.[47] Although most lesions occur on exposed root surfaces, around 15% of all root lesions have been found on surfaces without gingival recession, although of course there is loss of periodontal attachment.[13,33,47] It is not yet clear whether these root lesions form in periodontal pockets or whether an exposed root surface later becomes covered by the overgrowth of inflamed gingiva. Problems in locating the cemento-enamel junction because of obliteration by restorations or calculus can add to the diagnostic difficulties.[27]

The extent of root caries can be expressed as a simple prevalence figure, meaning the proportion of a defined population with at least one root lesion, and as the mean number of carious or restored root lesions per person (i.e., a DFS count). To provide the most complete profile of root caries activity, however, these values should be accompanied by the number of missing teeth and by Root Caries Index (RCI) scores.

The RCI, first described in 1980,[26] was intended to make the simple prevalence measures more specific by including the concept of teeth at risk (in contrast to the DMF index). A tooth was considered to be at risk of root caries if enough gingival recession had occurred to expose part of the cemental surface to the oral environment. The RCI is computed by scoring root lesions and restorations and noting teeth with gingival recession, according to the following formula:

$$\frac{(\text{Root surfaces: decayed} + \text{filled}) \times 100}{(\text{Root surfaces with loss of periodontal attachment: decayed} + \text{filled} + \text{sound})}$$

Table 15-1 Proposed case definitions of early childhood caries and severe early childhood caries[15]

Age in Months	Early Childhood Caries*	Severe Early Childhood Caries*
<12	1 or more dmf surfaces	1 or more smooth dmf surfaces
12-23	1 or more dmf surfaces	1 or more smooth dmf surfaces
24-35	1 or more dmf surfaces	1 or more smooth dmf surfaces
36-47	1 or more dmf surfaces	1 or more cavitated, filled, or missing (due to caries) smooth surfaces in primary maxillary anterior teeth *or* dmfs ≥4
48-59	1 or more dmf surfaces	1 or more cavitated, filled, or missing (due to caries) smooth surfaces in primary maxillary anterior teeth *or* dmfs ≥5
60-71	1 or more dmf surfaces	1 or more cavitated, filled, or missing (due to caries) smooth surfaces in primary maxillary anterior teeth *or* dmfs ≥6

*Any carious lesion, whether noncavitated (d1) or cavitated (d2-d4), tooth missing due to caries (m), or filled surface (f). Primary teeth only.

The index can be computed for an individual, for particular tooth types, or for a population at large. An RCI of 7% means that, of all teeth with gingival recession, 7% were decayed or filled on the root surfaces. As with any index scores, results are most useful if a distribution measure is also presented. The RCI does not take into account the time at risk of an exposed root surface; a root surface that has been exposed for years is obviously at more risk than one just recently exposed.

The original description of the RCI acknowledged the chance of underestimation due to exclusion of subgingival lesions,[26] but at the time these were considered unusual. As noted earlier, however, some 15% or more of root lesions since recorded are subgingival. Accordingly, it is now recommended that the RCI be applied to both supragingival and subgingival lesions but that the scores for each type of lesion be recorded separately.[28]

EARLY CHILDHOOD CARIES

Early childhood caries (ECC) is the name given to extensive carious attack in infants and young children that seems to be associated with regular exposure to sugar, often from fluid in a bottle. Its dietary associations have resulted in a plethora of names for the condition: baby bottle tooth decay, nursing caries, labial caries, and others.[24] This proliferation of names, some of which include the presumed etiology, has not helped our understanding of the condition, and for that reason the name *early childhood caries* is recommended.

A practical case definition of ECC has been slow to develop, and measurement cannot be validly carried out without a case definition. In an effort to bring some order out of chaos, a 1999 workshop set age-related criteria for ECC. The workshop took the view that *any* caries in children was ECC, and to define the severe categories (i.e., obvious caries in incisors and molars) that most dental people think of, the workshop introduced the term *severe early childhood caries* (S-ECC). The suggested criteria for these conditions are shown in Table 15-1.

These guidelines are a step in the right direction. Although some confusion may arise from application of the term *ECC* to *any* caries in children up to 6 years of age, the view that caries in young children is not normal is one to be encouraged. The inclusion of the age relationship also helps to clarify our view of the condition. These guidelines will probably be refined over time, but for now they are clearly a step forward in research on the subject, and their use is to be recommended.

CARIES TREATMENT NEEDS

Assessment of the caries treatment needs of a group, at first glance, appears to be nothing more than the D segment of a mean DMF score assessed from a survey. This approach, however, has been shown not to work for the following reasons:

- Criteria used to diagnose caries in a survey usually are not the same as those used by practitioners in forming a patient's treatment plan.

- Patients' own perceived needs, level of interest in their dental conditions, and ability or willingness to pay all influence the level of treatment carried out.
- A practitioner has to judge whether a minor lesion will develop into a major lesion over time, and whether a lesion in a primary tooth can safely remain untreated for the life of the tooth. A survey scores a tooth by how it appears at the time of the survey.
- Treatment philosophies change with expanding knowledge and technologic developments; a treatment that is standard today may not be so tomorrow.

Because surveys are usually conducted under less than ideal conditions, relative to the dental office, surveys would be expected to detect fewer carious lesions than practitioners do.[5] However, that begs the question of which assessment is "correct." Field surveys can miss early lesions, but practitioners can also overtreat. To add to the uncertainty, treatment plans for the same patients have been shown to vary drastically from dentist to dentist.[4,17,39,40]

The difficulties in determining treatment need through survey were illustrated in an important series of reports from Scotland. They began with a 1978 national dental survey in Britain, in the course of which 720 dentate adults in Scotland agreed to permit their dental records to be followed over subsequent years. After 3 years, records showed that, although 863 teeth in this group had been assessed as needing restorative care in the survey, 3108 actually had been restored. One might think that this finding could be explained by lesions missed under the poorer survey conditions, but if that explanation is accepted then the next finding has no logic: of the 863 teeth classified as needing restorative treatment in the survey, only 271 (31%) were among the 3108 restored.[39] This shows that the care carried out, rather than being an extension of the survey results, in fact bore no relation to them. Findings were similar for prosthetic treatment.[16]

Dental needs in the United States were assessed by examiners in the first National Health and Nutrition Examination Survey (NHANES I) of 1971-74, and 65% of the population were judged as being in need of care.[48] A similar assessment was made in the first national survey of schoolchildren in 1979-80, in which 37% of

schoolchildren were judged to be in need of restorative care.[49] The validity of these figures is debatable, and they have received little use. In later national surveys treatment needs assessments were not carried out.[50,51]

WHO includes a subjective treatment need assessment by the examiner as part of its Pathfinder survey method,[55] although it has not been determined how well these estimates approximate treatment actually carried out. WHO also has developed a broad-based approach to determining needs in low-income countries through what it calls a *situation analysis*, an enhancement of Pathfinder survey data with information on population trends, school enrollment figures, per capita income, and health care resources.[56]

REFERENCES

1. Ainsworth NJ. Mottled teeth. Br Dent J 1933;55:233-50, 274.
2. Anttonen V, Seppä L, Hausen H. Clinical study on the use of the laser fluorescence device DIAGNOdent for detection of occlusal caries in children. Caries Res 2003;37:17-23.
3. Backer Dirks O, Houwink B, Kwant GW. The results of 6½ years of artificial drinking water in the Netherlands; the Tiel-Culemborg experiment. Arch Oral Biol 1961;5:284-300.
4. Bader JD, Shugars DA. Agreement among dentists' recommendations for restorative treatment. J Dent Res 1993;72:891-6.
5. Bader JD, Shugars DA, Rozier RG. Relationship between epidemiologic coronal caries assessments and practitioners' treatment recommendations in adults. Community Dent Oral Epidemiol 1993;21:96-101.
6. Banting DW. Diagnosis and prediction of root caries. Adv Dent Res 1993;7:80-6.
7. Banting DW, Ellen RP, Fillery ED. Prevalence of root surface caries among institutionalized older persons. Community Dent Oral Epidemiol 1980;8:84-8.
8. Billings RJ, Banting DW. Future directions for root caries research. Gerodontology 1993;10:114-9.
9. Bjarnason S, Kohler B, Ranggard L. Dental caries in a group of 15- to 16-year-olds from Göteborg. Part I. Swed Dent J 1992;16:143-9.
10. Bodecker CF, Bodecker HWC. A practical index of the varying susceptibility to dental caries in man. Dent Cosmos 1931;73:707-16.
11. Bratthall D. Introducing the Significant Caries Index together with a proposal for a new oral health goal for 12-year-olds. Int Dent J 2000;50:378-84.
12. Burt BA. How useful are cross-sectional data from surveys of dental caries? Community Dent Oral Epidemiol 1997;25:36-41.
13. Burt BA, Ismail AI, Eklund SA. Root caries in an optimally fluoridated and a high-fluoride community. J Dent Res 1986;65:1154-8.

14. Dean HT, Arnold FA Jr, Elvove E. Domestic water and dental caries. V. Additional studies of the relation of fluoride domestic waters to dental caries experience in 4,425 white children aged 12-14 years of age in 13 cities in 4 states. Public Health Rep 1942;57:1155-79.

15. Drury TF, Horowitz AM, Ismail AI, et al. Diagnosing and reporting early childhood caries for research purposes. J Public Health Dent 1999;59:192-7.

16. Eddie S, Elderton RJ. Comparison of dental status determined in an epidemiological survey with prosthetic treatment need. Community Dent Oral Epidemiol 1983;11:271-7.

17. Espelid I, Tveit AB, Haugejorden O, Riordan PJ. Variation in radiographic interpretation and restorative treatment decisions on approximal caries among dentists in Norway. Community Dent Oral Epidemiol 1985;13:26-9.

18. Grainger RM. Epidemiological data. In: Chilton NW. Design and analysis in dental and oral research. 1st ed. Philadelphia: Lippincott, 1967:311-53.

19. Gruebbel AO. A measure of dental caries prevalence and treatment service for deciduous teeth. J Dent Res 1944;23:163-8.

20. Horowitz HS. Clinical trials of preventives for dental caries. J Public Health Dent 1972;32:229-33.

21. Hyatt TP. Report of an examination made of two thousand one hundred and one high school pupils. Dent Cosmos 1920;52:507-11.

22. Hyatt TP. Prophylactic odontotomy. Dent Cosmos 1923;65:234-41.

23. Ismail AI, Brodeur JM, Gagnon P, et al. Prevalence of non-cavitated and cavitated carious lesions in a random sample of 7-9-year-old schoolchildren in Montreal, Quebec. Community Dent Oral Epidemiol 1992;20:250-5.

24. Ismail AI, Sohn W. A systematic review of clinical diagnostic criteria of early childhood caries. J Public Health Dent 1999;59:171-91.

25. Kaste LM, Selwitz RH, Oldakowski RJ, et al. Coronal caries in the primary and permanent dentition of children and adolescents 1-17 years of age: United States, 1988-1991. J Dent Res 1996;75(Spec Issue):631-41.

26. Katz RV. Assessing root caries in populations: The evolution of the Root Caries Index. J Public Health Dent 1980;40:7-16.

27. Katz RV. The clinical diagnosis of root caries: Issues for the clinician and the researcher. Am J Dent 1995;8:335-41.

28. Katz RV. The RCI revisited after 15 years: Used, reinvented, modified, debated, and natural logged. J Public Health Dent 1996;56:28-34.

29. Katz RV, Meskin LH. Testing the internal and external validity of a simplified dental caries index on an adult population. Community Dent Oral Epidemiol 1976;4:227-31.

30. Kidd EA, Ricketts DNJ, Pitts NB. Occlusal caries diagnosis; a changing challenge for clinicians and epidemiologists. J Dent 1993;21:323-31.

31. Kingman A. A method of utilizing the subject's initial caries experience to increase efficiency in caries clinical trials. Community Dent Oral Epidemiol 1979;7:87-90.

32. Klein H, Palmer CE, Knutson JW. Studies on dental caries: I. Dental status and dental needs of elementary school children. Public Health Rep 1938;53:751-65.

33. Locker D, Slade GD, Leake JL. Prevalence of and factors associated with root decay in older adults in Canada. J Dent Res 1989;68:768-72.

34. Lussi A. Validity of diagnostic and treatment decisions of fissure caries. Caries Res 1991;25:296-303.

35. Lussi A. Comparison of different methods for the diagnosis of fissure caries without cavitation. Caries Res 1993;27:409-16.

36. Lussi A, Firestone A, Schoenberg V, et al. In vivo diagnosis of fissure caries using a new electrical resistance monitor. Caries Res 1995;29:81-7.

37. Machiulskiene V, Nyvad B, Baelum V. A comparison of clinical and radiographic caries diagnoses in posterior teeth of 12-year-old Lithuanian children. Caries Res 1999;33:340-8.

38. Nishi M, Stjernsward J, Carlsson P, Bratthall D. Caries experience of some countries and areas expressed by the Significant Caries Index. Community Dent Oral Epidemiol 2002;30:296-301.

39. Nuttall NM. Capability of a national epidemiological survey to predict General Dental Service treatment. Community Dent Oral Epidemiol 1983;11:296-301.

40. Nuttall NM, Pitts NB, Fyffe HE. Assessment of reports by dentists of their restorative treatment thresholds. Community Dent Oral Epidemiol 1993;21:273-8.

41. Nyvad B, Machiulskiene V, Baelum V. Reliability of a new caries diagnostic system differentiating between active and inactive caries lesions. Caries Res 1999;33:252-60.

42. Pitts NB. Clinical diagnosis of dental caries: A European perspective. J Dent Educ 2001;65:972-8.

43. Pitts NB. Current methods and criteria for caries diagnosis in Europe. J Dent Educ 1993;57:409-14.

44. Pitts NB, Fyffe HE. The effect of varying diagnostic thresholds upon clinical caries data for a low prevalence group. J Dent Res 1988;67:592-6.

45. Poulsen S, Horowitz H. An evaluation of a hierarchical method of describing the pattern of dental caries attack. Community Dent Oral Epidemiol 1974;2:7-11.

46. Sheiham A, Maizels J, Maizels A. New composite indicators of dental health. Community Dent Health 1987;4:407-14.

47. Stamm JW, Banting DW, Imrey PB. Adult root caries survey of two similar communities with contrasting natural water fluoride levels. J Am Dent Assoc 1990;120:143-9.

48. US Public Health Service, National Center for Health Statistics. Basic data on dental examination findings of persons aged 1-74 years; United States. DHEW Publication No. (PHS) 79-1662, Series 11 No. 214. Washington DC: Government Printing Office, 1979.

49. US Public Health Service, National Institute of Dental Research. Dental treatment needs of United States children. NIH Publication No. 83-2246. Washington DC: Government Printing Office, 1982.

50. US Public Health Service, National Institute of Dental Research. Oral health of United States adults; national findings. NIH Publication No. 87-2868. Washington DC: Government Printing Office, 1987.

51. US Public Health Service, National Institute of Dental Research. Oral health of United States children. NIH Publication No. 89-2247. Washington DC: Government Printing Office, 1989.

52. Weerheijm KL, Groen HJ, Bast AJ, et al. Clinically detected occlusal dentine caries: A radiographic comparison. Caries Res 1992;26:305-9.

53. Weerheijm KL, Gruythuysen RJ, van Amerongen WE. Prevalence of hidden caries. ASDC J Dent Child 1992;59:408-12.

54. World Health Organization. A guide to oral health epidemiological investigations. Geneva: WHO, 1979.

55. World Health Organization. Oral health surveys; basic methods. 4th ed. Geneva: WHO, 1997.

56. World Health Organization. Planning oral health services. WHO Offset Publication No. 53. Geneva: WHO, 1980.

57. World Health Organization. The Significant Caries Index (SiC), website: http://www.whocollab.od.mah.se/expl/sic.html. Accessed December 11, 2003

16

Measuring Periodontal Diseases

MEASURING GINGIVITIS
MEASURING PERIODONTITIS
PERIODONTAL TREATMENT NEEDS

PLAQUE AND CALCULUS
PARTIAL-MOUTH PERIODONTAL
  MEASUREMENTS

Although the DMF (decayed, missing, and filled teeth) index for caries has remained stable over a 50-year period, the philosophical basis for measuring periodontal diseases has changed several times over a shorter time span. In the early days of modern periodontal research (i.e., the 1950s and 1960s), "periodontal disease" was viewed as a single entity that began with gingivitis and progressed to periodontitis and tooth loss. This view is now obsolete (see Chapter 21), so that indexes based on it are considered invalid. The separate clinical measures now used for gingivitis and periodontitis were first described some 40 years ago, and they are still important. They will likely be joined soon by some measures based on molecular biology as knowledge in this area continues to grow rapidly.

MEASURING GINGIVITIS

Gingivitis is inflammation of the gingivae without involvement of the deeper supporting tissues. The oldest reversible index is the P-M-A (standing for Papillary-Marginal-Attached), which dates from immediately after World War II.[41] As the inflammatory process became better understood, it gave way to the Gingival Index (GI) of Löe and Silness[38] in the early 1960s, an index that is still used. The GI grades the gingiva on the mesial, distal, buccal, and lingual surfaces of the teeth. Each area is scored on an ordinal scale of 0-3 according to the criteria shown in Box 16-1. The GI has been used to score selected teeth in the mouth[56] as well as all

erupted teeth.[37] The GI, an index of gingivitis that takes no account of deeper changes in the periodontium, is sufficiently sensitive to distinguish between groups with little and with severe gingivitis, although it may not discriminate as well between groups in the middle ranges.

Gingival bleeding after gentle probing has become a standard measure of gingivitis in clinical trials. Although visual assessments of inflammation (color, swelling) are subjective, the appearance of spots of blood after the probe is gently run around the gingival margin is more sensitive[21] and more objective in those sites that are difficult to view directly.[22] Validity against the GI has also been demonstrated.[43] The major area of subjectivity with use of a gingival bleeding index is the "gentle probing," which has been shown to vary between 3 and 130 g for different examiners.[49]

A further refinement of the bleeding indexes came with the Eastman Interdental Bleeding Index,[14] which may be more sensitive than other measures of papillary bleeding.[15] Gingival bleeding measures that do not carry any particular name are collectively designated by the acronym *BOP* (bleeding on probing).

The use of gingival bleeding indexes, as opposed to visual determination of gingivitis, is not recommended in public health programs for three reasons:

1. This degree of sensitivity is rarely required in surveys, surveillance, or screening; it may be needed in cohort and case-control studies.

0: Normal gingiva
1: Mild inflammation—slight change in color, slight edema; no bleeding on probing
2: Moderate inflammation—redness, edema, and glazing; bleeding on probing
3: Severe inflammation—marked redness and edema; ulceration; tendency to spontaneous bleeding

2. Such indexes have uncertain discriminatory power in field conditions.[39]
3. Concerns about infection control make the deliberate inducement of gingival bleeding outside the clinic hard to justify.

The Modified Gingival Index (MGI) was developed to eliminate the use of bleeding on probing while still providing high visual sensitivity for incipient gingivitis.[36] Gingivitis is an area in which the development of valid nonclinical measures would be highly beneficial.

MEASURING PERIODONTITIS

Periodontitis is a family of related diseases that differ in natural history, and response to therapy but that are characterized by a common underlying chain of events.[48] These commonalities, and their clinical expression, permit valid clinical measurement by similar procedures, basically measurement of clinical attachment loss (CAL) and probing depth. Periodontitis is a bacterially induced inflammation of the gingival tissues together with some loss of both the attachment of the periodontal ligament and bony support. The clinical manifestations of periodontitis come from the interaction between bacterial infection and the host response.

Many early epidemiologic studies of periodontal diseases were based on radiographic surveys of alveolar bone loss.[16,54,55] However, radiography, although a standard diagnostic procedure in periodontitis clinical trials and patient care, is impractical and probably unethical in field studies. The attempt was therefore made to develop reversible indexes that were both sensitive and clinically manageable in field conditions. In this group, the most widely used periodontal index for many years was the Periodontal Index (PI), first described by Russell in 1956.[53]

The PI was a composite index, meaning that it scored both gingivitis and periodontitis on the same scale. This represented the thinking of the time, but modern understanding has shown the PI to be invalid because it does not include evaluation of CAL, grades all pockets of 3 mm or more equally, and scores gingivitis and periodontitis on the same weighted scale. Its compression of all information into a group mean also fails to illuminate the disease distribution, and a primary research interest today is why some people have no disease and others have severe disease. However, in the 1960s, the PI was viewed as an ideal field index and was used in a series of epidemiologic studies that correlated disease scores with clinical and social determinants. These correlations (see Chapter 21) soon became accepted as basic knowledge.

The same fundamental problem of a composite index was evident in the Periodontal Disease Index (PDI), intended as a more sensitive version of the PI for use in clinical trials.[51] Although the PDI is also no longer used, the indirect method of measuring CAL that Ramfjord described then is still employed today. The PDI also gave us the "Ramfjord teeth," a set of six teeth taken to represent the whole mouth during examination. The Ramfjord teeth are the maxillary right first molar, left central incisor, and left first bicuspid, and the mandibular left first molar, right central incisor, and right first bicuspid. Ramfjord chose this group of teeth to save time in clinical examinations. (Partial-mouth recording is discussed later in this chapter.)

In field studies today periodontitis is still measured by Ramfjord's technique for the indirect measurement of CAL.[51] The approach is shown graphically in Fig. 16-1. First, the examiner measures probing depth from the gingival crest to the base of the pocket. Second, the cemento-enamel junction is located and the depth from this junction to the gingival crest is recorded. The difference between these values gives an indirect measure of CAL. These measurements are usually carried out at between two and six sites per tooth, depending on the pur-

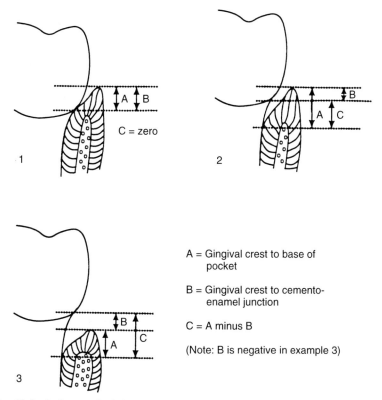

A = Gingival crest to base of
pocket

B = Gingival crest to cemento-
enamel junction

C = A minus B

(Note: B is negative in example 3)

Fig. 16-1 Indirect method of measuring loss of periodontal attachment and pocket depth.[51]

pose of the study, either for selected teeth or for the whole dentition. It is an exacting process: measuring six sites per tooth for an intact dentition can take 30-40 minutes per examination, even for an experienced examiner.

The Extent and Severity Index (ESI) records the percentage of sites with a CAL greater than 1 mm and the mean CAL for those affected sites.[13] When amended to set a cutoff value of 2 mm, it has yielded some useful summary information.[9] Despite its name, the ESI is a method of summarizing data rather than a true index. Its measurements are made by the Ramfjord method.

Measurement of any disease is based on a case definition, and the uncertainty in the case definition for periodontitis is clearly part of the reason we still use a recording procedure that is almost 50 years old. A case definition for periodontitis needs to establish the following:

- What depth of CAL at any one site constitutes evidence of disease processes

- How many such sites need to be present in a mouth to establish disease presence
- How probing depth and BOP are to be included in the case definition

In addressing the first issue, allowance also must be make for examiner variation, which can confuse efforts to measure CAL progression. Even though measurements of pocket depth are repeatable to within 1 mm more than 90% of the time,[29] the standard deviation of repeated CAL measurements of the same site by an experienced examiner with a manual probe is around 0.8 mm.[24] Accordingly, change in attachment level in a clinical study must be at least 2 mm (i.e., two to three times the standard deviation) before the investigators can be confident that they are seeing real change rather than measurement error.[25,34] CAL progression of at least 3 mm over a given time period has been the criterion for change in some studies.[11,24,26]

Even the introduction of computerized, constant-force probes[28] has not changed these issues much. Computerized probes are widely used in clinical studies,[52] but there is little difference in the reliability of measurements taken with manual and with computerized probes for most examiners.[23,45]

The problems inherent in clinical measurement have led researchers to look for *markers* of periodontitis. The most promising candidates are the inflammatory cytokines expressed in gingival crevicular fluid (GCF) as part of the host response to inflammation, a number of which have been associated with active disease.[44,46] These cytokines include prostaglandin E_2, tumor necrosis factor-α, interleukin-1α, interleukin-1β, and others. Although it has been documented for some time that these and other constituents of GCF are associated with inflammatory response,[31-33] actually quantifying these associations and determining the sensitivity of the measures (i.e., the extent to which the quantity of expressed cytokine increases or decreases as inflammation increases or decreases) is proving difficult. To date, measurement of periodontitis by means of inflammatory cytokines in GCF is still experimental, but this field is developing rapidly, and practical and efficient tests are likely to emerge.

PERIODONTAL TREATMENT NEEDS

Any assessment of periodontal treatment needs in a population has the same limitations that are seen with caries. Treatment plans are subjective, often depending on some dentist-patient factors that are not part of a clinical examination, and standard treatment for a given condition can change quickly as knowledge develops (e.g., treatment of periodontal pockets has substantially shifted from surgical removal of pockets to scaling and root planing). Even so, a number of methods aimed at assessing periodontal treatment needs have been developed over the years,[10,58] culminating in the Community Periodontal Index of Treatment Needs (CPITN).

The CPITN was first described in 1982,[3] and with some promotion by the World Health Organization (WHO) it received worldwide use.[2] It differs from earlier indexes in several ways. The most obvious is that it requires use of a special periodontal probe, which has a 0.5 mm diameter ball at its tip, a black band for visibility between 3.5 mm and 5.5 mm, and circular markings at 8.5 mm and 11.5 mm. The purpose of the ball is to assist in feeling subgingival calculus and to help prevent the probe from being pushed through inflammatory tissue at the base of a pocket. Probing pressure is recommended to be no more than 20 g (described as the pressure at which the probe can be inserted under a fingernail without discomfort). Another difference is that the CPITN originally was used to categorize people into treatment-need groups rather than to compute mean values. Codes to be used with the index are shown in Box 16-2.

Widespread use of the CPITN has produced substantial contributions to WHO's Global Oral Health Data Bank (see Chapter 21), and a number of national dental associations have encouraged use of the CPITN by its practitioner members. In the United States, the Indian Health Service used the CPITN in its treatment planning for some years. Then the American Dental Association began to promote a slightly modified version known as the Periodontal Screening Record (PSR).[42] Another modification of the CPITN appeared in Britain, called the British Periodontal Examination, or BPE.[47] The validity of the CPITN/PSR continues to be debated; it appears that the index underestimates in some areas and overestimates in others.[5-7] The CPITN/PSR is not a research tool and thus should not be used as a measure of periodontitis in research studies.[8]

The index is now referred to as the Community Periodontal Index, or CPI. This

---

BOX 16-2 Codes and Criteria for the Community Periodontal Index Described by the World Health Organization[59]

0: Healthy gingiva.
1: Bleeding observed, directly or by using the mouth mirror, after "sensing" (i.e., gentle probing).
2: Calculus felt during probing but all the black area of the probe visible (3.5-5.5 mm from ball tip).
3: Pocket 4 or 5 mm (gingival margin situated on black area of probe, i.e., 3.5-5.5 mm from probe tip).
4: Pocket >6 mm (black area of probe not visible).
X: Excluded segment (less than two teeth present).
9: Not recorded.

change followed a workshop on the index in Manila in 1994.[2,30,47] The workshop recommended that the CPI remain the global standard for data on health planning but that the treatment need codes be eliminated because they had become obsolete in view of current treatment methods.[47] Hence the metamorphosis of the CPITN into the CPI. The current version of the CPI even includes optional use of CAL measurements.[59]

PLAQUE AND CALCULUS

Plaque and calculus are still measured in terms of quantity rather than quality, so most indexes are variations on that theme. These indexes have been around for some years.

The Simplified Oral Hygiene Index (OHI-S)[19,20] had wide use in surveys. It is quick and practical to apply, although it lacks sensitivity. The OHI-S scores calculus and plaque together, both supragingivally and subgingivally. The current focus on subgingival, rather than supragingival, plaque and calculus renders this index obsolete for most purposes today. A spin-off index is the Patient Hygiene Performance (PHP), in which plaque deposits are recorded in five different tooth surface zones after use of a disclosing tablet.[50]

Silness and Löe[56] developed the Plaque Index (PlI) to be used along with their GI. The same surfaces of the same teeth are scored as in the GI and a 0-3 ordinal scale is again used. The principal difference in approach between the PlI and the OHI-S is that the PlI scores plaque according to its thickness at the gingival margin rather than its coronal extent, a measure claimed to be more valid.[4] The PlI is still used; codes and criteria for this index are shown in Box 16-3.

WHO, after several earlier efforts to develop a simple measure of oral hygiene status,[58] settled for the measure of subgingival calculus that is part of the CPI.[59] Soft plaque deposits are ignored in the CPI. Because calculus appears to be the aspect of oral hygiene most closely associated with periodontitis,[40] a simple measure of its presence or absence, such as WHO uses in the CPI, is sufficient for many purposes. As always, however, the index chosen depends on the purpose of the given survey and the way the data are to be used.

> **BOX 16-3** Scores and Criteria for the Plaque Index[37]
>
> 0: No plaque in the gingival area.
> 1: A film of plaque adhering to the free gingival margin and adjacent area of the tooth. The plaque may only be recognized by running a probe across the tooth surface.
> 2: Moderate accumulation of soft deposits within the gingival pocket, on the gingival margin and/or adjacent tooth surface, which can be seen by the naked eye.
> 3: Abundance of soft matter within the gingival pocket and/or on the gingival margin and adjacent tooth surface.

The Volpe-Manhold Index, or VMI,[57] has been widely used in the United States in trials to test agents for plaque control and calculus inhibition.[35] It is intended to score new deposits of supragingival calculus, following a prophylaxis to remove all calculus, in clinical trials. (The reasoning is that all new calculus over a 3-month period, the approximate length of a clinical trial to test calculus-inhibiting products, will be supragingival.) The VMI scores calculus deposits on three planes (lingual, distal, and mesial) of each of the lower six anterior teeth. A probe is used to measure the linear extent of calculus in increments of 0.5 mm, from 0 to 5 mm. The tooth score is the sum of the scores in the three planes; patient total score is the sum of the tooth scores.

PARTIAL-MOUTH PERIODONTAL MEASUREMENTS

Because full-mouth examinations for gingival bleeding, CAL, plaque, and calculus can be time consuming, investigators have tried using various indexes on a subset of teeth to save time. The expectation is that the subset of teeth will act as a representative sample of all teeth in the mouth, yielding information that can be applied to the whole mouth but taking much less time to examine. Partial-mouth recording was pioneered by Ramfjord with the Ramfjord teeth subset in 1959,[51] and the CPI uses it today.

There is agreement that partial-mouth recording is valid for assessing plaque formation and gingivitis,[1,17,18,27] both of which are generalized conditions. Partial-mouth recording is less satisfactory for the site-specific conditions of CAL and pocketing, for which systematic underreporting occurs with this method.[1,6,17,27] Partial-mouth recording is adequate for surveys in which a degree of underestimation is an acceptable trade-off for lower costs, but it is not recommended for use in clinical trials or in any other situation that demands a high degree of precision in the data.

The National Institute of Dental and Craniofacial Research was criticized for the method it chose for measuring periodontitis in the National Survey of Employed Adults and Seniors in 1985-86. Two randomly chosen quadrants were examined, one maxillary and one mandibular, and probing depth and CAL were measured at two sites, the mesiobuccal and buccal. Critics thought this method would underestimate the true prevalence of periodontitis for the following reasons:

- The site specificity of periodontitis meant that severity would be underestimated if only two quadrants instead of the whole mouth were measured.
- Severity would be further underestimated by measurement of only two sites per tooth, and no lingual site at that.

That underestimation may be real, but the same method was used for measuring periodontitis in the third National Health and Nutrition Examination Survey (NHANES III) of 1988-94.[12] In fairness, the method may be sufficiently valid for the purposes of the survey, and it represents a great savings of time (and hence cost). It is a pragmatic measure, not recommended for analytic research but adequate for surveillance.

REFERENCES

1. Ainamo J, Ainamo A. Partial indices as indicators of the severity and prevalence of periodontal disease. Int Dent J 1985;35:322-6.
2. Ainamo J, Ainamo A. Validity and relevance of the criteria of the CPITN. Int Dent J 1994;44(Suppl 1):527-32.
3. Ainamo J, Barmes D, Beagrie G, et al. Development of the World Health Organization (WHO) Community Periodontal Index of Treatment Needs (CPITN). Int Dent J 1982;32:281-91.
4. Ainamo J, Bay I. Problems and proposals for recording gingivitis and plaque. Int Dent J 1975;25:229-35.
5. Almas K, Bulman JS, Newman HN. Assessment of periodontal status with CPITN and conventional periodontal indices. J Clin Periodontol 1991;18:654-9.
6. Aucott DM, Ashley FP. Assessment of the WHO partial recording approach in identification of individuals highly susceptible to periodontitis. Community Dent Oral Epidemiol 1986;14:152-5.
7. Baelum V, Manji F, Wanzala P, Fejerskov O. Relationship between CPITN and periodontal attachment loss findings in an adult population. J Clin Periodontol 1995;22:146-52.
8. Baelum V, Papapanou PN. CPITN and the epidemiology of periodontal disease. Community Dent Oral Epidemiol 1996;24:367-8.
9. Beck JD, Koch GG, Rozier RG, Tudor GE. Prevalence and risk indicators for periodontal attachment loss in a population of older community-dwelling blacks and whites. J Periodontol 1990;61:521-8.
10. Bellini HT, Gjermo P. Application of the Periodontal Treatment Need System (PTNS) in a group of Norwegian industrial employees. Community Dent Oral Epidemiol 1973;1:22-9.
11. Brown LJ, Beck JD, Rozier RG. Incidence of attachment loss in community-dwelling older adults. J Periodontol 1994;65:316-23.
12. Brown LJ, Brunelle JA, Kingman A. Periodontal status, 1988-91: Prevalence, extent, and demographic variation. J Dent Res 1996;75(Spec Issue):672-83.
13. Carlos JP, Wolfe MD, Kingman A. The Extent and Severity Index: A simple method for use in epidemiological studies of periodontal disease. J Clin Periodontol 1986;13:500-5.
14. Caton J, Polson AM. The Interdental Bleeding Index: A simplified procedure for monitoring gingival health. Compend Contin Educ Dent 1985;6:88-92.
15. Caton J, Polson A, Bouwsma O, et al. Associations between bleeding and visual signs of interdental gingival inflammation. J Periodontol 1988;59:722-7.
16. Dunning JM, Leach LB. Gingival-bone count: A method for epidemiological study of periodontal disease. J Dent Res 1960;39:506-13.
17. Fleiss JL, Park MH, Chilton NW, et al. Representativeness of the "Ramfjord teeth" for epidemiologic studies of gingivitis and periodontitis. Community Dent Oral Epidemiol 1987;15:221-4.
18. Goldberg P, Matsson L, Anderson H. Partial recording of gingivitis and dental plaque in children of different ages and in young adults. Community Dent Oral Epidemiol 1985;13:44-6.
19. Greene JC, Vermillion JR. The oral hygiene index: A method for classifying oral hygiene status. J Am Dent Assoc 1960;61:172-9.
20. Greene JC, Vermillion JR. The simplified oral hygiene index. J Am Dent Assoc 1964;68:7-13.
21. Greenstein G. The role of bleeding upon probing in the diagnosis of periodontal disease. J Periodontol 1984;55:684-8.
22. Greenstein G, Caton J, Polson AM. Histologic characteristics associated with bleeding after probing and visual signs of inflammation. J Periodontol 1981;52:420-5.

23. Grossi SG, Dunford RG, Ho A, et al. Sources of error for periodontal probing measurements. J Periodontal Res 1996;31:330-6.
24. Haffajee AD, Socransky SS. Attachment level changes in destructive periodontal diseases. J Clin Periodontol 1986;13:461-75.
25. Haffajee AD, Socransky SS, Goodson JM. Clinical parameters as predictors of destructive disease activity. J Clin Periodontol 1983;10:257-65.
26. Haffajee AD, Socransky SS, Smith C, Dibart S. Relation of baseline microbial parameters to future periodontal attachment loss. J Clin Periodontol 1991;18:744-50.
27. Hunt RJ. Efficiency of half-mouth examinations in estimating the prevalence of periodontal disease. J Dent Res 1987;66:1044-8.
28. Jeffcoat MK, Jeffcoat RL, Jens SC, Captain K. A new periodontal probe with automated cemento-enamel junction detection. J Clin Periodontol 1986;13:276-80.
29. Jeffcoat MK, Reddy MS. Advances in measurements of periodontal bone and attachment loss. Monogr Oral Sci 2000;17:56-72.
30. Khocht A, Zohn H, Deasy M, Chang KM. Assessment of periodontal status with PSR and traditional clinical periodontal examination. J Am Dent Assoc 1995;126:1658-65.
31. Kjeldsen M, Holmstrup P, Bendtzen K. Marginal periodontitis and cytokines: A review of the literature. J Periodontol 1993;64:1013-22.
32. Lamster IB. The host response in gingival crevicular fluid: Potential applications in periodontitis clinical trials. J Periodontol 1992;63(12 Suppl):1117-23.
33. Lee HJ, Kang IK, Chung CP, Choi SM. The subgingival microflora and gingival crevicular fluid cytokines in refractory periodontitis. J Clin Periodontol 1995;22:885-90.
34. Lindhe J, Haffajee AD, Socransky SS. Progression of periodontal disease in adult subjects in the absence of periodontal therapy. J Clin Periodontol 1983;10:433-42.
35. Lobene RR. A clinical comparison of the anticalculus effect of two commercially-available dentifrices. Clin Prev Dent 1987;9(4):3-8.
36. Lobene RR, Mankodi SM, Ciancio SG, et al. Correlation among gingival indices: A methodology study. J Periodontol 1989;60:159-62.
37. Löe H. The Gingival Index, the Plaque Index, and the Retention Index systems. J Periodontol 1967;38(Suppl):610-6.
38. Löe H, Silness J. Periodontal disease in pregnancy. I. Prevalence and severity. Acta Odontol Scand 1963;21:533-51.
39. Macaulay WR, Taylor GO, Lennon MA, et al. The suitability of three periodontal indices for epidemiological studies conducted for planning purposes. Community Dent Health 1988;5:113-9.
40. Mandel ID, Gaffar A. Calculus revisited. J Clin Periodontol 1986;13:249-57.

41. Massler M, Schour I, Chopra B. Occurrence of gingivitis in suburban Chicago schoolchildren. J Periodontol 1950;21:146-64.
42. Nasi JH. Background to, and implementation of, the Periodontal Screening and Recording (PSR) procedure in the USA. Int Dent J 1994;44(Suppl 1):585-8.
43. Nowicki D, Vogel RI, Melcer S, Deasy MJ. The gingival bleeding time index. J Periodontol 1981;52:260-2.
44. Offenbacher S, Collins JG, Yalda B, Haradon G. Role of prostaglandins in high-risk periodontitis patients. In: Genco R, et al, eds: Molecular pathogenesis of periodontal disease. Washington DC: American Society for Microbiology, 1994:203-13.
45. Osborn J, Stoltenberg J, Huso B, et al. Comparison of measurement variability using a standard and constant force periodontal probe. J Periodontol 1990;61:497-503.
46. Page RC. Host response tests for diagnosing periodontal disease. J Periodontol 1992;63(4 Suppl):356-66.
47. Page RC, Morrison EC. Summary of outcomes and recommendations of the workshop on CPITN. Int Dent J 1994;44(Suppl 1):589-94.
48. Page RC, Offenbacher S, Schroeder HE, et al. Advances in the pathogenesis of periodontitis: Summary of developments, clinical implications and future directions. Periodontol 2000 1997;14:216-48.
49. Polson AM, Caton JG. Current status of bleeding in the diagnosis of periodontal diseases. J Periodontol 1985;56(Spec Issue):1-3.
50. Podshadley AG, Haley JV. A method for evaluating oral hygiene performance. Public Health Rep 1968;83:259-64.
51. Ramfjord SP. Indices for prevalence and incidence of periodontal disease. J Periodontol 1959;30:51-9.
52. Reddy MS, Geurs NC, Jeffcoat RL, et al. Periodontal disease progression. J Periodontol 2000;71:1583-90.
53. Russell AL. A system of scoring for prevalence surveys of periodontal disease. J Dent Res 1956;35:350-9.
54. Sandler HC, Stahl SS. Measurement of periodontal disease prevalence. J Am Dent Assoc 1959;58:93-7.
55. Schei O, Waerhaug J, Lovdal A, Arno A. Alveolar bone loss as related to oral hygiene and age. J Periodontol 1959;30:7-16.
56. Silness J, Löe H. Periodontal disease in pregnancy. II. Correlation between oral hygiene and periodontal condition. Acta Odontol Scand 1964;22:112-35.
57. Volpe AR, Kupczak LJ, King WJ. In vivo calculus assessment. Part III. Scoring techniques, rate of calculus formation, partial mouth exams vs. full mouth exams, and intra-examiner reproducibility. Periodontics 1967;5:184-93.
58. World Health Organization. Oral health surveys; basic methods. 2nd ed. Geneva: WHO, 1977.
59. World Health Organization. Oral health surveys; basic methods. 4th ed. Geneva: WHO, 1997.

17 Measuring Dental Fluorosis

DEAN'S FLUOROSIS INDEX
TOOTH SURFACE INDEX OF FLUOROSIS
THYLSTRUP-FEJERSKOV INDEX

FLUOROSIS RISK INDEX
DEVELOPMENTAL DEFECTS OF DENTAL
  ENAMEL INDEX

This chapter describes methods for measuring dental fluorosis. Dental fluorosis is a hypomineralization of the dental enamel caused by excessive ingestion of fluoride during tooth development.[13] Depending on the quantity and timing of fluoride ingestion during this period, the clinical appearance of fluorosis can range from barely noticeable changes to an ugly brown stain with pitting and flaking of friable enamel.

DEAN'S FLUOROSIS INDEX

An index of fluorosis was needed when the initial investigations of fluorosis began in the 1930s (see Chapter 22). Dean's first Fluorosis Index set criteria for categorizing dental fluorosis on a seven-point ordinal scale: normal, questionable, very mild, mild, moderate, moderately severe, and severe. Dean used this seven-point scale for his Fluorosis Index for some years,[3,8] but by 1939 his experience led him to combine the "moderately severe" and "severe" categories into a single "severe" category.[9] By 1942 Dean had revised his Fluorosis Index into a six-point scale, including normal or unaffected enamel,[4] that still finds some use today. Dean's criteria for his revised version of the Fluorosis Index are shown in Box 17-1.

A spin-off of the Fluorosis Index was the Community Fluorosis Index (CFI), which Dean defined in 1935 by assigning arbitrary numerical values to his seven-point ordinal scale, again ranging from no fluorosis and borderline to severe and very severe.[6] Fig. 17-1 shows the dis-

tributional data from 10 communities[7] on which he based the CFI. Dean related this index to the concentration of fluoride in a water supply and was able to show a linear correlation, as one of his original charts demonstrates (Fig. 17-2). Dean also stated, although only in a footnote, that CFI scores below 0.4 were of "no public health significance."[5] With cosmetic awareness likely to be greater now than it was in the 1930s, however, Dean's personal assessment of the public health significance of fluorosis may be less relevant today.

TOOTH SURFACE INDEX OF FLUOROSIS

Fluorosis was the subject of surprisingly little study after the initial investigations of controlled water fluoridation[21] until the 1980s, when research was spurred by suggestions that its prevalence might be increasing.[16] During the 1980s, the Tooth Surface Index of Fluorosis (TSIF) was developed and used by researchers at the National Institute of Dental Research.[10,15] Criteria for the TSIF are shown in Box 17-2. The TSIF scale is probably more sensitive than Dean's index in identifying the mildest forms of fluorosis. The TSIF ascribes a score on a scale of 0-7 to each tooth surface in the mouth, whereas Dean's index applies only to the two most affected teeth in the mouth. The World Health Organization, however, still recommends use of Dean's Fluorosis Index in its basic survey manual.[26] TSIF results are given as an ordinal distribution rather than as mean scores.

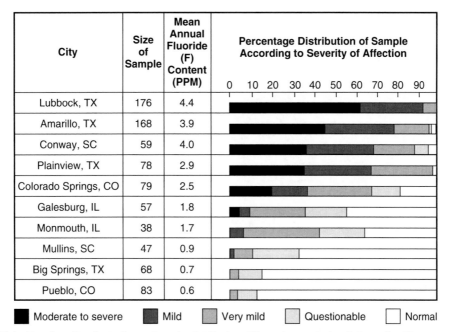

City	Size of Sample	Mean Annual Fluoride (F) Content (PPM)	Percentage Distribution of Sample According to Severity of Affection
Lubbock, TX	176	4.4	
Amarillo, TX	168	3.9	
Conway, SC	59	4.0	
Plainview, TX	78	2.9	
Colorado Springs, CO	79	2.5	
Galesburg, IL	57	1.8	
Monmouth, IL	38	1.7	
Mullins, SC	47	0.9	
Big Springs, TX	68	0.7	
Pueblo, CO	83	0.6	

■ Moderate to severe ■ Mild ▨ Very mild ▢ Questionable □ Normal

Fig. 17-1 Data from Dean's studies to show the distribution of fluorosis severity in relation to fluoride concentration of the drinking water in 10 communities.[8]

BOX 17-1 Criteria for Dean's Fluorosis Index[4]

Normal:
The enamel represents the usual translucent semivitriform type of structure. The surface is smooth, glossy, and usually of a pale creamy white color.
Questionable:
The enamel discloses slight aberrations from the translucency of normal enamel, ranging from a few white flecks to occasional white spots. This classification is utilized in those instances in which a definite diagnosis of the mildest form of fluorosis is not warranted and a classification of "normal" not justified.
Very mild:
Small, opaque, paper-white areas scattered irregularly over the tooth but not involving as much as approximately 25% of the tooth surface. Frequently included in this classification are teeth showing no more than about 1-2 mm of white opacity at the tip of the summit of the cusps of the bicuspids or second molars.
Mild:
The white opaque areas in the enamel of the teeth are more extensive but do not involve as much as 50% of the tooth.
Moderate:
All enamel surfaces of the teeth are affected, and surfaces subject to attrition show marked wear. Brown stain is frequently a disfiguring feature.
Severe:
Includes teeth formerly classified as "moderately severe" and "severe." All enamel surfaces are affected and hypoplasia is so marked that the general form of the tooth may be altered. The major diagnostic sign of this classification is the discrete or confluent pitting. Brown stains are widespread and teeth often present a corroded appearance.

The TSIF is viewed as a public health index rather than as a research tool. It does not call for drying of the teeth prior to scoring, on the grounds that when the appearance of teeth is judged in everyday life it is done so with the teeth wet. The very mildest forms of fluorosis are therefore likely to be missed with the TSIF.

The previous discussions of fluorosis indexes concern fluorosis in the permanent dentition, because fluorosis was for a long time thought not to occur at all in the primary teeth. It does, however, and the TSIF has also been used to record fluorosis in the primary dentition.[17,25]

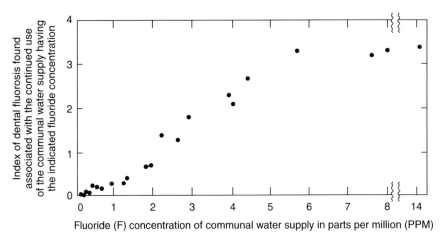

Fig. 17-2 Data from Dean's studies to show the relation between mean Fluorosis Index scores and the fluoride concentration of the drinking water.[4]

BOX 17-2 Clinical Criteria and Categorizations for the Tooth Surface Index of Fluorosis[15]

0: Enamel shows no evidence of fluorosis.

1: Enamel shows definite evidence of fluorosis, namely, areas with parchment-white color that total less than one third of the visible enamel surface. This category includes fluorosis confined only to incisal edges of anterior teeth and cusp tips of posterior teeth ("snowcapping").

2: Parchment-white fluorosis totals at least one third of the visible surface, but less than two thirds.

3: Parchment-white fluorosis totals at least two thirds of the visible surface.

4: Enamel shows staining in conjunction with any of the preceding levels of fluorosis. Staining is defined as an area of definite discoloration that may range from light to very dark brown.

5: Discrete pitting of the enamel exists, unaccompanied by evidence of staining of intact enamel. A pit is defined as a definite physical defect in the enamel surface with a rough floor that is surrounded by a wall of intact enamel. The pitted area is usually stained or differs in color from the surrounding enamel.

6: Both discrete pitting and staining of the intact enamel exist.

7: Confluent pitting of the enamel surface exists. Large areas of enamel may be missing and the anatomy of the tooth may be altered. Dark brown stain is usually present.

THYLSTRUP-FEJERSKOV INDEX

With studies of fluorosis being carried out in many regions of the world, Dean's Fluorosis Index inevitably became modified to meet specific needs; for example, its sensitivity at the higher end of the scale was increased to handle situations in which fluorosis was more severe than any with which Dean had to deal.[24] The resulting Thylstrup-Fejerskov (TF) index has a stronger biologic basis than Dean's more or less arbitrary index, because the index scores were developed by relating them to histologic features of affected enamel. The criteria for the TF index are shown in Box 17-3. Because its use necessitates drying of the teeth, the TF index is the most sensitive of existing indexes. At the same time, it requires assessment of only one surface per tooth because fluorosis affects all tooth surfaces equally.[14] It can be used on selected teeth or the whole dentition, and results again are expressed as distributions rather than as mean scores. An example of a TF distribution is shown in Fig. 17-3.

FLUOROSIS RISK INDEX

The Fluorosis Risk Index (FRI)[19] is designed for use in analytic studies that seek to identify risk factors for fluorosis; it explicitly recognizes that the risk of fluorosis is related to fluoride exposure at particular stages of dentition development. It divides the buccal and occlusal surfaces

---

BOX 17-3   Clinical Criteria and Scoring for the Thylstrup-Fejerskov Fluorosis Index[24]

0: Normal translucency of enamel remains after prolonged air-drying.

1: Narrow white lines located corresponding to the perikymata.

2: *Smooth surfaces:*
   More pronounced lines of opacity that follow the perikymata. Occasionally confluence of adjacent lines.
   Occlusal surfaces:
   Scattered areas of opacity <2 mm in diameter and pronounced opacity of cuspal ridges.

3: *Smooth surfaces:*
   Merging and irregular cloudy areas of opacity. Accentuated drawing of perikymata often visible between opacities.
   Occlusal surfaces:
   Confluent areas of marked opacity. Worn areas appear almost normal but usually circumscribed by a rim of opaque enamel.

4: *Smooth surfaces:*
   The entire surface exhibits marked opacity or appears chalky white. Parts of surface exposed to attrition appear less affected.
   Occlusal surfaces:
   Entire surface exhibits marked opacity. Attrition is often pronounced shortly after eruption.

5: *Smooth and occlusal surfaces:*
   Entire surface displays marked opacity with focal loss of outermost enamel (pits) <2 mm in diameter.

6: *Smooth surfaces:*
   Pits are regularly arranged in horizontal bands <2 mm in vertical extension.
   Occlusal surfaces:
   Confluent areas <3 mm in diameter exhibit loss of enamel. Marked attrition.

7: *Smooth surfaces:*
   Loss of outermost enamel in irregular areas involving <½ of entire surface.
   Occlusal surfaces:
   Changes in the morphology caused by merging pits and marked attrition.

8: *Smooth and occlusal surfaces:*
   Loss of outermost enamel involving >½ of surface.

9: *Smooth and occlusal surfaces:*
   Loss of main part of enamel with change in anatomic appearance of surface. Cervical rim of almost unaffected enamel is often noted.

---

of each permanent tooth into four zones based on the age at which calcification begins and selectively classifies each zone into one of two categories.[18] There is also a tight case definition of fluorosis. When related to the history of fluoride exposure, fluorosis that develops during the maturation phase of enamel can be differentiated from that which develops earlier. Wider use of this index is likely in studies on fluorosis risk factors.

DEVELOPMENTAL DEFECTS OF DENTAL ENAMEL INDEX

The intent of the Developmental Defects of Dental Enamel (DDE) index was to avoid the need to diagnose fluorosis before recording enamel opacities, a requirement that some think may introduce measurement bias.[12] The DDE index has been used a number of times since its introduction,[2,11,22,23] but the large amount of data generated has led to problems in presenting results in a meaningful fashion. Following a national survey of children in Ireland, modifications to the DDE index were suggested to make it simpler.[1]

Russell[20] addressed the same issue of distinguishing between milder forms of fluorosis and nonfluoride enamel opacities, and provided a description of differential diagnostic features as shown in Table 17-1. An accurate history of drinking water sources, as well as of the use of

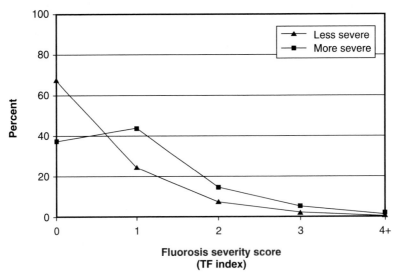

Fig. 17-3 Hypothetical data to show the distribution of fluorosis in two U.S. child populations, as measured by the Thylstrup-Fejerskov (TF) index.

Table 17-1 Differential diagnosis between milder forms of dental fluorosis (questionable, very mild, and mild) and nonfluoride opacities of enamel[20]

Characteristic of Enamel Opacities	Milder Forms of Fluorosis	Nonfluoride Opacities
Area affected	Usually seen on or near tips of cusps or incisal edges.	Usually centered in smooth surface; may affect entire crown.
Shape of lesion	Resembles line shading in pencil sketch; lines follow incremental lines in enamel, form irregular caps on cusps.	Often round or oval.
Demarcation	Shades off imperceptibly into surrounding normal enamel.	Clearly differentiated from adjacent normal enamel.
Color	Slightly more opaque than normal enamel; paper white. Incisal edges, tips of cusps may have frosted appearance. Does not show stain at time of eruption (in these milder degrees, rarely at any time).	Usually pigmented at time of eruption; often creamy yellow to dark reddish orange.
Teeth affected	Most frequent on teeth that calcify slowly (cuspids, bicuspids, second and third molars). Rare on lower incisors. Usually seen on six or eight homologous teeth. Extremely rare in deciduous teeth.	Any tooth may be affected. Frequent on labial surfaces of lower incisors. May occur singly. Usually one to three teeth affected. Common in deciduous teeth.
Gross hypoplasia	None. Pitting of enamel does not occur in the milder forms. Enamel surface has glazed appearance, is smooth to point of explorer.	Absent to severe. Enamel surface may seem etched, be rough to explorer.
Detection	Often invisible under strong light; most easily detected by line of sight tangential to tooth crown.	Seen most easily under strong light on line of sight perpendicular to tooth surface.

fluoride tablets, toothpaste, and rinses, should be sought by practitioners as an aid to diagnosing the nature of enamel disturbances in patients.

REFERENCES

1. Clarkson J, O'Mullane D. A modified DDE index for use in epidemiological studies of enamel defects. J Dent Res 1989;68:445-50.
2. Cutress TW, Suckling GW, Pearce EIF, Ball BE. Defects of tooth enamel in children in fluoridated and nonfluoridated water areas of Auckland. N Z Dent J 1985;81:12-9.
3. Dean HT. Chronic endemic dental fluorosis (mottled enamel). In: Gordon SM, ed: Dental science and dental art. Philadelphia: Lea and Febiger, 1938:387-414.
4. Dean HT. The investigation of physiological effects by the epidemiological method. In: Moulton FR, ed: Fluorine and dental health. Washington DC: American Association for the Advancement of Science, 1942:23-71.
5. Dean HT. Epidemiological studies in the United States. In: Moulton FR, ed: Dental caries and fluorine. Washington DC: American Association for the Advancement of Science, 1946:5-31.
6. Dean HT, Dixon RM, Cohen C. Mottled enamel in Texas. Public Health Rep 1935;50:424-42.
7. Dean HT, Elvove E. Some epidemiological aspects of chronic endemic dental fluorosis. Am J Public Health 1936;26:567-75.
8. Dean HT, Elvove E. Further studies on the minimal threshold of chronic endemic dental fluorosis. Public Health Rep 1937;52:1249-64.
9. Dean HT, Elvove E, Poston RF. Mottled enamel in South Dakota. Public Health Rep 1939;54:212-28.
10. Driscoll WS, Horowitz HS, Meyers RJ, et al. Prevalence of dental caries and dental fluorosis in areas with negligible, optimal, and above-optimal fluoride concentrations in drinking water. J Am Dent Assoc 1986;113:29-33.
11. Dummer PM, Kingdon A, Kingdon R. Prevalence of enamel developmental defects in a group of 11- and 12-year-old children in South Wales. Community Dent Oral Epidemiol 1986;14:119-22.
12. Fédération Dentaire Internationale, Commission on Oral Research and Epidemiology. An epidemiological index of developmental defects of dental enamel (DDE index). Int Dent J 1982;32:159-67.
13. Fejerskov O, Manji F, Baelum V. The nature and mechanisms of dental fluorosis in man. J Dent Res 1990;69(Spec Issue):692-700.
14. Fejerskov O, Manji F, Baelum V, Møller IJ. Dental fluorosis: A handbook for health workers. Copenhagen: Munksgaard, 1988.
15. Horowitz HS, Driscoll WS, Meyers RJ, et al. A new method for assessing the prevalence of dental fluorosis—the Tooth Surface Index of Fluorosis. J Am Dent Assoc 1984;109:37-41.
16. Leverett DH. Fluorides and the changing prevalence of dental caries. Science 1982;217:26-30.
17. Levy SM, Hillis SL, Warren JJ, et al. Primary tooth fluorosis and fluoride intake during the first year of life. Community Dent Oral Epidemiol 2002;30:286-95.
18. Pendrys DG. The Fluorosis Risk Index: A method for investigating risk factors. J Public Health Dent 1990;50:291-8.
19. Pendrys DG, Katz RV. Risk of enamel fluorosis associated with fluoride supplementation, infant formula, and fluoride dentifrice use. Am J Epidemiol 1989;130:1199-1208.
20. Russell AL. The differential diagnosis of fluoride and nonfluoride enamel opacities. Public Health Dent 1961;21:143-6.
21. Russell AL. Dental fluorosis in Grand Rapids during the seventeenth year of fluoridation. J Am Dent Assoc 1962;65:608-12.
22. Suckling GW, Brown RH, Herbison GP. The prevalence of defects of enamel in nine-year-old children in New Zealand in a health and development study. Community Dent Health 1985;2:303-13.
23. Suckling GW, Pearce EIF. Developmental defects of enamel in a group of New Zealand children. Community Dent Oral Epidemiol 1984;12:177-84.
24. Thylstrup A, Fejerskov O. Clinical appearance of dental fluorosis in permanent teeth in relation to histologic changes. Community Dent Oral Epidemiol 1978;6:315-28.
25. Warren JJ, Levy SM, Kanellis MJ. Prevalence of dental fluorosis in the primary dentition. J Public Health Dent 2001;61:87-91.
26. World Health Organization. Oral health surveys; basic methods. 4th ed. Geneva: WHO, 1997.

Measuring Other Conditions in Oral Epidemiology

Other conditions have been studied in oral epidemiology with varying amounts of success. Some, like temporomandibular disorders, present so many inherent difficulties that they will probably always be extremely difficult to measure. Others such as soft tissue lesions other than oral cancer and precancers (e.g., oral pemphigus, lichen planus) have simply not attracted much attention.

MALOCCLUSION

Malocclusion is a difficult entity to define because individuals and cultures vary widely in perceptions of what constitutes a malocclusion problem. Quite a number of malocclusion indexes have been devised, but probably because of this perceptual problem, none has ever emerged as a standard. These issues have not changed over the years, and there are thoughtful, still valid commentaries from the 1970s on the problems of classifying and scoring malocclusions.[13,15]

Angle's classification, which dates from the nineteenth century,[1] may still be useful in treatment planning but is of no use in epidemiology because it is a nominal categorization. Most other indexes suffer from the limitation that they record specific conditions (e.g., overbite, posterior crossbite) rather than the status of the whole occlusion. The Malalignment Index[31] assesses rotation and tooth displacement, whereas the Occlusal Feature Index[24] records crowding, cuspal interdigitation, and vertical and horizontal overbite. The Handicapping Labio-Lingual Deviations (HLD, which, interestingly enough, is also the developer's initials)

Index[11] received considerable public health use when it was applied to assess treatment needs for a public orthodontic program in New York State. Grainger developed the Treatment Priority Index (TPI) for assessing treatment needs, an index that was used once, but only once, in a national study of orthodontic needs of children.[30] None of these indexes has seen much use in the years beyond its introduction. One modestly successful measure is the Occlusal Index, or OI,[29] which measures nine characteristics: dental age, molar relation, overbite, overjet, posterior crossbite, posterior open bite, tooth displacement, midline relations, and missing permanent maxillary incisors. Its use demands a fair degree of examiner skill and training, but it is probably closer to a complete malocclusion index than those listed earlier.

In Europe the Index of Orthodontic Treatment Need (IOTN) has received some use since it was first introduced in 1989.[4] It was modified from an existing Swedish scale and combines both a functional and an esthetic measure. Functional occlusion is categorized into five different grades, whereas the esthetic measure uses a 10-point ordinal scale that allows the individual to determine his own esthetic perception of the dentition. The IOTN has shown some promise for use in public health[19] but has not been widely adopted. The Peer Assessment Rating (PAR) index is designed to capture all the occlusal anomalies that might be found in malocclusion in a single score.[25] This sounds ambitious, but the PAR index has been found to equal the OI in reliability.[5] The search still continues for an omnibus measure, and the Index of Complexity, Outcome, and Need (ICON) arrived with the new millennium.[10] It has been shown to correlate well with patients' perceptions of esthetics, speech, function, and need for treatment.[17]

The very proliferation of these indexes underlines the difficulties in measuring this complex issue. The Fédération Dentaire Internationale jumped on the bandwagon with its attempt to develop an internationally accepted index and simplified method of determining malocclusion.[12] It was not successful; the result was a carefully qualified method of measuring occlusal traits. The index has been used[9] but seems to offer no more value than the other indexes described.

The complexities of malocclusion, and the frustrations that have grown up with the inadequacies of these indexes, have led many researchers to believe that functional malocclusion is virtually unmeasurable for epidemiologic purposes. In terms of trying to interpret group data on overbites, crowding, and other clinical conditions, that may well be true. Orthodontic indexes developed in the late 1980s, however, take a different philosophical approach in that they assess esthetic rather than clinical aspects of function. One is the Dental Aesthetic Index (DAI), published in 1986 after years of testing.[8] The DAI starts from the premise that the impact of malocclusion on other oral pathology is doubtful and that the main benefit of orthodontic treatment is its effect on the individual's social and psychological well-being. The DAI makes objective measurements of aesthetic acceptability according to social norms, and it has been validated for this use in a number of different countries. As noted earlier, the IOTN also includes an esthetic component measured on a 10-point ordinal scale.

The World Health Organization, in its Pathfinder survey protocol,[32] suggests using DAI criteria to record malocclusion in the following categories:
- Missing incisor, canine, and bicuspid teeth
- Incisal crowding in the maxillary and mandibular anterior segments
- Spacing in the maxillary and mandibular anterior segments
- Diastema between the two maxillary central incisors

- Largest irregularity in the front four maxillary anterior incisors (rotations or displacement from normal alignment)
- Largest irregularity in the front four mandibular anterior incisors
- Anterior maxillary and mandibular overjet
- Vertical anterior open bite
- Anteroposterior molar relation

ORAL CANCER

As with other cancers, occurrence of oral cancer is usually expressed as a proportion or rate. The age-adjusted rate of years of life lost from oral cancer, for example, dropped from 23.1 per 100,000 population in 1970 to 19.9 per 100,000 in 1985.[21] Five-year survival rates are also useful cancer measures: a 5-year survival rate of 67%, for example, means that 67% of persons in whom the condition was diagnosed 5 years earlier are still alive.

Cancer data are maintained in registries in most (but not all) states; information is reported to the registry by physicians and hospitals. Some 11 of these population-based registries in the United States participate in the Surveillance, Epidemiology, and End Results (SEER) program, which is conducted by the National Cancer Institute (see Chapter 4). The SEER program is the nation's principal source of national estimates of site-specific cancer incidence and trends, and is the primary source of the research data used in epidemiologic studies.

CLEFT LIP AND PALATE

The occurrence of cleft lip and palate is also usually expressed as a proportion; about 1 infant in 700 births exhibits this condition.[14] Soft tissue abnormalities of various kinds, as well as the more rare types of oral pathoses, are also most suitably expressed as proportions or rates. Cleft lip and palate, as a congenital abnormality, is supposed to be recorded on birth certificates in the United States, although such recording is unfortunately far from universal.

ORAL HEALTH AND QUALITY OF LIFE

Although philosophically it is desirable to measure health rather than disease, in practice epidemiology concerns itself with measuring disease because health is so difficult to define in operational terms (see Chapter 4). When a concept is difficult to define, it is also difficult to measure. Several extensive research efforts have been made to develop an index of oral health.[6,7,16,20,22,23] These approaches have been largely empiric, meaning that they have been based on what dentists consider oral health to be, and they require some form of weighting of conditions to reflect their relative seriousness. They do not take any subjective measures into account.

Given that health is more than the absence of disease, several commentators have argued that an individual's subjective assessment of his or her own oral health is at least as valid as a dentist's, and probably more so. This is a different philosophical approach to disease measurement, because subjective indicators and clinical indicators of oral health are poorly correlated.[18]

The Oral Health Impact Profile (OHIP) measures the social impact of oral conditions as perceived by the individual and was derived initially from statements given by dental patients in interviews. It was later refined and tested extensively for validity and reliability.[28] The OHIP was originally developed as a 49-item scale but later was shortened to a 14-item scale, which measured oral health quality of life as validly as the initial version[26] and was easier to work with.

Another index that has received widespread use is the General Oral Health Assessment Index (GOHAI), originally the Geriatric Oral Health Assessment Index. The GOHAI is a 12-item scale that assesses physical functions, psychosocial functions, and pain or discomfort.[2,3] Indexes like these have considerable potential for ranking oral disorders in terms of their impacts on peoples' daily lives, thus broadening our perspectives of oral health and aiding both clinical treatment planning and research.

Objective measurement of caries or periodontitis appears relatively simple compared to assessing the subjective impacts of oral disease and disabilities on peoples' lives. A 1996 conference at Chapel Hill, North Carolina, explored the various measures currently existing for assessing quality of life.[27] This conference was exploratory and came to no general conclusions. It is likely to be a baseline against which further developments in this complex area are measured.

REFERENCES

1. Angle EH. Classification of malocclusion. Dent Cosmos 1899;41:248-64.
2. Atchison KA. The General Oral Health Assessment Index (GOHAI). In: Slade GD, ed: Measuring oral health and quality of life. Chapel Hill NC: University of North Carolina, Department of Dental Ecology, 1997.
3. Atchison KA, Dolan TA. Development of the geriatric oral health assessment index. J Dent Educ 1990;54:680-7.
4. Brook PH, Shaw WC. The development of an index of orthodontic treatment priority. Eur J Orthod 1989;11:309-20.
5. Buchanan IB, Shaw WC, Richmond S, et al. A comparison of the reliability and validity of the PAR Index and Summers' Occlusal Index. Eur J Orthod 1993;15:27-31.
6. Bulman JS, Richards ND, Slack GL, Willcocks AJ. Demand and need for dental care; a socio-dental study. London: Oxford University Press, 1968.
7. Burke FJ, Wilson NH. Measuring oral health: An historical view and details of a contemporary oral health index (OHX). Int Dent J 1995;45:358-70.
8. Cons NC, Jenny J, Kohaut FJ. DAI: The Dental Aesthetic Index. Iowa City IA: University of Iowa, 1986.
9. Cons NC, Mruthyunjaya YC, Pollard ST. Distribution of occlusal traits in a sample of 1,337 children, ages 15-18, residing in upstate New York. Int Dent J 1978; 28:154-64.
10. Daniels C, Richmond S. The development of the index of complexity, outcome, and need (ICON). J Orthod 2000;27:149-62.
11. Draker HL. Handicapping labio-lingual deviations proposed for public health purposes. Am J Orthod 1960;46:295-305.
12. Fédération Dentaire Internationale. Commission on Classification and Statistics for Oral Conditions. A method for measuring occlusal traits. Int Dent J 1973;23:530-7.
13. Foster TD. The public health interest in assessment for orthodontic treatment. J Public Health Dent 1979;39:137-42.
14. Greene JC. Epidemiology of congenital clefts of the lip and palate. Public Health Rep 1963;78:589-602.
15. Jago JD. The epidemiology of dental occlusion; a critical appraisal. J Public Health Dent 1974;34:80-93.
16. Koch AL, Gershen JA, Marcus M. A children's oral health status index based on dentists' judgment. J Am Dent Assoc 1985;110:36-42.
17. Koochek AR, Yeh MS, Rolfe B, Richmond S. The relationship between Index of Complexity, Outcome and Need, and patients' perceptions of malocclusion: A study in general dental practice. Br Dent J 2001; 191:325-9.
18. Locker D, Slade GD. Association between clinical and subjective indicators of oral health status in an older adult population. Gerodontology 1994;11:108-14.
19. Lunn H, Richmond S, Mitropoulos C. The use of the Index of Orthodontic Treatment Need (IOTN) as a public health tool: A pilot study. Community Dent Health 1993;10:111-21.
20. Marcus M, Koch AL, Gershen JA. Construction of a population index of adult oral health status derived from

dentists' preferences. J Public Health Dent 1983;43: 284-94.

21. Myers MH, Glockler Ries LA. Cancer patient survival rates: SEER program results for 10 years of follow-up. CA Cancer J Clin 1989;39:21-32.

22. Nikias MK, Sollecito WA, Fink R. An empirical approach to developing multidimensional oral status profiles. J Public Health Dent 1978;38:148-58.

23. Nikias MK, Sollecito WA, Fink R. An oral health index based on ranking of oral status profiles by panels of dental professionals. J Public Health Dent 1979;39: 16-26.

24. Poulton DR, Aaronson SA. The relationship between occlusion and periodontal status. Am J Orthod 1961; 47:690-9.

25. Richmond S, Shaw WC, O'Brien KD, et al. The development of the PAR Index (Peer Assessment Rating): Reliability and validity. Eur J Orthod 1992;14:125-39.

26. Slade GD. Derivation and validation of a short-form oral health impact profile. Community Dent Oral Epidemiol 1997;25:284-90.

27. Slade GD, ed. Measuring oral health and quality of life. Chapel Hill NC: University of North Carolina, 1997.

28. Slade GD, Spencer AJ. Development and evaluation of the Oral Health Impact Profile. Community Dent Health 1994;11:3-11.

29. Summers CJ. The Occlusal Index; a system for identifying and scoring occlusal disorders. Am J Orthod 1971;59:552-67.

30. US Public Health Service, National Center for Health Statistics. Orthodontic treatment priority index. PHS Publication No. 1000, Series 2 No. 25. Washington DC: Government Printing Office, 1967.

31. Van Kirk LE Jr, Pennell EH. Assessment of malocclusion in population groups. Am J Orthod 1959;45:752-8.

32. World Health Organization. Oral health surveys; basic methods. 4th ed. Geneva: WHO, 1997.

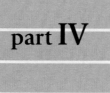

part **IV**

The Distribution of Oral Diseases and Conditions

19 Tooth Loss

Tooth loss, especially total tooth loss or edentulism, is the dental equivalent of death. Tooth loss diminishes the quality of life, often substantially, and tooth loss is also related to poorer general health.[44] If retaining teeth were just a matter of preventing disease conditions then the issue would be reasonably straightforward, but it is more complicated than that. Although loss of teeth is an end product of oral disease, it is also a reflection of patient and dentist attitudes, the dentist-patient relationship, the availability and accessibility of care, and the prevailing philosophies of care. This chapter reviews the issues and trends in tooth loss, and the reasons why people lose teeth.

THE HISTORICAL PICTURE

For centuries, tooth loss was considered an inevitable part of the human condition and was thus generally accepted with resignation. Long before dentistry emerged as a true profession (see Chapter 1) the tooth-puller was a necessary part of most cultures, sometimes based in a village and sometimes plying an itinerant trade. As the profession of dentistry evolved during the nineteenth century, much of the work of dentists was still devoted to tooth extraction. Caries was rampant at this time (see Chapter 20), restorative techniques crude and painful, prevention unknown. As a result, people expected to lose teeth and dentists expected to extract them.

Appalling oral health status marked by extensive loss of teeth extended well into the twentieth century in high-income countries. The oral condition of the millions drafted into the armies of many countries during World War I (1914-18) was generally dreadful. The response of authorities was to extract more teeth, so that troops preparing to bayonet each other would not be bothered by toothache. Right after the war, surveys in New York found that schoolgirls ages 13-17 years had lost 13.5% of first molars and 2.5% of second molars, whereas adults of different ages had lost 22%-47% of first molars.[31,32] Things improved only slowly. In the Hagerstown studies of 1938, 15-year-old children averaged 1.1 lost permanent teeth per child, 94% of which were first molars.[37] Age-specific tooth loss among white-collar working adults in a large insurance office showed only mild improvement between 1927 and 1942,[20] and extensive tooth loss was still common among World War II (1939-45) draftees in the United States.[49,53]

By the beginning of the twenty-first century tooth retention was much improved in all the high-income nations. Change came about with improvements in restorative dentistry (especially the development of the air-turbine dental engine in the late 1950s), increasing affluence and its accompanying positive attitudes toward tooth retention, and significant research advances in preventing oral diseases. In that latter context, the advent of water fluoridation (see Chapter 25) was probably the most profound influence, because it demonstrated to individuals and their families, in a way that dental treatment could not, that dental caries and subsequent tooth loss were not inevitable.

EDENTULISM

The sight of grandfather's false teeth in a glass of water was a familiar one to several generations of Americans; the acquisition of false teeth was thought to go along with rheumatics, constipation, sensory diminution, and loss of memory as a normal part of growing old.[13]

That editorial comment from the mid-1980s conjured up an image that is fast becoming unknown to the present generation, because edentulism continues to decline steadily in the United States[12] and in other economically developed nations.[36,50,54] Table 19-1 shows the proportion of persons ages 65 and over who are edentulous in 10 countries, along with the national income category for each country. Fig. 19-1 shows the proportion of adults, by age, who are edentulous, as measured in national surveys in the United States in 1957-58, 1971, 1985-86, and 1988-94. These data indicate that edentulism has declined consistently in each age-group with each succeeding survey. The relative decline in edentulism has been sharpest in the younger age-groups, which suggests that edentulism will become even rarer as today's younger cohorts grow older.

Table 19-1 Percentage of persons ages 65 and older who are edentulous in 10 countries classified by national income status[68]

Country	Percent Edentulous	National Income Category*
Canada	58	High
Finland	41	High
Slovenia	16	High
United Kingdom	46	High
United States	24	High
Malaysia	57	Upper middle
Albania	69	Lower middle
Egypt	7	Lower middle
Thailand	16	Lower middle
Indonesia	24	Low

*As defined by the World Bank in World Bank Group, Data and statistics, Country groups, website: http://www.worldbank.org/data/countryclass/classgroups.htm. Accessed December 19, 2003.

The third National Health and Nutrition Examination Survey (NHANES III) was conducted between 1988 and 1994, and collected data from a representative sample of the population of the United States. In NHANES III,

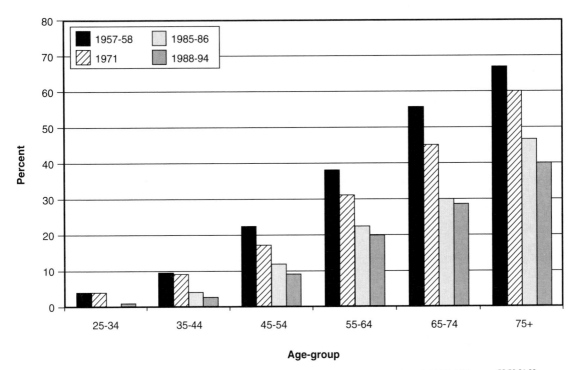

Fig. 19-1 Proportion of the U.S. population edentulous in 1957-58, 1971, 1985-86, and 1988-94 by age.[58,59,61,63]

10.5% of Americans ages 18 or older were found to be edentulous.[19] There were sharply defined age-cohort differences: only some 1% of 25- to 34-year-olds were edentulous compared to 44% of those ages 75 years or older.[43] One estimate of the decline in edentulism suggested that by the year 2024 only 10% of Americans ages 65-74 would be edentulous,[67] compared to 28% edentulous in that age-group in 1988-91.[43] Those who will be in the 65-74 age-cohort in 2024 were in the 25- to 34-year-old group from 1988 to 1991, a cohort benefiting from the postfluoride age of prevention (see Chapter 20). This steady decline in edentulism among United States adults is expected to continue in spite of the aging of the population (see Chapter 2).

Many people are puzzled by the apparently slow rate of progress in decreasing edentulism when we constantly hear of rapid improvements in oral health status. The reason lies in the nature of the condition. When the data in Fig. 19-1 are considered, it can be noted that the youngest individuals in the 75-and-older cohort for 1988-94 were born in 1919, and most were born earlier. The early adult years for this group were during the Great Depression of the 1930s, and many of them then served in World War II. Indeed, it is probable that a good proportion of this cohort first became edentulous during that war, and they have been influencing the statistics ever since. In time, these aging cohorts will be replaced by the baby boomers, who grew up in a totally different world of affluence and modern disease prevention, and with fundamentally more positive attitudes toward tooth retention. Already the emerging elderly cohorts (i.e., the 55-64 and 65-74 cohorts from the two most recent surveys in Fig. 19-1) represent the *new elderly*, a term coined to describe the post-World War II group who have experienced material affluence, higher education than their predecessors, and more of the benefits of modern preventive health care.[24] The level of total tooth loss among these age-groups in 1985-86 and 1988-94 was already sharply lower than that in the 75-and-over groups in Fig. 19-1.

The importance of nondisease factors in edentulism emerges from Table 19-1, which shows that the proportion of edentulous individuals among the elderly bears little relationship to national income, and from Table 19-2, which shows the extent of total tooth loss among adults ages 35-44 in nine high-income countries in the 1968-77 period. The data in Table 19-2, most of them coming from the first International Collaborative Survey (ICS I) of the mid-1970s,[4] show a range in the proportion of edentulous persons from one country to another that is too high to be explained solely in terms of dental disease; health beliefs and societal attitudes must be operating here. At the time the data in Table 19-2 were collected, there was still quite a high proportion of adults in New Zealand, for example, who attached no stigma to wearing full dentures.[18] In developing countries, where access to Western-type dental care is limited, edentulism is uncommon.[5,22,41]

We introduced the National Oral Health Surveillance System in Chapter 4 and noted that total tooth loss was one of the eight indicators of oral health. The information is collected by interview as part of the Behavioral Risk Factor Surveillance System (see Chapter 4), and some of the differences between states in proportion of older people who are edentulous give us food for thought. Data for a selection of 10 states, chosen more or less arbitrarily to highlight the interstate contrasts, are shown in Table 19-3.

Historically, there has been a higher degree of edentulism among women than among men, and women have tended to become edentulous at a younger age.[18,26,57,61] These historical gender differences are not easy to explain; many think they reflected dentist-patient relationships more than disease occurrence. Data from the 1980s and later, however, suggest that these gender differences are fading, because there was

Table 19-2 Percentage of persons ages 35-44 who were edentulous in nine countries, 1968-77[7,8,26,57]

Community/Country	Percent Edentulous
Yamanashi, Japan	0.0
Hannover, Germany	1.6
Trøndelag, Norway	6.4
Ontario, Canada	8.7
Baltimore, USA	10.6
Sydney, Australia	13.2
England and Wales	22.0
Scotland	35.0
Canterbury, New Zealand	35.7

Table 19-3 Percentage of persons in 10 of the United States, ages 65 and older, who are edentulous[60]

State	Percent Edentulous
United States	24.4
Hawaii	15.9
Nevada	16.5
California	18.5
Michigan	21.8
Georgia	28.9
Arkansas	29.2
Maine	35.0
Indiana	36.2
West Virginia	43.2
Kentucky	44.3

no pattern of difference between men and women in the various age-groups among the 4.2% of employed U.S. adults who were edentulous in 1985-86.[64] In the more representative sample seen in NHANES III, there again was virtually no difference between men and women in the proportion edentulous.[43]

In the United States, there has historically been a greater degree of edentulism among whites than among African-Americans,[61] perhaps because whites have traditionally had better access to dental care (see Chapter 2) and thus were at greater risk of having teeth extracted (see Dental Care and Tooth Loss later this chapter). Like gender differences, however, differences between the races have become less distinct since the 1980s, perhaps because edentulism overall is becoming so uncommon among younger cohorts. In both the national survey of 1985-86 and that of 1988-94, only a slightly higher proportion of whites than African-Americans were edentulous.[43,64] Fig. 19-2 shows the proportions of edentulous people by age in the various racial and ethnic groups in the 1988-94 national survey. It can be seen that only Mexican-Americans had notably less edentulism than the other groups.

Edentulism is tightly related to socioeconomic status (SES). These SES-related differences are found consistently in many societies and probably reflect expectations and health attitudes at least as much as occurrence of oral diseases.[23,25] Unpublished data from the 1985-86 U.S. survey show that the strongest risk indicator for edentulism in employed adults (other

than age) was SES: 10.2% of those with fewer than 8 years of education were edentulous compared to 1.6% of those with 13 or more years. Fig. 19-3 shows the proportions of edentulous persons in three income-level groupings, and clear and predictable differences are seen among them. Similar SES-related differences have been demonstrated in regional studies in the United States[14,29] and in Europe.[34] Edentulous people have also been found to have more risk factors for cardiovascular disease than dentate people,[33] and it should not be surprising that older people in good health enjoy greater tooth retention than do people of the same age in poor health.[40,45]

PARTIAL TOOTH LOSS

Like edentulism, the extent of partial tooth loss has been diminishing in the United States as caries comes under control, more and better treatment becomes available, and attitudes toward tooth retention improve with increasing affluence. In contrast to edentulism, in which attitudes are a major factor in a person's decision to have all the teeth removed, partial tooth loss appears to be more closely related to oral disease.[14]

For the same reasons as found for edentulism, the sharpest improvement in reducing tooth loss is evident in younger age-groups. As an illustration of the extent of the improving trend, in the first National Health and Nutrition Examination Survey (NHANES I) of 1971-74,[62] young people ages 12-17 years on average had each lost 0.6 permanent teeth. Estimates from the 1986-87 national survey of schoolchildren,[65] however, showed that average loss of permanent teeth in 12-17-year-olds had been reduced to 0.05, a remarkable 12-fold decrease over some 14 years.

The change is naturally not as sharp among adults, because those adults who lost first molars to caries when they were young will continue to influence the data for a while yet. However, comparison of data from the NHANES I survey[62] of 1971-74 with those from the 1985-86 adult survey[64] showed a sharp improvement in tooth retention among dentate persons. In 1971-74, 59.5% of adults ages 18-74 had lost six or fewer teeth, whereas in

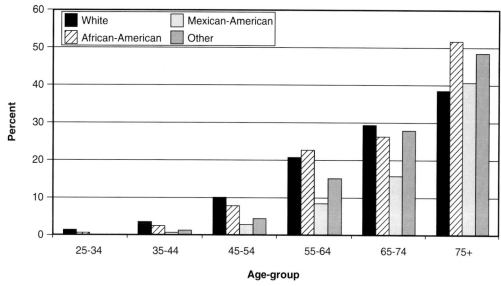

Fig. 19-2 Proportion of the U.S. population edentulous by age and racial/ethnic group in the third National Health and Nutrition Examination Survey, 1988-94.[58]

1985-86, 80.6% of employed adults ages 18-64 had lost six or fewer. Fig. 19-4 shows mean tooth loss among U.S. adults in 1971-74, in 1985-86, and in the NHANES III survey of 1988-94. The bias toward higher SES of the sample in the 1985-86 survey means that the national extent of tooth loss projected from

that survey is most likely an underestimate; the true extent of the improvement in tooth retention can be seen in comparing the 1971-74 data with that from 1988-94. Tooth retention is improving at all ages.

Fig. 19-5 shows the mean number of lost teeth according to income level among dentate

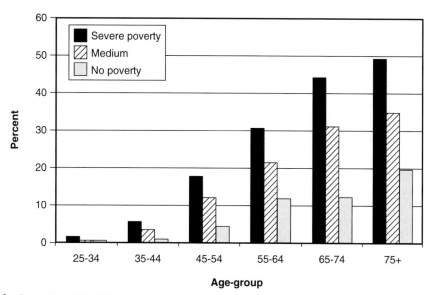

Fig. 19-3 Proportion of the U.S. population edentulous by age and poverty status in the third National Health and Nutrition Examination Survey, 1988-94.[58]

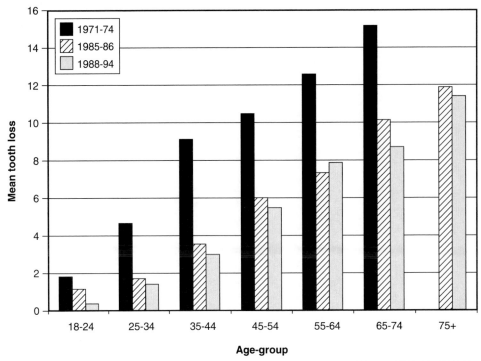

Fig. 19-4 Mean number of missing teeth in dentate adults and seniors in the United States, 1971-74, 1985-86, and 1988-94.[58,61,64]

adults in 1988-94. As was seen with edentulism, income (which reflects SES) is an important risk indicator for tooth loss. Also as with edentulism, gender differences in partial tooth loss have diminished. Fig. 19-6 shows the mean number of teeth remaining in dentate men and women as found in the NHANES III survey.

Longitudinal studies to identify risk factors that lead to tooth loss, either total or partial, have not been very successful.[27,30] Smoking, not surprisingly, has been identified as a risk indicator,[23,25,28,39] and early tooth loss was found to be a strong predictor of subsequent edentulism.[23] SES in early life is also a demonstrated predictor of tooth loss in early adulthood.[56]

REASONS FOR TOOTH LOSS

Conventional wisdom for many years was that caries was the main reason for tooth loss before age 35 and periodontal disease the main reason after age 35. This belief was based on some ancient and rather dubious data.[11,51] The older of these reports stated that "periclasia" was the

main reason for tooth loss "after maturity." Even as late as 1978 there was a report that 8%-10% of teeth are lost to periodontal disease by age 40 and that such loss increases rapidly after that age.[38]

Whether or not such historical views were accurate, the picture has changed considerably. From around the mid-1980s, studies in a number of countries and among different types of populations have been consistent in finding that caries is the principal cause of tooth loss at most ages, with the possible exception of the oldest (i.e., persons over 80 years).[66] Data on which these conclusions were based came from surveys of practitioners,[1,2,9,10,15,17,35] reviews of dental records,[6,16,48,55] and examinee questioning or diagnosis during survey examinations.[5,21,41,42,46] One exception to this trend was reported in Canada, where an Ontario survey found that periodontal diseases were the main reason given for extraction of most teeth in patients over 40 years of age, although multiple extractions in a relatively small number of patients can skew such data.[47] It is interesting to note that data

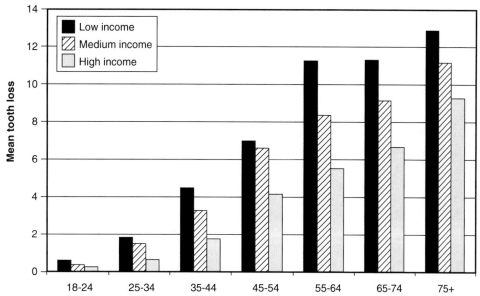

Fig. 19-5 Mean number of missing teeth in dentate adults by income level and age in the United States, 1988-94.[58]

were published as long ago as 1944 showing that most teeth were extracted for caries.[3]

A slight twist on this view came from a study of dental records of 1877 insured patients ages 40-69 years in the Kaiser Permanente health system in the western United States. Of all teeth extracted in 1992, 51% were extracted for periodontal diseases and 35% for caries. When the patient was taken as the analytical unit, however, 58% of patients had an extraction for caries and 40% for periodontal diseases.[52] Caries tends to result in extraction of one aching tooth, whereas periodontal diseases (real or presumed) can lead to a treatment decision for a full clearance.

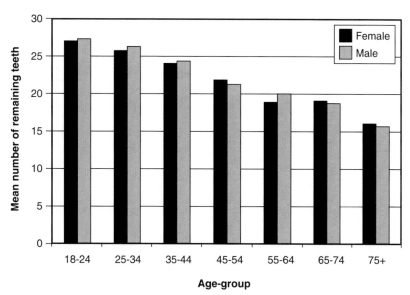

Fig. 19-6 Mean number of teeth remaining in dentate men and women by age in the United States, 1988-91.[43]

DENTAL CARE AND TOOTH LOSS

At the risk of stating the obvious, it is worth reminding ourselves that the main reason teeth are lost is because dentists extract them. To expand on that profound thought, "periodontal disease" may have been the chief reason for extraction in the era of "focal infection" (see Chapter 1), because no doubt many teeth with no more than severe gingivitis were extracted in the name of periodontal disease. The reasons given for the extractions were honest, but it seems likely that in many cases the disease was probably not what today would be considered severe. With the better understanding of periodontal diseases now prevailing, most such extractions have now ended. There are two major reasons for continuing improvement in tooth retention: (1) the modern preventive philosophy governing dental treatment, so that most present-day dentists extract teeth only when there is no practical alternative; and (2) positive attitudes among today's adults, both younger and older. Tooth loss for many of them is like smoking in the sense that both are simply unacceptable.

In summary, tooth retention is improving because of better prevention and control of the oral diseases, more positive attitudes toward tooth retention, and more conservative dental treatment philosophies. The result is that the proportion of people who are edentulous will continue to diminish until it bottoms out, probably at around 3%-4% of the population. Dentate persons will continue to retain more teeth as extractions for all reasons become less common. The greater retention of teeth will continue despite the aging of society, so the older dentate patient will become more and more common in dental practice.

REFERENCES

1. Agerholm DM, Sidi AD. Reasons given for extraction of permanent teeth by general dental practitioners in England and Wales. Br Dent J 1988;164:345-8.
2. Ainamo J, Sarkki L, Kuhalampi ML, et al. The frequency of periodontal extractions in Finland. Community Dent Health 1984;1:165-72.
3. Allen EF. Statistical study of the primary causes of extractions. J Dent Res 1944;23:453-8.
4. Arnljot HA, Barmes DE, Cohen LK, et al. Oral health care systems; an international collaborative study. London: Quintessence/World Health Organization, 1985.
5. Baelum V, Fejerskov O. Tooth loss as related to dental caries and periodontal breakdown in adult Tanzanians. Community Dent Oral Epidemiol 1986;14:353-7.
6. Bailit HL, Braun R, Maryniuk GA, Camp P. Is periodontal disease the primary cause of tooth extraction in adults? J Am Dent Assoc 1987;114:40-5.
7. Barmes DE. A progress report on adult data analysis in the WHO/USPHS International Collaborative Study. Int Dent J 1978;28:348-60.
8. Bonito AJ. The United States study of dental manpower systems in relation to oral health status: The private practice system. Final report for USPHS contract No. NO1-DH-34051. Baltimore: University of Maryland Dental School, 1977.
9. Bouma J, Schaub RM, van de Poel F. Periodontal status and total tooth extraction in a medium-sized city in the Netherlands. Community Dent Oral Epidemiol 1985;13:323-7.
10. Bouma J, Schaub RM, van de Poel F. Relative importance of periodontal disease for full mouth extractions in the Netherlands. Community Dent Oral Epidemiol 1987;15:41-5.
11. Brekhus PJ. Dental disease and its relation to the loss of human teeth. J Am Dent Assoc 1929;16:2237-47.
12. Brown LJ. Trends in tooth loss among U.S. employed adults from 1971 to 1985. J Am Dent Assoc 1994; 125:533-40.
13. Burt BA. The oral health of older Americans [editorial]. Am J Public Health 1985;75:1133-4.
14. Burt BA, Ismail AI, Morrison EC, Beltran ED. Risk factors for tooth loss over a 28-year period. J Dent Res 1990;69:1126-30.
15. Cahen PM, Frank RM, Turlot JC. A survey of the reasons for dental extractions in France. J Dent Res 1985; 64:1087-93.
16. Chauncey HH, Glass RL, Alman JE. Dental caries. Principal cause of tooth extraction in a sample of US male adults. Caries Res 1989;23:200-5.
17. Corbet EF, Davies WIR. Reasons given for tooth extraction in Hong Kong. Community Dent Health 1991;8:121-30.
18. Cutress TW, Hunter PBV, Davis PB, et al. Adult oral health and attitudes to dentistry in New Zealand 1976. Wellington NZ: Medical Research Council, 1979.
19. Drury TF, Brown LJ, Zion GR. Tooth retention and tooth loss in the permanent dentition of adults: United States, 1988-91. J Dent Res 1996;75(Spec Issue): 684-95.
20. Dunning JM, Klein H. Saving teeth among home office employees of the Metropolitan Life Insurance Company. J Am Dent Assoc 1944;31:1632-42.
21. Eckerbom M, Magnusson T, Martinsson T. Reasons for and incidence of tooth mortality in a Swedish population. Endod Dent Traumatol 1992;8:230-4.
22. Ekanayaka A. Tooth mortality in plantation workers and residents in Sri Lanka. Community Dent Oral Epidemiol 1984;12:128-35.
23. Eklund SA, Burt BA. Risk factors for total tooth loss in the United States; longitudinal analysis of national data. J Public Health Dent 1994;54:5-14.
24. Ettinger RL, Beck JD. The new elderly: What can the dental profession expect? Spec Care Dentist 1982;2:62-9.

25. Gilbert GH, Duncan RP, Crandall LA, et al. Attitudinal and behavioral characteristics of older Floridians with tooth loss. Community Dent Oral Epidemiol 1993;21:384-9.

26. Gray PG, Todd JE, Slack GL, Bulman JS. Adult dental health in England and Wales 1968. London: Her Majesty's Stationery Office, 1970.

27. Hand JS, Hunt RJ, Kohout FJ. Five-year incidence of tooth loss in Iowans aged 65 and older. Community Dent Oral Epidemiol 1991;19:48-51.

28. Holm, G. Smoking as an additional risk for tooth loss. J Periodontol 1994;65:996-1001.

29. Hunt RJ, Beck DJ, Lemke JH, et al. Edentulism and oral health problems among elderly rural Iowans: The Iowa 65+ rural health study. Am J Public Health 1985;75:1177-81.

30. Hunt RJ, Drake CW, Beck JD. Eighteen-month incidence of tooth loss among older adults in North Carolina. Am J Public Health 1995;85:561-3.

31. Hyatt TP. Report of an examination made of two thousand one hundred and one high school girls. Dent Cosmos 1920;52:507-11.

32. Hyatt TP. Prophylactic odontotomy. Dent Cosmos 1923;65:234-41.

33. Johansson I, Tidehag P, Lundberg V, Hallmans G. Dental status, diet and cardiovascular risk factors in middle-aged people in northern Sweden. Community Dent Oral Epidemiol 1994;22:431-6.

34. Kalsbeek H, Truin GJ, Burgersdijk R, van't Hof M. Tooth loss and dental caries in Dutch adults. Community Dent Oral Epidemiol 1991;19:201-4.

35. Kay EJ, Blinkhorn AS. The reasons underlying the extraction of teeth in Scotland. Br Dent J 1986;160:287-90.

36. Klock KS, Haugejorden O. Primary reasons for extraction of permanent teeth in Norway: Changes from 1968 to 1988. Community Dent Oral Epidemiol 1991;19:336-41.

37. Knutson JW, Klein H. Studies on dental caries. IV. Tooth mortality in elementary school children. Public Health Rep 1938;53:1021-32.

38. Löe H, Ånerud A, Boysen H, Smith M. The natural history of periodontal disease in man. Tooth mortality rates before 40 years of age. J Periodont Res 1978;13:563-72.

39. Locker D. Smoking and oral health in older adults. Can J Public Health 1992;83:429-32.

40. Loesche WJ, Abrams J, Terpenning MS, et al. Dental findings in geriatric populations with diverse medical backgrounds. Oral Surg Oral Med Oral Pathol Oral Radiol Endod 1995;80:43-54.

41. Luan WM, Baelum V, Chen X, Fejerskov O. Tooth mortality and prosthetic treatment patterns in urban and rural Chinese aged 20-80 years. Community Dent Oral Epidemiol 1989;17:221-6.

42. Manji F, Baelum V, Fejerskov O. Tooth mortality in an adult rural population in Kenya. J Dent Res 1988;67:496-500.

43. Marcus SE, Drury TF, Brown LJ, Zion GR. Tooth retention and tooth loss in the permanent dentition of adults: United States, 1988-1991. J Dent Res 1996;75(Spec Issue):684-95.

44. Marshall TA, Warren JJ, Hand JS, et al. Oral health, nutrient intake and dietary quality in the very old. J Am Dent Assoc 2002;133:1369-79.

45. Miller Y, Locker D. Correlates of tooth loss in a Canadian adult population. J Can Dent Assoc 1994;60:549-55.

46. Mosha HJ, Lema PA. Reasons for tooth extraction among Tanzanians. East Afr Med J 1991;68:10-4.

47. Murray H, Locker D, Kay EJ. Patterns of and reasons for tooth extractions in general dental practice in Ontario, Canada. Community Dent Oral Epidemiol 1996;24:196-200.

48. Niessen LC, Weyant RJ. Causes of tooth loss in a veteran population. J Public Health Dent 1989;49:19-23.

49. Nizel AE, Bibby BG. Geographic variations in caries prevalence in soldiers. J Am Dent Assoc 1944;31:1619-26.

50. Osterberg T, Carlsson GE, Sundh W, Fyhrlund A. Prognosis of and factors associated with dental status in the adult Swedish population, 1975-1989. Community Dent Oral Epidemiol 1995;23:232-6.

51. Pelton WJ, Pennell EH, Druzina A. Tooth morbidity experience of adults. J Am Dent Assoc 1954;49:439-45.

52. Phipps KR, Stephens VJ. Relative contribution of caries and periodontal disease in adult tooth loss for an HMO dental population. J Public Health Dent 1995;55:250-2.

53. Schlack CA, Restarski JS, Dochterman EF. Dental status of 71,015 naval personnel at first examination in 1942. J Am Dent Assoc 1946;33:1141-6.

54. Steele JG, Walls AW, Ayatollahi SM, Murray JJ. Major clinical findings from a dental survey of elderly people in three different English communities. Br Dent J 1996;180:17-23.

55. Stephens RG, Kogon SL, Jarvis AM. A study of the reasons for tooth extraction in a Canadian population sample. J Can Dent Assoc 1991;57:501-4.

56. Thomson WM, Poulton R, Kruger E, Boyd D. Socio-economic and behavioural risk factors for tooth loss from age 18 to 26 among participants in the Dunedin Multidisciplinary Health and Development Study. Caries Res 2000;34:361-6.

57. Todd JE, Whitworth A. Adult dental health in Scotland, 1972. London: Her Majesty's Stationery Office, 1974.

58. US Department of Health and Human Services, National Center for Health Statistics. Third National Health and Nutrition Examination Survey, 1988-94. Public Use Data File No. 7-0627. Hyattsville MD: Centers for Disease Control and Prevention, 1997.

59. US Public Health Service. Loss of teeth, United States June 1957-June 1958. PHS Publication No. 584-B22, Series B No. 22. Washington DC: Government Printing Office, 1960.

60. US Public Health Service, Centers for Disease Control and Prevention. National Oral Health Surveillance System, Complete tooth loss, website: http://www2a.cdc.gov/nohss/ListV.asp?qkey=4. Accessed December 19, 2003.

61. US Public Health Service, National Center for Health Statistics. Edentulous persons, United States 1971. DHEW Publication No. (HRA) 74-1516, Series 10 No. 89. Washington DC: Government Printing Office, 1974.

62. US Public Health Service, National Center for Health Statistics. Decayed, missing, and filled teeth among persons 1-74 years; United States. DHHS Publication No. (PHS) 81-1673, Series 11 No. 223. Washington DC: Government Printing Office, 1981.

63. US Public Health Service, National Center for Health Statistics. Use of dental services and dental health, United States 1986. DHHS Publication No. (PHS) 88-1593, Series 10 No. 165. Washington DC: Government Printing Office, 1988.

64. US Public Health Service, National Institute of Dental Research. Oral health of United States adults; national findings. NIH Publication No. 87-2868. Washington DC: Government Printing Office, 1987.

65. US Public Health Service, National Institute of Dental Research. Oral health of United States children. NIH Publication No. 89-2247. Washington DC: Government Printing Office, 1989.

66. Warren JJ, Watkins CA, Cowen HJ, et al. Tooth loss in the very old: 13-15-year incidence among elderly Iowans. Community Dent Oral Epidemiol 2002;30:29-37.

67. Weintraub JA, Burt BA. Tooth loss in the United States. J Dent Educ 1985;49:368-76.

68. World Health Organization. WHO oral health country/area profile programme, Caries for 12-year-olds by country/area, website: http://www.whocollab. odont. lu.se/countriesalphab.html. Accessed December 20, 2003.

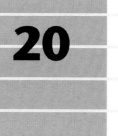

20 Dental Caries

Dental caries is an ancient disease, dating back to at least the time that agriculture replaced hunting and gathering as the principal source of food. Examination of skulls in Britain suggests that the moderate caries experience found in the Anglo-Saxon period (fifth to seventh centuries) had changed little by the end of the Middle Ages, approximately the year 1500.[154,155] Dental attrition in this period was extensive and occurred early in life; some lesions in young persons seem to have begun in the occlusal fissures but developed no further because attrition progressed faster than caries. Most lesions found in human remains from this period were cervical or root caries; coronal caries was relatively uncommon. The modern pattern of caries in the high-income nations, with lesions beginning in fissured surfaces and developing later on proximal surfaces, was not evident in Britain until the sixteenth century.[156]

Dietary changes that began during the eighteenth century, principally increased refinement of foods and greater availability of sugar, are considered chiefly responsible for the development of the modern pattern of caries. Import duties on sugar in Britain were relaxed in 1845 and completely removed by 1875, a period during which the severity of caries greatly increased.[51,119] By the end of the nineteenth century, dental caries was well established as an endemic disease of massive proportions in most developed countries.[35]

This chapter examines the distribution of dental caries in populations and the factors that influence that distribution. Although there is a rare disease known as bone caries, we use the term *caries* in this chapter to refer to dental caries.

GLOBAL DISTRIBUTION OF CARIES

Although some of the historic patterns of high attrition, little coronal caries, and moderate prevalence of root caries could still be found in remote places in the twentieth century,[184-186] they are fast disappearing as once-isolated populations become infected with cariogenic bacteria and increasingly adopt the cariogenic diets and lifestyles of the developed world.

For most of the twentieth century, caries was seen as a disease of the high-income countries, with low prevalence in poorer countries. The most obvious reason for this pattern is diet. The high level of consumption of refined carbohydrates in the wealthier countries led to selective proliferation of cariogenic bacteria.[52] Poorer societies, on the other hand, survived by hunting and subsistence farming, both of which provided diets low in fermentable carbohydrates.

By the late twentieth century, there were signs of change in this traditional pattern. First, there was some evidence that caries experience in some low-income countries had risen sharply in the years after World War II (1939-45).[151] However, this change was by no means universal, and caries incidence in many such countries, especially those in Africa, remains relatively low.[12,50,144,158-160] The second change is the marked reduction in caries experience among children and young adults in high-income countries, a trend that first became evident in the late 1970s.[35] This change, which has already had a marked impact on dental practice, will affect oral conditions among the whole population in due course as today's younger cohorts progress through the life span.

The World Health Organization (WHO) maintains the Global Oral Health Data Bank, a collection of surveillance data from almost all countries in the world. The most extensive data set in the data bank is for DMFT values (number of decayed, missing, or filled permanent teeth) for 12-year-olds, a response to the global goal set by WHO in 1982 (see Chapter 5). Table 20-1 shows the trends in these values in 11 high-income countries over a recent period of some 10-20 years. In most of these countries the decline in caries levels has been substantial, even spectacular in some cases. It is not universal, however, because both Korea and Kuwait have seen a rise in DMFT scores. This could be because preventive measures have lagged behind growing affluence in these two countries, whereas preventive measures have become established, at least to some extent, in the other nine.

Table 20-2 shows the same trends for middle-income countries, those without the resources of the countries in the previous table, and here the pattern is different. Only Cuba, which has had a school dental service for years, and Estonia, where caries levels were very high, have shown a substantial drop in caries levels over the same 10-20 years. Of the others, four have shown a minor decline, and four have had an increase. These countries are arbitrarily chosen from many in WHO's Global Oral Data Bank, but they do show a picture that is fairly representative—nations with better-developed public health prevention generally have shown most success in caries prevention. However, among countries of all income levels there are distinct differences in caries experience from one country to another, and from region to region within a country. Intercountry differences are illustrated by the results of the first International Collaborative Study (ICS I), promoted by WHO with funding and cooperation from the U.S. Public Health Service and the participating countries. These data were collected during the mid-1970s,[9] and the mean DMFT values for children ages 13-14 in the first seven

Table 20-1 Trends in dental caries experience, as measured by mean DMFT values in 12-year-old children, in 11 high-income countries[*] in the late twentieth century[233]

Country	Initial DMFT	Latest DMFT	Initial Year	Latest Year
Australia	3.0	0.8	1982	1999
Denmark	5.0	0.9	1980	2001
Finland	4.0	1.1	1982	1997
France	4.2	1.9	1987	1998
Iceland	8.3	1.5	1982	1996
Ireland	3.3	1.3	1984	2002
Korea	2.5	3.1	1979	1995
Kuwait	2.0	2.6	1982	1993
Japan	5.4	2.4	1981	1999
Spain	4.2	2.3	1984	1994
USA	1.8	1.3	1987	1994

[*]As defined by the World Bank in World Bank Group, Data and statistics, Country groups, website: http://www.worldbank.org/data/countryclass/classgroups.htm. Accessed December 18, 2003.

participating countries are shown in Fig. 20-1. These data were not from nationally representative population samples but rather from selected communities. The data for the United States, for instance, came from the metropolitan area of Baltimore, a city with fluoridated water since 1952. The areas chosen for examination in Australia (Sydney) and Canada (Ontario) also had had fluoridated water for some years.

The data in Fig. 20-1 provide some food for thought regarding both caries treatment and its measurement. The two highest mean DMF values are found in Norway (Trøndelag) and New Zealand (Canterbury), both countries with extensive school dental services. The same two countries, it will be noticed, have the lowest mean D values, virtually no tooth loss, and by far the highest mean F values. As noted in the

Table 20-2 Trends in dental caries experience, as measured by mean DMFT values in 12-year-old children, in 11 lower-middle- and upper-middle-income countries[*] in the late twentieth century[233]

Country	Initial DMFT	Latest DMFT	Initial Year	Latest Year
China	0.8	1.0	1983	1996
Cuba	2.9	1.4	1989	1998
Estonia	4.1	2.7	1992	1998
Lithuania	3.6	4.9	1986	1994
Malaysia	2.4	1.6	1988	1997
Morocco	2.3	2.5	1991	1999
Poland	4.4	3.8	1985	2000
Saudi Arabia	2.0	1.7	1985	1995
Sri Lanka	1.9	1.4	1984	1995
Thailand	1.5	1.6	1984	2001
Trinidad Tobago	4.9	5.2	1989	1998

[*]As defined by the World Bank in World Bank Group, Data and statistics, Country groups, website: http://www.worldbank.org/data/countryclass/classgroups.htm. Accessed December 18, 2003.

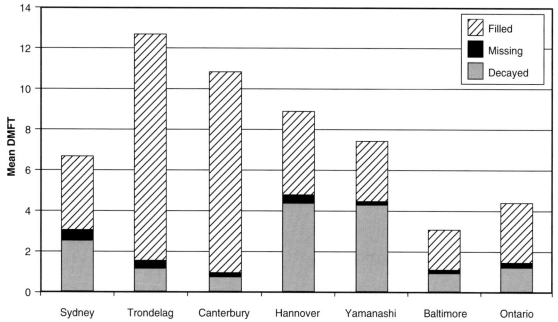

Fig. 20-1 Decayed, missing, and filled permanent teeth in children ages 13-14 in seven countries. Data from the first International Collaborative Study, 1973-75.[15,25,67]

discussion of the DMF index in Chapter 15, data such as those in Fig. 20-1 reflect dental treatment as much as disease.

SECULAR VARIATIONS IN CARIES EXPERIENCE

When caries was more prevalent and severe than at present, affected teeth were attacked within 2-4 years after eruption. By the early 1980s, there were reports from local surveys to suggest that the average prevalence and severity of caries among children in the United States was declining from its previously high levels.[34,72,87,200] Similar information from other high-income countries around the same time[7,88,89,143,182] indicated that this reduction in caries experience was widespread.

The decline in caries experience among children was confirmed for the United States by results of the National Dental Caries Prevalence Survey of U.S. schoolchildren in 1979-80.[219] This survey showed that mean DMF scores among children ages 5 to17 years were some 32% lower than those found in the first National Health and Nutrition Examination Survey (NHANES I) of 1971-74.[217] The next national survey of U.S. schoolchildren in 1986-87 found that the decline was continuing,[221] with mean DMF scores for 5- to

17-year-olds again 36% lower than those from 7 years earlier, and further decline was seen in the third National Health and Nutrition Examination Survey (NHANES III) of 1988-94.[213] Mean DMFS scores (number of decayed, missing, or filled permanent tooth surfaces) for schoolchildren ages 9-17 in 1979-80 and 1988-94 are shown in Fig. 20-2, and the reduction in caries experience is obvious. In the 1988-94 data there were few missing teeth, and the highest mean value for decayed surfaces was 1.14 for the 17-year-olds. The index bars for 1988-94 data in Fig. 20-2 are made up predominantly of the F component. The decline has also been documented in primary teeth: mean dfs scores (number of decayed or filled primary tooth surfaces) for 6-year-olds in the 1979-80 survey was 4.76;[219] this was down to 3.73 in 1986-87.[221]

The seemingly sudden caries decline among children in high-income nations was documented at a conference in Boston in 1982, the proceedings of which were published in a special issue of the *Journal of Dental Research* in November 1982. The caries decline in the permanent dentition among children of high-income nations has continued since then,[10,23,37,47,56,117,140,195,211] although caries experience in the primary dentition may have leveled out by the early 1990s.[33,37,79,98,140,194,211]

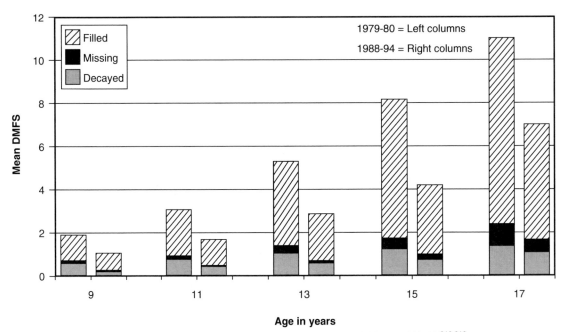

Fig. 20-2 DMFS values for U.S. children ages 9-17, in 1979-80 and 1988-94.[213,219]

Although the downward trend in caries experience (permanent teeth) among American and Canadian children was continuing through the 1990s, the rate of decrease must get slower as overall caries experience approaches an irreducible minimum level. The main caries problem in the United States and some other countries today is not so much overall caries levels as the disparities in disease experience and treatment between different socioeconomic and racial-ethnic groups.

The reduction in caries has not occurred evenly for all kinds of tooth surfaces; it has been proportionately greater for free smooth surfaces and proximal surfaces than for pit-and-fissure surfaces.[24,110,196] An unexpected outcome in a 3-year longitudinal study in Michigan in the early 1980s was that 81% of all new lesions were on pit- and-fissure surfaces. No lesions at all were found on free smooth surfaces.[38]

As caries prevalence falls, the least susceptible sites (proximal and smooth surfaces) reduce by the greatest proportion, while the most susceptible sites (occlusal) reduce by the smallest proportion.[142]

The net result is that, although the total number of new carious lesions has been declining, an increasing proportion of them is made up of pit- and-fissure lesions. This trend has enhanced the attractiveness of fissure sealants as a preventive measure (see Chapter 27).

History has many examples of diseases that have waxed and waned without precise knowledge of why, and the caries decline is one of these. No clear reasons for the caries decline have been identified, although most researchers view the various uses of fluoride as the main cause.[30] Sugar consumption in the United States has increased (see Chapter 28) rather than diminished, and it is difficult to ascribe the decline to better oral hygiene or to changes in the bacterial ecology of the oral cavity, whereas an influential role for fluoride is hard to reject.[36] Even the effect of widespread use of pediatric antibiotics on oral bacteria has been suggested as a contributory factor.[128] However, as with other diseases that show a cyclical nature over time, it is quite likely that factors are operating that have not been identified.

UNEVEN DISTRIBUTION OF CARIES

For many years, the results of surveys and even research studies were presented only as mean DMF values, usually with only a standard deviation to indicate the distribution. Although means are useful, they compress extreme values (i.e., absence of caries and caries in many teeth in the same mouth) into an average figure that sometimes can be misleading. A landmark break from this convention came with the results of the National Preventive Dentistry Demonstration Program (NPDDP) in the mid-1980s. The NPDDP studied the effects of a series of preventive procedures in children in grades 1, 2, and 5 in five cities with and five cities without fluoridated water. The NPDDP drew attention to the fact that, although average caries experience in children was lower than the researchers had originally expected, there was still a significant minority with severe caries.[74] This type of distribution is illustrated in Fig. 20-3, which provides data from the national surveys of schoolchildren in 1979-80 and 1988-94. Whereas Fig. 20-2 illustrates the decline in mean DMFS scores that occurred between the two surveys, Fig. 20-3 shows the distributional changes. It is evident that in the more recent survey the proportion of "caries-free" children (Box 20-1) had increased, whereas the proportion with severe caries had decreased. Even so, the shape of the distribution remained much the same: highly skewed toward zero or few DMFS teeth, but with a persistent "tail," meaning that there were still children at the severe end of the scale.

Although there is no established definition of "severe" caries, DMFS values of 7.0 or higher today can be considered to indicate severe disease in children up to age 17. Of all U.S. children, 27.3% fell into this category in 1979-80; this number had dropped to 17.3% by 1986-87. To pick a round figure, 20% is a fair estimate of the proportion of U.S. children who suffer from severe caries.

Fig. 20-4 is a cumulative frequency curve demonstrating that most caries occurs in a relatively small number of children. This figure is restricted to children of the same age (in this case, 15 years) so that the curve does not reflect age differences. When the values in Fig. 20-4 are read off, it can be seen that 60% of all affected

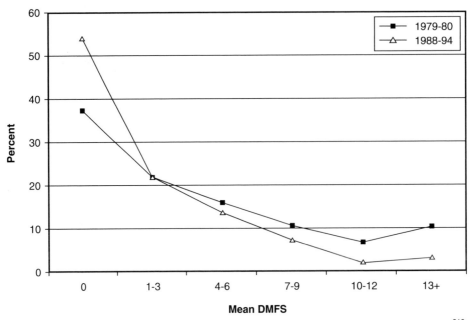

Fig. 20-3 Distribution of mean DMFS values in U.S. schoolchildren ages 5-17, 1979-80 and 1988-94.[213]

BOX 20-1 What Does *Caries Free* Mean?

The term *caries free* has traditionally been used to describe people with a DMF score (number of decayed, missing, or filled teeth) of 0, usually when the presence of a dentinal, or D3, lesion is the stated or implied criterion for caries. As the understanding of caries has increased, it has become evident that very few people are literally caries free. Just about everyone, at any given time, has some level of carious activity taking place. Most of this activity consists of early demineralization-remineralization cycles or a white spot or stained fissure that does not progress. In a healthy mouth, the bulk of this activity does not reach the stage where restorative dental treatment is needed, although preventive intervention may be called for. But this still means that the term *caries free* is not correct. Perhaps more importantly, use of this term can tend to promote a mindset that caries does not matter, or perhaps does not even exist, until it involves the dentin. That is clearly incorrect, for preventive treatment at this stage can forestall the need for later restorative treatment. A more accurate term would be *free of caries requiring restorative treatment*, but that is much too clumsy for everyday use.

The term *caries free* will continue to be used in this context because it has history and ease of use on its side. It must be remembered, however, that rarely is it a strictly correct term. It is used to mean that caries has not reached a stage where operative dental treatment is needed.

---

teeth are found in about 20% of children, and three fourths of all affected teeth are found in about one fourth of the children. This concentration of disease in relatively few children has led to the concept of *targeting* public health prevention programs toward that highly affected minority, and it has stimulated research into methods of predicting which children are likely to be in the 20% or so that is most affected (see Chapter 14).

REGIONAL VARIATIONS IN CARIES DISTRIBUTION IN THE UNITED STATES

Regional variations in caries experience within the United States were first documented with the examination of young men in the armed forces during World War II.[104,164,188,190] It is of interest to note that regional differences in caries prevalence among different tribes of Native Americans were demonstrated in the

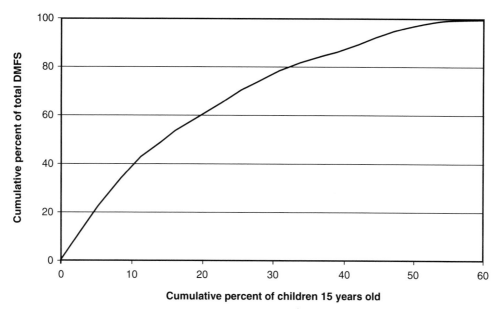

Fig. 20-4 Cumulative frequency curve of the proportion of total DMF teeth in U.S. schoolchildren ages 15 years, 1988-94.[213]

early 1930s,[106] with more severe disease among tribes in the Northwest than among those in the Southwest. This regional pattern is still seen today in the general American population.

The World War II surveys were in general agreement that the most severe caries experience was seen in recruits from New England, the Pacific Northwest, and the Great Lakes area, with distinctly less caries in young men from the South, the Southwest, and the mountain states. In the years since World War II, some of these differences have been obscured by the spread of water fluoridation, but they were still apparent in the late 1960s.[130] The regional differences in a representative sample of youths ages 12-17 years in a national survey conducted in 1966-70 are illustrated for whites and African-Americans in Fig. 20-5.

Regional differences in caries experience are not unique to the United States, for just about every country exhibits similar variations. For example, in Britain, despite an overall decline in caries experience that parallels that seen in the United States, children's oral health is still poorer in Scotland and northern England than in southern England.[170,171]

CARIES DISTRIBUTION: DEMOGRAPHIC RISK FACTORS

Age

Mean DMF scores increase with age, as shown in Fig. 20-2 for schoolchildren and Fig. 20-6 for adults. It can be seen that the increase with age for the children's' cohorts comes largely from an increase in numbers of restored teeth, whereas for the adults (see Fig. 20-6) most of the increase with age comes from missing teeth. Both figures are from cross-sectional data, so as younger cohorts replace today's older people, the M component will decrease (see Chapter 19). With fewer restorations now also being placed in younger people,[60] the overall DMF values in older people are also likely to decline with time. The impact of the caries decline naturally takes longer to become evident in adults than in children, because many of those who were adults when the data in Fig. 20-6 were collected had already experienced much of their caries activity before the modern age of prevention.

Caries used to be considered a childhood disease, a perception that arose in days of high caries severity when most susceptible surfaces were usually affected by adulthood. With younger people now reaching adulthood with

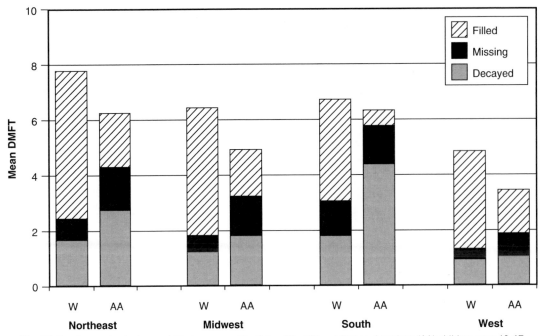

Fig. 20-5 Decayed, missing, and filled permanent teeth in white (W) and African-American (AA) children ages 12-17 in four geographic areas of the United States, 1966-70.[216]

many surfaces free of caries, the carious attack is spread out more throughout life. Adults of all ages can develop new coronal lesions,[57,77] and caries has to be viewed as a lifetime disease. Even the disease distribution seen in youth—

that is, the clustering of most disease in a relatively small number of people (see Fig. 20-4)—is seen in the elderly.[145]

In populations in which caries experience is severe, the disease starts early in life and is com-

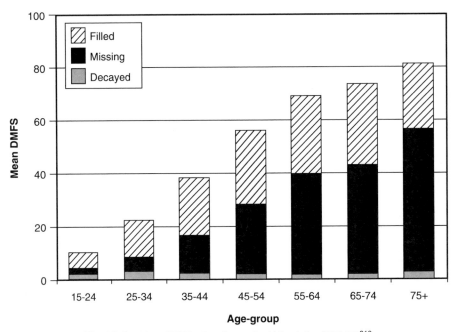

Fig. 20-6 Mean DMFS values by age for U.S. adults, 1988-94.[213]

mon in the young. A more even occurrence of new lesions throughout life is characteristic of communities with a lower attack rate.

Gender

Females have usually demonstrated higher DMF scores than do males of the same age,[215,220,221] although this finding is not universal. When observed in children, the difference has been attributed to the earlier eruption of teeth in females,[108,207] but this explanation is hard to support when the differences are seen in older age-groups. In those instances a treatment factor is more likely to be contributing to the differences. In national survey data, males usually have more untreated decayed surfaces than females, and females have more restored teeth. Females visit the dentist more frequently (see Chapter 2), so this observation is perhaps to be expected. In NHANES III, females ages 12-17 years had the same mean number of decayed and missing surfaces as their male counterparts but 25% more filled surfaces.[98] We cannot conclude from these figures that females are more susceptible to caries than are males; a combination of earlier tooth eruption plus a treatment factor is a more likely explanation for the observed differences.

Race and Ethnicity

Long-held contentions that certain races enjoy a high degree of resistance to dental caries probably came with early observations that some non-European races, such as those in Africa and India, enjoyed a greater freedom from caries than did Europeans. Today, however, we accept that global variations in caries experience result more from environment than from inherent racial attributes. To illustrate that point, there is evidence that certain racial groups once thought to be resistant to caries quickly developed the disease when they migrated to areas with different cultural and dietary patterns.[17,152,179] In the United States, most surveys before the 1970s found that whites had higher DMF scores than African-Americans, although the latter usually had more decayed teeth because of poorer access to care. The National Health Survey of 1960-62 showed that whites had higher DMF scores than did African-American adults of the same age-group, a difference that remained even

when the groups were standardized for income and education.[214] Fig. 20-5, showing regional differences in caries severity, also illustrates the differences in DMF status between whites and African-Americans in the 1960s. It can be seen in Fig. 20-5 that overall DMF scores are higher among whites, although big differences in dental treatment are obvious. This difference was still evident in NHANES I in 1971-74,[217] although other studies from around that time were finding little difference in DMF scores between whites and African-Americans of the same age.[13,85]

By the time of NHANES III in 1988-94, however, there was little difference in total DMF scores between whites and African-Americans, although whites still had a higher filled component and lower scores for decayed and missing surfaces. Fig. 20-7 shows data for children ages 13, 15, and 17 for illustration. DMF values for Mexican-Americans were in the midrange, and those in the "Other" racial-ethnic category had the highest overall DMF scores of all. This turnaround could indicate improving access to care for African-Americans, although it most likely reflects socioeconomic differences: the caries decline, as previously noted, is sharpest in the higher socioeconomic groups. The summary of relative DMFT scores for 12- and 15-year-old white and African-American children in five national surveys given in Fig. 20-8 illustrates the relative changes down the years.

The caries status of Hispanic Americans has not been as well studied, although valuable information came from the Hispanic Health and Nutrition Examination Survey (HHANES) of 1982-84. Data showed that DMF scores of Mexican-American adults were lower than the national average, but the D component was higher.[90] Among children, a similar picture emerged in Mexican-Americans of the Southwest, Cuban communities of Miami, and Puerto Rican groups in New York.[92]

The overall pattern gives no reason to believe that inherent differences exist in caries susceptibility among African-Americans, people of Hispanic origin, and whites. Socioeconomic differences—that is, differences in education, self-care practices, attitudes, values, available income, and access to health care—appear to be far more important.

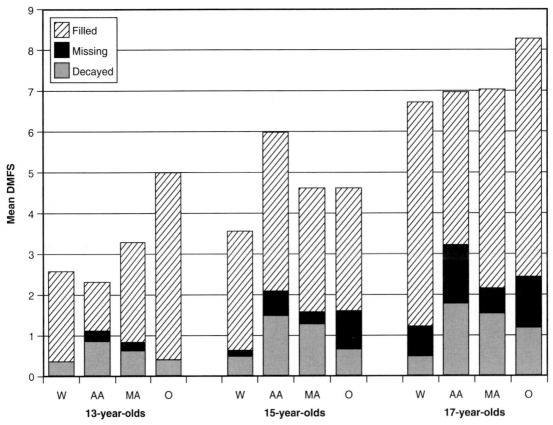

Fig. 20-7 Mean DMFS values for 13-, 15-, and 17-year-old children in white (W), African-American (AA), Mexican-American (MA), and other (O) racial and ethnic groups in the United States, 1988-94.[213]

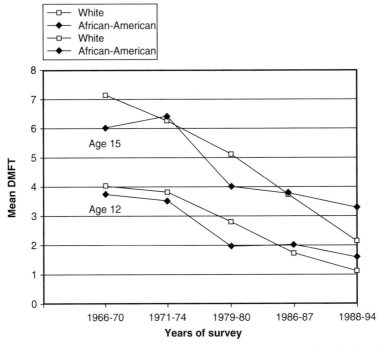

Fig. 20-8 Mean DMFT scores for 12- and 15-year-old white and African-American children in five national surveys in the United States, 1966-70 to 1988-94.[213]

Socioeconomic Status

Socioeconomic status (SES), called *social class* in Britain, is a broad recording of an individual's attitudes and values as measured by such factors as education, income, occupation, and place of residence. Attitudes toward health are often part of the set of values that follow from an individual's prestige in society and may explain some of the observed differences in health between SES groups. However, obtaining a valid measure of SES is always a problem because of its complexity. In the United States SES is usually measured by annual income or years of education, despite acknowledged shortcomings in these measures.[76]

SES is inversely related to the incidence of many diseases and to characteristics thought to affect health.[136] The reasons seem obvious in many cases, but not all.[123] For example, differences in infant mortality by SES can be explained partly by the fact that higher SES women have better access to prenatal care, more ability to afford such care, the time to get it, probably less fatalistic attitudes, and perhaps some other factors.[68] However, even after all these likely variables have been factored into explaining the differences, there is still a considerable gap that defies explanation. In dental health, a similar finding was reported in Finland,[148] where differences in caries experience between children in the higher and lower social classes still remained after accounting for age, sex, reported frequency of toothbrushing, consumption of sugars, and ingestion of fluoride tablets. Children in Finland also have virtually equal access to publicly funded dental care, regardless of SES, which is not the case in the United States. Measurements used in science cannot always pick up all the subtleties embedded in SES.

As part of his landmark research in caries epidemiology during the 1930s and 1940s, Klein observed that overall DMF values did not differ between SES groups, but aspects of treatment certainly did.[109] Lower SES groups had higher values for D and M, and lower values for F. In the first national survey of U.S. children in 1963-65, white children in the higher SES strata actually had higher DMF scores than did white children in the lower strata, but African-American children showed the opposite pattern.[215] In both white and African-American children, the mean number of D teeth diminished with increasing SES, and the mean number of M teeth showed little change. In white children, however the F component ballooned so much with increasing SES that it lifted the whole DMF index. By contrast, the F component in the African-American children did not change, with the net result that DMF diminished with increasing SES. As mentioned earlier, these results from 1963-65 showed that a "treatment effect" (see Chapter 15) was artificially inflating the DMF data in the white children, whereas the values for the African-American children were likely to be a more valid measure of the carious attack.

With the lower overall caries experience of today, however, the position has been reversed. The NPDDP showed that the higher SES groups have enjoyed the sharpest decline in caries experience,[74] so that the DMF values of children in the higher SES strata are now considerably below those of children in the lower SES strata. This is illustrated in Fig. 20-9, which graphs the components of the DMFS index for 15-year-old children in low, medium, and high SES groups as measured in NHANES III in 1988-94. Fig. 20-10 shows the same components for adults in three age-groups, and the same patterns can be seen relative to SES. Among the older adults, those in the higher SES groups had fewer missing and more filled surfaces. In the younger group, however, both total DMFS scores and the values of all of its components were lower in the higher SES groups. These data in Fig. 20-10 suggest that there may be a treatment effect in older age-groups that grew up before the preventive era, but among the 15- to 24-year-olds the higher SES groups clearly have lower caries experience.

Relationships between caries status and a broad range of SES measures (e.g., residence in private versus public housing, car ownership, quality of neighborhoods) have also been reported in Britain[44-46,73,166] and elsewhere in Europe.[83,141] When measures of social status appropriate for a nonindustrialized society have been used, such patterns have also been observed in Africa.[146] The British studies noted that, although fluoridation of water supplies (see Chapter 25) reduces the difference between the social classes, it does not entirely remove it.

These studies collectively demonstrate that dental caries today can be looked upon as a

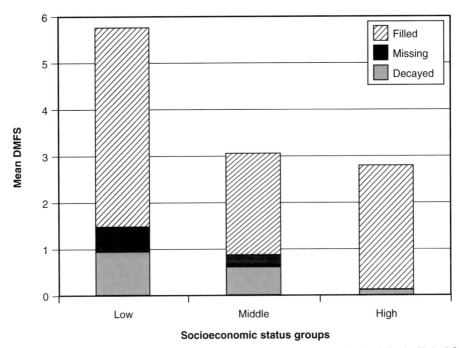

Fig. 20-9 Mean DMFS scores for 15-year-old children at three socioeconomic levels in the United States, 1988-94.[213]

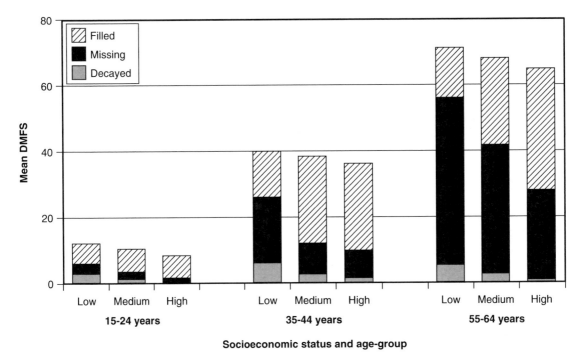

Fig. 20-10 Mean DMFS scores in adults ages 15-24 years, 35-44 years, and 55-64 years at three socioeconomic levels in the United States, 1988-94.[213]

disease of poverty or deprivation. The greatest reductions in caries experience have been enjoyed by the upper social groups, whereas reductions in the lower social groups have been more modest. When treatment programs are planned, caries experience can be expected to be more extensive and severe among lower SES populations.

Familial and Genetic Patterns

Familial tendencies ("bad teeth run in families") are noted by many dentists and have been clearly demonstrated.[70,107,111,174] However, these studies do not pin down whether such tendencies have a genetic basis or whether they stem from bacterial transmission or continuing familial dietary or behavioral traits. Husband-wife similarities clearly have no genetic origin, and intrafamilial transmission of cariogenic flora, especially from mother to infant, is accepted as a primary way for cariogenic bacteria to become established in children.[113,114,175] The lack of a genetic influence by race, discussed earlier, weakens the case for genetic inheritance of a susceptibility or resistance to caries, although Klein concluded that the similarities within families involved "strong familial vectors which very likely have a genetic basis, perhaps sex-linked."[105] Studies of identical twins have concluded that, although genetic factors could have affected caries experience to some extent, the influence of environmental variables was stronger.[135]

With the explosion of research discoveries of genetic influences in many diseases, dental caries is being viewed in a different light. It is likely that host attributes which could affect an individual's caries experience, such as salivary flow and composition, tooth morphology, and arch width, are genetically determined, and the genetics of the cariogenic bacteria themselves must have an effect. The rapid growth of research technology and interest in genetics holds promise that a new view of caries will emerge in the future.

CARIES DISTRIBUTION: RISK FACTORS AND RISK INDICATORS

Many factors are considered to be part of the causal web in dental caries: bacteria, diet, plaque deposits, saliva quantity and quality, enamel quality, and tooth morphology have all

been so considered. We do not attempt to detail the role of all of these factors in caries development; instead the reader is referred to texts such as *Dental caries: the disease and its clinical management*.[63] However, the role of bacteria and diet as risk factors (according to the definition given in Chapter 13) for development of caries is worth considering here.

Bacterial Infection

Caries is a bacterial disease. Bacteria are a necessary condition for its occurrence; that is, regardless of any other factor, caries cannot occur in the absence of bacteria.[62,127] The bacteria principally involved, the mutans streptococci and lactobacilli, are normal constituents of the flora in most mouths, so in that sense caries can be seen as an ecologic imbalance rather than an exogenous infection. It has been described as a carbohydrate-modified bacterial infectious disease, in which a cariogenic diet selectively favors cariogenic bacteria.[223] Cariogenic bacteria are transmissible, usually passed along from mother to child.[114,116,175] The complexity of bacterial interactions in caries development is illustrated by the finding that establishment of *Streptococcus sanguinis* during a "window of infectivity" in an infant appears to be antagonistic to the colonization of *Streptococcus mutans*.[48]

When caries experience is studied in groups, it usually is inversely related to counts of mutans streptococci in saliva or plaque,[20,26,112] although this relationship is not strong. At the individual level, however, bacterial counts by themselves are a poor predictor of future caries.[3,81,192] Although negative predictive values can be high (i.e., low bacterial counts predict the nondevelopment of caries fairly well), positive predictive values are not (i.e., high bacterial counts do not predict the development of future caries).[101]

The evidence is not yet clear enough to permit quantification of the risk attributable to specific bacteria, which in any case may vary in different populations. However, because infection with cariogenic bacteria is a necessary condition for caries to occur, it is obviously a risk factor for caries.

Nutrition and Caries

The term *diet* refers to the total oral intake of substances that provide nourishment and energy, whereas *nutrition* refers to the absorption of nutrients. In view of nutrition's fundamental role in human health, it is natural that its etiologic function in caries should have received a lot of attention. The suggestion that a deficiency of vitamin D is a causative factor in subsequent hypoplasia and development of dental caries[147] dates from 1934 and was most likely influenced by contemporary findings on vitamin-deficient diseases. There is evidence from studies of children in Peru that chronic and severe malnutrition during the first year of life is associated with increased caries years later, although this association is difficult to demonstrate because malnutrition delays eruption and exfoliation of the primary teeth.[5] Chronic malnutrition among children in India has been shown to reduce salivary flow, which could be one reason for a causative link.[94]

The epidemiologic evidence shows that, before the development of modern preventive methods, the prevalence of caries was lowest in those countries in which living standards were also lowest: even where generalized malnutrition was the norm, dental caries was uncommon.[1,58,133,139,178-180,206] This pattern is unlikely to have arisen because of protective factors in the unprocessed diet in poor societies, for it is very hard to identify any such factors that actually function in humans.[27] It is far more likely that the observed pattern came from nonexposure to the cariogenic foods found in high-income countries. Even in those countries in which caries prevalence is rising, this increase is largely confined to urban populations in which both dietary and cultural changes are occurring rapidly. Traditional village populations in Africa still show little sign of dental caries, although many of them suffer from some degree of malnutrition.[2,12,50,151,158-160,165,182] In the United States, no relation between nutritional adequacy and DMF scores could be found in NHANES I in 1971-74.[218]

The limited epidemiologic evidence thus favors the conclusion that severe, chronic malnutrition during infancy can predispose people to later dental caries. This situation is found in countries where malnourishment during early childhood is common but where there is later exposure to cariogenic foods; the malnutrition itself does not produce caries without the later cariogenic challenge. In the high-income nations, this degree of severe malnutrition is rare and is seen only in highly unusual circumstances.

Diet and Caries

In contrast to nutrition, diet has a clear influence on caries development. In particular, the relation between the intake of refined carbohydrates, especially sugars, and the prevalence and severity of caries is so strong that sugars are clearly a major etiologic factor in the causation of caries. This link has been recognized for many years.[29,39,64,131,161,162,176,191] Added sugars are the primary culprit, although a limited degree of caries occurs in populations for whom the only sugars consumed are naturally occurring.[183]

Although the evidence that consumption of sugars is a major risk factor for caries can be described as overwhelming, sugars are not the only food sources involved in the carious process. Cooked or milled starches can be broken down to low-molecular-weight carbohydrates by the salivary enzyme amylase and thus act as a substrate for cariogenic bacteria. It has been asserted that sugar-starch mixtures are more cariogenic than sugars alone,[22] and there is some animal evidence to support that view.[65] The issue may never be totally clarified in humans, but it is reasonable and prudent to view all sugar-containing food and drinks, as well as cooked or milled starches, as potentially cariogenic. By contrast, the high-molecular-weight carbohydrates in lightly cooked vegetables are considered noncariogenic because so little breakdown of these foods occurs in the mouth.[115,163]

Early Theories on Diet and Caries

The great exploratory voyages of the seventeenth and eighteenth centuries led to the discovery of peoples previously unknown to Europeans, such as the islanders of the South Pacific, who appeared to live an idyllic life free of the diseases that afflicted Europe at the time. The concept of the "noble savage"[59] thus developed during the latter part of the eighteenth century. An understandable offshoot of this ideal was the belief that the apparent freedom from caries enjoyed by so-called primitive races could be attributed to the "natural" diet on which they subsisted. Eating hard, fibrous, and unprocessed food, so the theory went, led to better development of the jaws and teeth and helped to clear food debris from the teeth. By contrast, Europeans were even then eating a lot of processed food, high in fermentable carbohydrates, which was thought to exercise the masticatory apparatus insufficiently and lead eventually to tooth decay. Against the background of these beliefs, Miller, in the late nineteenth century, put forward his chemoparasitic theory of the development of dental caries. Miller's theory, developed during the "golden age of bacteriology," was based on the action of microorganisms on fermentable carbohydrates that adhered to the tooth's surface.[149] Modern research shows that Miller's view of the overall picture was reasonably correct.

Theories about the preventive value of consumption of hard and fibrous foods became more widespread in the early twentieth century and became established dogma in many places. One such article of faith stated that accumulations of fermentable carbohydrates could be removed by eating hard and fibrous foods,[228] the so-called cleansing or detersive foods. Another view was that, if a meal were finished with a salivary stimulant such as an apple, the mouth would be kept free of fermentation both by the physical cleansing effect of the fibrous food and also by the salivary flow induced by it.[169]

As noted in the previous section, "protective" factors in an unrefined diet have proven hard to identify. High-fiber diets with a good proportion of unprocessed vegetables are today recommended by all health authorities. The low cariogenicity of these diets, however, is attributable less to the presence of hard and fibrous foods than to the relative absence of fermentable carbohydrates.

Some Major Epidemiologic Studies on Diet and Caries

World War II Studies

Strict food rationing in Japan made sugar virtually unobtainable during World War II. After the war, the mean DMF for 10-year-old children in 1950 was considerably below values recorded in 1940. However, by 1957 DMF values had returned to just higher than 1940 levels.[205]

Norway was occupied by German forces for much of World War II, a 5- to 6-year period during which strict food rationing was enforced. Among children 8-14 years of age, average height and weight were reduced, which indicated nutritional inadequacies. Dental effects during the occupation included delayed eruption of teeth, which began to be seen 1-2 years after rationing began and reached a peak after the war, returning to normal only in the 1950s.[208] Caries in the permanent dentition was drastically reduced, even after allowance was made for the effects of delayed eruption, and the number of children ages 7-8 who were free of detectable caries increased threefold to fourfold between 1941 and 1946.[209] Caries prevalence returned to 1941 levels by 1949, after rationing had ended.[210] Perhaps the most fascinating part of these Norwegian studies is the fact that they were done at all, given the conditions of the occupation.

Tristan da Cunha

The people on the remote island of Tristan da Cunha in the South Atlantic are mostly of European descent. The island's limited contacts with the outside world were gradually increasing when a volcanic eruption in the early 1960s led to the temporary evacuation of the entire community to England. The people returned when the island was habitable again, after which the establishment of some industry modernized the economy and created a demand for consumer goods. Much of the diet now consists of processed food. The Tristan da Cunha residents were given dental examinations on the island in 1932, 1937, and 1953; in England in 1962; and again on the island in 1966. The results show that the prevalence of caries in the first permanent molars of 6- to 19-year-olds was 0% in 1932 and 1937 but was 50% in 1962 and 80% in 1966.[66] More recent data will indicate if Tristan da Cunha has shared in the caries decline of more recent years.

Hopewood House

The Hopewood House institution in Australia provided an opportunity for a 15-year study of a group of children living on a basically vegetarian diet with severely restricted sucrose intake. The study began with 81 children, ages 4-9 years, of whom 63 (77.8%) had no detectable caries.[122] At age 13, 53% of the children still had no detectable caries, compared with 0.4%

of the local noninstitutionalized population of the same age.[201] Over the years some of the dietary restrictions at the institution were relaxed, but at the conclusion of the study the caries prevalence among 13-year-olds was still only 65.3%.[80] Although this study used small numbers and lacked a rigid research design, the differences between the Hopewood House children and the nearby population were so profound that the dental effects of dietary control were difficult to question.

Anthropologic Studies

There are numerous reports of the disastrously rapid increase in caries that occurs when an indigenous society comes in contact with the diet and lifestyle of high-income nations. Although the changes in such people's lives are often so culturally profound and abrupt that it is difficult to be sure that all changes in caries prevalence are due to diet, there is little question that the dietary factors are important. Examples of such instances have been reported in Polynesia,[16] Ghana,[114] and Greenland,[93,153,168] among the Inuit people of Canada's Northwest,[53] among Australian aborigines,[185,186] and among children on a remote Scottish island where a modern lifestyle replaced traditional ways.[78,79]

Hereditary Fructose Intolerance

The rare disease of hereditary fructose intolerance (HFI) requires that people who have it greatly minimize their sugar intake on a lifelong basis. Studies of persons with HFI, hard to conduct because of the rarity of the condition, show that they experience virtually no caries compared with normal subjects without HFI.[163] Although the numbers of people studied are necessarily small, the differences in the intake of sugars and in caries experience are extreme and obvious.

Vipeholm

The best-known attempt to conduct an experimental study on the effect of diet on dental decay in humans was the Vipeholm study, carried out in Sweden between 1945 and 1952.[75] The study was conducted in a mental institution, and by today's standards it would be considered unethical because it fed high quantities of sugars to people unable to give their informed consent to this regimen. Be that as it may, its conclusions profoundly influenced the views on the role of sugars in dental decay. The study design was complicated and not free of flaws. Briefly, inmates of the institution were divided into groups with controlled consumption of refined sugars that varied in amount, frequency, physical form, and time of consumption (with or between meals). The extremes of intake were (1) no added sugars at all, and (2) daily between-meal consumption of 24 sticky toffees, each of which was too large to be swallowed and so had to be sucked and chewed. The differences in caries incidence between the groups were pronounced. Some of the conclusions of the Vipeholm study can be challenged in light of more recent research, but they are listed in Box 20-2 because of the historical importance of this study.

Sugars-Caries Relationships in Today's Low-Caries Environment

The major studies described earlier were all conducted in the prefluoride era when caries was widespread and severe in high-income countries. In light of modern research protocols, design and analysis can be criticized in virtually all of them: all studies except the Vipeholm investigation were cross-sectional, and analysis considered only sugar intake (measured in various ways) and caries status. In the period of caries decline, however, we have to think that the "Vipeholm rules" have changed. Are all the children with no

---

BOX 20-2 Summarized Conclusions of the Vipeholm Study, 1946-52[75]

- Sugar consumption increases caries activity.
- The risk of increased caries activity is greater if the sugar is in sticky form.
- The risk is greatest if the sugar is taken between meals and in a sticky form.
- The increase in caries under uniform conditions shows great individual variation.
- The increase in caries disappears on withdrawal of sticky foodstuffs from the diet.
- Caries can still occur in the absence of refined sugar, natural sugars, and high total dietary carbohydrates.

Reprint by permission of Taylor & Francis AS.

detectable caries we see today not consuming sugar, or are other factors having a major influence? Studies such as those suggesting that oral hygiene is an important covariable in the sugars-caries relationship[82,103,203] have raised questions about the validity of the Vipehölm findings.

Two prospective studies reported in the 1980s, one in Britain and one in the United States, measured diet and caries incidence concurrently and included more analytical detail than did any previous research. The British study followed 405 children with an average initial age of 11.5 years for 2 years.[177] The children, all from a low-fluoride area near Newcastle, completed five food diaries, each for a 3-day period, for a total of 15 days of recorded diet over the 2 years. Interviews with a dietitian followed each 3-day period to clarify uncertainties and to quantify amounts. The mean DMFS incidence of the group was 3.63 over the 2 years, with 57% of new lesions in pits and fissures, a lower caries increment than the authors had expected. Average consumption of all sugars was 118 g/day, providing 21% of energy intake. The results showed that caries increment was weakly but significantly correlated with total intake of sugars, but poorly correlated with frequency of intake. The authors stated that, because of the lower than expected caries increment, more clear-cut results would have been likely if the study had been extended for another year.

The second study was based in the low-fluoride area of Coldwater, Michigan. It followed 499 children, initially ages 11-15, for 3 years.[38] The majority completed four 24-hour dietary recall interviews with a dietitian, although 27% completed more interviews. The boys in the study averaged 156 g of sugar intake per day from all sources, the girls 127 g; sugars accounted for 26% of total energy intake. Both of these measures are higher than was found in the British group. Caries incidence was lower than in the British group, however, averaging 2.9 DMF surfaces over the 3 years, of which 81% were pit-and-fissure lesions (buccal pits and lingual extensions as well as occlusal lesions). Nearly 30% of the group developed no caries at all over the 3 years, and only 51 children (10.2%) developed two or more proximal lesions during the study. Only in this latter

"high-caries" group was caries experience related to total intake of sugars, and that relationship was weak. No relationship was found between caries experience and frequency of consumption. The relative risk of caries from high sugar consumption compared with low sugar consumption was small[42]; each additional 5 g of sugar ingested daily was associated with a 1% increase in the probability of developing caries.[204]

Despite some differences in study protocols, findings in these two independent studies were generally similar. Between them, the studies indicated that consumption of sugars is not a major risk factor for many children (i.e., those with no caries despite consumption of a lot of sugar), but it is for those who are still clearly susceptible to caries (broadly defined here as the minority who got proximal-surface caries). A similar conclusion was reached in a systematic review of the caries-sugar relationship in countries where there is widespread exposure to fluoride.[41]

The much-stressed role of frequency of consumption of sugars ("it's not how much you eat, it's how often you eat it") is clearly called into question by the studies in Newcastle and Michigan, as it has been by others in Sweden.[21,198,202] The importance of frequency of consumption was a major finding of the Vipehölm study, and it has dominated dental health education ever since. However, the importance of frequency in Vipehölm was based principally on the caries experience of the group that consumed 24 large toffees between meals each day, a frequency of consumption that was not even approached in either the British or the Michigan study. The results from the highly artificial circumstances of the Vipehölm study thus may be misleading when generalized to the population. (The implications of these findings for dental health education are discussed in Chapter 28.)

Caries and Soft Drinks

As discussed earlier, sugar in liquid form is cariogenic. Sugar in liquid form served well to induce demineralization in landmark experimental caries studies.[226] There is more recent evidence to show that soft drink consumption is related to caries: the more soft drinks consumed, the greater the extent and severity of caries.[95,121,138,229] Soft drinks have also been implicated as part of the cause of the global epidemic of obesity in children,[134] because it is now common to find soft drinks and juices replacing formula and milk for children up to 2 years of age.[137] Therefore the subject has serious health implications that go beyond dentistry and is yet another example of a public general health problem that has clear dental overtones. (This issue is discussed further in Chapter 28.)

ROOT CARIES

Root caries is defined as caries that begins on cemental root surfaces below the cervical margin. It thus is found only where loss of periodontal attachment has led to exposure of the roots to the oral environment and hence to the accumulation of bacterial plaque around these exposed roots. Root caries appears to be polymicrobial,[189,223] with the bacterial composition of dental plaque in root lesions apparently little different from that of plaque found in coronal lesions.[32,61,69] As with coronal caries, sugars are part of the etiology.[167]

Root caries has been with humankind since our earliest days; indeed, most of the caries found in skulls dating from the Stone Age or earlier is root caries.[99,100,154] A similar pattern can be found today in some low-income coun-

tries.[129,132,187] In high-income countries, general awareness of root caries only increased in the early 1980s with the realization that older adults were retaining more teeth than they had previously. Subsequent studies have confirmed that root caries is highly prevalent among older persons in high-income countries.[14,18,49,71,84,124,126,157,181]

In NHANES III, the prevalence of root caries among American adults ages 18 or older was 25.1%.[232] Prevalence reached over 50% in men ages 65 or older and in women ages 75 or older. Prevalence varies in more localized surveys according to the age and nature of the population examined. Localized surveys in parts of the United States and Canada have found that incidence can range from 0.3 to 0.6 surfaces per person per year.[77,118,120]

Fig. 20-11 shows the prevalence of root caries by age among dentate adults in NHANES III. Males appear to be more affected than females. Although the condition is more prevalent in older age-groups, it is not uncommon among younger people. It is not yet clear whether these data represent a cohort pattern or whether the younger age-groups will look like the current older cohorts in the years ahead. One argument is that, as more teeth are retained, the number of surfaces at risk of root caries will increase. But if gingival recession becomes less common, then the overall prevalence and severity may not change much.

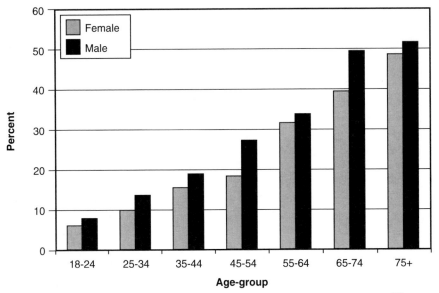

Fig. 20-11 Prevalence of root caries in U.S. adults and seniors by gender, 1988-94.[213]

Root caries, by definition, is strongly associated with the loss of periodontal attachment.[118,125,173,193,224,231] Other factors found to be associated with root caries are primarily socioeconomic, such as years of education, number of remaining teeth, use of dental services, oral hygiene levels, and preventive behavior.[18,54,86,225] An important risk factor is also the use of multiple medications among the elderly,[102] a common practice in nursing homes and one that can promote xerostomia (salivary diminution). Xerostomia has long been known as a major risk factor for caries among people of any age and is particularly prevalent among those who have received radiation treatment for cancer.[8] Other risk factors identified in a representative British sample of people ages 65 or older were practicing poor oral hygiene, wearing partial dentures, sucking candies in a dry mouth, and living in an institution.[199] People who suffer from coronal caries also seem likely to be at risk of root caries when gingival recession occurs,[19,225] and root caries is less prevalent in high-fluoride areas than it is in low-fluoride communities.[40,197] Smokers exhibit more root caries than nonsmokers, and severity tends to be inversely related to the number of teeth remaining.[18,125]

With regard to racial distribution, Fig. 20-12 shows the average number of root lesions in whites, African-Americans and Mexican-Americans as found in NHANES III. This graph suggests that African-Americans of most ages average more root lesions per person than do the other groups.

Root caries seems to be a particular problem among older people of lower SES, those who have lost some teeth, those who do not maintain good oral hygiene, and those who do not visit the dentist regularly. Because of the aging of the population and increasing retention of teeth, the dimensions of the root caries problem are likely to continue to grow in the future, even if the number of lesions per person shows little change. The attention of dental practitioners should be increasingly devoted to treating and preventing root caries in adults, as less time is needed to deal with coronal caries in children.

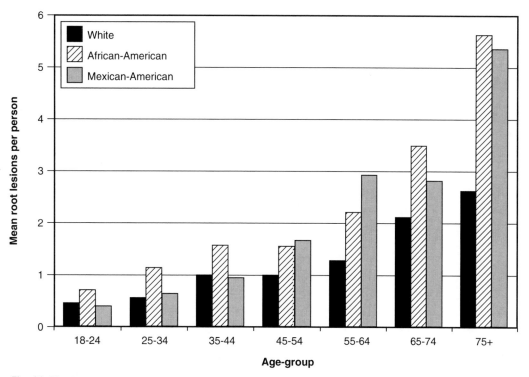

Fig. 20-12   Mean number of root lesions in whites, African-Americans, and Mexican-American by age in the United States, 1988-94.[213]

EARLY CHILDHOOD CARIES

Early childhood caries (ECC) is a distressing syndrome characterized by severe caries in the primary maxillary incisors of infants, typically those 1-3 years old. Total destruction of tooth crowns is common, other teeth in the mouth are usually involved, and ECC is difficult and expensive to treat.[227] There has long been confusion over the name of the condition,[91] which has variously been called *nursing caries, labial caries,* and *baby bottle tooth decay,* among other things, because the condition was seen to arise from prolonged infant feeding by either bottle or breast. Now it is understood that broader exposure to cariogenic diets can also be a factor.[55,212] The role of prolonged feeding with milk, either human or cow's, to which no further sugar has been added is uncertain. A systematic review of breastfeeding as a risk factor for ECC could reach no conclusions because the literature was marked by inconsistent study methods and case definitions.[222] Milk does not promote caries in laboratory studies,[28] and another systematic review concluded that the evidence for even prolonged use of the bottle as a risk factor in ECC is weak.[172] Prolonged exposure to liquids with added sugars or to high-sugar fluids such as soft drinks or fruit juices is considered the main culprit, but, again, precise evidence is elusive.

In the United States prevalence of ECC at the national level is extremely low, but in particular groups in which ECC is concentrated, prevalence can be as high as 70%.[150] A cursory visual inspection of children ages 12-23 months in NHANES III found a 2% prevalence, with most cases among children of Mexican-American heritage.[96] ECC is prevalent among immigrants to the United States and among Native Americans,[31,230] as well as among indigenous peoples elsewhere.[4,6] It is more prevalent in lower SES populations and among infants who are being cared for by persons with little education.[150] ECC has been associated with lower than average growth among affected infants,[11] and children with the condition seem to be at greater risk for caries in the permanent dentition later in life.[97] These latter observations may reflect chronically poor and cariogenic diets rather than direct cause and effect.

Research into the condition has been hampered by absence of a clear case definition.

Caries of the primary maxillary incisors, often with little if any caries of primary molars, is the most common case definition, but some investigators have defined it as generalized rampant caries or the presence of caries on the buccal and lingual surfaces of the incisors. In an effort to reach a clear case definition, a workshop group in 1999 took the view that *any* caries before 6 years of age is ECC and that there are degrees of severity above that, referred to as *severe early childhood caries,* or S-ECC (see Chapter 15). Whether this approach to the problem will clarify the issue remains to be seen.

Prevention of ECC has been based largely on education, but it is clear that simply pointing out to parents the dangers of excessive feeding with sugary liquids is by itself ineffective.[230] A better understanding of the social and cultural factors involved among the population groups most affected is clearly needed if the prevalence of ECC is to be seriously reduced among affected groups.

REFERENCES

1. Afonsky D. Some observations on dental caries in central China. J Dent Res 1951;30:53-61.
2. Akpata ES. Pattern of dental caries in urban Nigerians. Caries Res 1979;13:242-9.
3. Alaluusua S, Kleemola-Kujala E, Gronroos L, Evalahti M. Salivary caries-related tests as predictors of future caries increment in teenagers. A three-year longitudinal study. Oral Microbiol Immunol 1990;5:77-81.
4. Albert RJ, Cantin RY, Cross HG, Castaldi CR. Nursing caries in the Inuit children of the Keewatin. J Can Dent Assoc 1988;54:751-8.
5. Alvarez JO. Nutrition, tooth development, and dental caries. Am J Clin Nutr 1995;61:410S-416S.
6. Amaratunge A. Rampant dental caries in Papua New Guinean children. Odontostomatol Trop 1989;12:14-6.
7. Anderson RJ, Bradnock G, James PMC. The changes in the dental health of 12-year-old school children in Shropshire. Br Dent J 1981;150:278-81.
8. Anneroth G, Holm LE, Karlsson G. The effect of radiation on teeth. A clinical, histologic and microradiographic study. Int J Oral Surg 1985;14:269-74.
9. Arnjlot HA, Barmes DE, Cohen LK, et al. Oral health care systems; an international collaborative study. London: Quintessence/World Health Organization, 1985.
10. Athanassouli I, Mamai-Homata E, Panagopoulos H, et al. Dental caries changes between 1982 and 1991 in children aged 6-12 in Athens, Greece. Caries Res 1994;28:378-82.
11. Ayhan H, Suskan E, Yildirim S. The effect of nursing or rampant caries on height, body weight and head circumference. J Clin Pediatr Dent 1996;20:209-12.

12. Baelum V, Fejerskov O, Manji F. The "natural history" of dental caries and periodontal diseases in developing countries: Some consequences for health care planning. Tandlaegebladet 1991;95:139-48.
13. Bagramian RA, Russell AL. Epidemiologic study of dental caries experience and between-meal eating patterns. J Dent Res 1973;52:342-7.
14. Banting DW. Epidemiology of root caries. Gerodontology 1986;5:5-11.
15. Barmes DE. Features of oral health care across cultures. Int Dent J 1976;26:353-68.
16. Baume LJ. Caries prevalence and caries intensity among 12,344 schoolchildren of French Polynesia. Arch Oral Biol 1969;14:181-205.
17. Beal JF. The dental health of five-year-old children of different ethnic origins resident in an inner Birmingham area and a nearby borough. Arch Oral Biol 1973;18:305-12.
18. Beck JD. The epidemiology of root surface caries: North American studies. Adv Dent Res 1993;7:42-51.
19. Beck JD, Drake CW. Do root lesions tend to develop in the same people who develop coronal lesions? J Public Health Dent 1997;57:82-8.
20. Beighton D, Manji F, Baelum V, et al. Associations between salivary levels of *Streptococcus mutans*, *Streptococcus sobrinus*, lactobacilli, and caries experience in Kenyan adolescents. J Dent Res 1989;68:1242-6.
21. Bergendal B, Hamp SE. Dietary pattern and dental caries in 19-year-old adolescents subjected to preventive measures focused on oral hygiene and/or fluorides. Swed Dent J 1985;9:1-7.
22. Bibby BG. The cariogenicity of snack foods and confections. J Am Dent Assoc 1975;90:121-32.
23. Bjarnason S, Finnbogason SY, Holbrook P, Kohler B. Caries experience in Icelandic 12-year-old urban children between 1984 and 1991. Community Dent Oral Epidemiol 1993;21:195-7.
24. Bohannan HM. Caries distribution and the case for sealants. J Public Health Dent 1983;43:200-4.
25. Bonito AJ. The United States study of dental manpower systems in relation to oral health status: The private practice system. Final report for USPHS contract NO1-DH-34051. Baltimore: University of Maryland, 1977.
26. Bowden GH. Mutans streptococci caries and chlorhexidine. J Can Dent Assoc 1996;62:700, 703-7.
27. Bowen WH. Food components and caries. Adv Dent Res 1994;8:215-20.
28. Bowen WH. Response to Seow: Biological mechanisms of early childhood caries. Community Dent Oral Epidemiol 1998;26(1 Suppl):28-31.
29. Bowen WH. Role of carbohydrates in dental caries. In: Shaw JH, Roussos GG, eds: Sweeteners and dental caries. Washington DC: IRL Press, 1978:147-52.
30. Bratthall D, Hänsel Petersson G, Sundberg H. Reasons for the caries decline: What do the experts believe? Eur J Oral Sci 1996;104:416-22.
31. Broderick E, Mabry J, Robertson D, Thompson J. Baby bottle tooth decay in Native American children in Head Start centers. Public Health Rep 1989;104:50-4.
32. Brown LR, Billings RJ, Kaster AG. Quantitative comparisons of potentially cariogenic microorganisms cultured from noncarious and carious root and coronal tooth surfaces. Infect Immun 1986;51:765-70.
33. Brown LJ, Kingman A, Brunelle JA, Selwitz RH. Most US schoolchildren are caries free in their permanent teeth: This is no myth. Public Health Rep 1995;110:531-3.
34. Bryan ET, Collier DR, Vancleave ML. Dental health status of children in Tennessee; a 25-year comparison. J Tenn Dent Assoc 1982;62:31-3.
35. Burt BA. Influences for change in the dental health status of populations: An historical perspective. J Public Health Dent 1978;38:272-88.
36. Burt BA. The future of the caries decline. J Public Health Dent 1985;45:261-9.
37. Burt BA. Trends in caries prevalence in North American children. Int Dent J 1994;44(Suppl 1):403-13.
38. Burt BA, Eklund SA, Morgan KJ, et al. The effects of sugars intake and frequency of ingestion on dental caries increment in a three-year longitudinal study. J Dent Res 1988;67:1422-9.
39. Burt BA, Ismail AI. Diet, nutrition, and food cariogenicity. J Dent Res 1986;65(Spec Issue):1475-84.
40. Burt BA, Ismail AI, Eklund SA. Root caries in an optimally fluoridated and a high-fluoride community. J Dent Res 1986;65:1154-8.
41. Burt BA, Pai S. Sugar consumption and caries risk: A systematic review. J Dent Educ 2001;65:1017-23.
42. Burt BA, Szpunar SM. The Michigan Study: The relationship between sugars intake and dental caries over three years. Int Dent J 1994;44:230-40.
43. Carlos JP, Gittelsohn AM. Longitudinal studies of the natural history of caries. II. A life-table study of caries incidence in the permanent teeth. Arch Oral Biol 1965;10:739-51.
44. Carmichael CL, French AD, Rugg-Gunn AJ, Furness JA. The relationship between social class and caries experience in five-year-old children in Newcastle and Northumberland after twelve years' fluoridation. Community Dent Health 1984;1:47-54.
45. Carmichael CL, Rugg-Gunn AJ, Ferrell RS. The relationship between fluoridation, social class and caries experience in 5-year-old children in Newcastle and Northumberland in 1987. Br Dent J 1989;167:57-61.
46. Carmichael CL, Rugg-Gunn AJ, French AD, Cranage JD. The effect of fluoridation upon the relationship between caries experience and social class in 5-year-old children in Newcastle and Northumberland. Br Dent J 1980;149:163-7.
47. Carvalho JC, Van Nieuwenhuysen JP, D'Hoore W. The decline in dental caries among Belgian children between 1983 and 1998. Community Dent Oral Epidemiol 2001;29:55-61.
48. Caufield PW, Dasanayake AP, Li Y, et al. Natural history of *Streptococcus sanguinis* in the oral cavity of infants: Evidence for a discrete window of infectivity. Infect Immun 2000;68:4018-23.
49. Chalmers JM, Carter KD, Fuss JM, et al. Caries experience in existing and new nursing home residents in Adelaide, Australia. Gerodontology 2002;19:30-40.
50. Chironga L, Manji F. Dental caries in 12-year-old urban and rural children in Zimbabwe. Community Dent Oral Epidemiol 1989;17:31-3.
51. Corbett ME, Moore WJ. Distribution of dental caries in ancient British populations. IV. The 19th century. Caries Res 1976;10:401-14.

52. Coykendall AL. On the evaluation of *Streptococcus mutans* and dental caries. In: Stiles HM, Loesche WJ, O'Brien TC, eds: Proceedings of microbial aspects of dental caries. Microbiol Abstr 1976;3(Spec Suppl): 703-12.

53. Curzon ME, Curzon JA. Dental caries in Eskimo children of the Keewatin District in the Northwest Territories. J Can Dent Assoc 1970;36:342-4.

54. DePaola PF, Soparkar PM, Tavares M, Kent RL Jr. The clinical profiles of individuals with and without root caries. Gerodontology 1989;8:9-16.

55. Douglass JM, Tinanoff N, Tang JM, Altman DS. Dental caries patterns and oral health behaviors in Arizona infants and toddlers. Community Dent Oral Epidemiol 2001;29:14-22.

56. Downer MC. Caries prevalence in the United Kingdom. Int Dent J 1994;44(Suppl 1):365-70.

57. Drake CW, Hunt RJ, Beck JD, Koch GG. Eighteen-month coronal caries incidence in North Carolina older adults. J Public Health Dent 1994;54:24-30.

58. Dreizen S, Mann AW, Spies TD, Hunt FM. Prevalence of dental caries in malnourished children. Am J Dis Child 1947;74:265-73.

59. Dubos R. The mirage of health. New York: Doubleday, 1959.

60. Eklund SA, Pittman JL, Smith RC. Trends in dental care among insured Americans: 1980 to 1995. J Am Dent Assoc 1997;128:171-8.

61. Ellen RP, Banting DW, Fillery ED. *Streptococcus mutans* and *Lactobacillus* detection in the assessment of dental root surface caries risk. J Dent Res 1985;64:1245-9.

62. Emilson CG, Krasse B. Support for and implications of the specific plaque hypothesis. Scand J Dent Res 1985;93:96-104.

63. Fejerskov O, Kidd EA, eds. Dental caries: The disease and its clinical management. Malden MA: Blackwell, 2003.

64. Finn SB, Glass RB. Sugar and dental decay. World Rev Nutr Diet 1975;22:304-26.

65. Firestone AR, Schmid R, Mühlemann HR. Effect on the length and number of intervals between meals on caries in rats. Caries Res 1984;18:128-33.

66. Fisher FJ. A field survey of dental caries, periodontal disease and enamel defects in Tristan da Cunha. Br Dent J 1968;125:447-53.

67. Foster MK, Hunt AM. A study of dental manpower systems in relation to oral health status. Part 1: Ontario. Final report for Health and Welfare grant 606-1334-43. Toronto: University of Toronto, 1978.

68. Fuchs V. Who shall live? Health, economics, and social choice. New York: Basic Books, 1974.

69. Fure S, Romaniec M, Emilson CG, Krasse B. Proportions of *Streptococcus mutans*, lactobacilli and *Actinomyces* spp in root surface plaque. Scand J Dent Res 1987;95: 119-23.

70. Garn SM, Rowe NH, Cole PE. Husband-wife similarities in dental caries experience. J Dent Res 1977;56: 186.

71. Gilbert GH, Duncan RP, Dolan TA, Foerster U. Twenty-four month incidence of root caries among a diverse group of adults. Caries Res 2001;35:366-75.

72. Glass RL. Secular changes in caries prevalence in two Massachusetts towns. Caries Res 1981;15:445-50.

73. Gratrix D, Holloway PJ. Factors of deprivation associated with dental caries in young children. Community Dent Health 1994;11:66-70.

74. Graves RC, Bohannan HM, Disney JA, et al. Recent dental caries and treatment patterns in US children. J Public Health Dent 1986;46:23-9.

75. Gustafsson BE, Quensel C-E, Swenander Lanke L, et al. The Vipehölm dental caries study. The effect of different levels of carbohydrate intake on caries activity in 436 individuals observed for five years. Acta Odont Scand 1954;11:232-364.

76. Hadden WC. The use of educational attainment as an indicator of socioeconomic position. Am J Public Health 1996;86:1525-6.

77. Hand JS, Hunt RJ, Beck JD. Incidence of coronal and root caries in an older adult population. J Public Health Dent 1988;48:14-19.

78. Hargreaves JA. Changes in diet and dental health of children living in the Scottish Island of Lewis. Caries Res 1972;6:355-76.

79. Hargreaves JA, Wagg BJ, Thompson GW. Changes in caries prevalence of Isle of Lewis children, a historical comparison from 1937 to 1984. Caries Res 1987;21:277-84.

80. Harris R. Biology of the children of Hopewood House, Bowral, Australia. 4. Observations on dental caries experience extending over five years (1957-1961). J Dent Res 1963;42:1387-99.

81. Hausen H. Caries prediction—state of the art. Community Dent Oral Epidemiol 1997;25:87-96.

82. Hausen H, Heinonen OP, Paunio I. Modification of occurrence of caries in children by toothbrushing and sugar exposure in fluoridated and nonfluoridated areas. Community Dent Oral Epidemiol 1981;9:103-7.

83. Hausen H, Milen A, Heinonen OP, Paunio I. Caries in primary dentition and social class in high and low fluoride areas. Community Dent Oral Epidemiol 1982;10:33-6.

84. Hawkins RJ, Main PA, Locker D. Oral health status and treatment needs of Canadian adults aged 85 years and over. Special Care Dent 1998;18:164-9.

85. Heifetz SB, Horowitz HS, Korts DC. Prevalence of dental caries in white and black children in Nelson County, Virginia, a rural southern community. J Public Health Dent 1976;36:79-87.

86. Hix JO, O'Leary TJ. The relationship between cemental caries, oral hygiene status and fermentable carbohydrate intake. J Periodontol 1976;47:398-404.

87. Hughes JT, Rozier RG. The survey of dental health in the North Carolina population; selected findings. In: Bawden JW, De Friese GH, eds: Planning for dental care on a statewide basis; the North Carolina dental manpower project. Chapel Hill NC: Dental Foundation of North Carolina, 1981:21-37.

88. Hugoson A, Koch G, Hallonsten A-L, et al. Dental health 1973 and 1978 in individuals aged 3-20 years in the community of Jonkopping, Sweden. Swed Dent J 1980;150:217-29.

89. Hunter PBV. The prevalence of dental caries in 5-year-old New Zealand children. N Z Dent J 1979;75:154-7.

90. Ismail AI, Burt BA, Brunelle JA. Prevalence of total tooth loss, dental caries, and periodontal disease in Mexican-American adults: Results from the Southwestern HHANES. J Dent Res 1987;66:1183-8.

91. Ismail AI, Sohn W. A systematic review of clinical diagnostic criteria of early childhood caries. J Public Health Dent 1999;59:171-91.

92. Ismail AI, Szpunar SM. The prevalence of dental caries and periodontal disease among Mexican-Americans, Cubans, and Puerto Ricans. Findings from HHANES, 1982-84. Am J Public Health 1990;80(Suppl):66-70.

93. Jakobsen J. Recent reorganization of the Public Dental Health Service in Greenland in favor of caries prevention. Community Dent Oral Epidemiol 1979;7:75-81.

94. Johansson I, Saellstrom AK, Rajan BP, Parameswaran A. Salivary flow and dental caries in Indian children suffering from chronic malnutrition. Caries Res 1992;26:38-43.

95. Jones C, Woods K, Whittle G, et al. Sugar, drinks, deprivation and dental caries in 14-year-old children in the north west of England in 1995. Community Dent Health 1999;16:68-71.

96. Kaste LM, Drury TF, Horowitz AM, Beltran E. An evaluation of NHANES III estimates of early childhood caries. J Public Health Dent 1999;59:199-200.

97. Kaste LM, Marianos D, Chang R, Phipps KR. The assessment of nursing caries and its relationship to high caries in the permanent dentition. J Public Health Dent 1992;52:64-8.

98. Kaste LM, Selwitz RH, Oldakowski RJ, et al. Coronal caries in the primary and permanent dentition of children and adolescents 1-17 years of age: United States, 1988-1991. J Dent Res 1996;75(Spec Issue):631-41.

99. Keene HJ. Dental caries prevalence in early Polynesians from the Hawaiian Islands. J Dent Res 1986;65:935-8.

100. Kerr NW. The prevalence and pattern of distribution of root caries in a Scottish medieval population. J Dent Res 1990;69:857-60.

101. Kingman A, Little W, Gomez I, et al. Salivary levels of *Streptococcus mutans* and lactobacilli and dental caries experiences in a US adolescent population. Community Dent Oral Epidemiol 1988;16:98-103.

102. Kitamura M, Kiyak HA, Mulligan K. Predictors of root caries in the elderly. Community Dent Oral Epidemiol 1986;14:34-8.

103. Kleemola-Kujala E, Rasanen L. Relationship of oral hygiene and sugar consumption to risk of caries in children. Community Dent Oral Epidemiol 1982;10:224-33.

104. Klein H. The dental status and dental needs of young adult males, rejectable or acceptable for military service, according to Selective Service dental requirements. Public Health Rep 1941;56:1369-87.

105. Klein H. The family and dental disease. IV. Dental disease (DMF) experience in parents and offspring. J Am Dent Assoc 1946;33:735-43.

106. Klein H, Palmer CE. Dental caries in American Indian children. Public Health Bulletin No. 239. Washington DC: Government Printing Office, 1937.

107. Klein H, Palmer CE. Studies on dental caries. V. Familial resemblance in the caries experience of siblings. Public Health Rep 1938;53:1353-64.

108. Klein H, Palmer CE. Studies on dental caries. VII. Sex differences in dental caries experience of elementary school children. Public Health Rep 1938;53:1685-90.

109. Klein H, Palmer CE. Community economic status and the dental problem of school children. Public Health Rep 1940;55:187-205.

110. Klein H, Palmer CE. Studies on dental caries. XII. Comparison of the caries susceptibility of the various morphological types of permanent teeth. J Dent Res 1941;20:203-16.

111. Klein H, Shimizu T. The family and dental disease. I. DMF experience among husbands and wives. J Am Dent Assoc 1945;32:945-55.

112. Kohler B, Bjarnason S, Finnbogason SY, Holbrook WP. Mutans streptococci, lactobacilli and caries experience in 12-year-old Icelandic urban children, 1984 and 1991. Community Dent Oral Epidemiol 1995;23:65-8.

113. Kohler B, Bratthall D. Intrafamilial levels of *Streptococcus mutans* and some aspects of the bacterial transmission. Scand J Dent Res 1978;86:35-42.

114. Kohler B, Bratthall D, Krasse B. Preventive measures in mothers influence the establishment of the bacterium *Streptococcus mutans* in their infants. Arch Oral Biol 1983;28:225-31.

115. Krasse B. Oral effects of other carbohydrates. Int Dent J 1982;32:24-32.

116. Krasse B. Biological factors as indicators of future caries. Int Dent J 1988;38:219-25.

117. Kumar J, Green E, Wallace W, Bustard R. Changes in dental caries prevalence in upstate New York schoolchildren. J Public Health Dent 1991;51:158-63.

118. Lawrence HP, Hunt RJ, Beck JD. Three-year root caries incidence and risk modeling in older adults in North Carolina. J Public Health Dent 1995;55:69-78.

119. Lennon MA, Davies RM, Downer MC, Hull PS. Tooth loss in a 19th century British population. Arch Oral Biol 1974;19:511-6.

120. Leske GS, Ripa LW. Three-year root caries increments: An analysis of teeth and surfaces at risk. Gerodontology 1989;8:17-22.

121. Levy SM, Warren JJ, Broffitt B, et al. Fluoride, beverages and dental caries in the primary dentition. Caries Res 2003;37:157-65.

122. Lilienthal B, Goldsworthy NE, Sullivan HR, Cameron DA. The biology of the children of Hopewood House, Bowral, NSW. I. Observations on dental caries extending over five years (1947-1952). Med J Aust 1953;1:878-81.

123. Link BG, Phelan JC. Understanding sociodemographic differences in health; the role of fundamental social causes [editorial]. Am J Public Health 1996;86:471-3.

124. Lo EC, Schwarz E. Tooth and root conditions in the middle-aged and the elderly in Hong Kong. Community Dent Oral Epidemiol 1994;22:381-5.

125. Locker D, Leake JL. Coronal and root decay experience in older adults in Ontario, Canada. J Public Health Dent 1993;53:158-64.

126. Locker D, Slade GD, Leake JL. Prevalence of and factors associated with root decay in older adults in Canada. J Dent Res 1989;68:768-72.

127. Loesche WJ. Dental caries: A treatable infection. 2nd ed. Grand Haven MI: ADQ Publications, 1993.

128. Loesche WJ, Eklund SA, Mehlisch D, Burt BA. Possible effect of medically administered antibiotics on the mutans streptococci: Implications for reductions in decay. Oral Microbiol Immunol 1989;4:77-81.

129. Luan WM, Baelum V, Chen X, Fejerskov O. Dental caries in adult and elderly Chinese. J Dent Res 1989;68:1771-6.

130. Ludwig TG, Bibby BG. Geographic variations in the prevalence of dental caries in the United States of America. Caries Res 1969;3:32-43.

131. Mandel ID. Dental caries. Am Sci 1979;67:680-8.

132. Manji F, Fejerskov O, Baelum V. Pattern of dental caries in an adult rural population. Caries Res 1989;23:55-62.

133. Mann AW, Dreizen S, Spies TD, Hunt FM. A comparison of dental caries activity in malnourished and well-nourished patients. J Am Dent Assoc 1947;34:244-52.

134. Mann J. Sugar revisited—again [editorial]. Bull World Health Organ 2003;81:552.

135. Mansbridge JN. Heredity and dental caries. J Dent Res 1959;38:337-47.

136. Marmot M, Wilkinson RG, eds. Social determinants of health. New York: Oxford University Press, 1999.

137. Marshall TA, Levy SM, Broffitt B, et al. Patterns of beverage consumption during the transition stage of infant nutrition. J Am Diet Assoc 2003;103:1350-3.

138. Marshall TA, Levy SM, Broffitt B, et al. Dental caries and beverage consumption in young children. Pediatr 2003;112(3 Pt 1):184-91.

139. Marshall Day CD. Nutritional deficiencies and dental caries in Northern India. Br Dent J 1944;76:115-22.

140. Marthaler TM, O'Mullane DM, Vrbic V. The prevalence of dental caries in Europe 1990-1995. Caries Res 1996;30:237-75.

141. Martinsson T. Socio-economic investigation of school children with high and low caries frequency. III. A dietary study based on information given by the children. Odontol Revy 1972;23:93-113.

142. McDonald SP, Sheiham A. The distribution of caries on different tooth surfaces at varying levels of caries—a compilation of data from 18 previous studies. Community Dent Health 1992;9:39-48.

143. McEniery TM, Davies GN. Brisbane dental survey 1977. A comparative study of caries experience of children in Brisbane, Australia, over a 20-year period. Community Dent Oral Epidemiol 1979;7:42-50.

144. McGregor AB. Changing diet and its effect on caries prevalence in Ghana [abstract]. J Dent Res 1963;42:1086-7.

145. McGuire SM, Fox CH, Douglass CW, et al. Beneath the surface of coronal caries: Primary decay, recurrent decay, and failed restorations in a population-based survey of New England elders. J Public Health Dent 1993;53:76-82.

146. McNulty JA, Fos PJ. The study of caries prevalence in children in a developing country. ASDC J Dent Child 1989;56:129-36.

147. Mellanby M. Diet and the teeth. Part III. The effect of diet on dental structure and disease in man. London: His Majesty's Stationery Office, 1934.

148. Milen A. Role of social class in caries occurrence in primary teeth. Int J Epidemiol 1987;16:252-6.

149. Miller WD. Agency of micro-organisms in decay of human teeth. Dent Cosmos 1883;25:1-12.

150. Milnes AR. Description and epidemiology of nursing caries. J Public Health Dent 1996;56:38-50.

151. Møller IJ. Impact of oral diseases across cultures. Int Dent J 1978;28:376-80.

152. Møller IJ, Pindborg JJ, Roed-Petersen B. The prevalence of dental caries, enamel opacities and enamel hypoplasia in Ugandans. Arch Oral Biol 1972;17:9-22.

153. Møller IJ, Poulsen S, Nielsen VO. The prevalence of dental caries in Godhavn and Scoresbysund districts, Greenland. Scand J Dent Res 1972;80:169-80.

154. Moore WJ, Corbett ME. The distribution of dental caries in ancient British populations. I. Anglo-Saxon period. Caries Res 1971;5:151-68.

155. Moore WJ, Corbett ME. The distribution of dental caries in ancient British populations. II. Iron Age, Romano-British and Mediaeval periods. Caries Res 1973;7:139-53.

156. Moore WJ, Corbett ME. The distribution of dental caries in ancient British populations. III. The 17th century. Caries Res 1975;9:163-75.

157. Morse DE, Holm-Pedersen P, Holm-Pedersen J, et al. Dental caries in persons over the age of 80 living in Kungsholmen, Sweden: Findings from the KEOHS project. Community Dent Health 2002;19:262-7.

158. Mosha HJ, Ngilisho LA, Nkwera H, et al. Oral health status and treatment needs in different age groups in two regions of Tanzania. Community Dent Oral Epidemiol 1994;22:307-10.

159. Mosha HJ, Robison VA. Caries experience of the primary dentition among groups of Tanzanian urban preschoolchildren. Community Dent Oral Epidemiol 1989;17:34-7.

160. Mosha HJ, Scheutz F. Dental caries in the permanent dentition of schoolchildren in Dar es Salaam in 1979, 1983 and 1989. Community Dent Oral Epidemiol 1992;20:381-2.

161. Newbrun E. Dietary carbohydrates: Their role in cariogenicity. Med Clin North Am 1979;63:1069-86.

162. Newbrun E. Sugar and dental caries: A review of human studies. Science 1982;217:418-23.

163. Newbrun E, Hoover C, Mettraux G, Graf H. Comparison of dietary habits and dental health of subjects with hereditary fructose intolerance and control subjects. J Am Dent Assoc 1980;101:619-26.

164. Nizel AE, Bibby BG. Geographic variations in caries prevalence in soldiers. J Am Dent Assoc 1944;31:1619-26.

165. Ojofeitimi EO, Hollist NO, Banjo T, Adu TA. Effect of cariogenic food exposure on prevalence of dental caries among fee and non-fee-paying Nigerian schoolchildren. Community Dent Oral Epidemiol 1984;12:274-7.

166. Palmer JD, Pitter AFV. Differences in dental caries levels between 8-year-old children in Bath from different

socio-economic groups. Community Dent Health 1988;5:363-7.

167. Papas AS, Joshi A, Palmer CA, et al. Relationship of diet to root caries. Am J Clin Nutr 1995;61:423S-429S.

168. Pedersen PO. Dental disease in Europe and Greenland. J R Soc Health 1971;91:88-91.

169. Pickerill HP. The prevention of dental caries and oral sepsis. 3rd ed. London: Baillière, Tindall and Cox, 1923.

170. Pitts NB, Evans DJ. The dental caries experience of 5-year-old children in the United Kingdom. Surveys coordinated by the British Association for the Study of Community Dentistry in 1995/96. Community Dent Health 1997;14:47-52.

171. Pitts NB, Evans DJ, Nugent ZJ. The dental caries experience of 12-year-old children in the United Kingdom. Surveys coordinated by the British Association for the Study of Community Dentistry in 1996/97. Community Dent Health 1998;15:49-54.

172. Reisine ST, Psoter W. Socioeconomic status and selected behavioral determinants as risk factors for dental caries. J Dent Educ 2001;65:1009-16.

173. Ringelberg ML, Gilbert GH, Antonson DE, et al. Root caries and root defects in urban and rural adults: The Florida Dental Care Study. J Am Dent Assoc 1996;127:885-91.

174. Ringelberg ML, Matonski GM, Kimball AW. Dental caries-experience in three generations of families. J Public Health Dent 1974;34:174-80.

175. Rogers AH. Evidence for the transmissibility of dental caries. Aust Dent J 1977;22:53-56.

176. Rugg-Gunn AJ, Edgar WM. Sugar and dental caries; a review of the evidence. Community Dent Health 1984;1:85-92.

177. Rugg-Gunn AJ, Hackett AF, Appleton DR, et al. Relationship between dietary habits and caries increment assessed over two years in 405 English adolescent school children. Arch Oral Biol 1984;29:983-92.

178. Russell AL. International nutrition surveys: A summary of preliminary dental findings. J Dent Res 1963;42:233-44.

179. Russell AL. Dental caries and nutrition in Lebanon. J Dent Res 1966;45:957-63.

180. Russell AL, Leatherwood EC, Le Van Hien, Van Reen R. Dental caries and nutrition in South Vietnam. J Dent Res 1965;44:102-11.

181. Salonen L, Allander L, Bratthall D, et al. Oral health status in an adult Swedish population. Prevalence of caries. A cross-sectional epidemiological study in the Northern Alvsborg county. Swed Dent J 1989;13:111-23.

182. Sardo Infirri J, Barmes DE. Epidemiology of oral diseases; differences in national problems. Int Dent J 1979;29:183-90.

183. Schamschula RG, Adkins BL, Barmes DE, et al. WHO study of dental caries etiology in Papua New Guinea. WHO Offset Publication No. 40. Geneva: World Health Organization, 1978.

184. Schamschula RG, Barmes DE, Keyes PH, Gulbinat W. Prevalence and interrelationships of root surface caries in Lufa, Papua New Guinea. Community Dent Oral Epidemiol 1974;2:295-304.

185. Schamschula RG, Cooper MH, Adkins BL, et al. Oral conditions in Australian children of Aboriginal and Caucasian descent. Community Dent Oral Epidemiol 1980;8:365-9.

186. Schamschula RG, Cooper MH, Wright MC, et al. Oral health of adolescent and adult Australian Aborigines. Community Dent Oral Epidemiol 1980;8:370-4.

187. Schamschula RG, Keyes PH, Hornabrook KRW. Root surface caries in Lufa, New Guinea. I. Clinical observations. J Am Dent Assoc 1972;85:603-8.

188. Schlack CA, Restarske JS, Dochterman EF. Dental status of 71,015 naval personnel at first examination in 1942. J Am Dent Assoc 1946;33:1141-6.

189. Schupbach P, Osterwalder V, Guggenheim B. Human root caries: Microbiota in plaque covering sound, carious and arrested carious root surfaces. Caries Res 1995;29:382-95.

190. Senn WW. Incidence of dental caries among aviation cadets. Mil Surg 1943;93:461-4.

191. Shaw JH. Nutrition and dental caries. In: National Research Council, Committee on Dental Health. Survey of the literature on dental caries. National Research Council Publication No. 225. Washington DC: National Academy of Sciences, 1952:415-567.

192. Sigurjons H, Magnusdottir MO, Holbrook WP. Cariogenic bacteria in a longitudinal study of approximal caries. Caries Res 1995;29:42-5.

193. Slade GD, Spencer AJ, Gorkic E, Andrews G. Oral health status and treatment needs of non-institutionalized persons aged 60+ in Adelaide, South Australia. Aust Dent J 1993;38:373-80.

194. Speechley M, Johnston DW. Some evidence from Ontario, Canada, of a reversal in the dental caries decline. Caries Res 1996;30:423-7.

195. Spencer AJ, Davies M, Slade G, Brennan D. Caries prevalence in Australasia. Int Dent J 1994;44(Suppl 1):415-23.

196. Stamm JW. Is there a need for dental sealants? Epidemiological indications in the 1980s. J Dent Educ 1984;48:9-17.

197. Stamm JW, Banting DW, Imrey PB. Adult root caries survey of two similar communities with contrasting natural water fluoride levels. J Am Dent Assoc 1990;120:143-9.

198. Stecksen-Blicks C, Arvidsson S, Holm A-K. Dental health, dental care, and dietary habits in children in different parts of Sweden. Acta Odontol Scand 1985;43:59-67.

199. Steele JG, Sheiham A, Marcenes W, et al. Clinical and behavioural risk indicators for root caries in older people. Gerodontology 2001;18:95-101.

200. Stookey GK, Sergeant JW, Park KK, et al. Prevalence of dental caries in Indiana school children: Results of 1982 survey. Pediatr Dent 1985;7:8-13.

201. Sullivan HR, Harris R. The biology of the children of Hopewood House, Bowral, NSW. II. Observations extending over five years (1952-1956). 2. Observations on oral conditions. Austr Dent J 1958;3:311-7.

202. Sundin B, Birkhed D, Granath L. Is there not a strong relationship nowadays between caries and consumption of sweets? Swed Dent J 1983;7:103-8.

203. Sundin B, Granath L, Birkhed D. Variation of posterior approximal caries incidence with consumption of sweets with regard to other caries-related factors in 15-18 year-olds. Community Dent Oral Epidemiol 1992;20:76-80.

204. Szpunar SM, Eklund SA, Burt BA. Sugar consumption and caries risk in schoolchildren with low caries experience. Community Dent Oral Epidemiol 1995;23:142-6.

205. Takeuchi M. Epidemiological study on dental caries in Japanese children before, during, and after World War II. Int Dent J 1961;11:443-57.

206. Taylor GF, Marshall Day CD. Osteomalacia and dental caries. Br Dent J 1940;69:316.

207. Todd JE. Children's dental health in England and Wales, 1973. London: Her Majesty's Stationery Office, 1975.

208. Toverud G. The influence of war and post-war conditions on the teeth of Norwegian school children. I. Eruption of permanent teeth and status of deciduous dentition. Milbank Mem Fund Q 1956;34:354-430.

209. Toverud G. The influence of war and post-war conditions on the teeth of Norwegian school children. II. Caries in the permanent teeth of children aged 7-8 and 12-13 years. Milbank Mem Fund Q 1957;35:127-96.

210. Toverud G. The influence of war and post-war conditions on the teeth of Norwegian school children. III. Discussion of food supply and dental condition in Norway and other European countries. Milbank Mem Fund Q 1957;35:373-459.

211. Truin GJ, Konig KG, Bronkhorst EM, et al. Time trends in caries experience of 6- and 12-year-old children of different socioeconomic status in The Hague. Caries Res 1998;32:1-4.

212. Tsubouchi J, Tsubouchi M, Maynard RJ, et al. A study of dental caries and risk factors among Native American infants. ASDC J Dent Child 1995;62:283-7.

213. US Department of Health and Human Services, National Center for Health Statistics. Third National Health and Nutrition Examination Survey, 1988-94. Public Use Data File No. 7-0627. Hyattsville MD: Centers for Disease Control and Prevention, 1997.

214. US Public Health Service, National Center for Health Statistics. Decayed, missing, and filled teeth in adults, United States, 1960-1962. PHS Publication No. 1000, Series 11 No. 23. Washington DC: Government Printing Office, 1967.

215. US Public Health Service, National Center for Health Statistics. Decayed, missing, and filled teeth among children; United States. DHEW Publication No. (HSM) 72-1003, Series 11 No. 106. Washington DC: Government Printing Office, 1971.

216. US Public Health Service, National Center for Health Statistics. Decayed, missing, and filled teeth among youths 12-17 years, United States. DHEW Publication No. (HRA) 75-1626, Series 11 No. 144. Washington DC: Government Printing Office, 1974.

217. US Public Health Service, National Center for Health Statistics. Decayed, missing, and filled teeth among persons 1-74 years, United States 1971-1974. DHHS Publication No. (PHS) 81-1678, Series 11 No. 223. Washington DC: Government Printing Office, 1981.

218. US Public Health Service, National Center for Health Statistics. Diet and dental health; a study of relationships. DHHS Publication No. (PHS) 82-1675, Series 11 No. 225. Washington DC: Government Printing Office, 1982.

219. US Public Health Service, National Institute of Dental Research. The prevalence of dental caries in United States children, 1979-80. NIH Publication No. 82-2245. Washington DC: Government Printing Office, 1981.

220. US Public Health Service, National Institute of Dental Research. Oral health of United States adults; national findings. NIH Publication No. 87-2868. Washington DC: Government Printing Office, 1987.

221. US Public Health Service, National Institute of Dental Research. Oral health of United States children. NIH Publication No. 89-2247. Washington DC: Government Printing Office, 1989.

222. Valaitis R, Hesch R, Passarelli C, et al. A systematic review of the relationship between breastfeeding and early childhood caries. Can J Public Health 2000;91:411-7.

223. van Houte J, Lopman J, Kent R. The predominant cultivable flora of sound and carious human root surfaces. J Dent Res 1994;73:1727-34.

224. Vehkalahti MM. Relationship between root caries and coronal decay. J Dent Res 1987;66:1608-10.

225. Vehkalahti MM, Paunio IK. Occurrence of root caries in relation to dental health behavior. J Dent Res 1988;67:911-4.

226. Von der Fehr FR, Löe H, Theilade E. Experimental caries in man. Caries Res 1970;4:131-48.

227. Wadhawan S, Kumar JV, Badner VM, Green EL. Early childhood caries-related visits to hospitals for ambulatory surgery in New York State. J Public Health Dent 2003;63:47-51.

228. Wallace JS. The cause and prevention of decay in teeth. 2nd ed. London: Churchill, 1902.

229. Watt RG, Dykes J, Sheiham A. Preschool children's consumption of drinks: Implications for dental health. Community Dent Health 2000;17:8-13.

230. Weinstein P. Research recommendations: Pleas for enhanced research efforts to impact the epidemic of dental disease in infants. J Public Health Dent 1996;56:55-60.

231. Whelton HP, Holland TJ, O'Mullane DM. The prevalence of root surface caries amongst Irish adults. Gerodontology 1993;10:72-5.

232. Winn DM, Brunelle JA, Selwitz RH, et al. Coronal and root caries in the dentition of adults in the United States, 1988-1991. J Dent Res 1996;75(Spec No.):642-51.

233. World Health Organization. WHO oral health country/area profile programme, Caries for 12-year-olds by country/area, website: http://www.whocollab.odont.lu.se/countriesalphab.html. Accessed December 18, 2003.

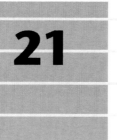

21 Periodontal Diseases

The term *periodontal disease* has long been recognized as a generic term used to describe a group of diseases, so it should more correctly be used in the plural form. It is generally more useful to refer specifically to gingivitis and periodontitis, with the term *periodontal diseases* reserved only for those situations in which the generic term is specifically intended.

This chapter describes the epidemiology of gingivitis and adult periodontitis, their distribution, and the risk factors and background characteristics associated with them. Periodontal diseases have been prevalent throughout human history, although without the obvious secular variations that characterize dental caries. Human remains from the early Christian era show clear evidence of periodontal bone loss.[156]

PERIODONTAL INFECTIONS AND HOST RESPONSE

Both gingivitis and periodontitis result from bacterial infections. The expression of clinical disease, however, is a function of both bacterial infection and the host response to that infection, mediated by environmental factors like smoking and oral hygiene. *Gingivitis* is an inflammatory process of the gingiva in which the junctional epithelium, although altered by the disease, remains attached to the tooth at its original level. There are initial, early, and established gingivitis lesions, and a sequential microbial colonization leads to bacteriologically more complex plaque as the lesions progress.[176]

Periodontitis is also an inflammatory condition of the gingival tissues, characterized by clinical attachment loss (CAL) of the periodontal ligament and loss of bony support of the tooth. Periodontitis develops as an extension of gingivitis, although only a small proportion of gingivitis sites make this transition.[112,124,139] What happens in this transition is that supragingival plaque serves as a reservoir for periodontopathogenic organisms,[71,201,251] and when this infection is strong enough to overwhelm the host defense, bacteria in supragingival plaque migrate subgingivally to form a subgingival biofilm.[180] Inflammatory mediators play an important role in the progression of periodontitis.[166,177] A number of microbial species have been associated with destructive periodontitis, although it is unlikely that all of these bacteria are essential players in the disease.[179] As is discussed later in this chapter, some of these species have been associated with serious systemic diseases.

Whether or not periodontitis develops after infection, and its severity if it does, are determined by the nature and extent of the host response to these infections. Only some 20% of periodontal diseases are now attributed to bacterial variance, 50% are attributed to genetic variance, and 20% to tobacco use,[180] although the contribution of tobacco use may be higher than that.[93] Only a small proportion of virtually any population is susceptible to severe, generalized periodontitis, even though most people have these infections to some degree. This has led to the hypothesis that there are two distinct types of periodontitis. One is the *plaque and local factors* type, the most common form, in which specific pathogens dominate the host response in controlling disease expression; the second is the *compromised host* type, in which severity and rate of progression are often rapid and are not well correlated with local factors like plaque deposits.[166] The compromised host type is less common, responds much less favorably to standard treatments, and is thought to be the type of disease found in aggressive and diabetes-associated periodontitis. Neutrophil abnormalities have been associated with the compromised host form of the disease,[178] and at least in aggressive periodontitis the compromised host response is thought to be of genetic origin.[50]

Many different classifications of periodontal diseases have been proposed; their evolution is well documented in the various world workshops held down the years. These workshops are international gatherings of experts to review the state of knowledge in the periodontal field and were held in 1966,[191] 1977,[110] 1989,[163] and 1996 (reported in the first issue of *Annals of Periodontology*). A subsequent workshop in 1999, held to review disease classifications, produced the list shown in Box 21-1. This classification is far more detailed than its predecessor.[163] It is becoming increasingly accepted that the periodontal diseases are a family of more or less related conditions, and advances in molecular biology will most likely provide new bases for classifying them in the future.

Although these different categories of periodontitis are widely recognized, there are no generally accepted definitions of *serious* or *moderate periodontitis*, terms widely used in clinical practice, epidemiology, and public health. Several definitions of serious periodontitis that have been used in epidemiologic studies are shown in Box 21-2. Two of these definitions use CAL plus the presence of pockets, whereas the third is based on a cutpoint on a statistical distribution. When the term *serious* or *severe periodontitis* is used in this chapter, the reference is to a degree of periodontitis severe enough to cause or threaten the loss of teeth. There is moderate agreement in the literature that CAL of 6 mm or more is a reasonable cutoff point to differentiate serious from moderate periodontitis; the latter term is usually applied to CAL of 4-5 mm or less. *Moderate periodontitis* is used in this chapter to mean periodontitis in which pocketing, CAL, or even some bone loss can be clinically or radiographically demonstrated, but the condition is not yet severe enough to threaten the loss of teeth.

CURRENT MODELS OF PERIODONTAL DISEASES

As mentioned in Chapter 16, perceptions of the nature of periodontal diseases changed radically as a result of research during the 1980s and 1990s. The old view of periodontal disease before that time is summarized in the following statement from a 1961 report by an expert committee of the World Health Organization (WHO):

Periodontal disease is one of the most widespread diseases of mankind. No nation and no area of the world is free from it and in most it has a high prevalence, affecting in some degree approximately half the child population and almost the entire adult population. Research and clinical evidence indicate that the damage caused to the supporting structures of the teeth by periodontal disease in early adult life is irreparable, while in the middle adult life it destroys a large part of the natural dentition and deprives many people of all their teeth long before old age. The total effect of periodontal disease on the general health of the populations is unassessable.[250]

BOX 21-1 Summarized Classification of Gingival and Periodontal Conditions[11]

Gingival Diseases
   Dental plaque–induced gingival diseases
      Gingivitis associated with dental plaque only
      Gingival diseases modified by systemic factors
      Gingival diseases modified by medications
      Gingival diseases modified by malnutrition
   Non–plaque-induced gingival lesions
      Gingival diseases of specific bacterial origin
      Gingival diseases of viral origin
      Gingival diseases of fungal origin
      Gingival diseases of genetic origin
      Gingival manifestations of systemic conditions
      Traumatic lesions
      Foreign body reactions
      Not otherwise specified

Chronic Periodontitis
   Localized
   Generalized

Aggressive Periodontitis
   Localized
   Generalized

Periodontitis As a Manifestation of Systemic Diseases
   Associated with hematologic disorders
   Associated with genetic disorders
   Not otherwise specified

Necrotizing Periodontal Diseases
   Necrotizing ulcerative gingivitis
   Necrotizing ulcerative periodontitis

Abscesses of the Periodontium
   Gingival abscess
   Periodontal abscess
   Pericoronal abscess

Periodontitis Associated With Endodontic Lesions
   Combined periodontic-endodontic lesions

Developmental or Acquired Deformities and Conditions
   Localized tooth-related factors that modify or predispose to plaque-induced gingival diseases/periodontitis
   Mucogingival deformities and conditions around teeth
   Mucogingival deformities and conditions on edentulous ridges
   Occlusal trauma

BOX 21-2 Some Definitions of "Serious" Periodontitis Used in Periodontal Studies

- Four or more sites with loss of periodontal attachment (CAL) of ≥5 mm, with pocket depth of ≥4 mm at one or more of those sites[26]
- Two or more teeth with CAL of ≥6 mm, plus one or more sites with pocket depth of ≥5 mm[137]
- Mean CAL in the top 20th percentile of the distribution[129]

This whole passage conjures up a vision of helpless peoples, all equally susceptible and suffering en masse. It was also accepted at that time that gingivitis invariably progressed to periodontitis, a view that has now changed to recognition that few gingivitis lesions actually make that transition.

Challenges to the concept of universal susceptibility came with epidemiologic studies in low-income countries. These surveys yielded broadly similar results in that they found massive deposits of plaque and calculus, and thus high levels of gingivitis.[21] But contrary to expectations, they also found that the prevalence of serious, generalized periodontitis in these poorer countries was little different from that in the highly treated populations of high-income countries.[16,17,19,122,131,170] Further substantial modification to the traditional perception of periodontitis came with the demonstration in the early 1980s that the periodontal tissues apparently had the capacity to repair themselves.[75] This finding was incorporated into what became known as the *burst theory* of periodontitis,[211] which essentially states that periodontitis progresses in a series of relatively short, acute bursts of rapid tissue destruction, followed by some tissue repair and long periods of remission.[125] This view was the converse of the hypothesis of linear progression that had been assumed until that time and resulted from analyzing measurements from individual sites rather than using pooled data as had been done before. The burst theory of periodontal destruction has been accepted by most researchers, and there is now good epidemiologic evidence to support it.[28]

Basic, clinical, and epidemiologic research from around the late 1970s onward (about the same time that the caries decline was recognized) has therefore led to a perception of the periodontal diseases that can be summarized as shown in Box 21-3.

Although periodontal diseases are constantly becoming better understood, the measurement problems described in Chapter 16 have not gone away. We are still not confident about how to separate susceptible from nonsusceptible people and active from inactive sites.[174] Until research finds a suitable way of measuring active disease, then CAL, pocket depth, radiographic bone loss, and gingival bleeding must serve as measures of periodontal diseases, cumbersome and inappropriate for some purposes though they are.

DISTRIBUTION OF PERIODONTAL DISEASES

Geographic Distribution

Over 70% of adults in all parts of the world have some degree of gingivitis or periodontitis.[20] Under the old perception of periodontal disease, it was considered that prevalence and severity were greater in low-income countries than in the higher-income world. However, data collected since 1980 in WHO's Global Oral Health Data Bank,[187,188] when added to the results of other epidemiologic studies,[15] suggest that, although gingivitis and calculus deposits are more prevalent and severe in low-income nations, there are fewer global differences in the prevalence of severe periodontitis. Gingivitis and calculus deposits can be controlled by personal oral hygiene and

---

BOX 21-3 A Current Model of Periodontal Diseases

- Only a small proportion of persons (5%-15%) exhibit severe periodontitis, where "severe" means that tooth loss occurs or is threatened. Mild gingivitis is common, as is mild to moderate periodontitis. Most adults exhibit some loss of bony support and loss of probing attachment while still maintaining a functioning dentition.
- Gingivitis and periodontitis are associated with bacterial flora that have some similarities but also some differences between the two conditions. Gingivitis precedes periodontitis, but only a fraction of sites with gingivitis later develop periodontitis.
- Although periodontitis is usually related to age in cross-sectional surveys, it is not a natural consequence of aging.
- Periodontitis is not the major cause of tooth loss in adults, except perhaps in the oldest age-groups in some populations.
- Periodontitis is usually a site-specific condition and is only occasionally seen in generalized forms. Generalized periodontitis is usually severe and of the early-onset type.
- Periodontitis is usually thought to proceed in bursts of destructive activity with quiescent periods between the bursts.

---

professional dental care, so it is to be expected that they are less severe in high-income nations. This geographic profile, in which severe periodontitis is not clearly dependent on the presence of plaque and calculus, is consistent with the compromised host model of periodontitis described earlier.

Prevalence of Gingivitis

At the population level, gingivitis is found in early childhood, is more prevalent and severe in adolescence, and tends to level off after that. The prevalence of gingivitis among schoolchildren in the United States has been around 40%-60% in various national surveys.[235] In a national survey of employed adults in 1985-86, 47% of males and 39% of females ages 18-64 had at least one site that bled on probing.[237] In the first national survey of adults that measured gingivitis, conducted in 1960-62, some 85% of men and 79% of women were affected.[234] Even with allowance for the differences between the two surveys in measurement techniques and the populations studied, it seems fairly clear that there has been an improvement in gingival health over that period.[171]

Gingivitis is closely correlated with plaque deposits, a relationship long considered one of cause and effect. Studies of the natural history of periodontal diseases in Norway and Sri Lanka found no increase in prevalence and severity of gingivitis between the late teen years and age 40. In Norwegian professionals and students, among whom oral hygiene was excellent,[8] and in Sri Lankan tea workers, among whom gingival conditions and oral hygiene were poorer, there was no age-related increase in gingivitis. Surveys in other low-income countries show that gingivitis, associated with extensive plaque and calculus deposits, is the norm among adults.[15]

Gingivitis is likely to have declined over recent years in the United States because of greater attention to oral hygiene as a part of personal grooming. The main research interest in gingivitis today is why some lesions progress to periodontitis and some do not, and what factors may predict these outcomes.

Prevalence of Periodontitis

Interpretation of epidemiologic data from before 1980 or so is difficult because the indexes used to measure the conditions before that time are no longer considered valid (see Chapter 16). The impression created by these data was that summed up in the WHO quotation given earlier: "periodontal disease" was uniformly extensive and serious in most populations. Later research, however, in which the use of disaggregated indexes in epidemiology played a prominent part, has led to an almost total reversal of that concept. Data from many parts of the world have now shown that the prevalence of generalized, severe periodontitis is in the range of 5%-15% in almost all populations, regardless of their state of economic development, conditions of oral hygiene, or availability of dental care.[15,51,112,229] This relatively low proportion supports a fundamental shift away from the old view of universal susceptibility, even though it still represents a lot of people with serious periodontitis.

Any assessment of the prevalence of a condition, and the form of its distribution in a population, must begin with a case definition of the disease. Here is the first difficulty, for as described earlier there is no clear agreement on how to define moderate and serious periodontitis. We stated earlier that 6-mm CAL is generally considered serious and 4- to 5-mm CAL moderate, but to many it seems reasonable to say that *any* CAL should be considered disease. Philosophically that may be true, but in practical terms considering all CAL as disease is not helpful. To illustrate this point, Fig. 21-1 graphs the proportion of adults in the United States with at least one site showing 2-mm CAL. A high proportion of even the younger age-groups is affected, and the condition soon becomes almost universal. CAL of at least 2 mm is so common, and is so often found in persons with functional dentitions, that one has to wonder whether philosophically it should be thought of as disease in a clinical sense. Certainly any criterion that is so commonly met is not useful in epidemiologic research in which risk factors are being sought.

CAL is considered to be the most valid measure of periodontitis,[74] even though it measures past disease rather than present activity. If CAL of 2 mm is too common to discriminate between people who are susceptible and those who are not susceptible to serious periodontitis, then where should the cutoff be? Fig. 21-2 graphs the proportion of adults with at least one site showing CAL of 2 mm, 4 mm, or 6 mm, and Fig. 21-3 shows the skewed distribution of CAL in three age-groups. If the use of a 2-mm measure is not sensitive enough (i.e., includes too many false negatives), a 6-mm cutoff may be not specific enough (i.e., it could exclude too many true positives). We stated earlier that CAL of 4-5 mm has generally been considered moderate periodontitis in the literature, so CAL of at least 3 mm, at the upper end of mild periodontitis, seems a reasonable basis for a case definition of periodontitis. In incidence studies, 3-mm CAL is usually taken as the criterion for incident periodontitis because this level is outside the change that could reasonably be attributed to error by a trained, experienced examiner.[25]

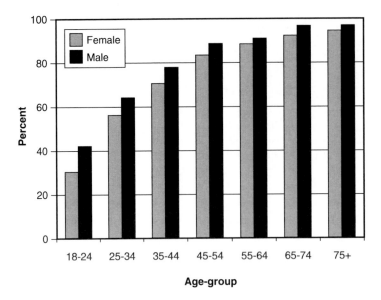

Fig. 21-1 Proportion of U.S. adults with at least one site showing clinical attachment loss of 2 mm or more by age and gender, 1985-86.[233]

Incidence of Periodontitis

Longitudinal studies of periodontitis onset and progression in community-dwelling populations are inherently expensive and difficult, so it is not surprising that only a few have been conducted. One was the Piedmont project in North Carolina, so named for the five-county geographic region in which a community-dwelling sample (i.e., neither institutionalized nor taken from patient lists at a dental school) ages 65-80 years, mostly rural and of low income, received a series of periodontal examinations in their own homes over 5 years. Periodontal conditions in

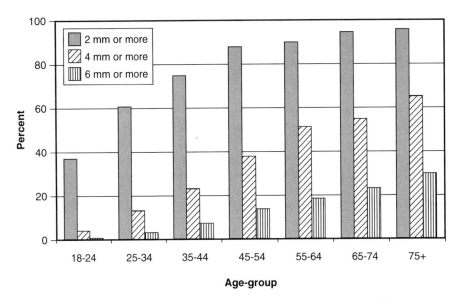

Fig. 21-2 Proportion of U.S. adults with at least one site showing clinical attachment loss of 2 mm or more, 4 mm or more, and 6 mm or more, by age, 1988-94.[233]

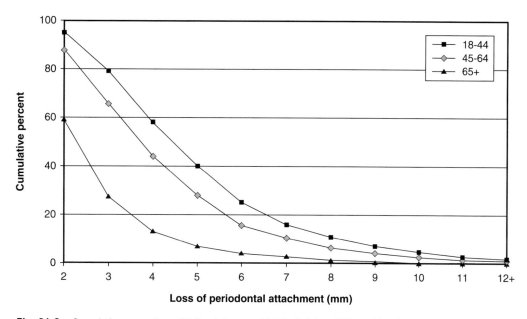

Fig. 21-3 Cumulative proportion of U.S. adults ages 18-44, 45-64, and 65 or older showing varying degrees of clinical attachment loss at most severely affected site, 1988-94.[233]

this group were generally not good. Although the mean number of affected sites at baseline was only a little more than that found in younger age-groups, the severity of disease at those sites was considerably greater.[26] When disease incidence (defined as an increase in CAL of at least 3 mm) was assessed for the first 18 months and for the second 18 months separately, CAL during the first period was positively related to CAL in the second period at the level of the individual but not at the site level.[24] These findings were confirmed at the 5-year examination: the presence of CAL in the first period did not put a site at risk for CAL in subsequent periods.[27] These findings support the episodic, randomized model of periodontitis in susceptible persons. At the mesiobuccal sites examined, increased pocket depth rather than gingival recession accounted for most disease incidence, whereas for buccal sites gingival recession accounted for most incidence.[23] The research team found that risk factors were not the same as *prognostic factors* (their term for risk factors related to the *progression* of existing disease). However, counted among both risk and prognostic factors were low income, tobacco use, presence of specific bacteria, and use of medications likely to result in soft tissue reactions.

A longitudinal project of major importance was the 15-year study of periodontitis among 480 tea workers in Sri Lanka.[131] The group studied had virtually no dental treatment of the type found in developed countries, so the data reflected the natural history of periodontitis. Based on tooth loss and interproximal CAL over the 15 years of the study, it was concluded that some 8% demonstrated rapid progression, 81% moderate progression, and 11% no progression beyond gingivitis. This study provided important evidence demonstrating the range of susceptibility to periodontitis. A subsequent finding on disease incidence in this group was that gingival recession progressed over time on virtually all surfaces, whereas in a comparison group of high-income Norwegians it was largely confined to the buccal surfaces. The buccal-only recession was thought to come from toothbrush abrasion, whereas the all-surfaces recession among the Sri Lankans was seen as plaque related.[130]

Clinical studies that have followed groups of patients over a period of time have contributed valuable information toward the understanding of periodontitis.[73,84,127] These should not be called epidemiologic studies, for when patients are followed then all participants, by definition, are susceptible to the disease. Although epidemiologic research is better for defining risk factors, clinical studies are valuable for studying disease progression in susceptible individuals.

DEMOGRAPHIC RISK FACTORS IN PERIODONTITIS
Gender and Race or Ethnicity

Surveys of periodontal conditions usually show that men have poorer periodontal health than women. This has long been observed and is still the case in the most recent national survey in the United States. Figs. 21-1, 21-4, and 21-5 show that, as measured by CAL, the presence of pockets, and subgingival calculus, women consistently look better than men. In older surveys[234,236] this finding was obscured by the greater tooth loss among women, tooth loss that was assumed to reflect the ravages of periodontal disease. More recently, however, differences in tooth loss between the sexes are no longer evident (see Chapter 19). Women usually exhibit better oral hygiene than do men,[237] which would explain the differences seen in gingivitis. The fact that women show less subgingival calculus (see Fig. 21-5) is likely to contribute toward their better periodontal conditions as measured by CAL and pocket depth. Current knowledge of the pathogenesis of periodontitis, when added to the epidemiologic evidence, indicates that there are no inherent differences between men and women in susceptibility to periodontitis.

There is also little evidence to suggest different susceptibility to periodontitis among different races. Early epidemiologic studies showed considerable differences between nations[190,198] but no consistent associations with race or ethnicity when persons of the same age and oral hygiene status were compared. Reviews presented at world workshops in 1966[243] and 1977[44] also found no differences in disease prevalence that could be attributed to race or ethnicity, and that view essentially still prevails.[15] On the other hand, in the 1986-87 national survey of schoolchildren, the prevalence of CAL (at least one site with attachment loss of 3+ mm) in 13- to 17-year-olds was 10% among African-Americans, 5% among Hispanics, and only 1.3% among whites.[3] These data did not account for socioeconomic differences, so the differences seen may not be attributable to race or ethnicity.

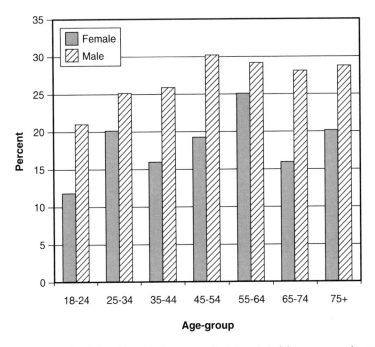

Fig. 21-4 Proportion of U.S. adults with at least one periodontal pocket of 4 mm or more by age and gender, 1988-94.[233]

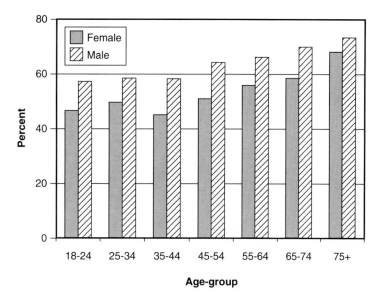

Fig. 21-5 Proportion of U.S. adults with at least one site showing subgingival calculus by age and gender, 1988-94.[233]

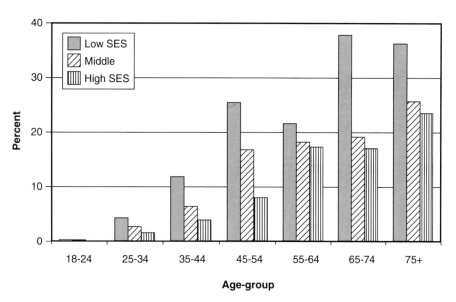

Fig. 21-6 Proportion of U.S. adults with at least one site showing clinical attachment loss of 6 mm or more by age and socioeconomic status (SES), 1988-94.[233]

Fig. 21-6 shows the extent of severe CAL in the United States by socioeconomic status (SES), and Fig. 21-7 shows the prevalence of severe periodontitis among four racial-ethnic groups in the United States in the third National Health and Nutrition Examination Survey (NHANES III) of 1988-94. Data in these charts are not con-sistent from one age-group to another except that prevalence is higher at all ages among African-Americans, and this pattern is likely to be associated with SES rather than to reflect true racial differences. The WHO Global Oral Health Data Bank, which maintains data from many nations collected using the Community

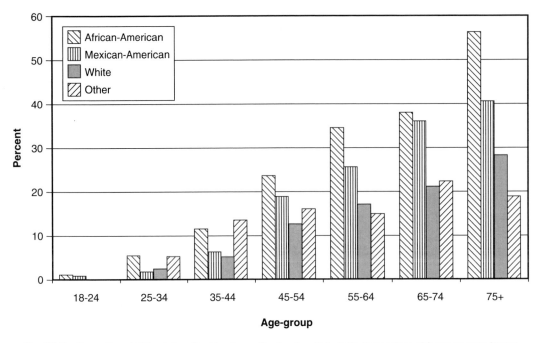

Fig. 21-7 Proportion of U.S. adults with at least one site showing clinical attachment loss of 6 mm or more by age and race or ethnicity, 1988-94.[233]

Periodontal Index, suggests a rather remarkable uniformity of conditions around the world.[187,188] Overall, the evidence indicates that race and ethnicity in themselves cannot be considered as demographic risk factors for periodontitis.

Age

The relationship between age and periodontitis is not always an easy one to understand. Much of the problem dates back to the older perception of the disease, in which the interpretation of cross-sectional survey data was generally that the severity of the disease increased with advancing age. However, today we do not view periodontitis as a disease of aging. The greater prevalence and severity of CAL in older people in cross-sectional surveys come not from a greater susceptibility in older people but from the cumulative progression of lesions over time.[35]

Fig. 21-2 shows the distribution of degree of CAL at the most affected site among adults as measured by NHANES III in United States during 1988-94. These cross-sectional data show that there is a linear relationship between

age and the proportion of people with at least one site with 4-mm or 6-mm CAL. By contrast, the proportion of people with at least one site with 2-mm CAL rises rapidly with age and then tends to flatten out at a high level. This suggests that people who get only this low level of periodontitis get it early in life, and as discussed previously it is too common to be of value in discriminating between disease and nondisease.

Fig. 21-4 shows that the relationship between age and the presence of at least one pocket of 4 mm or more is not as direct as that found with CAL. If pockets are taken to reflect active disease (as opposed to CAL, which is a "scar" of past disease), then this weak relationship with age is not surprising.

Age-related findings were a feature of the Sri Lankan studies described previously.[131] Earlier reports of these researchers compared the Sri Lankans with a group of college students and professors in Oslo, Norway, a dentally conscious group.[8,132,133] The oral hygiene status of the Oslo group was excellent, with no increase in the prevalence and severity of gingivitis from the late teenage years to around 40 years of age.

Mean annual CAL in the Oslo group was 0.07-0.13 mm. The Sri Lankan group was followed for 15 years, and as described earlier participants could be categorized into three groups in terms of rate of disease progression: rapid, moderate, and little to none. In the first two groups, periodontitis progressed with age, although naturally much more so in the rapid-progression group, virtually all of whom were edentulous by 40-45 years of age. In the moderate-progression group, the annual mean rate of CAL increased from 0.3 mm when the members were in their twenties to 0.5 mm 15 years later. By contrast, annual CAL in the rapid-progression group averaged 1.04 mm when they were ages 25-29. In the nonprogressing group, average annual CAL was around 0.05 mm and did not change with age.

Rather than showing an increased susceptibility to periodontitis with increasing age, post-1980 epidemiologic studies support the view that those who retain their teeth into old age are likely to be the less susceptible individuals. When periodontitis occurs in susceptible persons, it starts young.[*] None of these studies demonstrating moderate CAL in young people followed their subjects into later life. These young people may fit the compromised host disease model,[166] although without case-control studies or additional longitudinal data this cannot be stated for sure. It fits the pattern of many diseases, however, if the persons most susceptible to periodontitis are those who exhibit the disease in their youth. (We should note that we are not referring here to the specific condition of aggressive periodontitis, which is thought to affect some 0.1%-0.2% of the adolescent population.)[239]

The likelihood that older dentate people may be of low susceptibility is strengthened by the finding that serious disease is not as common among such groups as once thought. As shown in Fig. 21-3, the distribution of people by their most severe CAL site is skewed, and this skewed distribution is largely independent of age.[91] Other analyses of cross-sectional national survey data have also concluded that age is not a major determinant of periodontitis.[1,36]

Even though there are indications from clinical studies that the aging periodontium does not tolerate plaque as well as it used to, that the

nature of the plaque itself may change with age, and that the periodontium recovers from injury more slowly, these potential problems are overshadowed by the patient's susceptibility to disease.[238] This further supports the idea that, when a patient is susceptible to periodontitis, the tendency is seen early. Adult periodontitis in the elderly is characterized by infrequent and slow progression, and does not usually lead to tooth loss. Even in cases in which periodontitis is reported as a leading cause of tooth loss in the elderly (see Chapter 19), it is likely that a lot of the teeth extracted then have been seriously diseased for years rather than becoming that way in old age.

To summarize the data on age and periodontitis: cross-sectional survey data invariably show, on average, a greater extent of CAL among older than among younger persons. The apparent increase of CAL with age is more a lifetime accumulation of effects than a greater susceptibility in the older years. Limited longitudinal data suggest that CAL increases rapidly with age among the 5%-15% of any population that is susceptible to serious disease and to a lesser extent among the majority that exhibits moderate disease. Those susceptible to serious disease exhibit CAL and bone loss when young, often in the teenage years.

Socioeconomic Status

Generally, those who are better educated, wealthier, and live in better circumstances enjoy better health status than the less educated and poorer segments of society. Many disease conditions are associated with SES, a complex variable that can subsume a lot of cultural factors. Periodontal diseases are among this group[13,225] and have historically been related to lower SES.[234,236] The periodontal ill effects of living in deprived circumstances can start early in life.[206]

Gingivitis and poorer oral hygiene are clearly related to lower SES, but the relationship between periodontitis and SES is less direct. Fig. 21-8 shows that there are obvious SES differences only among younger people when CAL is 2 mm or more, but as we have stated several times already, CAL of 2 mm is not a sensitive measure. When those with CAL of at least 6 mm (see Fig. 21-6) are classified by SES, a more consistent difference is seen, especially at younger ages. As shown in Fig. 21-9, when the measure is the

---

[*]References 4,9,16,17,19,38,48,49,88,91,120,131,141,224, 227,249.

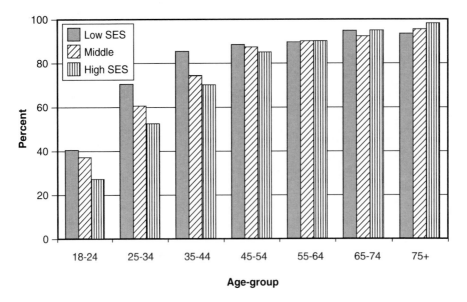

Fig. 21-8 Proportion of U.S. adults with at least one site showing clinical attachment loss of 2 mm or more by age and socioeconomic status (SES), 1988-94.[233]

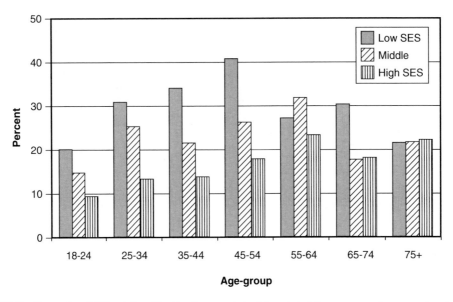

Fig. 21-9 Proportion of U.S. adults with at least one periodontal pocket of 4 mm or more by age and socioeconomic status (SES), 1988-94.[233]

prevalence of pockets of at least 4 mm, differences are also seen between SES strata and are most pronounced among the young. Subgingival calculus deposits are also more prevalent among lower SES groups (Fig. 21-10).

The widely observed association between SES levels and gingival health is a function of better oral hygiene among the more educated and a greater frequency of dental visits among the more dentally aware and those with dental insurance (who are more likely to be white-collar employees, i.e., those with more education). SES is a complex and multifaceted variable, and it is virtually impossible to remove the effect of SES as a confounder in the race-ethnicity associations seen in Fig. 21-7.

Genetics

The first report identifying a genetic component in periodontitis appeared in 1997.[113] Most of the research studies relating to genetics as a determinant of disease have been laboratory and clinical investigations rather than epidemiologic studies but they should still be briefly considered here.

The original 1997 report, based on data from patients in private practices, found that a specific genotype of the polymorphic interleukin-1 (IL-1) gene cluster was associated with more severe periodontitis. This relationship could only be demonstrated in nonsmokers, which indicated immediately that the genetic factor was not as strong a risk factor as was smoking. The IL-1 gene cluster has received a lot of research attention since then. This is appropriate, given that the proinflammatory cytokine IL-1 is a key regulator of the host response to microbial infection,[147] although IL-1 is unlikely to be the only genetic factor involved.[142] IL-1 has been identified as a contributory cause of periodontitis among some patient groups[53,61,116,119] and in an epidemiologic study.[224]

Although there is little doubt that periodontitis has a genetic component, the strength of that component is still to be determined. On the one hand, a study of 169 twin pairs concluded that about half of the variance in periodontitis was attributable to heredity.[153] On the other hand, there were no differences in tooth loss attributable to IL-1 variation over 10 years in a nonsmoking population with good periodontic maintenance treatment.[39] A combination of IL-1 genotyping and smoking history may provide a good risk profile for

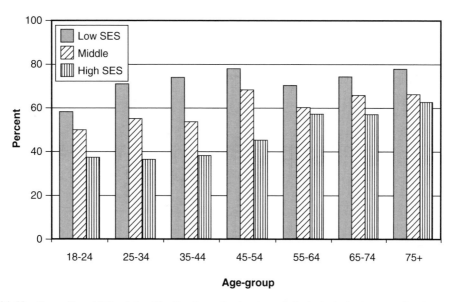

Fig. 21-10 Proportion of U.S. adults with at least one site showing subgingival calculus by age and socioeconomic status (SES), 1988-94.[233]

patients,[147] and an interaction between smoking and genetics may be a contributory factor in severity of periodontitis.[150,183] IL-1 has been described as playing a clear, but not essential, role in regulating host response to infection.[53,61] Further research, including epidemiologic studies of people with and without disease, are necessary before the genetic contribution to the initiation and progression of periodontitis can be specified. Current knowledge tells us that inducing periodontal patients to stop smoking should be a higher priority than genetic testing.

RISK FACTORS FOR PERIODONTITIS
Oral Hygiene, Plaque, and Microbiota

Although there is a clear causal relationship between poor oral hygiene and gingivitis, the relationship between oral hygiene status and periodontitis is less straightforward. Good oral hygiene can favorably influence the ecology of the microbial flora in shallow to moderate pockets, but it does not affect host response.

A simple but elegant study of experimental human gingivitis conducted in the mid-1960s[134] showed the relation between plaque deposits and gingivitis to be one of cause and effect. Gingivitis is a nonspecific infection caused by bacteria found in supragingival plaque. There is less gingivitis in high-income countries where good oral hygiene is a social norm than in poorer societies where oral hygiene activities are not a normal part of the daily routine. There is also less calculus, both supragingival and subgingival, as a result of better oral hygiene and more professional dental care. These differences are evident not only between countries but also between the genders and between socioeconomic strata within the United States, as illustrated in Figs. 21-5 and 21-10, although subgingival calculus is seen to be quite prevalent even among higher SES American adults.

The presence of plaque and calculus deposits is found to correlate poorly with severe periodontitis in population studies,[*] and the same is true for other measures of plaque quantity.[†] What these studies of populations

with poor oral hygiene and little dental treatment suggest is that, although gingivitis and calculus deposition are more severe,[7] the prevalence and severity of periodontitis is not all that different from conditions in developed nations.[15,76,187,188] Even among health professionals in the United States, oral hygiene practices seem unrelated to periodontitis.[152]

These poor correlations have all been obtained using various measures of plaque quantity (i.e., extent of plaque or calculus deposits). Qualitative measures of plaque (i.e., specification of microbiota) have also produced mixed results. In cross-sectional data, associations between putative periodontopathogenic organisms and clinical periodontitis have been reported,[26,212] and the presence of these organisms in subgingival plaque samples from susceptible patients has predicted CAL over the short term.[85] On the other hand, the presence of specific microbiota could not predict the development or progression of periodontitis in clinical longitudinal studies of up to 3 years.[126,127,244]

It has long been understood that gram-negative anaerobes and spirochetes are the main putative pathogens in periodontal pockets, but searches for the "cause" of periodontitis down the years have not been able to discriminate well between the various bacteria. More recently it has become clearer that, within the broad spectrum of gram-negative organisms found at diseased sites, several putative pathogens are consistently found. The predominant group includes *Actinomyces actinomycetemcomitans, Bacteroides forsythus, Porphyromonas gingivalis, Prevotella intermedia, Fusobacterium nucleatum, Campylobacter rectus,* and *Treponema denticola.*[3,82,86,87,138,182,194,251] The presence of different clonal types of these bacteria is recognized, and it is not known whether all clonal types are pathogenic. If they are not, that could well account for some of the inconsistent associations found between the bacterial presence in the periodontal crevice and clinical disease.[180]

Maintaining excellent oral hygiene affects only the plaque and not the host response, one reason why oral hygiene is not always effective in controlling periodontitis. Still, practicing good oral hygiene is a behavior whose value is supported by the evidence, mostly relating to the conversion of supragingival plaque to subgingival microfilm as discussed earlier in this chapter.

---

*References 16,17,19,55,99,122,130,131,145,170.
†References 14,77,78,84,124,137,185.

Local Factors

Cleaning under gingival overhangs is difficult, and the growth of pathogenic flora can be encouraged by inadequate hygiene. Although gingival overhangs are common, they have been found not to be associated with serious periodontitis, at least not in young people.[123] Although overhangs obviously should be treated, local factors of this nature are generally considered to be of minor importance in the etiology of periodontitis compared to the nature of the infection and the host response.[175]

Nutrition

Despite the centuries-old observation that sailors suffering from scurvy (severe deficiency of ascorbic acid, or vitamin C) had bleeding gums, no nutritional or dietary factors have been shown to be directly related to the prevalence or intensity of periodontitis. The possibility that generalized malnutrition may influence its severity, however, cannot be ignored.[37,199] In the well-fed societies of the high-income world, generalized malnutrition is not a public health problem, although malnutrition can be found in some individuals with eating disorders. Ascorbic acid is probably the nutrient most often thought to be a factor, but it has been shown to be associated with periodontitis only at the lowest levels of intake in the United States, that is, 25% or less of the recommended dietary allowance.[101]

A series of worldwide epidemiologic studies in the 1960s, although they used the Periodontal Index and lacked rigor in their measurement of nutritional deficiencies, found little evidence for a relationship between periodontal disease and poor nutrition.[197] These studies were important at the time, but their relevance today is questionable. Subsequent studies suggest that there may be an association between more extensive gingival bleeding and ascorbic acid deficiency,[103,121] but whether such a mechanism relates to bone loss or CAL is not known. Nutritional adequacy is of course a precondition for successful treatment of virtually any disease, but there is no evidence to support the use of ascorbic acid, or any other nutrient, in the treatment of periodontitis.

Tobacco Use

Smoking is clearly a risk factor for periodontitis, with relative risk on the order of 2.5-6.0 or even higher.[32] Exactly how smoking acts in the causal chain, however, is still a subject of research. Smoking was first identified as a risk factor for periodontal diseases in an analysis of data from the first National Health and Nutrition Examination Survey (NHANES I) in 1971-74 in the United States,[100] and the evidence has continued to mount since then.[6,30,41,72,77,78,83,102,128] Assessments of randomly chosen patient groupings invariably show a higher prevalence of periodontitis among smokers.[81,89,106] It has been stated that 90% of persons with refractory chronic periodontitis are smokers,[107] and healing following treatment is slower in smokers.[79,109] Slower healing could be due to the inhibition of growth and attachment of fibroblasts in the periodontal ligament of smokers and in their slower posttherapy reduction of white blood cells and neutrophils.[45]

Experimental studies of plaque accumulation in smokers compared to nonsmokers have given mixed results; some showed no difference,[41,56,81] whereas others found more plaque and calculus in smokers.[158,181] Evidence on whether smoking promotes the growth of periodontal pathogens is mixed. Earlier studies showed no difference in prevalence of these bacteria subgingivally,[189,215] but more recent investigations suggest that smokers may have higher prevalence, rather than higher counts or proportions, of pathogenic species subgingivally.[83] Smoking appears to promote a favorable habitat for these species in shallow pockets.[63,83,241]

Smoking suppresses the vascular reaction that follows gingivitis and compromises host response to infection in other ways. In experimental plaque-induced gingivitis, although the rate of plaque accumulation was equal in smokers and nonsmokers, the increase in gingival vascularity in smokers was only half of that seen in nonsmokers.[31] In effect, this is a masking of the signs of inflammation.[32] Further studies have confirmed that smoking suppresses hemorrhagic response as measured by bleeding on probing.[29,33] Others have found no difference in the extent of bleeding on probing between smokers and nonsmokers, despite the fact that smokers had deeper pockets[240] or more plaque and calculus.[181] In both instances more gingival bleeding would have been expected in the smokers.

With regard to other aspects of host response, smoking inhibits granulocyte function,[213] and interactions between smoking and the IL-1 gene cluster have also been indentified.[151] In this study, no difference in mean CAL could be detected between smokers and nonsmokers among those who were negative for the periodontitis-associated genotype, but among those who were positive for this genotype the smokers had considerably greater CAL than nonsmokers. Smoking aggravates all tissue-destructive diseases, periodontitis included, by priming the production of tumor necrosis factor-α,[80] and it also causes the release of cytokines.[66] Smoking has been shown to be a stronger risk factor for periodontitis than is insulin-dependent diabetes mellitus.[155]

In summary, the evidence is clear that smoking is a major risk factor for periodontitis. The first line of treatment for periodontitis should always be to induce patients who smoke to quit smoking.

Psychosocial Stress

Psychosocial stress seems to be associated with progressive periodontitis, whether assessed in a case-control study,[52] cross-sectionally,[69] or in a longitudinal design.[64] Because psychosocial distress is a well-documented risk factor for a number of different diseases,[143] the identification of its predictive role in periodontitis strengthens the hypothesis that periodontitis is related to systemic diseases. Our understanding of the mind-body connection in periodontitis, as well as in other diseases, is likely to expand and become more important with time.

PERIODONTITIS AND SYSTEMIC CONDITIONS

An emerging area of importance is that of the potential link between periodontitis and some serious systemic conditions. The periodontitis-diabetes link is already well established. If others become established, then prevention and treatment of periodontitis will be seen in a completely different light. Here we look briefly at the relationship between periodontitis and diabetes, human immunodeficiency virus (HIV) infection, cardiovascular conditions, osteoporosis, and adverse pregnancy outcomes.

Diabetes

Both type 1 diabetes mellitus (type 1 DM, formerly called insulin-dependent diabetes mellitus) and type 2 DM (formerly called non-insulin dependent diabetes mellitus) are risk factors for periodontitis. There is good evidence to believe that the most critical issue in managing periodontitis in diabetic patients is the degree of metabolic control achieved: generally, the poorer the metabolic control, the more severe the periodontitis.[2,42,172,200,219,220,231] The converse has also been proposed; that is, untreated periodontal disease has been suggested to diminish glycemic control and thus aggravate diabetes.[218]

Younger adult patients with type 1 DM, especially those in whom the disease is of long duration, have more gingivitis and more deep pockets than nondiabetic patients.[59,68,92,203] No essential difference in subgingival flora has been demonstrated between diabetics and nondiabetics. However, among diabetics mild periodontitis is a risk factor for more severe diabetes, because diabetic patients have an exaggerated host response to a given bacterial burden.[202] Diabetic patients with good metabolic control respond to conservative treatment for periodontitis as well as do nondiabetic individuals,[46] and conservative treatment can improve glycemic control in patients with less well-controlled diabetes.[214]

Periodontitis also progresses more rapidly in individuals with poorly controlled diabetes,[208] and early age of onset of diabetes also is considered a risk factor for more severe disease.[226] Persons with poorly controlled diabetes have also been found to exhibit higher levels of the enzyme β-glucuronidase in their gingival crevicular fluid than do those in whom the disease is well controlled.[173]

The most extensive studies among patients with type 2 DM have been conducted in the Gila River community in Arizona, where prevalence of type 2 DM is high. Patients with type 2 DM had substantially greater CAL, loss of alveolar bone, and tooth loss.[162,209] When age, gender, and oral hygiene level all were controlled for, type 2 DM was found to be associated with a two to three times higher risk of developing destructive periodontitis.[65] This degree of risk is similar to that found for severe CAL in diabetic as compared to nondiabetic individuals in an adult population in upstate New York.[78]

Studies of quantitative and qualitative aspects of microflora in individuals with diabetes (both type I DM and type 2 DM) reveal no notable differences between diabetics and non-diabetics.[222,254] Other suggested mechanisms by which diabetes may contribute to periodontitis include vascular changes, polymorphonuclear leukocyte dysfunction, abnormal collagen synthesis, cytokine production, and genetic predisposition.[34,54,108,115,172] Individuals with poorly controlled diabetes have also been shown to have impaired salivary flow.[40] Periodontal treatment should always be a standard feature of health care for diabetic patients.

HIV Infection

It was the loss of immune response in acquired immune deficiency syndrome (AIDS) that focused attention on the relationship between HIV infection and periodontitis. Most early reports of this relationship came from cross-sectional investigations studying convenience samples of homosexual men, many of whom were in late stages of the disease and severely immunosuppressed.[247,248] Most of these studies were not rigorously designed,[195] so interpretation of their results is uncertain. Studies of the HIV-periodontitis link remain limited, but those conducted with patients at earlier stages of HIV infection, and especially with patients receiving antiretroviral therapy, have raised questions about the nature of the HIV-periodontitis association.

Several studies examined the periodontal condition of patients taking part in clinical trials of the drug zidovudine (AZT). One reported the periodontal health of patients in the early stages of HIV disease to be generally good,[62] and a longitudinal study of 30 HIV-positive patients found a greater progression of periodontitis over 18 months in this group than in 10 HIV-negative controls.[253] However, in neither study was there analysis of periodontal disease in the patients taking AZT compared to the others. In another follow-up of 114 homosexual or bisexual men conducted over a period of 20 months, periodontal changes were found to be related to HIV-1 serostatus, immune status, age, and plaque deposits. The risk of CAL of 3 mm or more over the 20 months was 6.16 times higher in the more immunosuppressed patients (CD4+ counts of less than 200/μl) than in the

less immunosuppressed patients, and this finding was more pronounced in older subjects.[22] HIV-positive patients showed a more sensitive reaction to plaque than did the HIV-negative patients. This study concluded that immunosuppression, especially in combination with older age, was a risk factor for progression of CAL and that seropositivity, independent of immune status, was a risk factor for gingivitis.

In a cross-sectional study of HIV-positive military personnel, however, the relation between periodontal health and immune status was less clear.[216] A detailed follow-up of 474 patients from the same population, ages 18-49, found CAL of 5 mm or more in 20% of the patients. In this group, which was about 85% male, neither the clinical stage of the disease nor the CD4+ count was a good independent predictor of severe CAL when account was taken of other significantly associated variables (e.g., tobacco use).[228]

If HIV infection is really a risk factor for periodontitis, we would expect to see an inverse relation between severity of periodontitis and CD4+ counts. The evidence is mixed, however, except for those in the most severe stages of AIDS. One early comparison between men at different stages of HIV disease found little difference in terms of periodontal health.[67] The severity of periodontitis could not be related to CD4+ counts in an HIV-positive group of patients, none of whom was receiving antiretroviral therapy.[144] Even in an African population with no access to modern antiretroviral drugs, periodontitis among HIV-positive individuals was less prevalent and severe than had been expected.[205] The usual oral manifestations of AIDS (candidiasis, hairy leukoplakia, Kaposi's sarcoma) were less common than expected in a patient group receiving antiretroviral therapy,[217] and HIV-infected children whose disease was under good medical control had no more periodontal disease than did HIV-negative controls.[207] However, there are contrary findings as well. HIV-positive patients in North Carolina hospitals were found to have more severe periodontitis than uninfected persons, and these lesions were related to the degree of immunosuppression.[149] A British study found more periodontopathogenic bacteria in HIV-positive patients than in HIV-negative controls,[204] and greatly increased numbers of mast cells and neutrophils were found in the gingival tissue of HIV-positive patients.[161] There are few reports regarding levels of inflammatory cytokines in HIV-positive persons, although one found more total IL-1β in gingival crevicular fluid from HIV-positive persons than in that from unaffected persons.[117]

The microbiology of periodontitis in HIV-positive persons relative to those not infected is not clear, for both little difference[159,160,192] and significant differences[154] have been reported. None of these studies reported on the immunosuppression status of the subjects, although a later assessment of HIV-positive patients found the occurrence of necrotizing ulcerative periodontitis to be related to decreasing CD4+ counts.[70] Pathogenic bacteria have been reported as no more frequent in HIV-positive than in HIV-negative persons,[221,232] although the stage of immunosuppression of the patients in these studies was not reported.

Our understanding of the relationship between periodontitis and HIV/AIDS demands further research, especially since the success of highly active antiretroviral therapy has changed the outlook on HIV infection (see Chapter 10).

Cardiovascular Disorders

Biomedicine's recognition that chronic inflammation anywhere in the body might affect heart function[12] has been a spur for research into the way that periodontitis might affect cardiovascular disorders. An association between periodontitis and cardiovascular disorders has been shown fairly consistently, although by no means universally. The odds ratios have been in the range of 1.5-3.0; if confirmed, this means that periodontitis could be a causal factor of some consequence in the top-ranked cause of death in the United States. However, although an association between these factors is evident, cause and effect has not yet been demonstrated. Cardiovascular diseases are complex, and the research in this area has the challenge of disentangling a maze of confounding and correlated factors. Longitudinal studies with large numbers of participants are required to separate true risk factors from this "background noise." Clinical trials of interventions, that is, tests to see if periodontal treatment will reduce cardiovascular mortality, are also needed to establish causality.

One report drawing on the NHANES I database (1971-74) concluded that persons with periodontitis at baseline had a 25% greater risk of subsequent coronary heart disease than did those without periodontitis.[60] The risk was especially strong for men under age 50 at baseline. However, other analyses of the NHANES I data set have found the opposite. Two studies from the University of Washington (1) have failed to demonstrate any significant association between periodontal conditions and cardiovascular disease[94] and (2) have found that the edentulous were at no greater risk of a cardiovascular event than patients with periodontitis.[95] Using the data from NHANES I, this research group concluded that periodontitis does not increase the risk of a bad cardiovascular outcome among those with preexisting heart disease. They have also suggested that the associations between chronic periodontitis and cardiovascular conditions observed in smaller studies can be attributed to insufficient statistical control for lifestyle differences.[96] At the same time, it must be recognized that NHANES I recorded periodontal diseases by the now-defunct Periodontal Index (see Chapter 16), and this would tend to bias results toward showing no effect. There is also reason to believe that results can vary by the population studied,[146] which confirms the need for studies involving large numbers and representative samples. Self-reported periodontal conditions were not a risk factor for cardiovascular disease in a study of male physicians,[90] whereas periodontitis was related to self-reported heart conditions in NHANES III.[10]

Circumstantial evidence supports an association between periodontitis and cardiovascular conditions. The presence of C-reactive protein is a risk factor for cardiovascular disease, and the protein has been found at higher levels in persons with periodontitis both in clinical studies[135,164] and in NHANES III.[210] The NHANES III data, interestingly enough, showed C-reactive protein levels also to be high in edentulous people, for reasons unknown.

If causality is to be established, the sequence of events over time must be determined with some confidence. (This is a drawback of cross-sectional studies such as NHANES, because in cross-sectional studies the exposure and the outcome are both measured at the same time.

An example is when there is a follow-up of people examined, as in NHANES I.) The results of two studies using a retrospective cohort design are helpful here. One was conducted in Canada, where participants took part in a 1970-72 Nutrition Canada Survey that included a periodontal assessment. The cardiovascular mortality of participants was assessed in 1993, and significant associations were found between subsequent death from cardiovascular disease and (1) severe gingivitis at baseline and (2) edentulism at baseline.[157] The second study was done in Sweden, where mortality experience from 1970 to 1996 was assessed for 1393 participants in a 1970 dental epidemiologic study. Results of this study were essentially similar to those of the Canadian study.[104]

It is interesting to note that what is being discussed here is essentially the "focal infection" issue, which was first raised in 1911[97] and subsequently became the underlying rationale for mass extractions over subsequent decades. The focal infection theory faded in the 1950s, but its underlying principle seems to have reemerged.

Osteoporosis

Osteoporosis is a condition of bone fragility characterized by low bone mass and structural deterioration. It is common in old age, especially in postmenopausal women. *Osteopenia* is a less severe form of bone-mineral loss. Because alveolar bone loss is often seen with generalized osteoporosis, the question naturally arises as to how much alveolar bone loss is actually due to osteoporosis rather than to periodontitis. The issues can also be stated as follows:[43]

- Is generalized osteoporosis or osteopenia a risk factor for periodontitis?
- Does generalized osteoporosis or osteopenia lead to oral osteopenia?
- Does periodontitis lead to oral osteopenia?

It can be seen from these questions that getting the time sequence right in these slowly developing conditions is an inherent research problem, and that is probably the main reason why these questions remain incompletely answered.

Cross-sectional studies, not surprisingly, give conflicting results. A number of studies show an association between periodontitis and low bone mineral density at various locations in the body.[98,111,196,223] However, other cross-sectional studies have shown no association between periodontitis and systemic bone mineral density measured at eight points in the body[245] and no difference in periodontitis levels in postmenopausal women with osteoporosis and in those without.[136] A literature review concluded that CAL was greater in osteoporotic women than in nonosteoporotic women, although the body of literature available for review was rather sparse.[114]

Few longitudinal studies are available. One, conducted in Denmark, followed 20 young people with severe periodontitis over a 5- to 10-year period. Mandibular bone mineral content was significantly lower than bone mineral content elsewhere in the body, which essentially indicates that periodontitis is a local condition.[242] The remaining longitudinal studies were 1-2 years in duration and focused on the effect of estrogen supplementation in postmenopausal women. Low estrogen level is a factor in osteoporotic bone loss. Estrogen-sufficient women in this study gained in alveolar bone mineral density over a year, whereas the estrogen-insufficient women experienced a mean loss of bone.[184] Estrogen supplementation was also shown to reduce CAL in osteopenic and osteoporotic women in early menopause.[193]

More research is clearly needed in this area.

Adverse Pregnancy Outcomes

The inflammatory mediators that are seen in the periodontal diseases are the same ones that play an important part in the initiation of labor, so it is reasonable to hypothesize that there are biologic mechanisms linking the two conditions.[246]

A 1996 report concluded that mothers of premature, low-birth-weight infants were about 7.5 times more likely to have periodontitis during pregnancy than mothers of normal-weight infants.[168] A later case-control study conducted by the same research group found that levels of the inflammatory cytokine prostaglandin E_2 were significantly higher in mothers who had given birth to preterm low-birth-weight infants than in mothers whose infants were of normal birth weight.[167] A later case-control study by a different research group involving 448 women found that those who had given birth to low-birth-weight infants were four times as likely to have high *P. gingivalis*–specific maternal serum immunoglobulin G levels than did those who had infants of normal birth weight.[57] However, another case-control study found that the risk of having a preterm low-birth-weight infant decreased with increasing pocket depth; that is, periodontitis appeared to be protective.[58] This finding is not easy to explain in light of the other evidence.

Prospective studies are usually regarded as stronger evidence than case-control studies because the strength and extent of the exposure can be measured more exactly. In a cohort of 1313 women, the risk of a preterm birth (35 or fewer weeks' gestation) was some five times greater among women who had periodontitis at 21-24 weeks of pregnancy than among those who did not.[105] In another prospective study in North Carolina, 19.9% of preterm infants showed seropositivity for one or more periodontal pathogens in fetal cord blood, compared to 6.9% of full-term babies.[140]

Interim data from the first 814 deliveries in a projected 5-year prospective study demonstrate that the incidence or progression of periodontitis during pregnancy is significantly associated with a higher occurrence of preterm births.[169] The conclusions of this study were strengthened by the finding of a dose-response relationship: greater severity of the periodontal conditions was directly related to the increased risk of a preterm low-birth-weight outcome.

The evidence favors an association between maternal periodontitis and the risk of delivering a preterm low-birth-weight infant. It is too early yet to say that this link is causal, but it is strong enough to indicate that periodontal monitoring, and treatment when necessary, is a good idea during pregnancy.

PREDICTION OF PERIODONTITIS

Attempts to identify predictors of future disease go back some years. The aim is to identify the presence of some easily measured entity, one that clinicians can readily test for in a patient, that will predict with high reliability the risk of future disease. The research studies to identify these predictors must have longitudinal designs in which suspected predictors (e.g., plaque deposits, subgingival calculus deposits, tobacco use, diabetes, SES, specific cytokines in gingival crevicular fluid, psychic stress) are measured in participants at baseline, and development of

new periodontal lesions or progression of existing lesions is noted over a period of time. The disease outcome can then be related to the baseline measures. There are many complications in this type of research given the complexity of the host response to periodontal infections.[18] Models that fit past data often cannot be accurately extended to present conditions.[252]

The presence of visible plaque and calculus, as one example of a hypothesized marker, was long assumed to predict future CAL or bone loss, but it is now seen that clinical measures of plaque and calculus by themselves do not predict future disease to any useful extent.[14,47,85,118,186] Models that have included the subgingival presence of specific pathogens like *A. actinomycetemcomitans*, *P. intermedia*, *P. gingivalis*, and *B. forsythus* along with other indicators have shown a moderate degree of predictive value.[25,138,227,230] Host response must be worked into the equation, and it is now recognized that smoking and genetic predisposition are major players in this regard. When smoking and periodontitis-associated IL-1 genotype status (positive or negative) were included in a predictive model, none of the baseline clinical indicators added significantly to the ability of the model to predict subsequent tooth loss. The baseline clinical indicators performed much better in a model that included IL-1 genotype status in nonsmokers.[148] What this body of research has demonstrated is that multiple predictors work better than any single predictor by itself, and the nearest we can get to a universal predictor is tobacco use.[5,25,139,165]

REFERENCES

1. Abdellatif HM, Burt BA. An epidemiological investigation into the relative importance of age and oral hygiene status as determinants of periodontitis. J Dent Res 1987;66:13-8.
2. Ainamo J, Lahtinen A, Uitto VJ. Rapid periodontal destruction in adult humans with poorly controlled diabetes. A report of 2 cases. J Clin Periodontol 1990;17:22-8.
3. Albandar JM, Brown LJ, Löe H. Clinical features of early-onset periodontitis. J Am Dent Assoc 1997;128:1393-9.
4. Al-Kufaishi KA, Hirschmann PN, Lennon MA. The radiographic assessment of early periodontal bone loss in adolescents. Br Dent J 1984;157:91-3.
5. Alpagot T, Bell C, Lundergan W, et al. Longitudinal evaluation of GCF MMP-3 and TIMP-1 levels as prognostic factors for progression of periodontitis. J Clin Periodontol 2001;28:353-9.

6. Amarasena N, Ekanayaka AN, Herath L, Miyazaki H. Tobacco use and oral hygiene as risk indicators for periodontitis. Community Dent Oral Epidemiol 2002;30:115-23.

7. Ånerud A, Löe H, Boysen H. The natural history and clinical course of calculus formation in man. J Clin Periodontol 1991;18:160-70.

8. Ånerud A, Löe H, Boysen H, Smith M. The natural history of periodontal disease in man: Changes in gingival health and oral hygiene before 40 years of age. J Periodont Res 1979;14:526-40.

9. Ånerud KE, Robertson PB, Löe H, et al. Periodontal disease in three young adult populations. J Periodont Res 1983;18:655-68.

10. Arbes SJ, Slade GD, Beck JD. Association between extent of periodontal attachment loss and self-reported history of heart attack: An analysis of NHANES III data. J Dent Res 1999;78:1778-82.

11. Armitage GC. Development of a classification system for periodontal diseases and conditions. Ann Periodontol 1999;4:1-38.

12. Armitage GC. Periodontal infections and cardiovascular disease—how strong is the association? Oral Dis 2000;6:335-50.

13. Astrom AN, Rise J. Socio-economic differences in patterns of health and oral health behaviour in 25 year old Norwegians. Clin Oral Investig 2001;5:122-8.

14. Badersten A, Nilveus R, Egelberg J. Scores of plaque, bleeding, suppuration and probing depth to predict probing attachment loss. 5 years of observation following nonsurgical periodontal therapy. J Clin Periodontol 1990;17:102-7.

15. Baelum V, Chen X, Manji F, et al. Profiles of destructive periodontal disease in different populations. J Periodont Res 1996;31:17-26.

16. Baelum V, Fejerskov O, Karring T. Oral hygiene, gingivitis, and periodontal breakdown in adult Tanzanians. J Periodont Res 1986;21:221-32.

17. Baelum V, Fejerskov O, Manji F. Periodontal diseases in adult Kenyans. J Clin Periodontol 1988;15:445-52.

18. Baelum V, Luan W-M, Chen X, Fejerskov O. Predictors of destructive periodontal disease incidence and progression in adult and elderly Chinese. Community Dent Oral Epidemiol 1997;25:265-72.

19. Baelum V, Luan W-M, Fejerskov O, Xia C. Tooth mortality and periodontal conditions in 60-80-year-old Chinese. Scand J Dent Res 1988; 96:99-107.

20. Barmes DE. Epidemiology of dental disease. J Clin Periodontol 1977;4:80-93.

21. Barmes DE, Leous PA. Assessment of periodontal status by CPITN and its applicability to the development of long-term goals on periodontal health of the population. Int Dent J 1986;36:177-81.

22. Barr C, Lopez MR, Rua-Dobles A. Periodontal changes by HIV serostatus in a cohort of homosexual and bisexual men. J Clin Periodontol 1992;19:794-801.

23. Beck JD, Koch GG. Characteristics of older adults experiencing periodontal attachment loss as gingival recession or probing depth. J Periodont Res 1994;29:290-8.

24. Beck JD, Koch GG, Offenbacher S. Attachment loss trends over 3 years in community-dwelling older adults. J Periodontol 1994;65:737-43.

25. Beck JD, Koch GG, Offenbacher S. Incidence of attachment loss over 3 years in older adults—new and progressing lesions. Community Dent Oral Epidemiol 1995;23:291-6.

26. Beck JD, Koch GG, Rozier RG, Tudor GE. Prevalence and risk indicators for periodontal attachment loss in a population of older community-dwelling blacks and whites. J Periodontol 1990;61:521-8.

27. Beck JD, Sharp T, Koch GG, Offenbacher S. A 5-year study of attachment loss and tooth loss in community-dwelling older adults. J Periodont Res 1997;32:516-23.

28. Beck JD, Slade GD. Epidemiology of periodontal diseases. Curr Opin Periodontol 1996;3:3-9.

29. Bergstrom J, Bostrom L. Tobacco smoking and periodontal hemorrhagic responsiveness. J Clin Periodontol 2001;28:680-5.

30. Bergstrom J, Floderus-Myrhed B. Co-twin control study of the relationship between smoking and some periodontal disease factors. Community Dent Oral Epidemiol 1983;11:113-6.

31. Bergstrom J, Persson L, Preber H. Influence of cigarette smoking on vascular reaction during experimental gingivitis. Scand J Dent Res 1988;96:34-9.

32. Bergstrom J, Preber H. Tobacco use as a risk factor. J Periodontol 1994;65:545-50.

33. Biddle AJ, Palmer RM, Wilson RF, Watts TL. Comparison of the validity of periodontal probing measurements in smokers and non-smokers. J Clin Periodontol 2001;28:806-12.

34. Bulut U, Develioglu H, Taner IL, Berker E. Interleukin-1 beta levels in gingival crevicular fluid in type 2 diabetes mellitus and adult periodontitis. J Oral Sci 2001;43:171-7.

35. Burt BA. Periodontitis and aging: Reviewing recent evidence. J Am Dent Assoc 1994;125:273-9.

36. Burt BA, Ismail AI, Eklund SA. Periodontal disease, tooth loss, and oral hygiene among older Americans. Community Dent Oral Epidemiol 1985;13:93-6.

37. Carlos JP, Wolfe MD. Methodological and nutritional issues in assessing the oral health of aged subjects. Am J Clin Nutr 1989;50:1210-8.

38. Carlos JP, Wolfe MD, Zambon JJ, Kingman A. Periodontal disease in adolescents: Some clinical and microbiologic correlates of attachment loss. J Dent Res 1988;67:1510-4.

39. Cattabriga M, Rotundo R, Muzzi L, et al. Retrospective evaluation of the influence of the interleukin-1 genotype on radiographic bone levels in treated periodontal patients over 10 years. J Periodontol 2001;72:767-73.

40. Chavez EM, Borrell LN, Taylor GW, Ship JA. A longitudinal analysis of salivary flow in control subjects and older adults with type 2 diabetes. Oral Surg Oral Med Oral Pathol Oral Radiol Endodont 2001;91:166-73.

41. Chen X, Wolff L, Aeppli D, et al. Cigarette smoking, salivary/gingival crevicular fluid cotinine and periodontal status. A 10-year longitudinal study. J Clin Periodontol 2001;28:331-9.

42. Cherry-Peppers G, Ship JA. Oral health in patients with type II diabetes and impaired glucose tolerance. Diabetes Care 1993;16:638-41.

43. Chesnut CH. The relationship between skeletal and oral bone mineral density: An overview. Ann Periodontol 2001;6:193-6.

44. Chilton NW, Miller ME. Epidemiology. In: International Conference on Research in the Biology of Periodontal Disease. Chicago: University of Illinois School of Dentistry, 1977:119-43.

45. Christian C, Dietrich T, Hagewald S, et al. White blood cell count in generalized aggressive periodontitis after non-surgical therapy. J Clin Periodontol 2002;29: 201-6.

46. Christgau M, Palitzsch KD, Schmalz G, et al. Healing response to non-surgical periodontal therapy in patients with diabetes mellitus: Clinical, microbiological, and immunologic results. J Clin Periodontol 1998;25:112-24.

47. Claffey N, Nylund K, Kiger R, et al. Diagnostic predictability of scores of plaque, bleeding, suppuration and probing depth for probing attachment loss. 3½ years of observation following initial periodontal therapy. J Clin Periodontol 1990;17:108-14.

48. Clerehugh V, Lennon MA. The radiographic measurement of early periodontal bone loss and its relationship with loss of attachment. Br Dent J 1986;161:141-4.

49. Clerehugh V, Lennon MA. A two-year longitudinal study of early periodontitis in 14- to 16-year-old schoolchildren. Community Dent Health 1986;3: 135-41.

50. Consensus report. Periodontal diseases: Pathogenesis and microbial factors. Ann Periodontol 1996;1:926-32.

51. Consensus report. Periodontal diseases: Epidemiology and diagnosis. Ann Periodontol 1996;1:216-22.

52. Croucher R, Marcenes WS, Torres MC, et al. The relationship between life-events and periodontitis. A case-control study. J Clin Periodontol 1997;24:39-43.

53. Cullinan MP, Westerman B, Hamlet SM, et al. A longitudinal study of interleukin-1 gene polymorphisms and periodontal disease in a general adult population. J Clin Periodontol 2001;28:1137-44.

54. Cutler CW, Eke P, Arnold RR, Van Dyke TE. Defective neutrophil function in an insulin dependent diabetes mellitus patient. A case report. J Periodontol 1991;62: 394-401.

55. Cutress TW, Powell RN, Ball ME. Differing profiles of periodontal disease in two similar South Pacific island populations. Community Dent Oral Epidemiol 1982;10:193-203.

56. Danielsen B, Manji F, Nagelkerke N, et al. Effect of cigarette smoking on the transition dynamics in experimental gingivitis. J Clin Periodontol 1990;17:159-64.

57. Dasanayake AP, Boyd D, Madianos PN, et al. The association between Porphyromonas gingivalis-specific maternal serum IgG and low birth weight. J Periodontol 2001;72:1491-7.

58. Davenport ES, Williams CE, Sterne JA, et al. Maternal periodontal disease and preterm low birthweight: Case-control study. J Dent Res 2002;81:313-8.

59. de Pommereau V, Dargent-Pare C, Robert JJ, Brion M. Periodontal status in insulin-dependent diabetic adolescents. J Clin Periodontol 1992;19:628-32.

60. DeStefano F, Anda RF, Kahn HS, et al. Dental disease and risk of coronary heart disease and mortality. Br Med J 1993;306:688-91.

61. Diehl SR, Wang Y, Brooks CN, et al. Linkage disequilibrium of interleukin-1 genetic polymorphisms with early-onset periodontitis. J Periodontol 1999;70: 418-30.

62. Drinkard CR, Decher L, Little JW, et al. Periodontal status of individuals in early stages of human immunodeficiency virus infection. Community Dent Oral Epidemiol 1991;19:281-5.

63. Eggert FM, McLeod MH, Flowerdew G. Effects of smoking and treatment status on periodontal bacteria: Evidence that smoking influences control of periodontal bacteria at the mucosal surface of the gingival crevice. J Periodontol 2001;72:1210-20.

64. Elter JR, Beck JD, Slade GD, Offenbacher S. Etiologic models for incident periodontal attachment loss in older adults. J Clin Periodontol 1999;26:113-23.

65. Emrich LJ, Shlossman M, Genco RJ. Periodontal disease in non-insulin-dependent diabetes mellitus. J Periodontol 1991;62:123-31.

66. Fredriksson M, Bergstrom K, Asman B. IL-8 and TNF-alpha from peripheral neutrophils and acute-phase proteins in periodontitis. J Clin Periodontol 2002;29:123-8.

67. Friedman RB, Gunsolley J, Gentry A, et al. Periodontal status of HIV-seropositive and AIDS patients. J Periodontol 1991;62:623-7.

68. Galea H, Aganovic I, Aganovic M. The dental caries and periodontal disease experience of patients with early onset insulin dependent diabetes. Int Dent J 1986;36:219-24.

69. Genco RJ, Ho AW, Grossi SG, et al. Relationship of stress, distress and inadequate coping behaviors to periodontal disease. J Periodontol 1999;70:711-23.

70. Glick M, Muzyka BC, Salkin LM, Lurie D. Necrotizing ulcerative periodontitis: A marker for immune deterioration and a predictor for the diagnosis of AIDS. J Periodontol 1994;65:393-7.

71. Gmur R, Marinello CP, Guggenheim B. Periodontitis associated bacteria in supragingival plaque of dental hygienists: Stability of carrier state and clinical development. Eur J Oral Sci 1999;107:225-8.

72. Gonzalez YM, De Nardin A, Grossi SG, et al. Serum cotinine levels, smoking, and periodontal attachment loss. J Dent Res 1996;75:796-802.

73. Goodson JM, Haffajee AD, Socransky SS. The relationship between attachment level loss and alveolar bone loss. J Clin Periodontol 1984;11:348-59.

74. Goodson JM. Selection of suitable indicators of periodontitis. In: Bader JD, ed: Risk assessment in dentistry. Chapel Hill NC: University of North Carolina, 1990: 69-74.

75. Goodson JM, Tanner ACM, Haffajee AD, et al. Patterns of progression and regression of advanced destructive periodontal disease. J Clin Periodontol 1982;9:472-81.

76. Griffiths GS, Wilton JM, Curtis MA, et al. Detection of high-risk groups and individuals for periodontal diseases. Clinical assessment of the periodontium. J Clin Periodontol 1988;15:403-10.

77. Grossi SG, Genco RJ, Machtei EE, et al. Assessment of risk for periodontal disease. II. Risk indicators for alveolar bone loss. J Periodontol 1995;66:23-9.

78. Grossi SG, Zambon JJ, Ho AW, et al. Assessment of risk for periodontal disease. I. Risk indicators for attachment loss. J Periodontol 1994;65:260-7.

79. Grossi SG, Zambon J, Machtei EE, et al. Effects of smoking and smoking cessation on healing after mechanical periodontal therapy. J Am Dent Assoc 1997;128:599-607.

80. Gustafsson A, Asman B, Bergstrom K. Cigarette smoking as an aggravating factor in inflammatory tissue-destructive diseases. Increase in tumor necrosis factor-alpha priming of peripheral neutrophils measured as generation of oxygen radicals. Int J Clin Lab Res 2000;30:187-90.

81. Haber J, Wattles J, Crowley M, et al. Evidence for cigarette smoking as a major risk factor for periodontitis. J Periodontol 1993;64:16-23.

82. Haffajee AD, Cugini MA, Tanner A, et al. Subgingival microbiota in healthy, well-maintained elder and periodontitis subjects. J Clin Periodontol 1998;25:346-53.

83. Haffajee AD, Socransky SS. Relationship of cigarette smoking to attachment level profiles. J Clin Periodontol 2001;28:283-95.

84. Haffajee AD, Socransky SS, Dzink JL, et al. Clinical, microbiological and immunological features of subjects with destructive periodontal diseases. J Clin Periodontol 1988;15:240-6.

85. Haffajee AD, Socransky SS, Goodson JM. Clinical parameters as predictors of destructive disease activity. J Clin Periodontol 1983;10:257-65.

86. Hamlet SM, Cullinan MP, Westerman B, et al. Distribution of *Actinobacillus actinomycetemcomitans*, *Porphyromonas gingivalis* and *Prevotella intermedia* in an Australian population. J Clin Periodontol 2001;28:1163-71.

87. Haraszthy VI, Hariharan G, Tinoco EM, et al. Evidence for the role of highly leukotoxic *Actinobacillus actinomycetemcomitans* in the pathogenesis of localized juvenile and other forms of early-onset periodontitis. J Periodontol 2000;71:912-22.

88. Hoover JN, Ellegaard B, Attstrom R. Radiographic and clinical examination of periodontal status of first molars in 15-16 year-old Danish schoolchildren. Scand J Dent Res 1981;89:260-3.

89. Horning GM, Hatch CL, Cohen ME. Risk indicators for periodontitis in a military treatment population. J Periodontol 1992;63:297-302.

90. Howell TH, Ridker PM, Ajani UA, et al. Periodontal disease and risk of subsequent cardiovascular disease in U.S. male physicians. J Am Coll Cardiol 2001;37:445-50.

91. Hugoson A, Jordan T. Frequency distribution of individuals aged 20-70 years according to severity of periodontal disease. Community Dent Oral Epidemiol 1982;10:187-92.

92. Hugoson A, Thorstensson H, Falk H, Kuylenstierna J. Periodontal conditions in insulin-dependent diabetics. J Clin Periodontol 1989;16:215-23.

93. Hujoel PP, Bergstrom J, del Aguila MA, DeRouen TA. A hidden chronic periodontitis epidemic during the 20th century? Community Dent Oral Epidemiol 2003;31:1-6.

94. Hujoel PP, Drangsholt M, Spiekerman C, DeRouen TA. Periodontal disease and coronary heart disease risk. JAMA 2000;284:1410-6.

95. Hujoel PP, Drangsholt M, Spiekerman C, DeRouen TA. Examining the link between coronary heart disease and the elimination of chronic dental infections. J Am Dent Assoc 2001;132:883-9.

96. Hujoel PP, Drangsholt M, Spiekerman C, DeRouen TA. Pre-existing cardiovascular disease and periodontitis: A follow-up study. J Dent Res 2002;81:186-91.

97. Hunter W. The role of sepsis and antisepsis in medicine. Lancet 1911; Jan 14;79-86.

98. Inagaki K, Kurosu Y, Kamiya T, et al. Low metacarpal bone density, tooth loss, and periodontal disease in Japanese women. J Dent Res 2001;80:1818-22.

99. Ismail AI, Burt BA, Brunelle JA. Prevalence of total tooth loss, dental caries, and periodontal disease in Mexican-American adults: Results from the Southwestern NHANES. J Dent Res 1987;66:1183-8.

100. Ismail AI, Burt BA, Eklund SA. Epidemiologic patterns of smoking and periodontal disease in the United States. J Am Dent Assoc 1983;106:617-21.

101. Ismail AI, Burt BA, Eklund SA. Relation between ascorbic acid intake and periodontal disease in the United States. J Am Dent Assoc 1983;107:927-31.

102. Ismail AI, Morrison EC, Burt BA, et al. Natural history of periodontal disease in adults: Findings from the Tecumseh Periodontal Disease Study, 1959-87. J Dent Res 1990;69:430-5.

103. Jacob RA, Omaye ST, Skala JH, et al. Experimental vitamin C depletion and supplementation in young men. Nutrient interactions and dental health effects. Ann N Y Acad Sci 1987;498:333-46.

104. Jansson L, Lavstedt S, Frithiof L, Theobald H. Relationship between oral health and mortality in cardiovascular diseases. J Clin Periodontol 2001;28:762-8.

105. Jeffcoat MK, Geurs NC, Reddy MS, et al. Periodontal infection and preterm birth: Results of a prospective study. J Am Dent Assoc 2001;132:875-80.

106. Jette AM, Feldman HA, Tennstedt SL. Tobacco use: A modifiable risk factor for dental disease among the elderly. Am J Public Health 1993;83:1271-6.

107. Johnson GK, Slach NA. Impact of tobacco use on periodontal status. J Dent Educ 2001;65:313-21.

108. Katz PP, Wirthlin MR Jr, Szpunar SM, et al. Epidemiology and prevention of periodontal disease in individuals with diabetes. Diabetes Care 1991;14:375-85.

109. Kinane DF, Radvar M. The effect of smoking on mechanical and antimicrobial periodontal therapy. J Periodontol 1997;68:467-72.

110. Klavan B, Genco R, Löe H, et al, eds. International conference on research in the biology of periodontal disease. Chicago: University of Illinois, 1977.

111. Klemetti E, Collin HL, Forss H, et al. Mineral status of skeleton and advanced periodontal disease. J Clin Periodontol 1994;21:184-8.

112. Kornman KS. Patients are not equally susceptible to periodontitis: Does this change dental practice and the dental curriculum? J Dent Educ 2001;65:777-84.

113. Kornman KS, Crane A, Wang HY, et al. The interleukin-1 genotype as a severity factor in adult periodontal disease. J Clin Periodontol 1997;24:72-7.

114. Krejci CB, Bissada NF. Women's health issues and their relationship to periodontitis. J Am Dent Assoc 2002;133:323-9.

115. Kurtis B, Develioglu H, Taner IL, et al. IL-6 levels in gingival crevicular fluid (GCF) from patients with non-insulin dependent diabetes mellitus (NIDDM), adult periodontitis and healthy subjects. J Oral Sci 1999;41:163-7.

116. Laine ML, Farre MA, Gonzalez G, et al. Polymorphisms of the interleukin-1 gene family, oral microbial pathogens, and smoking in adult periodontitis. J Dent Res 2001;80:1695-9.

117. Lamster IB, Grbic JT, Mitchell-Lewis DA, et al. New concepts regarding the pathogenesis of periodontal disease in HIV infection. Ann Periodontol 1998;3: 62-75.

118. Lang NP, Joss A, Orsanic T, et al. Bleeding on probing: A predictor for the progression of periodontal disease? J Clin Periodontol 1986;13:590-6.

119. Lang NP, Tonetti MS, Suter J, et al. Effect of interleukin-1 gene polymorphisms on gingival inflammation assessed by bleeding on probing in a periodontal maintenance population. J Periodont Res 2000;35: 102-7.

120. Latcham NL, Powell RN, Jago JD, et al. A radiographic study of chronic periodontitis in 15-year-old Queensland children. J Clin Periodontol 1983;10: 37-45.

121. Leggott PJ, Robertson PB, Rothman DL, et al. The effect of controlled ascorbic acid depletion and supplementation on periodontal health. J Periodontol 1986;57:480-5.

122. Lembariti BS, Frencken JE, Pilot T. Prevalence and severity of periodontal conditions among adults in urban and rural Morogoro, Tanzania. Community Dent Oral Epidemiol 1988;16:240-3.

123. Lervik T, Riordan PJ, Haugejorden O. Periodontal disease and approximal overhangs on amalgam restorations in Norwegian 21-year-olds. Community Dent Oral Epidemiol 1984;12:264-8.

124. Lindhe J, Okamoto H, Yoneyama T, et al. Longitudinal changes in periodontal disease in untreated subjects. J Clin Periodontol 1989;16:662-70.

125. Listgarten MA. Pathogenesis of periodontitis. J Clin Periodontol 1986;13:418-30.

126. Listgarten MA. Microbiological testing in the diagnosis of periodontal disease. J Periodontol 1992;63: 332-7.

127. Listgarten MA, Slots J, Nowotny AH, et al. Incidence of periodontitis recurrence in treated patients with and without cultivable *Actinobacillus actinomycetemcomitans*, *Prevotella intermedia*, and *Porphyromonas gingivalis*: A prospective study. J Periodontol 1991;62: 377-86.

128. Locker D. Smoking and oral health in older adults. Can J Public Health 1992;83:429-32.

129. Locker D, Leake JL. Risk indicators and risk markers for periodontal disease experience in older adults living independently in Ontario, Canada. J Dent Res 1993;72:9-17.

130. Löe H, Ånerud A, Boysen H. The natural history of periodontal disease in man: Prevalence, severity, and extent of gingival recession. J Periodontol 1992;63: 489-95.

131. Löe H, Ånerud A, Boysen H, Morrison E. Natural history of periodontal disease in man; rapid, moderate, and no loss of attachment in Sri Lankan laborers 14 to 46 years of age. J Clin Periodontol 1986;13:431-40.

132. Löe H, Ånerud A, Boysen H, Smith M. The natural history of periodontal disease in man. Study design and baseline data. J Periodont Res 1978;13:550-62.

133. Löe H, Ånerud A, Boysen H, Smith M. The natural history of periodontal disease in man: The rate of periodontal destruction before 40 years of age. J Periodontol 1978;49:607-20.

134. Löe H, Theilade E, Jensen SB. Experimental gingivitis in man. J Periodontol 1965;36:177-87.

135. Loos BG, Craandijk J, Hoek FJ, et al. Elevation of systemic markers related to cardiovascular diseases in the peripheral blood of periodontitis patients. J Periodontol 2000;71:1528-34.

136. Lundstrom A, Jendle J, Stenstrom B, et al. Periodontal conditions in 70-year-old women with osteoporosis. Swedish Dent J 2001;25:89-96.

137. Machtei EE, Christersson LA, Zambon JJ, et al. Alternative methods for screening periodontal disease in adults. J Clin Periodontol 1993;20:81-7.

138. Machtei EE, Dunford R, Hausmann E, et al. Longitudinal study of prognostic factors in established periodontitis patients. J Clin Periodontol 1997; 24:102-9.

139. Machtei EE, Hausmann E, Dunford R, et al. Longitudinal study of predictive factors for periodontal disease and tooth loss. J Clin Periodontol 1999;26:374-80.

140. Madianos PN, Lieff S, Murtha AP, et al. Maternal periodontitis and prematurity. Part II: Maternal infection and fetal exposure. Ann Periodontol 2001;6:175-82.

141. Mann J, Cormier PP, Green P, et al. Loss of periodontal attachment in adolescents. Community Dent Oral Epidemiol 1981;9:135-41.

142. Mark LL, Haffajee AD, Socransky SS, et al. Effect of the interleukin-1 genotype on monocyte IL-1 beta expression in subjects with adult periodontitis. J Periodont Res 2000;35:172-7.

143. Marmot M, Wilkinson RG, eds. Social determinants of health. New York: OUP, 1999.

144. Martinez-Canut P, Guarinos J, Bagan JV. Periodontal disease in HIV seropositive patients and its relation to lymphocyte subsets. J Periodontol 1996;67:33-6.

145. Matthesen M, Baelum V, Aarslev I, Fejerskov O. Dental health of children and adults in Guinea-Bissau, West Africa, in 1986. Community Dent Health 1990;7: 123-33.

146. Mattila KJ, Asikainen S, Wolf J, et al. Age, dental infections, and coronary heart disease. J Dent Res 2000;79: 756-60.

147. McDevitt MJ, Wang HY, Knobelman C, et al. Interleukin-1 genetic association with periodontitis in clinical practice. J Periodontol 2000;71:156-63.

148. McGuire MK, Nunn ME. Prognosis versus actual outcome. IV. The effectiveness of clinical parameters and IL-1 genotype in accurately predicting prognoses and tooth survival. J Periodontol 1999;70:49-56.

149. McKaig RG, Patton LL, Thomas JC, et al. Factors associated with periodontitis in an HIV-infected southeast USA study. Oral Dis 2000;6:158-65.

150. Meisel P, Siegemund A, Dombrowa S, et al. Smoking and polymorphisms of the interleukin-1 gene cluster (IL-1α, IL-1β, and IL-1RN) in patients with periodontal disease. J Periodontol 2002;73:27-32.

151. Meisel P, Timm R, Sawaf H, et al. Polymorphism of the N-acetyltransferase (NAT2), smoking and the potential risk of periodontal disease. Arch Toxicol 2000;74:343-8.

152. Merchant A, Pitiphat W, Douglass CW, et al. Oral hygiene practices and periodontitis in health care professionals. J Periodontol 2002;73:531-5.

153. Michalowicz BS, Diehl SR, Gunsolley JC, et al. Evidence of a substantial genetic basis for risk of adult periodontitis. J Periodontol 2000;71:1699-707.

154. Moore LV, Moore WE, Riley C, et al. Periodontal microflora of HIV-positive subjects with gingivitis or adult periodontitis. J Periodontol 1993;64:48-56.

155. Moore PA, Weyant RJ, Mongelluzzo MB, et al. Type 1 diabetes mellitus and oral health: Assessment of periodontal disease. J Periodontol 1999;70:409-17.

156. Moore WJ, Corbett ME. The distribution of dental caries in ancient British populations. II. Iron Age, Romano-British and mediaeval periods. Caries Res 1973;7:139-53.

157. Morrison HI, Ellison LF, Taylor GW. Periodontal disease and risk of fatal coronary heart and cerebrovascular diseases. J Cardiovasc Risk 1999;6:7-11.

158. Muller HP, Stadermann S, Heinecke A. Longitudinal association between plaque and gingival bleeding in smokers and non-smokers. J Clin Periodontol 2002; 29:287-94.

159. Murray PA, Grassi M, Winkler JR. The microbiology of HIV-associated periodontal lesions. J Clin Periodontol 1989;16:636-42.

160. Murray PA, Winkler JR, Peros WJ, et al. DNA probe detection of periodontal pathogens in HIV-associated periodontal lesions. Oral Microbiol Immunol 1991;6:34-40.

161. Myint M, Steinsvoll S, Yuan ZN, et al. Highly increased numbers of leukocytes in inflamed gingiva from patients with HIV infection. AIDS 2002;16:235-43.

162. Nelson RG, Shlossman M, Budding LM, et al. Periodontal disease and NIDDM in Pima Indians. Diabetes Care 1990;13:836-40.

163. Nevins M, Becker W, Kornman K, eds. Proceedings of the world workshop in clinical periodontics. Chicago: American Academy of Periodontology, 1990.

164. Noack B, Genco RJ, Trevisan M, et al. Periodontal infections contribute to elevated systemic C-reactive protein level. J Periodontol 2001;72:1221-7.

165. Norderyd O, Hugoson A, Grusovin G. Risk of severe periodontal disease in a Swedish adult population. A longitudinal study. J Clin Periodontol 1999;26: 608-15.

166. Offenbacher S, Collins JG, Yalda B, Haradon G. Role of prostaglandins in high-risk periodontitis patients. In: Genco RJ et al, eds: Molecular pathogenesis of periodontal disease. Washington DC: American Society for Microbiology, 1994.

167. Offenbacher S, Jared HL, O'Reilly PG, et al. Potential pathogenic mechanisms of periodontitis associated pregnancy complications. Ann Periodontol 1998;3: 233-50.

168. Offenbacher S, Katz V, Fertik G, et al. Periodontal infection as a possible risk factor for preterm low birth weight. J Periodontol 1996;67(Suppl):1103-13.

169. Offenbacher S, Lieff S, Boggess KA, et al. Maternal periodontitis and prematurity. Part I: Obstetric outcome of prematurity and growth restriction. Ann Periodontol 2001;6:164-74.

170. Okamoto H, Yoneyama T, Lindhe J, et al. Methods of evaluating periodontal disease data in epidemiological research. J Clin Periodontol 1988;15:430-9.

171. Oliver RC, Brown LJ, Löe H. Periodontal diseases in the United States population. J Periodontol 1998;69:269-78.

172. Oliver RC, Tervonen T. Diabetes—a risk factor for periodontitis in adults? J Periodontol 1994;65:530-8.

173. Oliver RC, Tervonen T, Flynn DG, Keenan KM. Enzyme activity in crevicular fluid in relation to metabolic control of diabetes and other periodontal risk factors. J Periodontol 1993;64:358-62.

174. Page RC. Milestones in periodontal research and the remaining critical issues. J Periodont Res 1999;34: 331-9.

175. Page RC. Current understanding of the aetiology and progression of periodontal disease. Int Dent J 1986;36:153-61.

176. Page RC. Gingivitis. J Clin Periodontol 1986;13: 345-59.

177. Page RC. The role of inflammatory mediators in the pathogenesis of periodontal disease. J Periodont Res 1991;26(3 Pt 2):230-42.

178. Page RC. Host response tests for diagnosing periodontal diseases. J Periodontol 1992;63(Suppl 4):356-66.

179. Page RC. Critical issues in periodontal research. J Dent Res 1995;74:1118-28.

180. Page RC, Offenbacher S, Schroeder HE, et al. Advances in the pathogenesis of periodontitis: Summary of developments, clinical implications and future directions. Periodontol 2000 1997;14:216-48.

181. Paidi S, Pack AR, Thomson WM. An example of measurement and reporting of periodontal loss of attachment (LOA) in epidemiological studies: Smoking and periodontal tissue destruction. N Z Dent J 1999; 95:118-23.

182. Papapanou PN, Baelum V, Luan WM, et al. Subgingival microbiota in adult Chinese: Prevalence and relation to periodontal disease progression. J Periodontol 1997;68:651-66.

183. Parkhill JM, Hennig BJ, Chapple IL, et al. Association of interleukin-1 gene polymorphisms with early-onset periodontitis. J Clin Periodontol 2000;27:682-9.

184. Payne JB, Zachs NR, Reinhardt RA, et al. The association between estrogen status and alveolar bone density changes in postmenopausal women with a history of periodontitis. J Periodontol 1997;68:24-31.

185. Peretz B, Machtei EE, Bimstein E. Changes in periodontal status of children and young adolescents: A one year longitudinal study. J Clin Pediatr Dent 1993;18:3-6.

186. Persson RE, Persson GR, Kiyak HA, Powell LV. Oral health and medical status in dentate low-income older persons. Spec Care Dentist 1998;18:70-7.

187. Pilot T, Barmes DE, Leclercq MH, et al. Periodontal conditions in adults, 35-44 years of age: An overview of CPITN data in the WHO Global Oral Data Bank. Community Dent Oral Epidemiol 1986;14:310-2.

188. Pilot T, Barmes DE, Leclercq MH, et al. Periodontal conditions in adolescents, 15-19 years of age: An overview of CPITN data in the WHO Global Oral Data Bank. Community Dent Oral Epidemiol 1987;15:336-38.

189. Preber H, Bergstrom J, Linder LE. Occurrence of periodontopathogens in smoker and non-smoker patients. J Clin Periodontol 1992;19:667-71.

190. Ramfjord SP, Emslie RD, Greene JC, et al. Epidemiological studies of periodontal disease. Am J Public Health 1968;58:1713-22.

191. Ramfjord SP, Kerr DA, Ash MM. World workshop in periodontics. Ann Arbor MI: University of Michigan Press, 1966.

192. Rams TE, Andriolo M Jr, Feik D, et al. Microbiological study of HIV-related periodontitis. J Periodontol 1991;62:74-81.

193. Reinhardt RA, Payne JB, Maze CA, et al. Influence of estrogen and osteopenia/osteoporosis on clinical periodontitis in postmenopausal women. J Periodontol 1999;70:823-8.

194. Riggio MP, Lennon A, Roy KM. Detection of *Prevotella intermedia* in subgingival plaque of adult periodontitis patients by polymerase chain reaction. J Periodont Res 1998;33:369-76.

195. Robinson P. Periodontal diseases and HIV infection. A review of the literature. J Clin Periodontol 1992;19:609-14.

196. Ronderos M, Jacobs DR, Himes JH, Pihlstrom BL. Associations of periodontal disease with femoral bone mineral density and estrogen replacement therapy: Cross-sectional evaluation of US adults from NHANES III. J Clin Periodontol 2000;27:778-86.

197. Russell AL. International nutrition surveys: A summary of preliminary dental findings. J Dent Res 1963;42:233-44.

198. Russell AL. Epidemiology of periodontal disease. Int Dent J 1967;17:282-96.

199. Russell AL, Leatherwood EC, Consolazio CF, Van Reen R. Periodontal disease and nutrition in South Vietnam. J Dent Res 1965;44:775-82.

200. Safkan-Seppala B, Ainamo J. Periodontal conditions in insulin-dependent diabetes mellitus. J Clin Periodontol 1992;19:24-9.

201. Sakellari D, Belibasakis G, Chadjipadelis T, et al. Supragingival and subgingival microbiota of adult patients with Down's syndrome. Changes after periodontal treatment. Oral Microbiol Immunol 2001;16:376-82.

202. Salvi GE, Beck JD, Offenbacher S. PGE2, IL-1 beta, and TNF-alpha responses in diabetics as modifiers of periodontal disease expression. Ann Periodontol 1998;3:40-50.

203. Sandholm L, Swanjung O, Rytomaa I, et al. Periodontal status of Finnish adolescents with insulin-dependent diabetes mellitus. J Clin Periodontol 1989;16:617-20.

204. Scully C, Porter SR, Mutlu S, et al. Periodontopathic bacteria in English HIV-seropositive persons. AIDS Patient Care STDS 1999;13:369-74.

205. Scheutz F, Matee MI, Andsager L, et al. Is there an association between periodontal condition and HIV infection? J Clin Periodontol 1997;24:580-7.

206. Schou L, Wight C. Does dental health education affect inequalities in dental health? Community Dent Health 1994;11:97-100.

207. Schoen DH, Murray PA, Nelson E, et al. A comparison of periodontal disease in HIV-infected children and household peers: A two year report. Pediatr Dent 2000;22:365-9.

208. Seppala B, Seppala M, Ainamo J. A longitudinal study on insulin-dependent diabetes mellitus and periodontal disease. J Clin Periodontol 1993;20:161-5.

209. Shlossman M, Knowler WC, Pettitt DJ, Genco RJ. Type 2 diabetes mellitus and periodontal disease. J Am Dent Assoc 1990;121:532-6.

210. Slade GD, Offenbacher S, Beck JD, et al. Acute-phase inflammatory response to periodontal disease in the US population. J Dent Res 2000;79:49-57.

211. Socransky SS, Haffajee AD, Goodson JM, Lindhe J. New concepts of destructive periodontal disease. J Clin Periodontol 1984;11:21-32.

212. Socransky SS, Haffajee AD, Smith C, Dibart S. Relation of counts of microbial species to clinical status at the sampled site. J Clin Periodontol 1991;18:766-75.

213. Soder B, Jin LJ, Wickholm S. Granulocyte elastase, matrix metalloproteinase-8 and prostaglandin E_2 in gingival crevicular fluid in matched clinical sites in smokers and non-smokers with persistent periodontitis. J Clin Periodontol 2002;29:384-91.

214. Stewart JE, Wager KA, Friedlander AH, Zadeh HH. The effect of periodontal treatment on glycemic control in patients with type 2 diabetes mellitus. J Clin Periodontol 2001;28:306-10.

215. Stoltenberg JL, Osborn JB, Pihlstrom BL, et al. Association between cigarette smoking, bacterial pathogens, and periodontal status. J Periodontol 1993;64:1225-30.

216. Swango PA, Kleinman DV, Konzelman JL. HIV and periodontal health. A study of military personnel with HIV. J Am Dent Assoc 1991;12:49-54.

217. Tappuni AR, Fleming GJ. The effect of antiretroviral therapy on the prevalence of oral manifestations in HIV-infected patients: A UK study. Oral Surg Oral Med Oral Pathol Oral Radiol Endod 2001;92:623-8.

218. Taylor GW. Bidirectional interrelationships between diabetes and periodontal diseases: An epidemiologic perspective. Ann Periodontol 2001;6:99-112.

219. Taylor GW. Exploring interrelationships between diabetes and periodontal disease in African Americans. Compend Contin Educ Dent 2001;22:42-8.

220. Taylor GW, Burt BA, Becker MP, et al. Glycemic control and alveolar bone loss progression in type 2 diabetes. Ann Periodontol 1998;3:30-9.

221. Tenenbaum H, Elkaim R, Cuisinier F, et al. Prevalence of six periodontal pathogens detected by DNA probe

method in HIV vs non-HIV periodontitis. Oral Dis 1997;3(Suppl 1):S153-S155.

222. Tervonen T, Oliver RC, Wolff LF, et al. Prevalence of periodontal pathogens with varying metabolic control of diabetes mellitus. J Clin Periodontol 1994; 21:375-9.

223. Tezal M, Wactawski-Wende J, Grossi SG, et al. The relationship between bone mineral density and periodontitis in postmenopausal women. J Periodontol 2000;71:1492-8.

224. Thomson WM, Edwards SJ, Dobson-Le DP, et al. IL-1 genotype and adult periodontitis among young New Zealanders. J Dent Res 2001;80:1700-3.

225. Thomson WM, Locker D. Dental neglect and dental health among 26-year-olds in the Dunedin Multidisciplinary Health and Development Study. Community Dent Oral Epidemiol 2000;28:414-8.

226. Thorstensson H, Hugoson A. Periodontal disease experience in adult long-duration insulin-dependent diabetics. J Clin Periodontol 1993;20:352-8.

227. Timmerman MF, van der Weijden GA, Abbas F, et al. Untreated periodontal disease in Indonesian adolescents. Longitudinal clinical data and prospective clinical and microbiological risk assessment. J Clin Periodontol 2000;27:932-42.

228. Tomar SL, Swango PA, Kleinman DV, Burt BA. Loss of periodontal attachment in HIV-seropositive military personnel. J Periodontol 1995;66:421-8.

229. Tonetti MS, Muller-Campanile V, Lang NP. Changes in the prevalence of residual pockets and tooth loss in treated periodontal patients during a supportive maintenance care program. J Clin Periodontol 1998;25:1008-16.

230. Tran SD, Rudney JD, Sparks BS, Hodges JS. Persistent presence of *Bacteroides forsythus* as a risk factor for attachment loss in a population with low prevalence and severity of adult periodontitis. J Periodontol 2001;72:1-10.

231. Tsai C, Hayes C, Taylor GW. Glycemic control of type 2 diabetes and severe periodontal disease in the US adult population. Community Dent Oral Epidemiol 2002;30:182-92.

232. Tsang CS, Samaranayake LP. Predominant cultivable subgingival microbiota of healthy and HIV-infected ethnic Chinese. APMIS 2001;109:117-26.

233. US Department of Health and Human Services, National Center for Health Statistics. Third National Health and Nutrition Examination Survey, 1988-94. Public Use Data File No. 7-0627. Hyattsville MD: Centers for Disease Control and Prevention, 1997.

234. US Public Health Service, National Center for Health Statistics. Periodontal disease in adults, United States, 1960-62. PHS Publication No. 1000, Series 11 No. 12. Washington DC: Government Printing Office, 1965.

235. US Public Health Service, National Center for Health Statistics. Periodontal disease and oral hygiene among children, United States. DHEW Publication No. (HSM) 72-1060, Series 11 No. 117. Washington DC: Government Printing Office, 1972.

236. US Public Health Service, National Center for Health Statistics. Basic data on dental examination findings of persons 1-74 years, United States, 1971-1974. DHEW Publication No. (PHS) 79-1662, Series 11 No. 214. Washington DC: Government Printing Office, 1979.

237. US Public Health Service, National Institute of Dental Research. Oral health survey of United States adults; national findings. NIH Publication No. 87-2868. Washington DC: Government Printing Office, 1987.

238. Van der Velden U. Effect of age on the periodontium. J Clin Periodontol 1984;11:281-94.

239. Van der Velden U, Abbas F, Van Steenbergen TJ, et al. Prevalence of periodontal breakdown in adolescents and presence of *Actinobacillus actinomycetemcomitans* in subjects with attachment loss. J Periodontol 1989;60: 604-10.

240. van der Weijden GA, de Slegte C, Timmerman MF, van der Velden U. Periodontitis in smokers and non-smokers: Intra-oral distribution of pockets. J Clin Periodontol 2001;28:955-60.

241. van Winkelhoff AJ, Bosch-Tijhof CJ, Winkel EG, van der Reijden WA. Smoking affects the subgingival microflora in periodontitis. J Periodontol 2001;72:666-71.

242. von Wowern N, Westergaard J, Kollerup G. Bone mineral content and bone metabolism in young adults with severe periodontitis. J Clin Periodontol 2001;28:583-8.

243. Waerhaug J. Epidemiology of periodontal disease: A review of literature. In: Ramfjord SP, Kerr DA, Ash MM, eds: World workshop in periodontics. Ann Arbor MI: University of Michigan, 1966:181-271.

244. Wennstrom J, Dahlen G, Svensson J, Nyman S. *Actinobacillus actinomycetemcomitans, Bacteroides gingivalis,* and *Bacteroides intermedius:* Predictors of attachment loss? Oral Microbial Immunol 1987;2: 158-63.

245. Weyant RJ, Pearlstein ME, Churak AP, et al. The association between osteopenia and periodontal attachment loss in older women. J Periodontol 1999;70: 982-91.

246. Williams CE, Davenport ES, Sterne JA, et al. Mechanisms of risk in preterm low-birthweight infants. Periodontol 2000 2000;223:142-50.

247. Winkler JR, Grassi M, Murray PA. Clinical description and etiology of HIV-associated periodontal diseases. In: Robertson PB, Greenspan JS, eds: Perspectives on oral manifestations of AIDS. Littleton MA: PSG Publishing, 1988:49-70.

248. Winkler JR, Robertson PB. Periodontal disease associated with HIV infection. Oral Surg Oral Med Oral Pathol 1992;73:145-50.

249. Wolfson SM, Lewis MH. A survey of periodontal conditions in Saskatchewan adolescents. J Can Dent Assoc 1985;51:486-9.

250. World Health Organization. Periodontal disease. Technical Report Series No. 207. Geneva: WHO, 1961.

251. Ximenez-Fyvie LA, Haffajee AD, Socransky SS. Comparison of the microbiota of supra- and subgingival plaque in health and periodontitis. J Clin Periodontol 2000;27:648-57.

252. Yang MC, Marks RG, Clark WB, Magnusson I. Predictive power of various models for longitudinal

attachment level change. J Clin Periodontol 1992;19:77-83.

253. Yeung SC, Stewart GJ, Cooper DA, Sindhusake D. Progression of periodontal disease in HIV seropositive patients. J Periodontol 1993;64:651-7.

254. Yuan K, Chang CJ, Hsu PC, et al. Detection of putative periodontal pathogens in non-insulin-dependent diabetes mellitus and non-diabetes mellitus by polymerase chain reaction. J Dent Res 2001;36:18-24.

22 Dental Fluorosis

Dental fluorosis is a permanent hypomineralization of enamel that is characterized by greater surface and subsurface porosity than in normal enamel and that results from exposure of the immature tooth to excess fluoride (F) during developmental stages. Preeruptive enamel maturation consists of an increase in mineralization within the developing tooth and a concurrent loss of early-secreted matrix proteins. Excess F available to the enamel during maturation disrupts mineralization and results in excessive retention of enamel proteins.[5] Fluorosis is thought to result from the unerupted tooth's constant exposure to elevated plasma F concentrations rather than from periodic spikes in F concentration.[69] Although sufficiently high F concentrations might affect enamel at all developmental stages,[15] early preeruptive maturation appears to be the time when enamel is most sensitive to the effects of F, both in animals[16,53] and in humans.[19] Elegantly designed human studies have suggested that this critical period for the development of fluorosis in the human maxillary permanent central incisor begins around the age of 22 months and extends for periods of up to several years after that for later-developing teeth.[19]

In its mildest forms, fluorosis appears as barely discernible fine, lacy markings that follow the perikymata across the width of the enamel surface. At this very mild level, fluorosis can be detected only by an experienced dental examiner. At the opposite extreme, the most severe forms of fluorosis manifest as heavily stained, pitted, and friable enamel that can result in loss of dental function. Fluorosis is a dose-response condition; gradations between these two extremes range from more obvious white, lacy markings to a nontranslucent white coloration of the whole enamel surface. The brown stain that often accompanies moderate fluorosis is a posteruptive feature that results when certain dietary ingredients are picked up by proteins in the porous outer enamel[21]; it is seen only when porous enamel has formed prior to eruption.

Fluorosed surface enamel contains higher F concentrations than does unaffected enamel, and the F enamel content increases with the severity of the condition.[52] Teeth that mineralize later in life generally show more severe fluorotic disturbances than do those that mineralize earlier.[3,35-37] Fluorosis is less common in the primary than in the permanent dentition, although fluorosis of the primary teeth does occur.[66,67] It is common in the primary dentition in high-F areas of the world, such as East Africa.[34,45,46,62]

Because dental fluorosis is a dose-response condition, the higher the F intake during the critical period of tooth development, the more severe the fluorosis.[14,17,35] The threshold, if indeed there is one, is low: 0.03-0.1 mg F/kg body weight has been suggested as the borderline zone,[22] at least for European children. Because that range encompasses the so-called optimum intake range of 0.05-0.07 mg F/kg body weight per day (Chapter 24), it is not clear whether other factors (e.g., nutrition) lead to these differences in estimates or whether they merely reflect biologic variation. Studies in Kenya have found fluorosis with average intakes as low as 0.04 mg F/kg body weight.[3] Certainly a range of fluorosis severity is seen among individuals who appear to have similar exposures to F.

In those parts of the world where severe fluorosis is endemic, such as some regions of Africa, the condition can be seen when F levels in drinking water are low,[18] so that other, unknown exposure sources must be present. In other cases it occurs with ingestion of certain foods known to be high in F.[70] Studies in such localities have increased our understanding of fluorosis, but the living conditions in those areas differ greatly from those in the United States and other high-income countries.

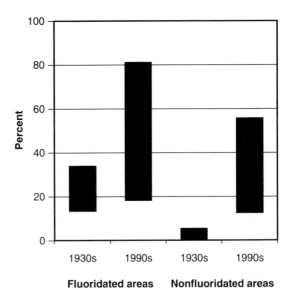

Fig. 22-1 Increase in dental fluorosis prevalence in North America since initial studies in the 1930s. The bars represent the prevalence ranges reported in Dean's studies and in those after 1990.[12,14]

PREVALENCE OF FLUOROSIS IN THE UNITED STATES

Fluorosis in the United States was first mapped by Dean during his classic studies of the 1930s and early 1940s. These studies are discussed in Chapter 24; they are an integral part of the story of how fluorosis and caries experience were first associated with F concentrations in drinking water.

One part of the United States that received a lot of attention from Dean was northern Illinois, where there is an extensive belt of naturally fluoridated drinking water. Seven of these communities, with water naturally fluoridated to varying degrees, were revisited by researchers from the National Institute of Dental and Craniofacial Research (NIDCR) in 1980, in 1985,[27] and again in 1990.[56] Relating age to fluorosis and tooth calcification, the NIDCR team concluded that F intake had increased during 1970-77 but had not increased subsequently. The 1990 follow-up found that the rise in age-standardized fluorosis prevalence observed in the optimally fluoridated areas over 1980-85 did not continue during 1985-90. At above-optimum water F concentrations, fluorosis either remained stable or showed no sustained increase over the decade between 1980 and 1990.

Although there are difficulties in comparing data obtained 60 years apart, it is clear that the prevalence of dental fluorosis in the United States has increased since the time of Dean.[12,60] Prevalence among children was reported to be 22.3% in the 1986-87 National Survey of Dental Caries in U.S. School Children, ranging by age from 18.5% of 17-year-olds to 25.8% of 9-year-olds.[7] This higher prevalence in the younger children hints that prevalence might still be increasing. Almost all of the fluorosis recorded in the 1986-87 survey was mild or very mild. Although there is little firm evidence, a slight increase in fluorosis severity may have accompanied the large increase in prevalence.[63]

The largest relative increase in fluorosis since Dean's time has been seen in nonfluorided areas (Fig. 22-1), which suggests that the F exposure from sources other than drinking water is driving the increase in fluorosis prevalence.

RISK FACTORS FOR DENTAL FLUOROSIS

Because fluorosis is a disturbance of enamel due to excessive F intake during the developmental period, risk factors are related to the ingestion and absorption of F at the critical periods of preeruptive tooth development. Age is a demographic risk factor in that fluorosis can only occur with preeruptive F exposure. There is no evidence for racial or ethnic differences, and socioeconomic status (SES) is a demographic risk factor only to the extent that F exposure from toothpaste and infant formula may vary by SES. There is no reason to believe that the use of F mouthrinses and the presence of professionally applied gels and varnishes are risk factors for fluorosis, although obviously the protocols for application of these products must be designed to minimize ingestion.

Fluoridated Drinking Water

Drinking fluoridated water is a minor risk factor for fluorosis. It was documented long ago that in the United States, even at around 1.0 parts per million (ppm) F, 7%-16% of children born and reared in areas with fluoridated water exhibit mild or very mild dental fluorosis in the permanent dentition.[1,14,55] This degree of prevalence was recorded at a time when drinking water was virtually the only source of exposure to F, and prevalence has risen relatively more in the nonfluoridated areas since then.[33,56] Even small changes in F concentrations in drinking water can lead to considerable change in fluorosis prevalence.[20,61]

Fluoride Dietary Supplements

F dietary supplements, in the form of tablets, drops, or F-vitamin combinations, have been used for years in nonfluoridated areas to prevent caries (see Chapter 26). Regardless of the role of F supplements in preventing caries, there is strong evidence that supplements are a risk factor for mild to moderate fluorosis. Case-control studies in nonfluoridated areas of New England found that exposure to F supplements during the first 6 years of life, together with higher SES, significantly increased the risk of developing fluorosis.[48,50] Later research, as would be expected, found the risk to be extremely high when supplements are used (inappropriately) in fluoridated areas.[49] Other studies have demonstrated the link between use of supplements and fluorosis risk,[2,32,34,51] and F supplementation was later confirmed as a risk factor for fluorosis in a comprehensive systematic review.[29] It was this evidence that led the American Dental Association in 1994 to reduce

the recommended F supplement dosage for caries prevention in children (see Chapter 26).

Early Use Of Fluoride Toothpaste

Young children in whom the swallowing reflex is not yet fully developed can ingest up to 0.3-0.5 g of toothpaste (0.3-0.5 mg F) at each brushing.[4,6,25] These findings naturally raise the issue of whether overzealous use of F toothpaste in young children is a risk factor for fluorosis. One study of a Toronto area with fluoridated water found that early use of F toothpaste (before 2 years of age) and prolonged use of infant formula produced with fluoridated water were strong risk factors for the later development of fluorosis.[47] Although most of the fluorosis seen in that Toronto study was very mild, later studies were able to confirm a clear risk of fluorosis with early use of F toothpaste.[*] The risk from early use of F toothpaste, however, was usually not as high as that seen with F supplements.

Infant Formula

Use of infant formula has been recognized as a risk factor for fluorosis, both because of its own F content and especially because it may be mixed with fluoridated water.[47,49] Soy-based formulas contain higher F concentrations than do milk-based formulas.[30,41]

DENTAL FLUOROSIS AND CARIES

Dean's studies in the 1930s and 1940s found that caries experience dropped sharply as the F concentration of drinking water rose from negligible to 1.0 ppm and that it tended to level off after that (see Chapter 24). But when F concentration reaches a point at which severe fluorosis is common and the enamel of affected individuals becomes friable and liable to fracture, caries experience has been observed to increase.[23] This phenomenon was demonstrated in the United States by the NIDCR studies in the seven communities in northern Illinois in 1980, 1985, and 1990 described earlier.[56] The results of the caries examinations in relation to several F concentrations in drinking water are shown in Fig. 22-2. Data for each year describe a u-shaped curve: with increasing F levels, caries experience diminishes to a cer-

---

*References 32,34,40,42,49,54,57.

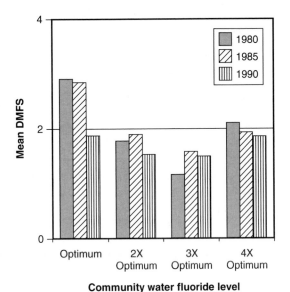

Fig. 22-2 Decayed, missing, and filled tooth surfaces (DMFS) in children in seven Illinois communities by level of fluoride in the drinking water in 1980, 1985, and 1990. Data are age-adjusted for comparability.[56]

tain point and then starts to rise again. Dean showed that caries experience in the 1930s continued to drop for water F levels at least as high as 2.6 ppm;[13] unfortunately he did not publish caries data from the communities with higher water F levels he studied earlier in his career.

Fig. 22-3 shows the relation between caries experience and water F levels, age standardized and restricted to data for permanent residents, among participants ages 5-17 in the 1986-87 National Survey of Dental Caries in U.S. Schoolchildren. It makes an interesting comparison with the corresponding data from Dean's studies (see Fig. 24-1); the absolute caries levels are much lower in Fig. 22-3, and there is a less pronounced association between caries and water F levels. These two factors together indicate the importance of F exposure from sources other than drinking water that has taken place since Dean's time. Fig. 22-4 shows fluorosis prevalence data from the same national survey, and here fluorosis seems to fall into three groups: the lowest prevalence from 0 to 0.5 ppm F, a plateau from 0.6 to 1.2 ppm F, and the highest prevalence at 1.3 ppm F and above.

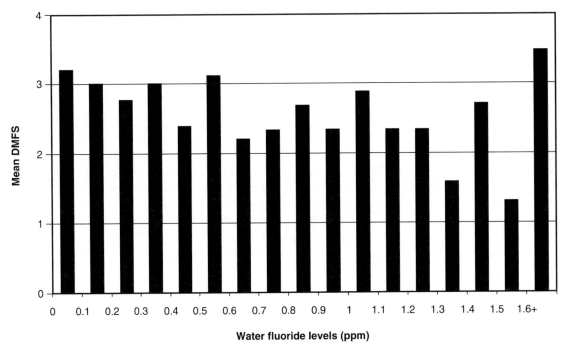

Fig. 22-3 Decayed, missing, and filled tooth surfaces (DMFS) in children ages 5-17 by fluoride level in the drinking water. Age-adjusted data for permanent residents from the 1986-87 National Survey of Dental Caries in U.S. Schoolchildren.[28]

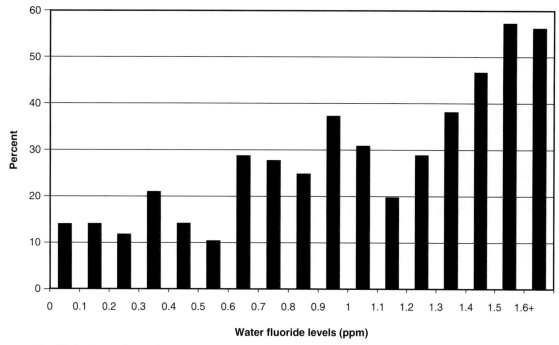

Fig. 22-4 Fluorosis prevalence among children ages 7-17 years by fluoride level in the drinking water. Age-adjusted data for permanent residents from the 1986-87 National Survey of Dental Caries in U.S. Schoolchildren.[28]

Caries could increase with higher F levels in drinking water either because restorative treatment is sought for fluorosed enamel or because pitted and friable enamel is diagnosed as caries. Although friable enamel can certainly lead to loss of function and require dental restoration, it is not caries. However, it is possible that broken enamel makes a tooth more vulnerable to caries. Whatever the link, severe fluorosis is obviously a condition to be avoided.

DENTAL FLUOROSIS AS A PUBLIC HEALTH PROBLEM

At what point does dental fluorosis become a public health problem? There is no reason to call it such in a community where it is found only in its mildest forms, even in U.S. communities where prevalence is around 50% in children. On the other hand, its high prevalence and severity make it a public health problem in the countries of East Africa[9,38,39,44,46,65,68] and in parts of India.[8,59] It is an urgent problem in those regions of Ethiopia and India where skeletal fluorosis, which can be a debilitating condition, is found.[24,31]

The relatively greater increase in fluorosis prevalence in nonfluoridated communities, compared to fluoridated areas (see Fig. 22-1), must be attributable largely to an increase in F ingestion from sources other than drinking water. The risk of fluorosis from dental products, notably toothpaste and F supplements, was described earlier, and F ingestion can be higher than expected from soft drinks and fruit juices processed with fluoridated water. For most people, drinking water is now just one of numerous exposures to F.

Dental fluorosis cannot be classed as a public health problem in the United States and other countries where controlled water fluoridation is extensive. It would be a mistake, however, to assume that it cannot become so. There is evidence from several parts of the world that people are quite aware of even the milder forms of fluorosis in their teeth.[10,11,26,43,54,58] If high-F toothpastes become widely marketed, and if the esthetic standards of the public regarding fluorosis become more stringent, then dental and public health authorities could be faced with demands to do something about it. This could include restricting exposure to F, so that possibility is best avoided by prudent use of F now. The U.S. Public Health Service recommendations[64] on use of F are a good place to start.

REFERENCES

1. Ast DB, Smith DJ, Wachs B, Cantwell KT. The Newburgh-Kingston caries-fluorine study. XIV. Combined clinical and roentgenographic dental findings after ten years of fluoride experience. J Am Dent Assoc 1956;52:314-25.
2. Awad MA, Hargreaves JA, Thompson GW. Dental caries and fluorosis in 7-9 and 11-14 year old children who received fluoride supplements from birth. J Can Dent Assoc 1994;60:318-22.
3. Baelum V, Fejerskov O, Manji F, Larsen MJ. Daily dose of fluoride and dental fluorosis. Tandlaegebladet 1987;91:452-6.
4. Barnhart WE, Hiller LK, Leonard GJ, Michaels SE. Dentifrice usage and ingestion among four age groups. J Dent Res 1974;53:1317-22.
5. Bawden JW, Crenshaw MA, Wright JT, LeGeros RZ. Concise review: Consideration of possible biologic mechanisms of fluorosis. J Dent Res 1995;74:1349-52.
6. Baxter PM. Toothpaste ingestion during toothbrushing by school children. Br Dent J 1980;148:125-8.
7. Brunelle JA. The prevalence of dental fluorosis in U.S. children, 1987 [abstract]. J Dent Res 1989;68(Spec Issue):995.
8. Chandra S, Sharma R, Thergaonkar VP, Chaturvedi SK. Determination of optimal fluoride concentration in drinking water in an area in India with dental fluorosis. Community Dent Oral Epidemiol 1980;8:92-6.
9. Chibole O. Epidemiology of dental fluorosis in Kenya. J R Soc Health 1987;107:242-3.
10. Chikte UM, Louw AJ, Stander I. Perceptions of fluorosis in northern Cape communities. S Afr Dent J 2001; 56:528-32.
11. Clark DC. Evaluation of aesthetics for the different classifications of the Tooth Surface Index of Fluorosis. Community Dent Oral Epidemiol 1995;23:80-3.
12. Clark DC. Trends in the prevalence of dental fluorosis in North America. Community Dent Oral Epidemiol 1994;22:148-52.
13. Dean HT. Endemic fluorosis and its relation to dental caries. Public Health Rep 1938;53:1443-52.
14. Dean HT. The investigation of physiological effects by the epidemiological method. In: Moulton FR, ed: Fluorine and dental health. Washington DC: American Association for the Advancement of Science, 1942: 23-31.
15. Den Besten PK, Crenshaw MA. Studies on the changes in developing enamel caused by ingestion of high levels of fluoride in the rat. Adv Dent Res 1987;1:176-80.
16. Den Besten PK, Thariani H. Biological mechanisms of fluorosis and level and timing of systemic exposure to fluoride with respect to fluorosis. J Dent Res 1992; 71:1238-43.
17. Eklund SA, Burt BA, Ismail AI, Calderone JJ. High-fluoride drinking water, fluorosis, and dental caries in adults. J Am Dent Assoc 1987;114:324-8.
18. El-Nadeef MA, Honkala E. Fluorosis in relation to fluoride levels in water in central Nigeria. Community Dent Oral Epidemiol 1998;26:26-30.
19. Evans RW, Stamm JW. An epidemiologic estimate of the critical period during which maxillary central incisors are most susceptible to fluorosis. J Public Health Dent 1991;51:251-9.
20. Evans RW, Stamm JW. Dental fluorosis following downward adjustment of drinking water. J Public Health Dent 1991;51:91-8.
21. Fejerskov O, Manji F, Baelum V, Møller IJ. Dental fluorosis—a handbook for health workers. Copenhagen: Munksgaard, 1988.
22. Fejerskov O, Stephen KW, Richards A, Speirs R. Combined effect of systemic and topical fluoride treatments on human deciduous teeth—case studies. Caries Res 1987;21:452-9.
23. Grobler SR, van Wyk CW, Kotze D. Relationship between enamel fluoride levels, degree of fluorosis and caries experience in communities with a nearly optimal and a high fluoride level in the drinking water. Caries Res 1986;20:284-8.
24. Haimanot RT, Fekadu A, Bushra B. Endemic fluorosis in the Ethiopian Rift Valley. Trop Geogr Med 1987;39: 209-17.
25. Hargreaves JA, Ingram GS, Wagg BJ. A gravimetric study of the ingestion of toothpaste by children. Caries Res 1972;6:236-43.
26. Hawley GM, Ellwood RP, Davies RM. Dental caries, fluorosis and the cosmetic implications of different TF scores in 14-year-old adolescents. Community Dent Health 1996;13:189-92.
27. Heifetz SB, Driscoll WS, Horowitz HS, Kingman A. Prevalence of dental caries and dental fluorosis in areas with optimal and above-optimal water-fluoride concentrations: A 5-year follow-up survey. J Am Dent Assoc 1988;116:490-5.
28. Heller KE, Eklund SA, Burt BA. Dental caries and dental fluorosis at varying water fluoride concentrations. J Public Health Dent 1997;57:136-43.
29. Ismail AI, Bandekar RR. Fluoride supplements and fluorosis: A meta-analysis. Community Dent Oral Epidemiol 1999;27:48-56.
30. Johnson J Jr, Bawden JW. The fluoride content of infant formulas available in 1985. Pediatr Dent 1987; 9:33-7.
31. Jolly SS, Singh BM, Mathur OC, Malhotra KC. Epidemiological, clinical, and biochemical study of endemic dental and skeletal fluorosis in Punjab. Br Med J 1968;4:427-9.
32. Kumar JV, Swango PA. Fluoride exposure and dental fluorosis in Newburgh and Kingston, New York: Policy implications. Community Dent Oral Epidemiol 1999;27:171-80.
33. Kumar J, Swango P, Lininger LL, et al. Intra-oral distribution of dental fluorosis in Newburgh and Kingston, New York. Am J Public Health 1998;88:1866-70.
34. Lalumandier JA, Rozier RG. The prevalence and risk factors of fluorosis among patients in a pediatric dental practice. Pediatr Dent 1995;17:19-25.
35. Larsen MJ, Kirkegaard E, Poulsen S. Patterns of dental fluorosis in a European country in relation to the

fluoride concentration of drinking water. J Dent Res 1987;66:10-2.

36. Larsen MJ, Richards A, Fejerskov O. Development of dental fluorosis according to age at start of fluoride administration. Caries Res 1985;19:519-27.

37. Larsen MJ, Senderovitz F, Kirkegaard E, et al. Dental fluorosis in the primary and the permanent dentition in fluoridated areas with consumption of either powdered milk or natural cow's milk. J Dent Res 1988;67:822-5.

38. Manji F, Baelum V, Fejerskov O. Dental fluorosis in an area of Kenya with 2 ppm fluoride in the drinking water. J Dent Res 1986;65:659-62.

39. Manji F, Kapila S. Fluorides and fluorosis in Kenya. Part III: Fluorides, fluorosis and dental caries. Odontostomatol Trop 1986;9:135-9.

40. Mascarenhas AK, Burt BA. Fluorosis risk from early exposure to fluoridated toothpaste. Community Dent Oral Epidemiol 1998;26:241-8.

41. McKnight-Hanes MC, Leverett DH, Adair SM, Shields CP. Fluoride content of infant formulas: Soy-based formulas as a potential factor in dental fluorosis. Pediatr Dent 1988;10:189-94.

42. Milsom K, Mitropolous CM. Enamel defects in 8-year-old children in fluoridated and non-fluoridated parts of Cheshire. Caries Res 1990;24:286-9.

43. Milsom KM, Tickle M, Jenner A, Peers A. A comparison of normative and subjective assessment of the child prevalence of developmental defects of enamel amongst 12-year-olds living in the North West Region, UK. Public Health 2000;114:340-4.

44. Møller IJ, Pindborg JJ, Gedalia I, Roed-Petersen B. The prevalence of dental fluorosis in the people of Uganda. Arch Oral Biol 1970;15:213-25.

45. Nair KR, Manji F. Endemic fluorosis in deciduous dentition. A study of 1276 children in typically high fluoride area (Kiambu) in Kenya. Odontostomatol Trop 1982;5:177-84.

46. Olsson B. Dental findings in high-fluoride areas in Ethiopia. Community Dent Oral Epidemiol 1979;7:51-6.

47. Osuji OO, Leake JL, Chipman ML, et al. Risk factors for dental fluorosis in a fluoridated community. J Dent Res 1988;67:1488-92.

48. Pendrys DG, Katz RV. Risk of enamel fluorosis associated with fluoride supplementation, infant formula, and fluoride dentifrice use. Am J Epidemiol 1989;130:1199-208.

49. Pendrys DG, Katz RV, Morse DE. Risk factors for enamel fluorosis in a fluoridated population. Am J Epidemiol 1994;140:461-71.

50. Pendrys DG, Katz RV, Morse DE. Risk factors for enamel fluorosis in a nonfluoridated population. Am J Epidemiol 1996;143:808-15.

51. Pendrys DG, Stamm JW. Relationship of total fluoride intake to beneficial effects and enamel fluorosis. J Dent Res 1990;69(Spec Issue):529-38.

52. Richards A, Fejerskov O, Baelum V. Enamel fluoride in relation to severity of human dental fluorosis. Adv Dent Res 1989;3:147-53.

53. Richards A, Kragstrup J, Josephsen K, Fejerskov O. Dental fluorosis developed in post-secretory enamel. J Dent Res 1986;65:1406-9.

54. Riordan PJ. Perceptions of dental fluorosis. J Dent Res 1993;72:1268-74.

55. Russell AL. Dental fluorosis in Grand Rapids during the seventeenth year of fluoridation. J Am Dent Assoc 1962;65:608-12.

56. Selwitz RH, Nowjack-Raymer RE, Kingman A, Driscoll WS. Prevalence of dental caries and dental fluorosis in areas with optimal and above-optimal water fluoride concentrations: A 10-year follow-up survey. J Public Health Dent 1995;55:85-93.

57. Skotowski MC, Hunt RJ, Levy SM. Risk factors for dental fluorosis in pediatric dental patients. J Public Health Dent 1995;55:154-9.

58. Stephen KW, Macpherson LM, Gilmour WH, et al. A blind caries and fluorosis prevalence study of school-children in naturally fluoridated and nonfluoridated townships of Morayshire, Scotland. Community Dent Oral Epidemiol 2002;30:70-9.

59. Subbareddy VV, Tewari A. Enamel mottling at different levels of fluoride in drinking water in an endemic area. J Indian Dent Assoc 1985;57:205-12.

60. Szpunar SM, Burt BA. Trends in the prevalence of dental fluorosis in the United States: A review. J Public Health Dent 1987;47:71-9.

61. Szpunar SM, Burt BA. Dental caries, fluorosis, and fluoride exposure in Michigan schoolchildren. J Dent Res 1988;67:802-6.

62. Thylstrup A. Distribution of dental fluorosis in the primary dentition. Community Dent Oral Epidemiol 1978;6:329-37.

63. US Public Health Service, Ad Hoc Subcommittee on Fluoride. Review of fluoride benefits and risks. Washington DC: Government Printing Office, 1991.

64. US Public Health Service, Centers for Disease Control and Prevention. Recommendations for using fluoride to prevent and control dental caries in the United States. MMWR 2001;50(RR-14):1-42.

65. Walvekar SV, Qureshi BA. Endemic fluorosis and partial defluoridation of water supplies—a public health concern in Kenya. Community Dent Oral Epidemiol 1982;10:156-60.

66. Warren JJ, Levy SM, Kanellis MJ. Prevalence of dental fluorosis in the primary dentition. J Public Health Dent 2001;61:87-91.

67. Weeks KJ, Milsom KM, Lennon MA. Enamel defects in 4- to 5-year old children in fluoridated and non-fluoridated parts of Cheshire, UK. Caries Res 1993;27:317-20.

68. Wenzel A, Thylstrup A, Melsen B, Fejerskov O. The relationship between water-borne fluoride, dental fluorosis and skeletal development in 11-15 year old Tanzanian girls. Arch Oral Biol 1982;27:1007-11.

69. Whitford G. Determinants and mechanisms of enamel fluorosis. Ciba Foundation Symposium No. 205. New York: Wiley, 1997:226-45.

70. Yoder KM, Mabelya L, Robison VA, et al. Severe dental fluorosis in a Tanzanian population consuming water with negligible fluoride concentration. Community Dent Oral Epidemiol 1998;26:382-3.

Oral Cancer and Other Oral Conditions

ORAL CANCER
  Occurrence and Distribution
  Risk Factors
  Dental Professionals and Oral Cancer

OTHER SOFT TISSUE LESIONS
CLEFT LIP AND PALATE
MALOCCLUSION
TEMPOROMANDIBULAR JOINT DISORDERS

With the decline in dental caries among children and the understanding that severe periodontal diseases are not as common as once thought, dental professionals are in a position to spend more time on the diagnosis and treatment of conditions that traditionally have not occupied much time in the dental office. This chapter looks at the distribution of some of these conditions and at the risk factors and risk indicators associated with them.

ORAL CANCER

Occurrence and Distribution

Of all conditions that dental professionals see and treat, oral cancer is the one that literally has life and death implications. Age-adjusted oral cancer mortality rates among males in the United States have shown a long-term reduction, most notably since the mid-1980s (Fig. 23-1). Mortality rates among American females, which have always been low, have shown only slight reduction over the 24-year period covered in Fig. 23-1.

The term *oral cancer* includes disease category numbers 140-149 of the International Classification of Diseases, ninth revision, known as ICD-9.[33] This group includes cancers of the lip, tongue, buccal mucosa, floor of the mouth, salivary glands, and pharynx. It does not include throat cancer. The occurrence of oral cancer and its site distribution within the mouth varies widely in different parts of the world,[61,65] presumably because of the environ-

mental factors with which these cancers are associated. Squamous cell carcinomas of the oral mucosa, tongue, and lip comprise 80% of all oral cancers on a global basis.[34]

In 2004 there were approximately 28,300 new oral cancer cases in the United States and some 7200 deaths from oral cancer. Table 23-1 shows the extent of oral cancer in the United States and compares incidence data for 2004 with that for 1988. There were more new cancers of all kinds in 2004 than in 1988, but the number of new oral cancers had actually dropped. As shown in the table, cancers of the oral cavity constituted some 2.1% of all new cases reported in 2004, down from 3.1% in 1988. Mortality from oral cancer has also dropped, both in absolute numbers and proportionately, and accounted for 1.3% of all cancer deaths in 2004. The proportionate drop in mortality rates is attributable both to the slight drop in absolute numbers of oral cancers and to the absolute increase in mortality from other types of cancer.

Although these overall trends in the United States are moving in the right direction, oral cancer remains twice as prevalent in males as in females (see Table 23-1), and annual incidence among males in 1992-99 remained more than twice the rate seen in females (Fig. 23-2). Twice as many deaths from oral cancer occur in males as in females. Some differences between the races are seen in the specific sites within the oral cavity in which oral cancer is found (Table 23-2), and there are no obvious explanations for these differences.

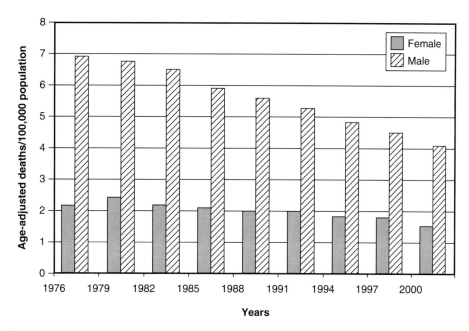

Fig. 23-1   Age-adjusted mortality from oral cancer per 100,000 population for males and females in the United States, selected years 1976-2000.[84]

Table 23-1   New cancer cases and deaths, by gender, for all cancers and for oral cancers, United States, 1988 and estimated for 2004[2,76]

Site	Year	Total	Males	Females
New Cases (Incidence)				
All cancers (thousands)	1988	985	495	490
	2004	1368	700	668
Oral cancers (thousands)	1988	30.2	20.5	9.7
	2004	28.3	18.6	9.7
Oral cancers as percentage of all cancers	1988	3.1	4.1	2.0
	2004	2.1	2.7	1.5
Deaths				
All cancers (thousands)	1988	494	263	231
	2004	564	291	273
Oral cancers (thousands)	1988	9.1	6.0	3.1
	2004	7.2	4.8	2.4
Oral cancer deaths as percentage of all cancer deaths	1988	1.8	2.3	1.3
	2004	1.3	1.6	0.9

Oral cancer is closely related to older age (Fig. 23-3), and peak age for mortality from oral cancer comes earlier for African-Americans than it does for whites. Overall annual mortality among African-Americans in the 1988-92 period was 5.2 per 100,000, nearly double the rate of 2.7 in whites.[82] However, by 2000, mortality among African-Americans had dropped to 4.1 per 100,000 and mortality among whites to 2.5 per 100,000.[85] Mortality is most likely related to low

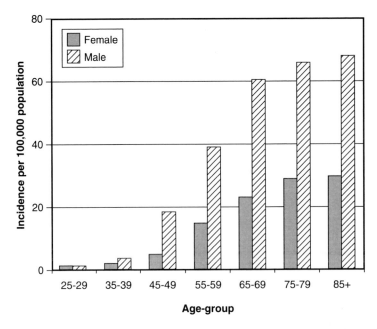

Fig. 23-2 Annual incidence of oral cancer per 100,000 population by age and gender in the United States, 1996-2000.[85]

Table 23-2 Site of occurrence of oral cancer for estimated new cases per 100,000 population, for all races, whites, African-Americans, and Asians/Pacific Islanders, United States, 2000[85]

Primary Site	All Races	Whites	African-Americans	Asians/Pacific Islanders
All cancers	464.2	462.7	464.0	298.2
All oral cancers	10.4	10.3	10.8	8.3
Lip	0.8	0.9	0.1	Negligible
Tongue	2.6	2.6	2.1	1.6
Salivary glands	1.2	1.2	0.7	0.9
Floor of the mouth	0.8	0.7	1.1	0.4
Gum and other mouth sites	1.6	1.6	1.8	1.2
Pharynx	3.2	3.0	4.3	3.9
Other sites	0.4	0.3	0.6	Negligible

socioeconomic status in the United States, as it has been shown to be in Britain.[64]

A standard measure of cancer severity is the 5-year relative survival rate, which is the percentage of people still alive 5 years after diagnosis, adjusted for those who died for some other reason over the 5 years. Fig. 23-4 shows these rates for men and women from 1974 to 1999, and it is evident that they have not changed much. Survival rates are much more favorable for whites than for African-Americans, and the disparity in survival rates between the races clearly had not improved by the turn of the century (Fig. 23-5). Survival rates have diminished in poorer parts of Europe over recent years, a

finding attributed to increasing alcohol consumption[4] and to social deprivation.[47]

The prospects for survival are considerably higher if diagnosis is made when the cancer is confined to a local lesion, rather than when there is regional or distant spread (Table 23-3). Five-year survival is four times greater when tumors are diagnosed at localized stages rather than after metastasis has occurred. It follows that cancers and precancerous lesions should be diagnosed as early as possible if treatment is to have a good prognosis, but there is nothing in the data to suggest that the proportion of oral cancers diagnosed at earlier, more localized stages has increased since 1973.[82]

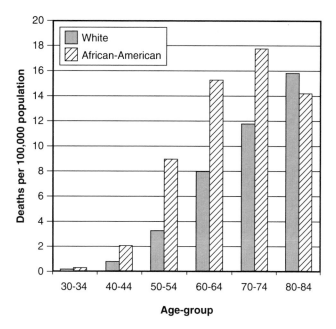

Fig. 23-3 Mortality from oral cancer per 100,000 population by age and race in the United States, 1996-2000.[85]

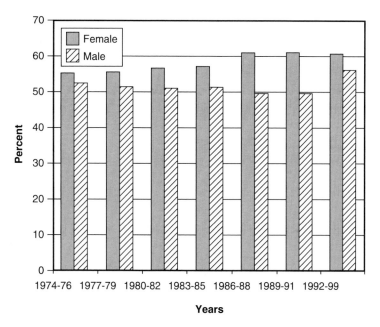

Fig. 23-4 Five-year relative survival rates for males and females diagnosed with oral cancer in the United States, 1974-99.[1,85]

Risk Factors

Worldwide, the combination of tobacco use, heavy alcohol use, and poor diet is responsible for 90% of all oral cancers.[35] The single risk factor most consistently associated with oral cancer on a global basis is the use of tobacco in its various forms.[65] For example, in India some 30%-40% of all reported cancers are oral cancers,[3,16] a remarkably high prevalence that is closely associated with several forms of tobacco smoking and chewing in that country. Elsewhere, smoking and other uses of tobacco are the most

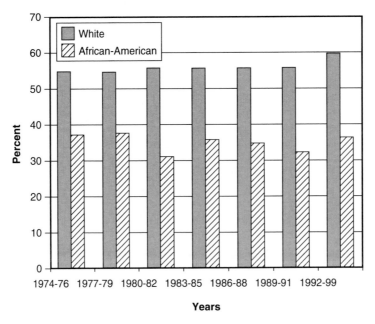

Fig. 23-5 Five-year relative survival rates for whites and African-Americans diagnosed with oral cancer in the United States, 1974-99.[85]

Table 23-3 Five-year survival rates for whites and African-Americans diagnosed with oral cancer by stage of metastatic spread from the primary site, United States, 1992-99[85]

	Localized (%)	Regional (%)	Distant (%)
Whites	82.7	49.9	26.7
African-Americans	68.8	30.6	21.5

consistently identified risk factors. High relative risks in the range of 6:1 to 14:1 for the development of oral cancers in smokers compared to nonsmokers continue to be reported in a number of countries.[20,21,36,51,53,60,80] The risk of developing oral cancer from smoking is just as high for women as for men,[37] and risk diminishes with time since quitting.[21,53] The risk of oral cancer in association with smoking is greatest for pharyngeal cancers and lowest for lip cancer.[51]

The extraordinarily high prevalence of oral cancer in India has naturally attracted research attention, especially in light of the widespread habit of chewing the areca nut (betel) in that country. Betel is usually chewed in a mix with tobacco, and lime and other ingredients are sometimes added. Some studies concluded that

the cancer risk comes largely from the tobacco with little role for betel.[28] However, other research has identified betel as a major etiologic factor in the development of oral submucous fibrosis,[58,83] a precancerous condition that has a high rate of malignant transformation.[58,77] Nodular leukoplakia, a precancerous condition that may be associated with oral submucous fibrosis, also shows a high rate of malignant transformation. Tobacco users with nodular leukoplakia are at especially high risk of oral cancer.[26] Intervention studies to curtail tobacco and betel chewing have had moderate success in reducing leukoplakia formation in India and confirm that chewing tobacco and betel are major risk factors for oral cancer.[27]

Over recent years, the resurgence in the use of smokeless tobacco has presented the United States with another risk factor for oral cancer. Because this recent increase in use is predominantly among young people,[11] it has so far had little impact on incidence and mortality data, but if widespread use continues, the incidence of oral cancer could rise sharply in the years ahead. The dimensions of smokeless tobacco use, its effects on human health, and what dental professionals can do about it are discussed in Chapter 30. Alcohol consumption, especially heavy consumption, has also been identified as a risk factor, although not all studies have found it to be a risk factor independent of tobacco use.[53,80]

The role of genetics in oral cancers is likely to be strong, although it requires further definition at present. Although mutation of the p53 cancer-suppression gene has been recognized as an etiologic factor in many forms of cancer for some years, its role in oral cancer is only starting to be well defined.[41,63] Further research in oral cancer is likely to focus on the genetic influences and molecular risk markers, but the importance of reducing the most common risk factors still remains.

Other risk factors have been identified, although the evidence is less consistent than it is for smoking and alcohol use. Painful and ill-fitting dentures are still often listed as a risk factor,[95] although supportive evidence is lacking. Long-term exposure to strong sunlight is seen as a risk factor for lip cancer; however, aside from the higher prevalence in sunnier climates, evidence for that contention is not easy to find.[79] Chronic inflammation, such as that found with lichen planus, has also been suggested as a possible risk factor.[14]

Dental Professionals and Oral Cancer

In terms of diagnosis, concern has been expressed that survival rates for oral cancer are unnecessarily low because of delays by patients in seeking attention for lesions and because of delays in diagnosis by health professionals.[25] Dentists and hygienists must be sensitive to the presence of leukoplakia and other precancerous conditions, especially in patients who present with known risk factors in their histories. Leukoplakia has long been known as a precancerous condition, meaning that it has been documented to precede the development of cancer. It has also been pointed out that mucosal erythroplakia, rather than leukoplakia, is often the first sign of cancerous change in a lesion.[51] A related issue here is the unusually high rate of second primary cancers among patients who have previously had oral cancer, a finding that is also correlated with higher tobacco use and alcohol consumption.[12]

OTHER SOFT TISSUE LESIONS

In general, the epidemiology of soft tissue lesions other than cancer has not been well studied. Precancerous conditions are obviously the lesions of most concern. A *precancerous lesion* is defined as morphologically altered tissue in which cancer is more likely to occur than in its apparently normal counterpart.[93] The principal precancerous conditions for oral cancer are generally recognized as leukoplakia and erythroplakia.

Leukoplakia, already mentioned as a risk factor in tobacco users, is generally defined as a white patch or plaque that cannot be characterized clinically or by pathologic examination as anything else,[42,89] a definition by default that is not very satisfactory. There is no general figure for the prevalence of leukoplakia in the population; it has been studied only in connection with known cancer risk factors such as smoking. The rate of transformation of leukoplakia lesions into oral cancer varies in different parts of the world but is generally on the order of 6%.[81]

Erythroplakia is a bright red or velvety plaque that cannot be characterized clinically or pathologically as being due to anything else,[93] another definition by default. When these lesions are found, or even suspected, immediate biopsy is called for and referral to an oral pathologist is recommended.

In general, little is known about the distribution of other soft tissue conditions, including papillary hyperplasia, candidiasis, pemphigus and pemphigoid, and lichen planus, or about the prevalence of herpes infections. Not surprisingly, risk factors have not been defined for these conditions (except that papillary hyperplasia is associated with ill-fitting dentures). There is a clear need for some basic epidemiologic research on all of these poorly understood conditions.

CLEFT LIP AND PALATE

The occurrence of cleft lip, cleft palate, or both in the United States each year was estimated some years ago as approximately 1 in 700 live births.[23] There is nothing to suggest that the rate has changed since then. Clefts are predominantly of genetic origin, and there is evidence of genetic-environmental interactions in their etiology.[8,32,45,57,75]

Attempts to isolate some of the potential environmental risk factors and the gene-environment interactions have proved difficult. Even the data on maternal smoking as a risk factor is inconsistent,[9,38,44,91,94] which seems odd considering the ubiquity of smoking as a risk factor for just about everything. There may be an interaction between maternal smoking during pregnancy and the infant's genotype.[32,75]

Maternal age seems not be a demographic risk factor,[88] and there also appears to be no link with socioeconomic status.[7] Among various ethnic groups in the United States, the lowest reported prevalence is among African-Americans and the highest is among persons of Japanese ancestry.[24] A correlation has been reported between late birth order and presence of clefts.[87]

Although problems with these studies are recognized, epidemiologic correlations reported from several studies[24,69,72] are the following:

- More facial clefts are found in boys, but more isolated cleft palates are found in girls.
- Cleft lip and palate appear more frequently in plural births than in single births.
- Babies with clefts generally are of lower birth weight, and an association has been found between clefts and prematurity. There is a higher infant mortality rate among children born with clefts,[31] and 35% of those born with clefts have associated malformations. The higher mortality rate is attributed more to these associated malformations; clefts without associated malformations do not present an increased risk of infant mortality.[19]

The occurrence of clefts is also associated with the following:

- Threatened spontaneous abortion during the first and second trimesters of pregnancy
- Influenza and fever in the first trimester
- Maternal drug use during the first trimester

The small number of studies on clefts means that the probability that the reported correlations are due to chance is moderately high. As a result, more study is needed to confirm the associations described.

MALOCCLUSION

The difficulties of quantifying malocclusion were described in Chapter 18. Differing cultural perceptions of what constitutes a malocclusion, differing perceptions of malocclusion on the part of orthodontic specialists and general dentists, and difficulties in achieving a sufficient degree of examiner consistency in use of malocclusion indexes all make summary statements difficult.

Malocclusion was measured on a nationally representative sample of U.S. youths ages 12-17 in the 1966-70 National Health Examination Survey.[86] This survey employed the Treatment Priority Index (see Chapter 18), and results showed that a higher proportion of African-American youths than white youths had either normal occlusion or only minor malocclusion. There was little difference in malocclusion between young white males and females; however, a notably higher proportion of African-American females than of African-American males had very severe malocclusion. Some occlusal traits were later measured in the third National Health and Nutrition Examination Survey (NHANES III, 1988-94), although no attempt was made to craft them into an index. The conditions recorded were diastema of more than 2 mm, alignment of lower and upper teeth, posterior crossbite, overbite, and overjet.[5]

A 1985 review of the prevalence of malocclusion in the United States[52] concluded that good epidemiologic evidence existed that there were significant departures from "normal occlusion" in American children and that a majority of American children "would benefit from orthodontic treatment." Unfortunately that conclusion remains as problematical as it always was, because normal occlusion was not defined, and in fact the authors seemed to be referring to ideal occlusion. Whether these children would really benefit, or whether orthodontic treatment would make no difference to their oral status, must remain a matter of conjecture.

TEMPOROMANDIBULAR JOINT DISORDERS

Disturbances of the temporomandibular joint, usually referred to as temporomandibular joint dysfunction (TMD) or temporomandibular pain and dysfunction syndrome (TMPDS), are a group of extremely painful and distressing conditions. Diagnosis is not easy because TMD is often accompanied by generalized pain in the head and neck region. There is no agreement on what constitutes standard treatment procedures, and treatment outcomes are mixed.[18] It is hardly surprising that the epidemiology of these conditions is poorly understood.[10,13]

The difficulty in defining risk factors in TMD stems from the absence of a suitable case definition of TMD. To put the problem in perspective, the disagreements on criteria for judging the presence of caries (see Chapter 15) exist over only a narrow range of clinical detection of an agreed-upon pathologic condition. The problems in defining TMD conditions, however, go far beyond these relatively restricted definitional problems; they are more akin to the problems in measuring malocclusion. When a condition cannot be defined, valid measurement is virtually impossible. Definitions of TMD exist,[67] but they tend to be all encompassing and nonspecific, and hence not of much operational value for research or treatment purposes. Conferences on TMD have generally agreed that a case definition should include elements of pain and dysfunction, but agreement on specifics beyond that is hard to find.

Epidemiologic studies of TMD have measured various signs and symptoms in various population groups, so summation of the state of knowledge is difficult. Commonly measured signs and symptoms include pain in the joint or masseter muscles with joint movement; limitations in mandibular movement; mandibular deviations on opening; and joint clicking or crepitus. Studies have used both self-report questionnaires and clinical examinations to obtain information. Many of what are referred to as epidemiologic studies in fact are clinical studies of patients receiving treatment, and thus their results must be interpreted cautiously. With regard to patients, there are three times as many women TMD patients as men patients, although no one knows why.[29]

There is general agreement that the prevalence of the commonly measured conditions just listed is quite high, even among people who do not perceive that they have a problem requiring treatment.[15,54,62,66,73,90] One study of a representative population in Toronto found that some 49% of adults responded positively to one or more of nine questions regarding symptoms, although a need for treatment was found in only 3%-10%, depending on the case

definition used.[46] However, it is very difficult to interpret what these data mean, for it is common to find prevalent symptoms that have no clinical significance.[54,68] Is a clicking joint, for example, a sign of impending trouble or is it of no consequence? A 20-year longitudinal study found that symptoms come and go over time but that progression to severe pain and dysfunction is rare.[49] Other longitudinal studies have obtained similar results.[17,48] It has been noted that signs and symptoms are as common in children and adolescents as they are in adults[54] and are even reported in preschool children,[92] although again the proper interpretation of these findings is unclear. Clicking joints in adolescents have been related to growth stages and come and go in response to "natural longitudinal fluctuations."[90] Cross-sectional studies can therefore give misleading information on prevalence and correlations.[40]

Although a great deal of TMD seems to have been treated by the use of orthodontic appliances, the current view is that occlusal discrepancies such as attrition and premature contacts are not a factor in TMD.[10,30,74] Moreover, there is no evidence that orthodontic treatment increases the risk of TMD.[39,43] It is widely thought that TMD should be treated as a medical orthopedic problem rather than a purely dental one.[13,22]

The need for a multidisciplinary approach to treatment is given weight by psychological studies of TMD patients. Such studies are essential in addressing the question of whether TMD is a discrete entity or whether it is part of broader psychological disturbances. Clinical depression is related to TMD.[78] Profiles of TMD patients have found that they tend to be of lower socioeconomic status,[6] that they tend to report their general health to be poorer than do nonpatients,[6,29,50] and that emotional distress and feelings of lack of control over their lives are common.[6] (The cause-and-effect relationship is not necessarily that emotional distress leads to TMD. On the contrary, it is entirely likely that the sequence is the other way around: continuing TMD, with lack of relief from treatment, could lead to emotional distress in an otherwise normal person.) Patients with complex orofacial pain conditions often do not respond as expected to dental care.[70] The state of the art with regard to psychological correlates of TMD is confused, and the results of a number of studies have been contradictory.[55,56,71]

Research into this highly distressing condition clearly has a long way to go before treatments with a firm scientific base, let alone prevention strategies, can be formulated. What is clear from the research to date is that the condition is highly complex and that multidisciplinary effort is required for its better comprehension.

REFERENCES

1. American Cancer Society. Cancer facts and figures, 1997. Atlanta: ACS, 1997.
2. American Cancer Society. Cancer incidence 2000, website: http://www.cancer.org/docrost/STT/stt_o. asp. Accessed January 9, 2004.
3. Binnie WH. Oral cancer. In: Dolby AE, ed: Oral mucosa in health and disease. Oxford: Blackwell, 1975:301-23.
4. Blot WJ, Devesa SS, McLaughlin JK, Fraumeni JF. Oral and pharyngeal cancers. Cancer Surv 1994; 19-20:23-42.
5. Brunelle JA, Bhat M, Lipton JA. Prevalence and distribution of selected occlusal characteristics in the US population, 1988-1991. J Dent Res 1996;75(Spec Issue): 706-13.
6. Carlsson GE, Kopp S, Wedel A. Analysis of background variables in 350 patients with TMJ disorders as reported in self-administered questionnaire. Community Dent Oral Epidemiol 1982;10:47-51.
7. Carmichael SL, Nelson V, Shaw GM, et al. Socioeconomic status and risk of conotruncal heart defects and orofacial clefts. Pediatr Perinat Epidemiol 2003;17: 264-71.
8. Christensen K, Fogh-Andersen P. Cleft lip (+/− cleft palate) in Danish twins, 1970-1990. Am J Med Genet 1993;47:910-6.
9. Chung KC, Kowalski CP, Kim HM, Buchman SR. Maternal cigarette smoking during pregnancy and the risk of having a child with cleft lip/palate. Plast Reconstr Surg 2000;105:485-91.
10. Clark GT. Etiologic theory and the prevention of temporomandibular disorders. Adv Dent Res 1991;5:60-6.
11. Cullen JW, Blot W, Henningfield J, et al. Health consequences of using smokeless tobacco: Summary of the Advisory Committee's report to the Surgeon General. Public Health Rep 1986;101:355-73.
12. Day GL, Blot WJ, Shore RE, et al. Second cancers following oral and pharyngeal cancers: Role of tobacco and alcohol. J Natl Cancer Inst 1994;86:131-7.
13. de Bont LG, Dijkgraaf LC, Stegenga B. Epidemiology and natural progression of articular temporomandibular disorders. Oral Surg Oral Med Oral Pathol Oral Radiol Endod 1997;83:72-6.
14. Deeb ZE, Fox LA, deFries HO. The association of chronic inflammatory disease in lichen planus with cancer of the oral cavity. Am J Otolaryngol 1989;10: 314-6.
15. Deng YM, Fu MK, Hagg U. Prevalence of temporomandibular joint dysfunction (TMJD) in Chinese children and adolescents. A cross-sectional epidemiological study. Eur J Orthod 1995;17:305-9.
16. Dharkar D. Oral cancer in India: Need for fresh approaches. Cancer Detect Prev 1988;11:267-70.
17. Dibbets JM, van der Weele LT. Prevalence of TMJ symptoms and x-ray findings. Eur J Orthod 1989;11:31-6.
18. Dolwick MF, Dimitroulis G. Is there a role for temporomandibular joint surgery? Br J Oral Maxillofac Surg 1994;32:307-13.
19. Druschel CM, Hughes JP, Olsen CL. First year-of-life mortality among infants with oral clefts: New York State, 1983-1990. Cleft Palate Craniofac J 1996; 33:400-5.
20. Franceschi S, Talamini R, Barra S, et al. Smoking and drinking in relation to cancers of the oral cavity, pharynx, larynx, and esophagus in northern Italy. Cancer Res 1990;50:6502-7.
21. Franco EL, Kowalski LP, Oliveira BV, et al. Risk factors for oral cancer in Brazil: A case-control study. Int J Cancer 1989;43:992-1000.
22. Greene CS. Orthodontics and temporomandibular disorders. Dent Clin North Am 1988;32:529-38.
23. Greene JC. Epidemiology of congenital clefts of the lip and palate. Public Health Rep 1963;78:589-602.
24. Greene JC, Vermillion JR, Hay S, et al. Epidemiologic study of cleft lip and cleft palate in four states. J Am Dent Assoc 1964;68:387-404.
25. Guggenheimer J, Verbin RS, Johnson JT, et al. Factors delaying the diagnosis of oral and oropharyngeal carcinomas. Cancer 1989;64:932-5.
26. Gupta PC, Bhonsle RB, Murti PR, et al. An epidemiologic assessment of cancer risk in oral precancerous lesions in India with special reference to nodular leukoplakia. Cancer 1989;63:2247-52.
27. Gupta PC, Mehta FS, Pindborg JJ, et al. Primary intervention trial of oral cancer in India: A 10-year follow-up study. J Oral Pathol Med 1992;21:433-9.
28. Gupta PC, Pindborg JJ, Mehta FS. Comparison of carcinogenicity of betel quid with and without tobacco: An epidemiological review. Ecol Dis 1982;1:213-9.
29. Helkimo M. Epidemiological surveys of dysfunction of the masticatory system. Oral Sci Rev 1976;7:54-69.
30. Houston F, Hanamura H, Carlsson GE, et al. Mandibular dysfunction and periodontitis. A comparative study of patients with periodontal disease and occlusal parafunctions. Acta Odont Scand 1987;45: 239-46.
31. Hujoel PP, Bollen AM, Mueller BA. First-year mortality among infants with facial clefts. Cleft Palate Craniofac J 1992;29:451-5.
32. Hwang SJ, Beaty TH, Panny SR, et al. Association study of transforming growth factor alpha (TGF alpha) TaqI polymorphism and oral clefts: Indication of gene-environment interaction in a population-based sample of infants with birth defects. Am J Epidemiol 1995;141: 629-36.
33. International Classification of Diseases, 9th revision, Clinical Modification, 4th ed. Los Angeles: Practice Management Information Corporation, 1994.
34. Johnson NW. Orofacial neoplasms: Global epidemiology, risk factors and recommendations for research. Int Dent J 1991;41:365-75.

35. Johnson NW. Tobacco use and oral cancer; a global perspective. J Dent Educ 2001;65:328-39.
36. Jones JB, Lampe HB, Cheung HW. Carcinoma of the tongue in young patients. J Otolaryngol 1989;18:105-8.
37. Kabat GC, Hebert JR, Wynder EL. Risk factors for oral cancer in women. Cancer Res 1989;49:2803-6.
38. Khoury MJ, Gomez-Farias M, Mulinare J. Does maternal cigarette smoking during pregnancy cause cleft lip and palate in offspring? Am J Dis Child 1989;143:333-7.
39. Kim MR, Graber TM, Viana MA. Orthodontics and temporomandibular disorder: A meta-analysis. Am J Orthod Dentofacial Orthop 2002;121:438-46.
40. Kirveskari P, Alanen P, Jamsa T. Association between craniomandibular disorders and occlusal interferences. J Prosthet Dent 1989;62:66-9.
41. Koch WM, Boyle JO, Mao L, et al. p53 gene mutations as markers of tumor spread in synchronous oral cancers. Arch Otolaryngol Head Neck Surg 1994;120:943-7.
42. Kramer I, El-Labban N, Lee K. The clinical features and risk of malignant transformation in sublingual keratosis. Br Dent J 1978;144:171-80.
43. Lagerstrom L, Egermark I, Carlsson GE. Signs and symptoms of temporomandibular disorders in 19-year-old individuals who have undergone orthodontic treatment. Swed Dent J 1998;22:177-86.
44. Lieff S, Olshan AF, Werler M, et al. Maternal cigarette smoking during pregnancy and risk of oral clefts in newborns. Am J Epidemiol 1999;150:683-94.
45. Lin YC, Lo LJ, Noordhoff MS, Chen YR. Cleft of the lip and palate in twins [English abstract]. Changgeng Yi Xue Za Zhi 1999;22:61-7.
46. Locker D, Slade G. Prevalence of symptoms associated with temporomandibular disorders in a Canadian population. Community Dent Oral Epidemiol 1988;16:310-3.
47. Macfarlane GJ, Sharp L, Porter S, Francheschi S. Trends in survival from cancers of the oral cavity and pharynx in Scotland: A clue as to why the disease is becoming more common? Br J Cancer 1996;73:805-8.
48. Magnusson T, Egermark-Eriksson I, Carlsson GE. Four-year longitudinal study of mandibular dysfunction in children. Community Dent Oral Epidemiol 1985;13:117-20.
49. Magnusson T, Egermark-Eriksson I, Carlsson GE. A longitudinal epidemiologic study of signs and symptoms of temporomandibular disorders from 15 to 35 years of age. J Orofac Pain 2000;14:310-9.
50. Marbach JJ, Lennon MC, Dohrenwend BP. Candidate risk factors for temporomandibular pain and dysfunction syndrome: Psychosocial, health behavior, physical illness and injury. Pain 1988;34:139-51.
51. Mashberg A, Samit AM. Early detection, diagnosis, and management of oral and oropharyngeal cancer. CA Cancer J Clin 1989;39:67-88.
52. McLain JB, Proffitt WR. Oral health status in the United States: Prevalence of malocclusion. J Dent Educ 1985;49:386-96.
53. Merletti F, Boffetta P, Ciccone G, et al. Role of tobacco and alcoholic beverages in the etiology of cancer of the oral cavity/oropharynx in Torino, Italy. Cancer Res 1989;49:4919-24.
54. Mintz SS. Craniomandibular dysfunction in children and adolescents: A review. Cranio 1993;11:224-31.
55. Moss RA, Adams HE. The assessment of personality, anxiety and depression in mandibular pain dysfunction subjects. J Oral Rehabil 1984;11:233-5.
56. Moss RA, Garrett JC. Temporomandibular joint dysfunction syndrome and myofascial pain dysfunction syndrome: A critical review. J Oral Rehabil 1984;11:3-28.
57. Murray JC. Gene/environment causes of cleft lip and/or palate. Clin Genet 2002;61:248-56.
58. Murti PR, Bhonsle RB, Gupta PC, et al. Etiology of submucous fibrosis with special reference to the role of areca nut chewing. J Oral Pathol Med 1995;24:145-52.
59. Murti PR, Gupta PC, Bhonsle RB, et al. Effect on the incidence of oral submucous fibrosis of intervention in the areca nut chewing habit. J Oral Pathol Med 1990;19:99-100.
60. Nandakumar A, Thimmasetty KT, Sreeramareddy NM, et al. A population-based case-control investigation on cancers of the oral cavity in Bangalore, India. Br J Cancer 1990;62:847-51.
61. Negri E, La Vecchia C, Levi F, et al. Comparative descriptive epidemiology of oral and oesophageal cancers in Europe. Eur J Cancer Prev 1996;5:267-79.
62. Nielsen L, Melsen B, Terp S. Prevalence, interrelation, and severity of signs of dysfunction from masticatory system in 14-16-year-old Danish children. Community Dent Oral Epidemiol 1989;17:91-6.
63. Nylander K, Dabelsteen E, Hall PA. The p53 molecule and its prognostic role in squamous cell carcinomas of the head and neck. J Oral Pathol Med 2000;29:413-25.
64. O'Hanlon S, Forster DP, Lowry RJ. Oral cancer in the North-East of England: Incidence, mortality trends and the link with material deprivation. Community Dent Oral Epidemiol 1997;25:371-6.
65. Pindborg JJ. Epidemiological studies of oral cancer. Int Dent J 1977;27:172-8.
66. Pullinger AG, Seligman DA, Solberg WK. Temporomandibular disorders. Part I: Functional status, dentomorphologic features, and sex differences in a nonpatient population. J Prosthet Dent 1988;59:228-35.
67. Ramfjord SP, Ash MM Jr. Occlusion. 3rd ed. Philadelphia: Saunders, 1983:175.
68. Riolo ML, TenHave TR, Brandt D. Clinical validity of the relationship between TMJ signs and symptoms in children and youth. ASDC J Dent Child 1988;55:110-3.
69. Robert E, Kallen B, Harris J. The epidemiology of orofacial clefts. I. Some general epidemiological characteristics. J Craniofac Genet Dev Biol 1996;16:234-41.
70. Rugh JD. Psychological components of pain. Dent Clin North Am 1987;31:579-94.
71. Rugh JD, Solberg WK. Psychological implications in temporomandibular pain and dysfunction. Oral Sci Rev 1976;7:3-30.
72. Saxen I. Epidemiology of cleft lip and palate; an attempt to rule out chance correlations. Br J Prev Soc Med 1975;29:103-10.

73. Schiffman EL, Fricton JR, Haley DP, Shapiro BL. The prevalence and treatment needs of subjects with temporomandibular disorders. J Am Dent Assoc 1990; 120:295-303.

74. Seligman DA, Pullinger AG, Solberg WK. The prevalence of dental attrition and its association with factors of age, gender, occlusion, and TMJ symptomatology. J Dent Res 1988;67:1323-33.

75. Shaw GM, Wasserman CR, Lammer EJ, et al. Orofacial clefts, parental cigarette smoking, and transforming growth factor-alpha gene variants. Am J Hum Genet 1996;58:551-61.

76. Silverberg E, Lubera JA. Cancer statistics, 1988. CA Cancer J Clin 1988;38:5-22.

77. Sinor PN, Gupta PC, Murti PR, et al. A case-control study of oral submucous fibrosis with special reference to the etiologic role of areca nut. J Oral Pathol Med 1990;19:94-8.

78. Sipila K, Veijola J, Jokelainen J, et al. Association between symptoms of temporomandibular disorders and depression: An epidemiological study of the Northern Finland 1966 birth cohort. Cranio 2001; 19:183-7.

79. Smith CJ, Pindborg JJ, Binnie WH, eds. Oral cancer: Epidemiology, etiology, and pathology. New York: Hemisphere, 1990.

80. Spitz MR, Fueger JJ, Goepfert H, et al. Squamous cell carcinoma of the upper aerodigestive tract. A case comparison analysis. Cancer 1988;61:203-8.

81. Squier CA. Smokeless tobacco and oral cancer: A cause for concern? CA Cancer J Clin 1984;34:242-7.

82. Swango PA. Cancers of the oral cavity and pharynx in the United States: An epidemiologic overview. J Public Health Dent 1996;56:309-18.

83. Trivedy CR, Craig G, Warnakulasuriya S. The oral health consequences of chewing areca nut. Addict Biol 2002;7:115-25.

84. US Public Health Service, Centers for Disease Control and Prevention. United States Cancer Statistics; 2000 incidence report, website: http://apps.nccd.cdc.gov/uscs/index.asp?, 2000. Accessed November 30, 2004.

85. US Public Health Service, National Cancer Institute. SEER program, website: http://www.seer.cancer.gov/faststats/html/inc_oralcav.html. Accessed November 30, 2004.

86. US Public Health Service, National Center for Health Statistics. An assessment of the occlusion of the teeth of youths 12-17 years, United States. DHEW Publication No. (HRA) 77-1644, Series 11 No. 162. Washington DC: Government Printing Office, 1977.

87. Vieira AR, Orioli IM. Birth order and oral clefts: A meta analysis. Teratology 2002;66:209-16.

88. Vieira AR, Orioli IM, Murray JC. Maternal age and oral clefts: A reappraisal. Oral Surg Oral Med Oral Pathol Oral Radiol Endod 2002;94:530-5.

89. Waldron C, Shafer W. Leukoplakia revisited. A clinicopathologic study of 3,256 oral leukoplakias. Cancer 1975;36:1386-92.

90. Wanman A, Agerberg G. Temporomandibular joint sounds in adolescents: A longitudinal study. Oral Surg Oral Med Oral Pathol 1990;69:2-9.

91. Werler MM, Lammer EJ, Rosenberg L, Mitchell AA. Maternal cigarette smoking during pregnancy in relation to oral clefts. Am J Epidemiol 1990;132:926-32.

92. Widmalm SE, Christiansen RL, Gunn SM. Crepitation and clicking as signs of TMD in preschool children. Cranio 1999;17:58-63.

93. World Health Organization, Collaborating Reference Centre for Oral Precancerous Lesions. Definition of leukoplakia and related lesions: An aid to studies on oral precancer. Oral Surg 1978;46:517-39.

94. Wyszynski DF, Wu T. Use of US birth certificate data to estimate the risk of maternal cigarette smoking for oral clefting. Cleft Palate Craniofac J 2002;39:188-92.

95. Young TB, Ford CN, Brandenburg JH. An epidemiologic study of oral cancer in a statewide network. Am J Otolaryngol 1986;7:200-8.

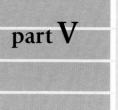

part V Prevention of Oral Diseases in Public Health

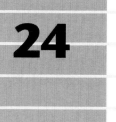

24 Fluoride: Human Health and Caries Prevention

It is hard for today's students to visualize what caries used to look like in prefluoride days. Periapical abscesses and gaping anterior lesions were common, extractions of first molars in young children were routine, and full extractions and complete dentures were virtually the norm for older people. Although higher educational levels, better technology, and the spread of middle-class standards have led to improvement of this situation, fluoride ranks as a primary influence in better oral health because its impact changed the way people thought about dental health. It demonstrated to patients and nonpatients alike that caries and subsequent tooth loss were not inevitable. Just as important, it helped dentists to reshape their attitudes toward tooth conservation.

This chapter deals with the issues of how fluoride's caries-inhibitory potential was first discovered, how the human body physiologically deals with fluoride when the material is ingested, how fluoride affects our health, and how it works to prevent caries. In this and subsequent chapters, we abbreviate the word *fluoride* to its chemical symbol F to make reading easier. It all begins with one of the great epidemiologic studies in the history of health research.

A CLASSIC EPIDEMIOLOGIC STUDY

Dr. Frederick McKay, as a new dental graduate in the early 1900s, headed west and opened a practice in Colorado Springs, Colorado. He soon noticed that many of his patients had a curious blotching of the enamel that he had not encountered before. People in the area called it "Colorado brown stain," and to them it was just a local oddity. It seemed harmless enough, though it was disfiguring in some cases. McKay was clearly a born scientist; he had an inquiring mind and fine powers of observation, and Colorado brown stain piqued his curiosity. In 1908 he began to investigate the extent of Colorado brown stain in the surrounding area.

In his travels over the next few years, McKay found that the condition was highly prevalent in the Colorado Springs area. It was found only in long-term residents, individuals who had been born there or who had come to the area as babies. Because the stain was difficult to polish off, McKay reasoned that it must be caused by an environmental agent that was active during the period of enamel formation. To ensure that his findings attracted some attention, McKay was shrewd enough to enlist the collaboration of G. V. Black, a major figure in dental history, in writing the first description of what then came to be called *mottled enamel*.[15] This detailed report, in the elegant prose of the time, is a tribute to McKay's investigative thoroughness.

McKay found that mottled enamel was endemic in many other communities along the Continental Divide and the plains to the east. It was most prevalent where deep artesian wells were the source of drinking water, and within any community the persons affected had almost invariably been users of the same water supply. By the 1920s McKay had reached the conclusion that the etiologic agent had to be a constituent of some community water supplies, despite the fact that chemical analyses all failed to identify likely constituents. In communities such as Andover and Britton, South Dakota, where he found severe mottling, he advised mothers to obtain their children's drinking water from sources other than the community supply. In Oakley, Idaho, McKay found that children living on the outskirts of the city, using water from a private spring, were free of mottling. He advised the citizens of Oakley to abandon their old supply and tap this spring for a new source, which the community did in 1925. McKay was right, for children born in Oakley subsequent to the change were free of mottled enamel.[128]

By 1930 new methods of spectrographic analysis of water had been developed. In 1931 McKay sent several samples of suspected water to an Alcoa Company chemist named Churchill, who was using these new methods. Churchill identified F in each of the samples, in amounts ranging up to 14 parts per million (ppm).[26] At around the same time, similar findings were reported by investigators at the University of Arizona[161] and by a veterinary group in Morocco, then still a French colony, that was studying *le darmous*, the local name given to an extreme degree of mottled enamel found in Moroccan sheep.[174]

The immediate reaction of the scientific community to the identification of F in drinking water was one of concern, because F in high concentrations was known to be a protoplasmic poison. The discovery led to the appointment in 1931 of the first dentist to the newly established National Institute of Health. This was H. Trendley Dean, who was transferred from elsewhere in the U.S. Public Health Service to

become the one-person Dental Hygiene Unit, an odd name for a unit formed to investigate mottled enamel (it subsequently became the National Institute of Dental Research in 1948).

Amidst this flurry of concern, however, McKay had also noted some benefits that seemed to accompany mottled enamel. In 1928, 3 years before F was identified in drinking water, he was confident enough to publish his view that caries experience was reduced by the same waters that produced mottled enamel.[127] A similar observation was made shortly afterward in England by Ainsworth,[2] who like McKay was an observant dentist with an inquiring mind. Although McKay was not the first to make this suggestion, none of the earlier observers took the idea any further. McKay, and Dean as well, are good examples of history's putting the right people in the right place at the right time.

The task of defining the relationship of F to mottled enamel now passed to Dean. His first job was to map out the prevalence of mottled enamel in the United States. Dean began like an investigative reporter, writing extensively to dental societies all around the country to ask for their experiences. He received a good response and published his first map on the distribution of mottled enamel in 1933.[32] His next step was to develop a seven-point ordinal-scale index to classify the full range of mottled enamel he had seen, from the finest of lacy markings to the stained and highly friable enamel seen with extreme hypomineralization.[33]

Dean began using the term *fluorosis* to replace *mottled enamel* in the mid-1930s.[39] He patiently surveyed children in many parts of the country, using his original fluorosis index, and built up a substantial body of information (what today we would call a database) for analysis. He devised his Community Fluorosis index based on his original seven grades of severity.[38] Studies through the mid-1930s analyzed many drinking water samples for minerals and other chemical constituents, but none apart from F could be related to fluorosis.[39,41] Dean chose his words carefully to define a desirable F concentration as follows:

For public health purposes, we have arbitrarily defined the minimal threshold of fluoride concentration in a domestic water supply as the highest concentration of fluoride incapable of producing a definite degree of mottled enamel in as much as 10 percent of the group examined.[39]

By the mid-1930s, Dean had concluded that this "minimal threshold" level was 1 ppm F,[34] and that fluorosis seen in communities with water below 1 ppm F was "of no public health significance."[40] Soon afterward he defined 1 ppm F as "the permissible maximum."[45] Later in that decade of the Great Depression, Dean condensed his original 1934 fluorosis index to one using a six-point ordinal scale (see Chapter 17) by combining the categories of "moderately severe" and "severe."[42] He then added numerical values to the categories to permit quantitative comparisons among populations. By 1942 Dean had documented the prevalence of fluorosis for most of the United States.[36]

Although he still documented fluorosis in his studies, the main theme of Dean's research from then on was the F-caries relationship. In the mid-1930s Dean matched his fluorosis data for children in parts of South Dakota, Colorado, and Wisconsin with the caries data from an earlier 26-state survey in what today would be called an ecologic study (see Chapter 13). Although he could hardly have failed to notice the low caries experience in communities with F-bearing water during his early surveys, this was his first report in which he commented on the inverse relationship between fluorosis and caries.[35]

Encouraged by these preliminary data, Dean chose four cities in central Illinois as study sites in which to test the hypothesis that consumption of F-containing water was associated with a reduced prevalence of caries. Galesburg and Monmouth, where Dean had already studied fluorosis,[40] used water from deep wells that averaged 1.8 and 1.7 ppm F. Macomb and Quincy used surface water averaging 0.2 ppm F. Clinical examinations of children ages 12-14 years, all with lifetime residence in their respective cities, showed that more than twice as many children in Galesburg and Monmouth were free of detectable caries than in the two cities with low-F water, and the mean number of permanent teeth affected by caries in Galesburg and Monmouth was half of that in the two cities with low-F water.[44] The evidence to support the F-caries hypothesis was now stronger.

Although caries prevalence and severity were low in Galesburg and Monmouth, fluorosis was an obvious problem in both communities.

Dean and the other investigators put it this way, in the flowing prose of the time:

[It is] obvious that whatever effect the waters with relatively high fluoride content (over 2.0 ppm of F) have on dental caries is largely one of academic interest; the resultant permanent disfigurement of many of the users far outweighs any advantage that might accrue from the standpoint of partial control of dental caries. On the other hand, the demonstration of such marked dental caries differences as were observed at Galesburg and Quincy made advisable a quantitative study of the influence on dental caries of waters with lower ranges of fluoride concentration. If marked inhibitory influences were operative at concentration levels as low as the minimal threshold of endemic fluorosis (1.0 ppm), the findings would be of considerable import.[43]

The next logical step was therefore to define the lowest F level at which caries was clearly inhibited. This was done through a series of investigations that have become known collectively as the 21 cities study and that are rightly considered a landmark in dental research. The first part consisted of the results of clinical examinations of children ages 12-14 with lifetime residence in eight suburban Chicago communities with various but stable mean F levels in their domestic water.[43] The project was later expanded by adding data from 13 additional cities in Illinois, Colorado, Ohio, and Indiana.[37] The collective findings of the 21 cities study are depicted graphically in Figs. 24-1 and 24-2. Fig. 24-1 shows that dental caries experience in different communities dropped sharply as F concentration rose toward 1 ppm, then leveled off. Fig. 24-2 shows the dental fluorosis experience that Dean found among the 12- to 14-year-olds in the 21 cities. Dean's practice was to show questionable fluorosis separately in his reports, as we have done in Fig. 24-2. The data in Fig. 24-2 suggest that, had "questionable" fluorosis been included in the prevalence figures, then the level for "acceptable" fluorosis might have been set at concentrations lower than 1 ppm F.

Because the 21 cities study had a cross-sectional design, the results confirmed the association but could not by themselves establish the cause-and-effect relationship between fluoridated water and reduced caries prevalence. But the data in Figs. 24-1 and 24-2 did lead to the adoption of 1.0-1.2 ppm as the appropriate concentration of F in drinking water in temperate climates, a standard that remains in place today

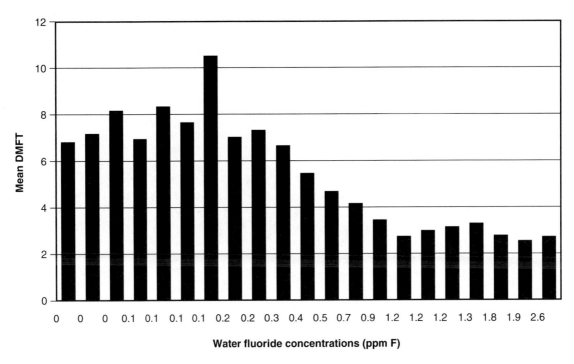

Fig. 24-1 Decayed, missing, and filled permanent teeth (DMFT) in children ages 12-14 in 21 cities in the late 1930s, related to the fluoride concentration.[37,43]

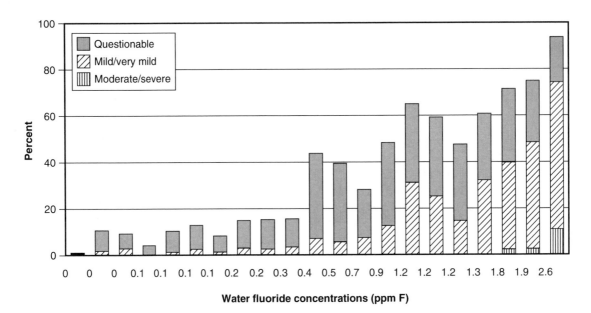

Fig. 24-2 Fluorosis experience of children ages 12-14 in 21 cities in the late 1930s, related to the fluoride concentration of drinking water.[37,43]

in the United States. These results also set the stage for a prospective test of the F-caries hypothesis, first suggested in 1943.[8] The years of study of people using water with F levels much higher than the proposed 1 ppm (detailed later in this chapter) were sufficient to convince public authorities that the prospective tests could be carried out in safety. These first prospective studies are described in Chapter 25.

Trendley Dean died in 1962. Those who knew him said that he could be autocratic, and the reverence he inspired in his colleagues may too often have been expressed as uncritical acceptance of all he did. But Dean had the researcher's virtues of dogged perseverance and remorseless logic as he progressed from one stage to the next. His grasp of the concept of "databasing" and his analytic mind make us wonder what he could have done with modern computer technology. Although knowledge of F's effects has advanced considerably since those days, we enjoy the benefits of F today because of the pioneering research of Dean and his colleagues. In time, it led to the substantial decline in dental caries in high-income nations, one of history's major public health success stories.

ENVIRONMENTAL FLUORIDE

Fluorine is one of the most reactive elements and therefore is never found naturally in its elemental form. The F ion, however, is abundant in nature and occurs almost universally in soils and waters in varying, but generally low, concentrations. Seawater contains 1.2-1.4 ppm F.[181] Fresh surface water generally has very low concentrations, 0.2 ppm F or less, whereas concentrations of up to 29.5 ppm F have been recorded in deep well water in Arizona[120] and concentrations of over 40 ppm in boreholes in Kenya.[112] F's ubiquity in soil and water means that all plants and animals contain F to some extent. Given this environmental omnipresence, it seems likely that all forms of life have evolved to thrive with continuous exposure to small amounts of F.

SOURCES AND AMOUNTS OF FLUORIDE INTAKE

Humans absorb F from air, food, and water. F intake from air is usually negligible, around 0.04 mg F/day.[180] Exceptions can occur around some industrial plants that work with F-rich material, such as aluminum smelters with inadequate safeguards to prevent the escape of F-containing compounds. Such environmental hazards should be controlled to the extent possible, an issue that has nothing whatever to do with the use of F to control caries.

F's abundance in soils and plants means that everyone consumes it to some extent. Studies to estimate the average daily intake of F from all sources have provided fairly consistent results, despite both the variability of the human diet and methodologic difficulties inherent in analyzing such minute amounts. Estimates for an adult North American male in an area with fluoridated water fall within the range of 1-3 mg F/day from food and beverages,[30,60,102,141,159,160,165] decreasing to 1 mg F/day or less in an area without fluoridation.[30,102,141,159,160] "Market basket" analyses indicated that 6-month-old infants ingested 0.21-0.54 mg F/day in four American cities with different F concentrations in the drinking water. For 2-year-olds in the same cities, the range was 0.41-0.61 mg F/day.[139,140]

F ingestion in infancy is a matter of some concern because of the risk of dental fluorosis. Methodical estimates of F intake by infants have come from the Iowa F studies, initiated in the 1990s, which showed that F exposure among infants is extensive and variable. The Iowa studies documented the F exposures of newborn infants at periodic intervals through extensive interviews about F exposure from drinking water, toothpaste, and dietary supplements. During the first 3 years of life, F ingestion from these sources averaged 0.37-0.45 mg daily from birth to 3 months, 0.5 mg at 6-9 months, 0.36 mg at 12 and 16 months, and 0.5-0.63 mg from 16 to 36 months.[107] Although mean intakes in Iowa were similar to those estimated in the earlier market basket surveys, there was a considerable range of intakes, with 90th percentile values well above the means and medians. When values were expressed as F intake per kilogram of body weight, nearly half of the children up to 6 months of age were found to be exceeding the desirable limits, although this proportion dropped considerably at later ages. The upper limit of intake for 12-month-old children, beyond which fluorosis risk is greatly increased, has been estimated at

0.43 mg F/day.[20] The 12-month-old children in the Iowa studies averaged 0.36 mg F/day,[107] but more than 25% of them were ingesting F above that upper limit.

The principal overall finding of the Iowa studies is the great variability of F intake during infancy, which is to be expected given the range of dietary choices for infants and the range of F concentrations in drinking waters. Despite the difficulty in conducting studies like these, the results are similar to those found in the market basket surveys described earlier and in studies from other countries.[70,115]

For most people, water and other beverages provide some 75% of F intake, whether or not the drinking water is fluoridated.[160] This may occur because many soft drinks and fruit juices are processed in cities with fluoridated water, or it may reflect variable F content of the ingredients. One brand of grape juice in North Carolina, for example, was found to contain more than 1.6 ppm F, even when reconstituted with deionized water.[143] Even in soft drinks of the same brand, F levels can vary considerably due to production at different sites.[76] Another source of high F intake for infants is powdered infant formula reconstituted with fluoridated drinking water.[22] The F content of some tested beverages is shown in Table 24-1.

FLUORIDE PHYSIOLOGY

Although the use of F is a contribution to the public's health of which dentistry can be proud, F compounds must be handled responsibly and with respect. Everyone in dentistry should understand how the human body handles ingested F so that the material can be used safely and efficiently.

Absorption, Retention, and Excretion

Ingested F is absorbed mainly from the upper gastrointestinal tract, and some 95% of ingested F is absorbed. Absorbed F is transported in the plasma and is either excreted or deposited in the calcified tissues. Most absorbed F is excreted in the urine; a single ingestion of 5 mg F by an adult is absorbed and cleared from the blood in 8-9 hours.[180] F ingested on an empty stomach produces a peak plasma level within 30 minutes. The time of the plasma peak is extended, and the level of the peak reduced, if the F is taken with food. This is probably because of the binding of some F with calcium and other divalent and trivalent cations. When F absorption is inhibited in this way, fecal excretion of F increases.[50]

Studies of what is called the *body burden* of F, meaning the amount that can be safely absorbed and the point at which F absorption

Table 24-1 Fluoride concentration (in ppm) of various beverages available in a nonfluoridated and a fluoridated community in Alberta, Canada, and in various communities in North Carolina and Iowa[28,96,143]

Beverage	Nonfluoridated, Canada	Fluoridated, Canada	North Carolina*	Iowa
Drinking water	0.23	1.08	—	—
Milk†	0.03	0.03	—	—
Juice (commercially prepared)‡	0.80	0.80	0.36	0.56
Juice (home reconstituted)	0.21	1.06	—	—
Apple-grape juice (commercially prepared)	—	—	—	0.64
Carbonated drinks‡	0.80	0.80	0.74	—
Gatorade	—	—	0.85	—
Soup	0.21	1.06	—	—
Tea	1.33	2.18	2.56	1.41
Coffee	0.23	1.08	—	—

*Means of samples from six cities.
†Available fluoride.
‡Commercially available prepared juice and the carbonated drinks in Canada both came from a fluoridated large city; for Iowa the figure is the mean for 532 juices.

become a health concern, have relied mostly on urinary volumes and plasma concentrations as the primary measures. Samples of both are relatively simple to obtain, although both measures reflect only recent F intake (i.e., during the previous 3-4 weeks) rather than lifetime intakes. Urinary concentrations can vary considerably with fluid intake during the period of F exposure,[49] and a 24-hour sample is required for accuracy. Accurate monitoring of plasma levels in individuals also requires frequent measurement because of normal hour-to-hour fluctuations. Plasma F concentrations are more closely correlated with urinary flow rates than with urinary F concentrations.[51] Although there is no absolute measure of lifetime F intake, even theoretically, the closest measure of long-term F intake would be based on bone F content. However, for research purposes, this is a theoretical concept only; people do not volunteer to give bone samples!

F balance is the net result from the accumulated effects of F ingestion, degree of F deposition in bones and teeth, mobilization rate of F from bone, and efficiency of the kidneys in clearing absorbed F.

Plasma F is found in ionic and nonionic forms. The biologic significance of the nonionic form has not yet been determined, and its concentration is independent of F intake. Absorbed F is transported by plasma as ionic F. It is the level of this ionic F that rises temporarily after F ingestion and then drops rapidly; ionic F levels are not homeostatically regulated. In a healthy adult male living in an area with fluoridated water, plasma F levels are around 0.019 ppm (1 μmol/L), although this level fluctuates throughout the day.[50] Plasma levels are generally higher in persons living in fluoridated communities than in those living in nonfluoridated communities. Plasma F levels in persons with chronic kidney failure can rise to 0.05-0.09 ppm F (2.6-4.7 μmol/L) without affecting health.[90] Nephrotoxic plasma F values in healthy individuals have been estimated at 0.95 ppm F (50 μmol/L).

F has an affinity for calcified tissues, that is, bone and developing teeth. F that is not excreted is deposited in these hard tissues, although storage is dynamic rather than inert. Bone F levels (from postmortem assays) range from 800 to 10,000 ppm, depending on many

factors, including age and F intake. F levels in the outer few microns of dental enamel range from 400 to 3000 ppm and decrease rapidly with greater enamel depth. F concentrations in soft tissue rise or fall in parallel with plasma F levels, but because healthy excretion and deposition mechanisms operate so rapidly, there is negligible retention of F in the fluids of soft tissues other than the kidney.[180] Some F has been found in the aorta, associated with calcification of that blood vessel. Deposition in the placenta is also associated with islets of calcified tissue.[55] A greater proportion of ingested F is excreted in older persons than in the young because the growing skeleton in young people absorbs more F[175,182] and probably because children have lower renal clearance rates than adults.[164]

Because of the importance of the kidneys in maintaining F balance, the only disease condition that requires medical consideration with regard to F ingestion is chronic kidney failure. Patients who receive renal dialysis for long periods with F-free water have maintained plasma levels of 0.06 ppm F, whereas in some inadvertently receiving dialysis with fluoridated water (definitely not a recommended procedure) levels as high as 0.24 ppm F have been recorded. Although a plasma level of around 0.09 ppm F had been suggested as the upper limit before a kidney patient undergoing dialysis should reduce F intake, evidence for this recommendation has come from only a few case studies.[90] With today's standards for dialysate fluid, current medical opinion is that even persons with severe renal impairment can consume fluoridated water without ill effects as long as they are receiving regular dialysis treatment.

Aluminum, iron, and other minerals create greater technical problems for the renal dialysis process than does F. The standard for dialysate water set by the Association for the Advancement of Medical Instrumentation is that the F content should not exceed 0.2 ppm.[94] Water used in renal dialysis should first be treated by reverse osmosis, which is superior to the older process of deionization in that it removes F and other minerals almost entirely.[166]

Optimal Fluoride Intake

Frank McClure, a biochemist with the U.S. Public Health Service, estimated in 1943 that the "average daily diet" contained 1.0-1.5 mg F, or about 0.05 mg F/kg body weight per day in children up to 12 years of age.[118] McClure's estimate somehow came to be interpreted as the lower limit of the range of "optimal" F intake. A widely quoted 1974 report[56] suggested that 0.06 mg F/kg body weight per day was optimal, although this estimate was based only on a number of personal opinions. The intake range of 0.05-0.07 mg F/kg body weight per day was suggested as optimal in 1980[139]; this is equivalent to 3.5-4.9 mg F/day for a 70-kg (154-lb) man. For a 10-kg infant (22 lb; i.e., a 12- to 18-month-old child), this optimal intake is equivalent to 0.45-0.64 mg F/day. (By comparison, in the Iowa studies described earlier, the 90th percentile of daily F ingestion for 16-month-old children was found to be 0.775 mg.)

The National Research Council, the body that establishes recommended dietary allowances for the United States, classified F as a "beneficial element for humans" because of its positive impact on dental health.[134] The council at one time considered F an essential nutrient,[133] but it backed away from that position because an essential role for F in human growth studies could not be confirmed and because the physiologic mechanism by which F would influence growth was unknown. Available evidence did not justify classifying F as an essential element by accepted standards.[134] Nutritional requirements became recorded as *dietary reference intakes* in the late 1990s, with an "adequate intake" level for F set at 0.01 mg/day for children 0-6 months. For all ages above 6 months the adequate intake was set at 0.05 mg F/kg/day, so the absolute intake amount increases with increasing weight to a maximum for adults age 19 or older of 4 mg/day for males and 3 mg/day for females.[85,86] It was not clear on what these intake levels were based.

The discussions about "optimal" intake are vague about what this intake is optimal for. The implication is that this degree of ingestion is optimal for caries resistance, but as will be described later in this chapter, ingested F plays only a minor role in caries control relative to intra-oral F. It is also worth noting that McClure's 1943 comment was observational, although it somehow was turned into a recommendation over time. Empirical evidence suggests that F intake of 0.05-0.07 mg/F/kg/day in

childhood is a broad upper limit if unesthetic fluorosis is to be avoided.[20] There is no evidence to link this range of F ingestion with caries inhibition, so we suggest that the term *optimal intake* be dropped from common usage.

FLUORIDE AND HUMAN HEALTH
Early Studies

Quite a lot was known about F at the time of Dean's appointment to the NIH Hygiene Unit in 1933,[117] but details of a safe range of F intake for humans were sketchy. The first study relating bone fracture experience to the F concentration in home water supplies (a subject revisited in the 1990s) concluded that there was no relationship.[119] McClure then demonstrated the close relationship between urinary F concentrations and the F levels of domestic water.[121] His balance studies during World War II, in which young men lived in rooms maintained at varying temperatures and humidity levels and received varying amounts of F in food and water, led to the conclusion that the elimination of absorbed F via urine and perspiration is almost complete when the quantity absorbed does not exceed 4-5 mg daily.[125] McClure suggested that this may be the limit of F that could be ingested without "appreciable hazard" of excessive F storage in the body.

Higher F intakes were likely in communities such as Bartlett, Texas, however, where community water carried about 8 ppm F. A long-term study of the residents of Bartlett, conducted by a U.S. Public Health Service team, began in 1943. Apart from severe dental fluorosis, the study found no adverse effects of long-term ingestion of this high-F water,[105] although postmortem bone F concentrations were high. Numerous animal studies in the early years of water fluoridation[104,109,116,122,124,186-188] supported the results from studies in human populations.

Although not every possible hypothesis regarding F and human health was tested prior to initiation of controlled fluoridation, there was sufficient research evidence to provide reasonable assurance that controlled fluoridation, with up to 1.2 ppm F in the drinking water, could be instituted in North America without creating any public health hazard.

Mortality

For the United States as a whole, no differences could be found in 1949-50 death rates between 32 cities with 0.7 ppm F or more and 32 randomly selected nearby cities with 0.25 ppm F or less in the drinking water. Mortality rates were similar for cancer, heart disease, intracranial lesions, nephritis, and cirrhosis of the liver.[71] In 1979 mortality rates for 478 cities with populations of 25,000 or more were examined for the periods 1949-50, 1959-61, and 1969-71. Data were collected on total deaths as well as those attributed to cardiovascular disease, renal conditions, and cancer. No differences between fluoridated and nonfluoridated communities were found.[157]

Cancer

The 1979 mortality study[157] was conducted as a response to testimony before a congressional committee in 1975 by Burk and Yiamouyiannis that fluoridation led to an increase in cancer deaths.[19] Their argument was based on a comparison of mortality data for the 10 largest fluoridated American cities between 1950 and 1970 and mortality data for 10 selected nonfluoridated cities over the same period. The crude mortality data, unadjusted for age, sex, or race, showed a greater increase in cancer deaths in the fluoridated cities over the 20-year period. Criticism of this analysis was based on the inappropriateness of using crude mortality data, because the populations of the big cities during that 20-year period had become older and poorer, and had changed their ethnic composition. Yiamouyiannis and Burk repeated their work in 1977, this time with some age adjustment,[185] and claimed that their data still showed an excess of cancer deaths in the fluoridated cities. But a number of independent analyses of the same data were conducted in both Britain and the United States and employed more detailed age-sex-race adjustments; none could find a link between cancer incidence and consumption of fluoridated water.[47,52,82,137,149,167]

One result of the Burk-Yiamouyiannis testimony was that a congressional committee directed the National Cancer Institute to carry out animal studies on the potential carcinogenicity of F. The National Toxicology Program (NTP) was responsible for conducting these studies, which were performed with several animal species and used four concentration of F in the drinking water: 0, 11, 45, and 79 ppm F. (Use of extremely high levels of the test material is standard practice in toxicology studies to avoid having to use huge populations of animals.) The studies, which tested the effects of the water on the animals over 2 years, took longer than expected, but the NTP finally issued an extensive draft report in 1990. Although a number of different cancers occurred in both test and control animals, the report found "equivocal evidence" of an excess incidence of osteosarcoma, a rare form of bone cancer, in male rats of a particular strain.[171] Three of the four osteosarcomas were in the rats ingesting 79 ppm F; the fourth was at 45 ppm F. Subsequent review of the data by statisticians, as well as a public hearing and considerable media attention, did not change this gray-zone conclusion.

In response, the Assistant Secretary for Health incorporated the NTP findings into a broader review of F and the environment, conducted by a special committee appointed by the U.S. Public Health Service. This committee reached the following conclusion on cancer risk:

Optimal fluoridation of drinking water does not pose a detectable cancer risk to humans as evidenced by extensive human epidemiological data available to date, including the new studies prepared for this report. While the presence of fluoride in sources other than drinking water reduces the ability to discriminate between exposure in fluoridated as compared to non-fluoridated communities, no trends in cancer risk, including the risk of osteosarcoma, were attributed to the introduction of fluoride into drinking water in these new studies. During two time periods, 1973-1980 and 1981-1987, there was an unexplained increase of osteosarcoma in males under age 20. The reason for this increase remains to be clarified, but an extensive analysis reveals that it is unrelated to the introduction and duration of fluoridation.[172]

The NTP report raised some interesting issues about risk assessment in the modern environment. Bone cancer is not common: of the 538,000 estimated cancer deaths in the United States in 1994, some 1075 (0.19%) were bone cancers of all kinds.[16] Case-control studies present the difficulty of documenting precisely all F exposure during a person's lifetime, which biases the results of such studies toward the null hypothesis (i.e., imprecise data make it more likely that the null hypothesis cannot be rejected). Risk assessment studies can be conducted with animals, but the question always remains: what is the relevance of health effects in rats drinking water with 79 ppm F to humans drinking water with 1-4 ppm F? The marginal nature of the findings makes answering the question even more difficult. In addition, a large number of tests were conducted in the NTP studies, and statistical logic tells us that false results will occur about five times in each 100 tests (see Chapter 13). In epidemiologic research involving humans, neither ecologic studies[63,130] nor case-control studies[64,126] have found any association between osteosarcoma and previous F exposure.

Down Syndrome

A claim that water fluoridation caused an increase in the congenital malformation known as Down syndrome was put forward in a series of papers in the mid-1950s.[145-147] The studies claimed to show from birth records in Wisconsin and Illinois that the incidence of Down syndrome was higher in fluoridated than in nonfluoridated areas, but there were errors in the research design.[153] The most serious error was the assumption that the city of birth was the place of residence of the mother, which is clearly not the case for hospitals serving a large rural population. More rigorous independent studies in the United States and Britain have subsequently failed to show any correlation between fluoridation and Down syndrome.[14,53,54,135] A systematic review in 2001 reached the same conclusion.[184]

Bone Density, Fracture Experience, and Osteoporosis

Bone fragility conditions (e.g., preventing spontaneous vertebral fracture in the elderly as a result of osteoporosis) have been treated for years with high doses of F combined with calcium, estrogen, and vitamin D. Controlled clinical trials have shown that high doses of F (30-60 mg/day), administered under medical supervision, can increase vertebral bone mass and reduce the vertebral fracture rate.[142] These favorable changes do not come without problems, however, for the new bone can be imperfectly mineralized, and a good proportion of patients do not respond to treatment.[74] Treatment also seems ineffective in preventing further fractures in patients who already have a fracture at first

presentation.[99] The main concern is that the positive effects seen in the vertebral column, which is mostly cancellous bone, are not seen in the appendicular skeleton, which is mostly cortical bone. Indeed, fracture rates in the appendicular skeleton have actually been shown to increase with intensive F treatment.[73,148] Although an international conference in 1988 recommended F treatment for vertebral crush syndrome,[74] high-dose F treatment (up to 80 mg F/day) for bone fragility conditions is no longer recommended in the United States,[78,98] nor is F therapy seen as a measure that can prevent fractures resulting from osteoporosis.[73,129]

These studies answer one prominent question about the health effects of F: they show that even frail elderly people can tolerate large F intakes (e.g., 30-60 mg F/day), vastly higher than anyone would experience with fluoridated drinking water. A more pertinent issue in dentistry is the effect of fluoridated water on bone fragility or fracture experience. Day-to-day use of fluoridated water obviously results in much lower daily intakes (1-3 mg F/day for adults, see earlier) than those seen at the therapeutic doses just described.

In the research by McClure mentioned earlier, McClure studied the relation between self-reported bone fracture experience and exposure to fluoridated water among young men during World War II and reported no association. As in other early studies,[13,66] no account was taken of confounding factors such as body mass, medication use, and dietary factors, and the radiographic techniques of that era have been shown to be insensitive. In more recent times, a series of ecologic studies (see Chapter 13) to assess the risk of bone fracture in those drinking fluoridated water have produced mixed results: decreased risk,[77,87,103,144,158] no association,[5,92,108,111,168] and increased risk.[29,31,88,89] The extent of increased risk in the latter group of studies was generally low, with relative risks in the range of 1.08-1.41. Given the lack of precision that is part of ecologic studies, it is not surprising that this body of research does not yield clear conclusions for either increased risk or a protective effect of F. Extensive reviews of the literature have also reached the conclusion that no relationship can be discerned between bone fracture experience and exposure to water with 1 ppm F.[3,46,78,91,97,98]

Results of research in which data are collected from individual study participants are likely to have higher validity than results of ecologic studies. Studies conducted in several rural Iowa communities found reduced radial bone mass and slightly higher fracture experience in a town where the drinking water contained 4.0 ppm F.[162,163] However, a study of some 2000 women in western Pennsylvania found no association between long-term exposure to water fluoridated at a lower level (1.0 ppm F) and bone mineral density and fracture experience.[24] A small Canadian study found only beneficial effects on skeletal growth from growing up in a fluoridated area.[6]

Research continues, but it can be stated that the evidence supports only marginal benefits to bone from fluoridated water, and there is no evidence that bone fracture experience is altered by exposure to drinking water containing 1.0 ppm F.[132]

Child Development

An important study of the effect of F on children was the Newburgh-Kingston fluoridation project, one of the original fluoridation field trials, which began in 1945. Participating children received a complete physical examination, selected physical measurements were taken, and laboratory and radiographic studies were performed. No significant differences in general health or body processes between children in the two cities were seen, and no radiographic differences in bone density could be demonstrated. There was essential similarity in vision and hearing test results and in measures of skeletal maturation, hemoglobin level, erythrocyte and leukocyte counts, and quantity of sugar, albumin, red blood cells, and casts in the urine. At the final examination, 19 of 476 children in fluoridated Newburgh (4.0%) and 20 of 405 children in non-fluoridated Kingston (4.9%) were referred to their family physicians for conditions including such minor ailments as plantar wart or ringworm. Long-term downward trends in stillbirths and maternal and infant mortality rates continued in each of the cities. The overall conclusion reached was that no differences of medical significance could be found between the two groups of children.[156]

As part of the main health study in the Newburgh-Kingston fluoridation project, 100 boys in each city, age 12 at final medical examination, were selected from the 881 participants in both cities for a substudy of specific urinary components.[155] Children who had recently been ill were excluded because results could otherwise have been confounded by a variety of unrelated conditions. No difference between the two populations was found.

FLUORIDE TOXICITY

There is a world of difference (literally!) between a single intake of 5.0 g F and constant intake of 1-3 mg F daily. F is thus like many other nutrients: beneficial in small amounts, toxic in high amounts. This gradation in response with variations in dose is a common pharmaceutical phenomenon and is known as a *dose-response relationship*.

Information on F toxicity levels cannot, of course, be taken from controlled studies with humans. Available data come from a mix of case studies of various kinds and research on workers in certain industrial processes. The classic work in occupational F toxicity is that of the Danish scientist Kaj Roholm, who studied cryolite workers in aluminum plants during the 1930s. Their daily absorption was estimated at 0.2-1.0 mg F/kg body weight (about 14-68 mg F/day for a 150-lb adult). Some workers had been employed as long as 31 years. Under these conditions a number of toxic effects were observed, principally gastric complaints and osteosclerosis.

Ingestion of a single dose of 5-10 g of NaF by an adult male (32-64 mg F/kg body weight) results in a rather unpleasant death in 2-4 hours if first aid is not rendered immediately. From that lower limit of 32 mg F/kg body weight, the estimated equivalent dose for a 10-kg child (12-18 months old) is 320 mg F.[75] Crippling skeletal fluorosis can eventually occur in an adult with daily ingestion of 10-25 mg F over a period of 10-20 years. The evidence on known toxic effects of F ingestion is summarized in Table 24-2.

If an individual is known or suspected to have taken a potentially toxic amount of F, first aid is to induce vomiting as quickly as possible or to have the person ingest a material to bind F: milk is usually the most readily available. The American Dental Association recommends, as a safety precaution, that F materials for home use contain no more than 264 mg F if packaged in a bulk container (tablets, mouthrinse) or up to 300 mg F if the F material is individually packaged.

At the other end of the toxicity spectrum, there are many instances of remarkable toleration of high quantities of F without ill effects, such as in osteoporosis patients as described earlier. Adverse effects in these patients are reported to be usually no worse than nausea, stomach pains, pain in the extremities, and occasional diarrhea. The greatly elevated levels of plasma F may also be associated with some arthritis-type joint pain, but it is not certain whether this pain comes from the treatment or the disease itself.

DENTAL FLUOROSIS

Dental fluorosis is a permanent hypomineralization of enamel that is characterized by greater surface and subsurface porosity than in normal enamel and that results from exposure of the developing tooth to excess F during maturational stages.[58] Its distribution and risk factors are described in Chapter 22.

FLUORIDE AND CARIES CONTROL: MECHANISMS OF ACTION

F works best to prevent caries when a constant, low level of F is maintained in the oral cavity.[27] Its most important caries-inhibitory action is posteruptive and takes place at the plaque-enamel interface.[57] The action of F in preventing caries is multifactorial; its effect comes from a combination of several mechanisms. Three major mechanisms of action have been identified, summarized in Box 24-1, although some possible additional mechanisms have been hypothesized.

It has long been held that preeruptive exposure to F inhibits caries to some degree. In this "preeruptive" model, F is said to act by becoming incorporated into the developing enamel hydroxyapatite crystal and thus reducing enamel solubility. It has been argued that preeruptive benefits are especially important for reducing pit-and-fissure lesions.[69] This caries-preventive action by F was assumed for many years to be F's primary effect, but the actual supportive evidence is largely associative. Any preeruptive effect on caries inhibition is likely to be minor; the evidence for posteruptive F action is much stronger.

Table 24-2 Degrees of potentially toxic ingestion of fluoride

Effect	Fluoride Intake and Time*
Acute fatal poisoning, adults[79]	2.5-5.0 g, in 2-4 hr
Acute fatal poisoning, 10-kg child[75]	320 mg, in 2-4 hr
Acute fatal poisoning, 3-year-old child[83]	Approximately 435 mg, in approximately 3 hr
Acute fatal poisoning, adult renal dialysis patient[61]	Dialysate fluid 35-50 ppm F, for 3 hr
Acute fatal poisoning, adult male[65]	17.9 mg F/kg body weight, for 24 hr
Short-term nonserious nausea in elementary school children[81]	93-375 ppm F in drinking water, small amounts; symptoms within 30 minutes
Nausea and vomiting in adults[176]	Nausea with ingestion of an estimated 80 mg F over a few hours, vomiting from ingestion of an estimated 143 mg F over a few hours
Severe skeletal fluorosis[79]	10-25 mg F daily, for 10-20 yr
Osteosclerosis, radiographic changes in human bone[80]	8-20 mg F daily, for 10-20 yr
Dental fluorosis[59]	<0.1 mg F/kg body weight/day during tooth development (i.e., the first 8 yr)
Acute fatal poisoning in animals[79]	Approximately 50 mg F/kg body weight
Interference with reproduction, thyroid disturbance, loss of body weight, and lameness in cattle[79]	40-60 ppm F in feed daily for several years

*With drinking water fluoridated at 1 ppm, an adult would have to drink 660 gal in 2-4 hr to reach the lower limit of a fatal dose. A 10-kg child (12-18 mo old) would have to drink 85 gal in 2-4 hr. Severe skeletal fluorosis could only result from drinking 2.6-6.6 gal of water daily for 10-20 yr if none of the fluoride were excreted.

BOX 24-1 Three Principal Mechanisms By Which Fluoride Inhibits the Development of Dental Caries

Posteruptive
1. Promotion of remineralization and inhibition of demineralization of early carious lesions.
2. Inhibition of glycolysis, the process by which cariogenic bacteria metabolize fermentable carbohydrates.

Preeruptive
3. Some reduction in enamel solubility in acid by preeruptive incorporation of fluoride into the hydroxyapatite crystal.

Fluoride and Plaque

The topical effect of a constant infusion of low-concentration F into the oral cavity, such as occurs with drinking fluoridated water or regularly brushing with a F toothpaste, is to inhibit demineralization and enhance remineralization during the repeated cycles of demineralization and remineralization (that awkward phrase is often shortened to *demin-remin*) in the early stages of the carious process. F introduced into the mouth is partly taken up by dental plaque, in which some 95% of it is held in bound form rather than as ionic F. Plaque contains 5-10 mg F/kg wet weight in low-F areas and some 10-20 mg F/kg wet weight in fluoridated areas. The bound F can be released in response to lowered pH,[169] and F is taken up more readily by demineralized enamel than by sound enamel.[179] The availability of plaque F to respond to the acid challenge leads to the gradual establishment of a well-crystallized and more acid-resistant apatite in the enamel surface during demin-remin.[25,95,170] This means that F can be incorporated into the enamel crystal, but more through cycles of demin-remin than through preeruptive absorption.

F in plaque also inhibits glycolysis, the process through which fermentable carbohydrate is metabolized by cariogenic bacteria to produce acid. F from drinking water and toothpaste concentrates in plaque, where its concentration is governed by the concentration of plaque calcium.[183] Plaque contains higher levels of F than does saliva.[72,160] There is also some evidence that plaque F can inhibit the production of extracellular polysaccharide by cariogenic bacteria, a necessary process for plaque adherence to smooth enamel surfaces.[72]

In addition to these mechanisms, high-concentration F gels may have a specific bactericidal action on cariogenic bacteria in the plaque. These gels also leave a temporary layer of a material resembling CaF_2 on the enamel surface, which is available for release when the pH drops at the enamel surface.[136] At lower concentrations, *Streptococcus mutans* has been shown under laboratory conditions to become less acidogenic through adaptation to an environment in which F is constantly present.[17,18,114,151] It is not yet known whether this ecologic adaptation reduces the cariogenicity of acidogenic bacteria in humans.[173]

Fluoride and Enamel

In the early days of F research, it was assumed that F's inhibition of caries depended on its preeruptive incorporation into developing dental enamel, which thus reduced enamel solubility in demineralizing acids.[38,123] In most of the early fluoridation studies, greater caries reductions were found in children who were born after fluoridation began than in those for whom fluoridation began after birth.[23,62,67,84,93] But it was also clear that caries inhibition occurred in teeth that had already erupted when fluoridation began[7,9,100,101,152] and in first molars that were erupting when fluoridation began.[10,12,154]

It became evident to researchers as early as the mid-1970s that a higher concentration of F in enamel could not by itself explain the extensive reductions in caries that F produced.[106] At a depth of 2 μm, enamel F concentrations averaged around 1700 ppm in nonfluoridated areas and 2200-3200 in areas fluoridated at 1 ppm. Even in areas with 5-7 ppm F, enamel F concentrations rose only to 4800 ppm,[1] which shows that enamel F is poorly correlated with water F levels. If the preeruptive hypothesis were true (i.e., preeruptive F uptake by developing enamel is the major factor in F's cariostatic effects), one would expect caries experience in a population to be inversely related to enamel F concentrations, but such is not the case.[27] The converse also holds; that is, it has been observed that higher concentrations of enamel F do not necessarily mean than caries will not occur.[4] The theoretical concentration of F in pure fluorapatite that would reduce its acid solubility is around 38,000 ppm,[177] a concentration that is not even approached in human dental enamel. So although some preeruptive effect of F can be inferred from field studies,[21,48] any such action is likely to be a minor part of the overall impact of F.

The most revealing epidemiologic study on the caries-inhibitory action of F came from the Tiel-Culemborg fluoridation study in the Netherlands,[68] in which caries was recorded as (1) incipient lesions confined to enamel, and (2) dentinal lesions. Although, as would be expected, there were considerably fewer dentinal lesions in fluoridated Tiel than in nonfluoridated Culemborg after 15 years of fluoridation, there was no difference between the two communities in lesions confined to enamel. This finding means that fewer enamel lesions progress to dentinal caries in a fluoridated area than in a nonfluoridated area. F does not prevent the *initial* carious attack, which would be expected if its presence in the enamel crystal increased enamel resistance to acid dissolution, but rather the F in the oral cavity acts to inhibit further demineralization of the lesion and to promote its remineralization.

Fluoride and Saliva

Resting salivary F concentrations are low, although they are some three times higher in fluoridated than in nonfluoridated areas. In a fluoridated area, salivary F levels averaged 0.016 ppm, whereas they were 0.006 ppm in a nonfluoridated area.[138] Fluctuation of salivary F levels is normal, and after toothbrushing with an F toothpaste or mouthrinsing with an F solution, salivary F levels can rise 100- to 1000-fold. This level rapidly drops back to normal, and the saliva is likely to be an important source of plaque F during this time.[150] The role of saliva in caries inhibition is still not well defined.

Effects on Different Tooth Surfaces

One of the observations from early fluoridation studies in the Netherlands and New Zealand was that caries reductions were greatest for the free smooth surfaces and proximal surfaces of teeth and were less pronounced for pit-and-fissure surfaces.[12,110] Murray's study of 15-year-olds in naturally fluoridated Hartlepool and nonfluoridated York, England, found that those

in Hartlepool had a mean DMF (decayed, missing, and filled) score of 4.96, whereas those in York had a mean DMF of 8.95. However, the number of carious approximal surfaces of molars was 11 times greater in York.[131] This pattern of more pronounced effect on smooth surfaces than on pit-and-fissure surfaces has since become a standard finding in studies in which caries is recorded for tooth surfaces.[11] It follows that when DMFS (decayed, missing, and filled surface) scores are declining in a population, the proportion of all decayed surfaces that are pit-and-fissure surfaces will increase, even though the absolute number may diminish.

EFFECTIVE USE OF FLUORIDE

Categorizing F compounds into "systemic fluorides" and "topical fluorides" is not easily done because the line between these categories gets blurred: "systemic" vehicles like water fluoridation and F supplements have been shown to have topical cariostatic action, and some "topical" vehicles like F toothpaste can be swallowed inadvertently and have systemic effects (fluorosis). As stated earlier, the evidence shows that the most effective community-wide use of F is in frequent, low-concentration intraoral exposures such as in drinking water or toothpaste.[4,57,113,178] Less frequent application of high-concentration gels has its place in the care of highly caries-susceptible patients.

The most cost-effective way of reaching an entire community with regular, low-concentration F is through water fluoridation. This is true public health action, and it is also one that has stirred public controversy. The unique position of water fluoridation as a public health action is the subject of the next chapter.

REFERENCES

1. Aasenden R. Fluoride concentrations in the surface tooth enamel of young men and women. Arch Oral Biol 1974;19:697-701.
2. Ainsworth NJ. Mottled teeth. Br Dent J 1933;55:233-50.
3. Allolio B, Lehmann R. Drinking water fluoridation and bone. Exp Clin Endocrinol Diabetes 1999;107:12-20.
4. Arends J, Christoffersen J. Nature and role of loosely bound fluoride in dental caries. J Dent Res 1990;69(Spec Issue):601-5.
5. Arnala I, Alhava EM, Kivivuori R, Kauranen P. Hip fracture incidence not affected by fluoridation. Osteofluorosis studies in Finland. Acta Orthop Scand 1986; 57:344-8.

6. Arnold CM, Bailey DA, Faulkner RA, et al. The effect of water fluoridation on the bone mineral density of young women. Can J Public Health 1997;88:388-91.

7. Arnold FA Jr, Dean HT, Knutson JW. Effect of fluoridated public water supplies on dental caries incidence. Results of the seventh year of study at Grand Rapids and Muskegon, Mich. Public Health Rep 1953;68:141-8.

8. Ast DB. The caries-fluorine hypothesis and a suggested study to test its application. Public Health Rep 1943;857-79.

9. Ast DB, Chase HC. The Newburgh-Kingston caries fluorine study. IV. Dental findings after six years of fluoridation. Oral Surg 1953;6:114-23.

10. Backer Dirks O. The relation between the fluoridation of water and dental caries experience. Int Dent J 1967;17:582-605.

11. Backer Dirks O. The benefits of water fluoridation. Caries Res 1974;8(Suppl 1):2-15.

12. Backer Dirks O, Houwink B, Kwant GW. The result of 6½ years of artificial drinking water in the Netherlands; the Tiel-Culemborg experiment. Arch Oral Biol 1961;5:284-300.

13. Bernstein DS, Sadowsky N, Hegsted DM, et al. Prevalence of osteoporosis in high- and low-fluoride areas in North Dakota. JAMA 1966;198:499-504.

14. Berry WTC. A study of the incidence of mongolism in relation to the fluoride content of water. Am J Ment Defic 1958;62:634-6.

15. Black GV, McKay FS. Mottled teeth—an endemic developmental imperfection of the teeth heretofore unknown in the literature of dentistry. Dent Cosmos 1916;58:129-56.

16. Boring CC, Squires TS, Tong T, Montgomery S. Cancer statistics, 1994. CA Cancer J Clin 1994;44:7-26.

17. Bowden GHW. Effects of fluoride on the microbial ecology of dental plaque. J Dent Res 1990;69(Spec Issue): 653-9.

18. Bowden GHW, Odlum O, Nolette N, Hamilton IR. Microbial populations growing in the presence of fluoride at low pH isolated from dental plaque of children living in an area with fluoridated water. Infect Immun 1982;36:247-54.

19. Burk D, Yiamouyiannis J. Fluoridation and cancer. 94th Congress, first session. Congress Record 1975 July 21;121:7172-6.

20. Burt BA. The changing patterns of systemic fluoride intake. J Dent Res 1992;71:1228-37.

21. Burt BA, Eklund SA, Loesche WJ. Dental benefits of limited exposure to fluoridated water in childhood. J Dent Res 1986;61:1322-5.

22. Buzalaf MA, Granjeiro JM, Damante CA, de Ornelas F. Fluoride content of infant formulas prepared with deionized, bottled mineral and fluoridated drinking water. ASDC J Dent Child 2001;68:37-41.

23. Carlos JP, Gittelsohn AM, Waddon W Jr. Caries in deciduous teeth in relation to maternal ingestion of fluoride. Public Health Rep 1962;77:658-60.

24. Cauley JA, Murphy PA, Riley TJ, Buhari AM. Effects of fluoridated drinking water on bone mass and fractures: The study of osteoporotic fractures. J Bone Miner Res 1995;10:1076-86.

25. Chow LC. Tooth-bound fluoride and dental caries. J Dent Res 1990;69(Spec Issue):595-600.

26. Churchill HV. Occurrence of fluorides in some waters of the United States. J Ind Eng Chem 1931;23:996-8.

27. Clarkson BH, Fejerskov O, Ekstrand J, Burt BA. Rational use of fluorides in caries control. In: Fejerskov O, Ekstrand J, Burt BA, eds: Fluorides in dentistry. 2nd ed. Copenhagen: Munksgaard, 1996:347-57.

28. Clovis J, Hargreaves JA. Fluoride intake from beverage consumption. Community Dent Oral Epidemiol 1988; 16:11-5.

29. Cooper C, Wickham CA, Barker DJ, Jacobsen SJ. Water fluoridation and hip fracture [letter]. JAMA 1991;266:513-4.

30. Dabeka RW, McKenzie AD, Lacroix GM. Dietary intakes of lead, cadmium, arsenic and fluoride by Canadian adults: A 24-hour duplicate diet study. Food Addit Contam 1987;4:89-101.

31. Danielson C, Lyon JL, Egger M, Goodenough GK. Hip fractures and fluoridation in Utah's elderly population. JAMA 1992;268:746-8.

32. Dean HT. Distribution of mottled enamel in the United States. Public Health Rep 1933;48:703-34.

33. Dean HT. Classification of mottled enamel diagnosis. J Am Dent Assoc 1934;21:1421-6.

34. Dean HT. Chronic endemic dental fluorosis (mottled enamel). JAMA 1936;107:1269-72.

35. Dean HT. Endemic fluorosis and its relation to dental caries. Public Health Rep 1938;53:1443-52.

36. Dean HT. The investigation of physiological effects by the epidemiological method. In: Moulton FR, ed: Fluorine and dental health. Washington DC: American Association for the Advancement of Science, 1942: 23-31.

37. Dean HT, Arnold FA Jr, Elvove E. Domestic water and dental caries. V. Additional studies of the relation of fluoride domestic waters to dental caries experience in 4,425 white children aged 12-14 years of 13 cities in 4 states. Public Health Rep 1942;57:1155-79.

38. Dean HT, Dixon RM, Cohen C. Mottled enamel in Texas. Public Health Rep 1935;50:424-42.

39. Dean HT, Elvove E. Studies on the minimal threshold of the dental sign of chronic endemic fluorosis (mottled enamel). Public Health Rep 1935;50: 1719-29.

40. Dean HT, Elvove E. Some epidemiological aspects of chronic endemic dental fluorosis. Am J Public Health 1936;26:567-75.

41. Dean HT, Elvove E. Further studies on the minimal threshold of chronic endemic dental fluorosis. Public Health Rep 1937;52:1249-64.

42. Dean HT, Elvove E, Poston RF. Mottled enamel in South Dakota. Public Health Rep 1939;54:212-28.

43. Dean HT, Jay P, Arnold FA Jr, Elvove E. Domestic water and dental caries. II. A study of 2,832 white children aged 12-14 years, of eight suburban Chicago communities, including *L. acidophilus* studies of 1,761 children. Public Health Rep 1941;56:761-92.

44. Dean HT, Jay P, Arnold FA Jr, et al. Domestic water and dental caries, including certain epidemiological aspects of oral *L. acidophilus*. Public Health Rep 1939;54: 862-88.

45. Dean HT, McKay FS. Production of mottled enamel halted by a change in common water supply. Am J Public Health 1939;29:590-6.

46. Demos LL, Kazda H, Cicuttini FM, et al. Water fluoridation, osteoporosis, fractures—recent developments. Aust Dent J 2001;46:80-7.

47. Doll R, Kinlen L. Fluoridation of water and cancer mortality in the U.S.A. Lancet 1977;1:1300-2.

48. Driscoll WS, Heifetz SB, Brunelle JA. Caries preventive effects of fluoride tablets in school children four years after discontinuation of treatments. J Am Dent Assoc 1981;103:878-81.

49. Ehrnebo M, Ekstrand J. Occupational fluoride exposure and plasma fluoride levels in man. Int Arch Occup Environ Health 1986;58:179-90.

50. Ekstrand J. Fluoride metabolism. In: Fejerskov O, Ekstrand J, Burt BA, eds: Fluoride in dentistry. Copenhagen: Munksgaard, 1996:55-68.

51. Ekstrand J, Ehrnebo M. The relationship between plasma fluoride, urinary excretion rate and urine fluoride concentration in man. J Occup Med 1983;25: 745-8.

52. Erickson JD. Mortality in selected cities with fluoridated and nonfluoridated water supplies. N Engl J Med 1978;298:112-6.

53. Erickson JD. Down syndrome, water fluoridation, and maternal age. Teratology 1980;21:177-80.

54. Erickson JD, Oakley GP Jr, Flynt JW Jr, Hay S. Water fluoridation and congenital malformations: No association. J Am Dent Assoc 1976;93:981-4.

55. Ericsson Y, Malmnas C. Placental transfer of fluorine investigated with F18 in man and rabbit. Acta Obstet Gynecol Scand 1962;41:144-58.

56. Farkas CS, Farkas EJ. Potential effect of food processing on the fluoride content of infant foods. Sci Total Environ 1974;2:399-405.

57. Featherstone JD. Prevention and reversal of dental caries: Role of low level fluoride. Community Dent Oral Epidemiol 1999;27:31-40.

58. Fejerskov O, Manji F, Baelum V. The nature and mechanisms of dental fluorosis in man. J Dent Res 1990;69 (Spec Issue):692-700.

59. Fejerskov O, Stephen KW, Richards A, Speirs R. Combined effect of systemic and topical fluoride treatments on human deciduous teeth—case studies. Caries Res 1987;21:452-9.

60. Filippo FA, Battistone GC. The fluoride content of a representative diet of the young adult male. Clin Chim Acta 1971;31:453-7.

61. Fluoride intoxication in a dialysis unit—Maryland. MMWR 1980;29:134-6.

62. Forrest JR, James PMC. A blind study of enamel opacities and dental caries prevalence after eight years of fluoridation of water. Br Dent J 1965;119:319-22.

63. Freni SC, Gaylor DW. International trends in the incidence of bone cancer are not related to drinking water fluoridation. Cancer 1992;70:611-8.

64. Gelberg KH, Fitzgerald EF, Hwang S, Dubrow R. Fluoride exposure and childhood osteosarcoma; a case-control study. Am J Public Health 1995;85:1678-83.

65. Gessner BD, Beller M, Middaugh JP, Whitford GM. Acute fluoride poisoning from a public water system. N Engl J Med 1994;330:95-9.

66. Goggin JE, Haddon W Jr, Hambly GS, Hoveland JR. Incidence of femoral fractures in postmenopausal women. Public Health Rep 1965;80:1005-11.

67. Grainger RM, Coburn CI. Dental caries of the first molars and the age of children when first consuming naturally fluoridated water. Can J Public Health 1955; 46:347-54.

68. Groeneveld A. Longitudinal study of the prevalence of enamel lesions in a fluoridated and a non-fluoridated area. Community Dent Oral Epidemiol 1985;13: 159-63.

69. Groeneveld A, Van Eck AAMJ, Backer Dirks O. Fluoride in caries prevention: Is the effect pre- or post-eruptive? J Dent Res 1990;69(Spec Issue):751-5.

70. Haftenberger M, Viergutz G, Neumeister V, Hetzer G. Total fluoride intake and urinary excretion in German children aged 3-6 years. Caries Res 2001;35:451-7.

71. Hagan TL, Pasternack M, Scholz G. Waterborne fluorides and mortality. Public Health Rep 1954;69:450-4.

72. Hamilton IR. Biochemical effects of fluoride on oral bacteria. J Dent Res 1990;69(Spec Issue):660-7.

73. Haguenauer D, Welch V, Shea B, et al. Fluoride for the treatment of postmenopausal osteoporotic fractures: A meta-analysis. Osteoporosis Int 2000;11:727-38.

74. Heaney RP, Baylink DJ, Johnston CC Jr, et al. Fluoride therapy for the vertebral crush fracture syndrome. A status report. Ann Intern Med 1989;111:678-80.

75. Heifetz SB, Horowitz HS. Amounts of fluoride in self-administered dental products: Safety considerations for children. Pediatrics 1986;77:876-82.

76. Heilman JR, Kiritsy MC, Levy SM, Wefel JS. Assessing fluoride levels of carbonated soft drinks. J Am Dent Assoc 1999;130:1593-9.

77. Hillier S, Cooper C, Kellingray S, et al. Fluoride in drinking water and risk of hip fracture in the UK: A case-control study. Lancet 2000;355:265-9.

78. Hillier S, Inskip H, Coggon D, Cooper C. Water fluoridation and osteoporotic fracture. Community Dent Health 1996;13(Suppl 2):63-8.

79. Hodge HC. The safety of fluoride tablets or drops. In: Johansen E, Taves DR, Olsen TO, eds: Continuing evaluation of the use of fluorides. AAAS Selected Symposium No. 11. Boulder CO: Westview, 1979:253-74.

80. Hodge HC, Smith FA. Fluorine chemistry. Vol 4 of a series, Simons JH, ed. New York: Academic Press, 1965.

81. Hoffman R, Mann J, Calderone J, et al. Acute poisoning in a New Mexico elementary school. Pediatrics 1980; 65:897-900.

82. Hoover RN, McKay FW, Fraumeni JF. Fluoridated drinking water and the occurrence of cancer. J Natl Cancer Inst 1976;57:757-68.

83. Horowitz HS. Abusive use of fluoride [editorial]. J Public Health Dent 1977;37:106-7.

84. Horowitz HS, Heifetz SB. Effects of prenatal exposure to fluoridation on dental caries. Public Health Rep 1967; 82:297-304.

85. Institute of Medicine, Food and Nutrition Board. Dietary reference intakes: Calcium, phosphorus, magnesium, vitamin D, and fluoride. Washington DC: National Academy Press, 1997:288-313.

86. Institute of Medicine, Food and Nutrition Board. Dietary reference intakes: Applications in dietary planning. Washington DC: National Academy Press, 2003.

87. Jacobsen SJ, O'Fallon WM, Melton LJ 3rd. Hip fracture incidence before and after the fluoridation of the public water supply, Rochester, Minnesota. Am J Public Health 1993;83:743-5.

88. Jacobsen SJ, Goldberg J, Cooper C, Lockwood SA. The association between water fluoridation and hip fracture among white women and men aged 65 years and older. A national ecologic study. Ann Epidemiol 1992;2:617-26.

89. Jacobsen SJ, Goldberg J, Miles TP, et al. Regional variation in the incidence of hip fracture: US white women aged 65 years and older. JAMA 1990;264:500-2.

90. Johnson WJ, Taves DR, Jowsey J. Fluoridation and bone disease in renal patients. In: Johansen E, Taves DR, Olsen TO, eds: Continuing evaluation of the use of fluorides. AAAS Selected Symposium No 11. Boulder CO: Westview, 1979:275-93.

91. Jones G, Riley M, Couper D, Dwyer T. Water fluoridation, bone mass and fracture: A quantitative overview of the literature. Aust N Z J Public Health 1999;23:34-40.

92. Karagas MR, Baron JA, Barrett JA, Jacobsen SJ. Patterns of fracture among the United States elderly: Geographic and fluoride effects. Ann Epidemiol 1996;6:209-16.

93. Katz S, Muhler JC. Prenatal and postnatal fluoride and dental caries experience in deciduous teeth. J Am Dent Assoc 1968;76:305-11.

94. Keshiviah P. Water treatment for hemodialysis. In: Henderson LW, Thuma RS, eds: Quality assurance in dialysis. Dordrecht: Kluwer, 1994:85-107.

95. Kidd EA, Thylstrup A, Fejerskov O, Bruun C. Influence of fluoride in surface enamel and degree of dental fluorosis on caries development in vitro. Caries Res 1980;14:196-202.

96. Kiritsy MC, Levy SM, Warren JJ, et al. Assessing fluoride concentrations of juices and juice-flavored drinks. J Am Dent Assoc 1996;127:895-902.

97. Kleerekoper M. Fluoride and the skeleton. Crit Rev Clin Lab Sci 1996;33:139-61.

98. Kleerekoper M. The role of fluoride in the prevention of osteoporosis. Endocrinol Metab Clin North Am 1998;27:441-52.

99. Kleerekoper M, Mendlovic DB. Sodium fluoride therapy of postmenopausal osteoporosis. Endocr Rev 1993;14:312-23.

100. Klein H. Dental caries in relocated children exposed to water containing fluorine. I. Incidence of new caries after 2 years of exposure among previously caries-free permanent teeth. Public Health Rep 1945;60:1462-7.

101. Klein H. Dental caries (DMF) experience in relocated children exposed to water containing fluorine. II. J Am Dent Assoc 1946;33:1136-41.

102. Kramer L, Osis D, Wiatrowski E, Spencer H. Dietary fluoride in different areas of the United States. Am J Clin Nutr 1974;27:590-4.

103. Lehmann R, Wapniarz M, Hofmann B, et al. Drinking water fluoridation: Bone mineral density and hip fracture incidence. Bone 1998;22:273-8.

104. Leone NC, Geever IF, Moran NC. Acute and subacute toxicity studies of sodium fluoride in animals. Public Health Rep 1956;71:459-67.

105. Leone NC, Shimkin MB, Arnold FA, et al. Medical aspects of excessive fluoride in the water supply. Public Health Rep 1954;69:925-36.

106. Levine RS. The action of fluoride in caries prevention; a review of current concepts. Br Dent J 1976;140:9-14

107. Levy SM, Warren JJ, Davis CS, et al. Patterns of fluoride intake from birth to 36 months. J Public Health Dent 2001;61:70-7.

108. Li Y, Liang C, Slemenda CW, et al. Effect of long-term exposure to fluoride in drinking water on risks of bone fractures. J Bone Miner Res 2001;16:932-9.

109. Likins RC, Scow R, Zipkin I, Steere AC. Deposition and retention of fluoride and radiocalcium in the growing rat. Am J Physiol 1959;197:75-80.

110. Ludwig TG. The Hastings Fluoridation Project. V. Dental effects between 1954 and 1964. N Z Dent J 1965;61:175-9.

111. Madans J, Kleinman JC, Cornoni-Huntley J. The relationship between hip fracture and water fluoridation: An analysis of national data. Am J Public Health 1983;73:296-8.

112. Manji F, Kapila S. Fluorides and fluorosis in Kenya. Part I: The occurrence of fluorides. Odontostomatol Trop 1986;9:15-20.

113. Margolis HC, Moreno EC. Physicochemical perspectives on the cariostatic mechanisms of systemic and topical fluorides. J Dent Res 1990;69(Spec Issue):606-13.

114. Marquis RE. Diminished acid tolerance of plaque bacteria caused by fluoride. J Dent Res 1990;69(Spec Issue):672-5.

115. Martinez-Mier EA, Soto-Rojas AE, Urena-Cirett JL, et al. Fluoride intake from foods, beverages and dentifrice by children in Mexico. Community Dent Oral Epidemiol 2003;31:221-30.

116. McCann HG, Bullock FA. The effect of fluoride ingestion on the composition and solubility of mineralized tissues of the rat. J Dent Res 1957;36:391-8.

117. McClure FJ. A review of fluorine and its physiological effects. Physiol Rev 1933;13:277-300.

118. McClure FJ. Ingestion of fluoride and dental caries. Quantitative relations based on food and water requirements of children 1 to 12 years old. Am J Dis Child 1943;66:362-9.

119. McClure FJ. Fluoride domestic waters and systemic effects. I. Relation to bone-fracture experience, height and weight of high school boys and young selectees of the armed forces of the United States. Public Health Rep 1944;59:1543-58.

120. McClure FJ. Water fluoridation; the search and the victory. Bethesda MD: National Institutes of Health, 1970:12-29.

121. McClure FJ, Kinser CA. Fluoride domestic waters and systemic effects. II. Fluorine content of urine in relation to fluorine in drinking water. Public Health Rep 1944;59:1575-91.

122. McClure FJ, Kornberg A. Blood hemoglobin and hematocrit results on rats ingesting sodium fluoride. J Pharmacol Exp Ther 1947;89:77-80.

123. McClure FJ, Likins RC. Fluorine in human teeth studied in relation to fluorine in the drinking water. J Dent Res 1951;30:172-6.

124. McClure FJ, Mitchell HH. The effect of fluorine on the calcium metabolism of albino rats and the composition of the bones. J Biol Chem 1931;60:297.

125. McClure FJ, Mitchell HH, Hamilton TS, Kinser CA. Balances of fluorine ingested from various sources in food and water by five young men. Excretion of fluorine through the skin. J Ind Hyg Toxicol 1945;27: 159-70.

126. McGuire SM, Vanable ED, McGuire MH, et al. Is there a link between fluoridated water and osteosarcoma? J Am Dent Assoc 1991;122:38-45.

127. McKay FS. The relation of mottled enamel to caries. J Am Dent Assoc 1928;15:1429-37.

128. McKay FS. Mottled enamel: The prevention of its further production through a change of water supply at Oakley, Idaho. J Am Dent Assoc 1933;20:1137-49.

129. Melton LJ 3rd. Fluoride in the prevention of osteoporosis and fractures. J Bone Miner Res 1990;5(Suppl 1):S163-S167.

130. Moss ME, Kanarek MS, Anderson HA, et al. Osteosarcoma, seasonality, and environmental factors in Wisconsin, 1979-1989. Arch Environ Health 1995;50:235-41.

131. Murray JJ. Caries experience of 15-year-old children from fluoride and non-fluoride communities. Br Dent J 1969;127:128-31.

132. National Research Council. Health effects of ingested fluoride. Washington DC: National Academy Press, 1993.

133. National Research Council, Food and Nutrition Board. Recommended dietary allowances. 8th ed. Washington DC: National Academy Press, 1974:98-9.

134. National Research Council, Food and Nutrition Board. Recommended dietary allowances. 10th ed. Washington DC: National Academy Press, 1989: 235-40.

135. Needleman HL, Pueschel SM, Rothman KJ. Fluoridation and the occurrence of Down's syndrome. N Engl J Med 1974;291:821-3.

136. Ogaard B. CaF_2 formation: Cariostatic properties and factors of enhancing the effect. Caries Res 2001;35 (Suppl 1):40-4.

137. Oldham PD, Newell DJ. Fluoridation of water supplies and cancer: A possible association? Appl Stat 1977;26:125-35.

138. Oliveby A, Twetman S, Ekstrand J. Diurnal fluoride concentration in whole saliva in children living in a high- and a low-fluoride area. Caries Res 1990; 24:44-7.

139. Ophaug RH, Singer L, Harland BF. Estimated fluoride intake of average two-year-old children in four dietary regions of the United States. J Dent Res 1980; 59:777-81.

140. Ophaug RH, Singer L, Harland BF. Estimated fluoride intake of 6-month-old infants in four dietary regions of the United States. Am J Clin Nutr 1980; 33:324-7.

141. Osis D, Kramer L, Wiatrowski E, Spencer H. Dietary fluoride intake in man. J Nutr 1974;104:1313-8.

142. Pak CY, Sakhaee K, Piziak V, et al. Slow-release NaF in the management of postmenopausal osteoporosis. A randomized controlled trial. Ann Intern Med 1994;120:625-32.

143. Pang DTY, Phillips CL, Bawden JW. Fluoride intake from beverage consumption in a sample of North Carolina children. J Dent Res 1992;71:1382-8.

144. Phipps KR, Orwoll ES, Mason JD, Cauley JA. Community water fluoridation, bone mineral density, and fractures: Prospective study of effects in older women. Br Med J 2000;321:860-4.

145. Rapaport I. Contribution a l'étude du mongolisme. Rôle pathogenique du fluor. Bull Acad Natl Med 1956;140:529-31.

146. Rapaport I. Nouvelles recherches sur le mongolisme. A propos du rôle pathogenique du fluor. Bull Acad Natl Med 1959;143:367-70.

147. Rapaport I. Oligophrénie mongolienne et caries dentaires. Revue Stomatol 1963;46:207-18.

148. Riggs BL, O'Fallon WM, Lane A, et al. Clinical trial of fluoride therapy in postmenopausal osteoporotic women: Extended observations and additional analysis. J Bone Miner Res 1994;9:265-75.

149. Rogot E, Sharrett AR, Feinlieb M, Fabsitz RR. Trends in urban mortality in relation to fluoridation status. Am J Epidemiol 1978;107:104-12.

150. Rölla G, Ekstrand J. Fluoride in oral fluids and dental plaque. In: Fejerskov O, Ekstrand J, Burt BA, eds: Fluoride in dentistry. Copenhagen: Munksgaard, 1996:215-29.

151. Rosen S, Frea JI, Hsu SM. Effect of fluoride-resistant microorganisms on dental caries. J Dent Res 1978; 57:180.

152. Russell AL. Dental effects of exposure to fluoride-bearing Dakota sandstone waters at various ages and for various lengths of time. II. Patterns of dental caries inhibition as related to exposure span, to elapsed time since exposure, and to periods of calcification and eruption. J Dent Res 1949;28:600-12.

153. Russell AL. Letters to Dr. Rapaport and Dr. Forrest. In: Crisp P. Report of the Royal Commission on the fluoridation of public water supplies. Hobart, Australia: Tasmanian Government Printing Office, 1968:262-5.

154. Russell AL, Hamilton PM. Dental caries in permanent first molars after eight years of fluoridation. Arch Oral Biol 1961;6:50-7.

155. Schlesinger ER, Overton DE. Study of children drinking fluoridated and nonfluoridated water. JAMA 1956;160:21-4.

156. Schlesinger ER, Overton DE, Chase HE, Cantwell KT. Newburgh-Kingston caries-fluorine study. XIII. Pediatric findings after ten years. J Am Dent Assoc 1956;52:296-306.

157. Schneiderman MA. Fluoridation and health: A short review of some evidence from the United States. Bethesda MD: National Cancer Institute, 1979.

158. Simonen O, Laitenen O. Does fluoridation of drinking water prevent bone fragility and osteoporosis? Lancet 1985;2(8452):432-4.

159. Singer L, Ophaug RH, Harland BF. Fluoride intake of young adult males in the United States. Am J Clin Nutr 1980;33:328-32.

160. Singer L, Ophaug RH, Harland BF. Dietary fluoride intake of 15-19-year-old male adults residing in the United States. J Dent Res 1985;64:1302-5.

161. Smith MC, Lantz EM, Smith HV. The cause of mottled enamel, a defect of human teeth. J Dent Res 1932;12:149-59. [Reprinted from: Technical Bulletin No. 32. Tucson AZ: University of Arizona College of Agriculture, 1931.]

162. Sowers MF, Clark MK, Jannausch ML, Wallace RB. A prospective study of bone mineral content and fracture in communities with differential fluoride exposure. Am J Epidemiol 1991;133:649-60.

163. Sowers MF, Wallace RB, Lemke JH. The relationship of bone mass and fracture history to fluoride and calcium intake: A study of three communities. Am J Clin Nutr 1986;44:889-98.

164. Spak CJ, Berg U, Ekstrand J. Renal clearance of fluoride in children and adolescents. Pediatrics 1985;75:575-9.

165. Spencer H, Osis D, Lender M. Studies of fluoride metabolism in man. A review and report of original data. Sci Total Environ 1981;17:1-12.

166. Stewart WK. The composition of dialysis fluid. In: Maher JF, ed: Replacement of renal function by dialysis. 3rd ed. Dordrecht: Kluwer, 1989:199-217.

167. Strassburg MA, Greenland S. Methodologic problems in evaluating the carcinogenic risk of environmental agents. J Environ Health 1979;41:214-7.

168. Suarez-Almazor ME, Flowerdew G, Saunders LD, et al. The fluoridation of drinking water and hip fracture hospitalization rates in two Canadian communities. Am J Public Health 1993;83:689-93.

169. Tatevossian A. Fluoride in dental plaque and its effects. J Dent Res 1990;69(Spec Issue):645-52.

170. Thylstrup A. Clinical evidence of the role of pre-eruptive fluoride in caries prevention. J Dent Res 1990;69(Spec Issue):742-50.

171. US Public Health Service. NTP technical report on the toxicity and cariogenesis studies of sodium fluoride in 344/N rats and B6C3F1 mice (drinking water studies). NIH Report No. 90-2848. Washington DC: Government Printing Office, 1990.

172. US Public Health Service, Ad Hoc Subcommittee on Fluoride. Review of fluoride benefits and risks. Washington DC: Government Printing Office, 1991.

173. Van Loveren C. Antimicrobial activity of fluoride and its in vivo importance: Identification of research questions. Caries Res 2001;35:65-70.

174. Velu H, Balozet L. Darmous (dystrophie dentaire) du mouton et solubilité du principé actif des phosphates naturels qui le provique. Bull Soc Pathol Exot 1931;24:848-51.

175. Villa A, Anabalon M, Cabezas L. The fractional urinary fluoride excretion in young children under stable fluoride intake conditions. Community Dent Oral Epidemiol 2000;28:344-55.

176. Vogt RL, Witherell L, LaRue D, Klaucke DN. Acute fluoride poisoning associated with an on-site fluoridator in a Vermont elementary school. Am J Public Health 1982;72:1168-9.

177. Wefel JS, Maharry G, Jensen ME, et al. In vivo demineralisation and remineralisation of enamel and root surfaces. In: Leach SA, ed: Factors relating to demineralisation and remineralisation of the teeth. Oxford: IRL Press, 1986:181-90.

178. Wefel JS. Effects of fluoride on caries development and progression using intra-oral models. J Dent Res 1990;69(Spec Issue):626-33.

179. White DJ, Nancollas GH. Physical and chemical considerations of the role of firmly and loosely bound fluoride in caries prevention. J Dent Res 1990;69(Spec Issue):587-94.

180. Whitford GM. Fluoride metabolism. In: Newbrun E, ed: Fluorides and dental caries. 3rd ed. Springfield IL: Thomas, 1986:174-98.

181. Whitford GM. The metabolism and toxicology of fluoride. Monogr Oral Sci 1989;13:1-160.

182. Whitford GM. Fluoride metabolism and excretion in children. J Public Health Dent 1999;99:224-8.

183. Whitford GM, Wasdin JL, Schafer TE, Adair SM. Plaque fluoride concentrations are dependent on plaque calcium concentrations. Caries Res 2002;36:256-65.

184. Whiting P, MacDonagh M, Kleijnan J. Association of Down's syndrome and water fluoride level: A systematic review of the evidence. BMC Public Health, website: http://www.biomedcentral.com/1471-2458/1/6. Accessed September 29, 2004.

185. Yiamouyiannis J, Burk D. Fluoridation and cancer: Age-dependence of cancer mortality related to artificial fluoridation. Fluoride 1977;10:102-23.

186. Zipkin I, Likins RC. The absorption of various fluorine compounds from the gastrointestinal tract of the rat. Am J Physiol 1957;191:549-50.

187. Zipkin I, McClure FJ. Cariostatic effect and metabolism of ammonium fluosilicate. Public Health Rep 1954;69:730-3.

188. Zipkin I, Scow RO. Fluoride deposition in different segments of the tibia of the young growing rat. Am J Physiol 1956;185:81-4.

Fluoridation of Drinking Water

Fluoridation is the controlled addition of a fluoride (F) compound to a public water supply to bring its F concentration up to a level that will best prevent dental caries while avoiding unsightly fluorosis. A related public health measure is defluoridation, the process of removing excess F naturally present in a water supply to prevent dental fluorosis (or even skeletal fluorosis in some parts of the world where the naturally occurring F concentration is high enough).

In our studies of F and its relationship to dental caries, water fluoridation deserves special attention. This is because the F-caries relationship was first discovered in studies of communities with naturally fluoridated water and because water fluoridation is the purest public health use of F. Fluoridation is not a targeted approach to caries prevention; its use means that F reaches everyone in the community. This feature is both the measure's greatest strength and its greatest problem in terms of social policy. This chapter describes the various issues specific to water fluoridation as a means of controlling caries at the community level.

The unit usually used in the United States for expressing the F concentration in drinking water is parts per million (ppm), although countries using metric measurements usually express it in milligrams per liter (mg/L). Fortunately the numerical values are the same in both measuring units; that is, 1.2 ppm is the same as 1.2 mg/L. We use parts per million in this book.

OPTIMAL FLUORIDE CONCENTRATIONS IN DRINKING WATER

Public policy for controlled water F levels in the United States takes the form of nonenforceable guidelines set by the U.S. Public Health Service (Box 25-1). Current policy is that these levels, for the United States, should be between 0.7 and 1.2 ppm F, depending on mean annual temperature of the locality. These guidelines, based on the assumption that people drink more water in a hotter climate than they do in a cooler one, are more than 40 years old and are shown in Table 25-1.

BOX 25-1   Who Watches Over How Much Fluoride Is in our Drinking Water?

Two agencies of the federal government are involved in overseeing levels of fluoride (F) in drinking water. At the regulatory level, the Environmental Protection Agency (EPA) sets the legal upper limit at 4.0 ppm F. No one adds fluoride to drinking water at that level, but it can occur naturally (although it is rare to find this high level in the United States). If such an F concentration is found in a public water supply, the excess F must be removed or a new water source found. Here the issue is human health. The EPA considers that 4.0 ppm F is the upper limit before the risk of skeletal fluorosis becomes too high. This regulation has nothing to do with what the best concentration for caries prevention might be.

In terms of guidelines for the best concentration for caries prevention, the U.S. Public Health Service recommends that drinking water in the United States be fluoridated to a level between 0.7 and 1.2 ppm F, depending on climate. This recommendation is nonenforceable.

The maximum contaminant level goal (MCLG) is the level of a contaminant in drinking water below which there is no known or expected risk to health. MCLGs allow for a margin of safety and are nonenforceable public health goals. The maximum contaminant level (MCL) is the highest level of a contaminant that is allowed in drinking water. MCLs are set as close to MCLGs as is feasible when the best available treatment technology and cost are taken into consideration. MCLs are enforceable standards. Both the MCLG and the MCL remain at 4.0 ppm F,[46] pending further review by the EPA.

Table 25-1   Fluoride levels recommended by the U.S. Public Health Service for cool and warm climates[122]

Annual Average of Maximum Daily Air Temperatures (Degrees F)*	Recommended Control Limits of Fluoride Concentrations (ppm)		
	Lower	Optimal	Upper
50.0-53.7	0.9	1.2	1.7
53.8-58.3	0.8	1.1	1.5
58.4-63.8	0.8	1.0	1.3
63.9-70.6	0.7	0.9	1.2
70.7-79.2	0.7	0.8	1.0
79.3-90.5	0.6	0.7	0.8

*Based on temperature data obtained for a minimum of 5 years.

These temperature-related guidelines were developed from a series of well-conducted epidemiologic studies performed in the American west during the 1950s[51-54]; from these data, the researchers produced an algebraic formula for determining a community's optimal water F level. This formula is based on Dean's conclusion (see Chapter 24) that 1.0 ppm F was the optimum concentration for the Chicago area. Regardless of how appropriate Dean's conclusion was in his time, the appropriateness of temperature-related guidelines is questionable given today's living conditions. The climate-related guidelines are widely ignored in the United States anyway.[80]

The temperature-related guidelines in Table 25-1, developed under American dietary and cultural conditions, have been found unsuit-able for Asian and African regions. Hong Kong, for example, reduced its water F levels to 0.5 ppm F by the mid-1990s because of increased fluorosis, and an expert committee of the World Health Organization has recommended a range of 0.5-1.0 ppm F for all parts of the world.[130] The recommended levels for the United States have been in place since 1962 and are due for revision, because much in our lifestyles and exposure to F has changed since then. For example:

- Air-conditioning is widespread and has been a major factor in promoting population growth in hotter parts of the country. Because we live in an increasingly climate-controlled environment, the original premise that people drink more water in hotter parts of the country becomes weaker.[65,113]

- There has been a huge increase in consumption of soft drinks and bottled waters (see Chapter 28). These may or may not be made with fluoridated water, and products from the same plant can be distributed to both fluoridated and nonfluoridated areas.
- An increase in the prevalence of fluorosis since the time the guidelines were developed (see Chapter 24) indicates that young people are ingesting more F than they used to. Increased use of commercial juice drinks in place of milk and water could be a factor.[83]

Like all guidelines for F use, the temperature-related recommendations for F levels in drinking water need periodic monitoring, because the world has changed since they were developed.

EARLY STUDIES OF FLUORIDATED WATER

The most important early studies of fluoridated water were described in Chapter 24. All the early research on the safety of F use and its impact on human health and function studied F in drinking water. By the time the first controlled fluoridation trials were begun in 1945, research had established the following facts:

- The healthy human body possesses a prompt and efficient excretory mechanism for F that, at least at the low F levels usually found naturally in drinking water in the United States, minimizes the danger of long-term accumulation.
- Although ingested F is partly deposited in bone, and although skeletal F concentrations increase with age, skeletal damage could not be demonstrated in users of F-bearing domestic water in the United States.
- No impairment in general health could be found among people who had drunk water with up to 8 ppm F for long periods of time.

Four independent studies of controlled fluoridation, in which the F concentration in the water supplies of the communities was brought up from negligible levels to 1.0-1.2 ppm, were begun in 1945 and 1946. They followed a long series of epidemiologic studies of caries experience related to F concentration in drinking water, which were summarized in Chapter 24. The four communities originally studied were the following:

1. Grand Rapids, Michigan. This study was begun in January 1945 with nearby Muskegon as the control city and was directed by Dean and his colleagues.[30]
2. Newburgh, New York, with Kingston as the control city.[4]
3. Evanston, Illinois, with Oak Park as control.[13]
4. Brantford, Ontario, with Sarnia as control. Naturally fluoridated Stratford, Ontario, was also included in this study.[68]

At the end of terms ranging up to 15 years, caries experience was shown to be sharply reduced in each of the study populations, despite some differences in study design and examination criteria.[2,5,12,69] These pioneer studies also found that dental fluorosis occurred to about the same extent[6,105] as Dean had described earlier[28]: namely, some 7%-16% of the population was found to have mild to very mild fluorosis when the F exposure came from drinking water containing 1.0 ppm F.

The four original studies in which F was added to drinking water are sometimes called "classic" studies, although "pioneering" might be a better term. By present-day standards of field trials they were rather crude. Although they are often referred to as "longitudinal" studies, none of them was; all were of sequential cross-sectional design. Sampling methods and dental examiners tended to vary from year to year,[1] which risked bias and unnecessary random error. Methods of statistical analysis were primitive by today's standards. Data from the control communities were largely neglected after the initial reports, and conclusions were based on the much weaker before-after analysis in the test cities. (Among the early studies, the only true longitudinal study of fluoridation's effects was the Tiel-Culemborg study in the Netherlands.)[8,9]

Perhaps too much emphasis has been given to these four pioneering studies, for they really just confirmed prospectively what had already been demonstrated through Dean's research, which still stands as a model of how to apply the epidemiologic method. But despite the design flaws in the original four studies, it is difficult for an open-minded observer to reject their conclusions that fluoridation was effective in reducing the prevalence and severity of caries.

Public policy on any issue usually has to be established without complete information, and water fluoridation is no exception. When one considers that adults, on average, ingest 1-3 mg F/day in their normal diets, that 9-10 million Americans (and many other peoples around the world) have been drinking naturally fluoridated water for a century or so, and that over 100 million Americans have been drinking F-supplemented water for generations, there is a lot of empirical evidence that fluoridation at 1 ppm is not harmful. Certainly there is no credible evidence that F in these amounts leads to serious ill health. The scientific method cannot prove a negative; we take inability to reject the null hypothesis for specific conditions (see Chapter 13) as evidence of safety. The occasional allegation of a sensitivity reaction should be investigated seriously, but with the passage of time the probability becomes greater that fluoridation at 1.0 ppm produces no undesirable side effects. We support the policy of the U.S. Public Health Service that F should be added to drinking water at the recommended concentrations.

WORLD STATUS OF FLUORIDATION

Unfortunately there is no central compendium for international data on populations receiving fluoridated water. The FDI World Dental Federation has some self-reported information for some countries on its website (http://www fdiworlddental.org), but the data are not collated. Older information from the FDI shows that in 1984 there were 34 countries reporting fluoridation projects reaching some 246 million people, not including areas with naturally occurring F in the drinking water. Both the British Fluoridation Society[16] and the World Health Organization[95] estimated that some 210 million people worldwide receive fluoridated water. The foregoing statements are all of uncertain validity. Some factual summary statements about the global distribution of fluoridation are shown in Box 25-2.

Ireland remains the only nation (apart from the city-state of Singapore) to have a mandatory fluoridation law. Enacted in 1960, it subsequently withstood a legal challenge that went to the Irish High Court. Most large Irish urban communities had fluoridated water in the period 1964-72; 71% of Ireland's population resided in fluoridated areas by 2004.[98] Information from the Pan American Health Organization shows that nine countries in South America and the Caribbean have water fluoridation; most notable are Brazil and Chile, with 42% of the population in each country receiving fluoridated water.

At the other end of the spectrum, fluoridation has made little headway in Europe, and it is not technically feasible for much of Asia and Africa because of the relative absence of municipal water systems there. In Europe, fluoridation in the socialist countries of Eastern Europe ended with the demise of the former Soviet Union in the early 1990s.[79] In Britain, the city of Birmingham, the second largest British city, has

---

BOX 25-2 Summary of Global Distribution of Water Fluoridation in 2000

- In 1984, the FDI World Dental Federation reported that 34 countries had some fluoridation projects, which reached a total of 246 million people.
- In the city-state of Singapore, fluoridation in 2004 reached virtually 100% of the population. The only other nation with a mandatory fluoridation law is Ireland, where over two thirds of the population now receives fluoridated water.
- Fluoridation reaches more than 50% of the population in Australia, Ireland, Malaysia, New Zealand, and the United States.
- In Europe, some 10% of the population of Spain and the United Kingdom receive fluoridated water. Principal cities fluoridated are Sevilla and Córdoba in Spain, and Birmingham and Newcastle in the United Kingdom.
- Previously reported fluoridation projects in eastern European countries are of uncertain status since the breakup of the Soviet Union in 1989-91. Those in the former East Germany are known to have ceased since German reunification in 1989.
- Extensive water fluoridation projects previously reported in South and Central America are of uncertain status.

been fluoridated since 1964, and there is a belt of fluoridated communities near Birmingham in the West Midlands. On the other hand, there is no water fluoridation at all in Austria, Belgium, Denmark, France, Germany, Italy, Norway, and Sweden. Specific bans are in place in Sweden and Denmark (where a law on additives is interpreted to exclude fluoridation), and for various reasons fluoridation is a dead political issue in the others.

In Europe a notable setback, as opposed to lack of progress, came in the Netherlands, where fluoridation at one point reached 3 million people but was halted by the government of the Netherlands in 1976. The long-fluoridated Finnish city of Kuopio also ceased fluoridating in 1992, as did the city of Basel in Switzerland in 2003.

FLUORIDATION IN THE UNITED STATES

The Division of Oral Health of the Centers for Disease Control and Prevention (CDC) in Atlanta maintains fluoridation surveillance for the United States. The Water Fluoridation Reporting System, a voluntary program, forwards data from the states to the CDC, which then publishes the information periodically on its website. Extent of fluoridation is one of the eight indicators used in the National Oral Health Surveillance System (see Chapter 4).

At the end of 2000, the CDC estimated that fluoridated water was reaching some 162 million people in the United States, 57% of the total population and 66% of those receiving municipal water.[125] About 10 million of these people were receiving water naturally fluoridated at 0.7 ppm F or more; the greatest concentrations of naturally fluoridated communities are found in Texas, Illinois, and New Mexico.[128] In the year 2000 there were over 10,000 water systems with controlled or natural fluoride levels of 0.7 ppm F or more; these represent 18% of all public water systems in the country. This may not sound like much, but a large majority of public water systems serve communities with fewer than 1000 people, so that fluoridation is not cost effective. Drinking water is fluoridated in 42 of the 50 largest American cities. Over 700 communities in the United States have been fluoridating the water

for 30 years or longer, and many of the naturally fluoridated communities have been using the same water source for more than three generations. The proportion of state populations reached by fluoridation ranges from close to 100% in Minnesota, Kentucky, Indiana, and Tennessee (plus the District of Columbia) to 2% in Utah and 9% in Hawaii.

Role of Federal, State, and Local Governments in Fluoridation

The decision to fluoridate is usually made by the local community, although a number of jurisdictions can be involved when water service district boundaries do not coincide with city and county boundaries. State laws requiring fluoridation now stand in 10 states; at the other end of the spectrum, there are three states that have laws requiring referenda. These states are shown in Table 25-2. The fluoridation laws have been generally successful, because in all states with them a high proportion of the population is receiving fluoridated water. Some of the states listed in Table 25-2, however, have provisions in their laws that can frustrate progress. These provisions reflect the political compromises necessary to get the law passed. For example, the California law, passed after a vigorous political battle in 1996, cannot be enforced unless outside funds (i.e., state or federal funds) are made available to the local community for the purchase, installation, and operation of the fluoridation system.

The U.S. Public Health Service, initially through its Division of Dental Health (now defunct) and later through the CDC, has provided funds and consultative expertise to promote fluoridation through several mechanisms. Federal funds were available through the Division of Dental Health in 1965-67, and 13 states used them to begin fluoridation projects. These funds were specifically earmarked for fluoridation but were cut repeatedly as the cost of the Vietnam War (1955-75) increased. Funding was revived from 1978 to 1981, when the CDC had a budget of up to $9 million per year for distribution to states and communities for fluoridation. Some 765 communities, with a population of nearly 11 million, benefited directly during this period.

In 1981 seven block grants were initiated as a method of distributing federal health funds to

Table 25-2 States of the United States with fluoridation laws requiring fluoridation in 2004*

State	Year Started	Size of Community Affected	Exemption Provision?	Maximum Natural F Level (ppm)	F Level to Be Maintained
CT	1965	20,000+	No	0.8	0.8-1.2
MN	1967	All	No	—	0.9-1.5
IL	1967	All	No	0.8	0.9-1.2
SD	1969	500+	No	0.9	0.9-1.7
OH	1969	5,000+	No	—	0.8-1.3
GA	1973	All incorporated	Public vote	—	No higher than 1.0 ppm
NE	1973	All political subdivisions	Public vote	0.7	0.8-1.5
CA	1996	10,000 service connections	No	0.7	0.7-1.2
DE	1998	All	No	—	0.8-1.2
NV	1999	Counties with 400,000+, with either a water system serving 100,000+ or a water authority	No	—	0.7-1.2

Data from the Centers for Disease Control and Prevention, personal communication, 2004.
*Three states have laws that require a favorable vote of the local community before fluoridation can be implemented; these are ME (1957), NH (1959), UT (1976, revised 2003).

BOX 25-3 Sources of Federal Government Funding for Fluoridation

- Preventive Health and Health Services Block Grant funds are awarded to states, although in 2002 only 2% of the $128 million granted to states was used for fluoridation.[126]
- Health Resources and Services Administration in 1998 funded six projects in six states for 3 years to develop their fluoridation programs and promote fluoridation. Four of these six awards were to state health departments, one was to a county health department, and one was to a nonprofit organization.[123]
- The Centers for Disease Control and Prevention (CDC) in 1999 awarded 3-year grants to 13 states or tribes for fluoridation. In 2001 and 2002, the CDC funded 5-year cooperative agreements with 12 states and one territory for state oral health program core capacity, including administration of state fluoridation programs. These jurisdictions were Alaska, Arkansas, Colorado, Illinois, Michigan, Nevada, New York, North Dakota, Oregon, Rhode Island, South Carolina, Texas, and the Republic of Palau. Four of these (Colorado, Illinois, Nevada, Texas) were also among the 1999 recipients. Two of these states received additional funds for fluoridation equipment.[127]

the states. The philosophy behind block grants is that funds to finance a host of federal categorical programs that have grown up over the years are lumped together in specific blocks, and recipient states can determine for themselves to which programs they will allocate the funds. The Preventive Health and Health Services Block Grant includes funds for fluoridation, but fluoridation projects then have to compete at the intrastate level against other worthy prevention causes such as hypertension control and emergency medical services. Recent sources of

federal funding for fluoridation are listed in Box 25-3. Future funding remains uncertain.

Drinking Water Standards

The U.S. Environmental Protection Agency (EPA) is the regulatory agency with responsibility for setting national standards for acceptable drinking water under the Safe Drinking Water Act (Public Law 93-523; see Box 25-1). This act was first passed in 1974 and has been renewed several times since. Most of these standards deal with defining acceptable levels of bacterial and chemical contaminants. In the 1975-76 National Interim Primary Drinking Water Regulations, in the standards promulgated soon after passage of the legislation, the EPA referred to naturally occurring F above 2 ppm as a "contaminant" requiring removal from drinking water. This latter requirement was intended to reduce dental fluorosis in affected areas, but it was criticized by many of the local authorities concerned on the grounds of cost (defluoridation is more expensive than fluoridation). Many communities that used drinking water naturally fluoridated at more than 2 ppm were small and could not afford the cost of meeting the standard. In addition, few of them seemed interested in defluoridating: the resulting fluorosis did not concern them and they were not aware of any other ill effects, so why bother?

The Interim Primary Drinking Water Regulations of 1980[40] left the *recommended maximum contaminant level* (RMCL) at 2 ppm F but included an explanatory statement that this standard did not contradict the beneficial effects of F in reducing dental decay. Whether this statement really helped clarify things, especially because that unfortunate word *contaminant* was retained, is doubtful. Public discussion on establishing the final standards became intense during the mid-1980s; the EPA was deluged with demands from both proponents and opponents of fluoridation. The state of South Carolina, for whom compliance with the RMCL of 2 ppm F would have been very expensive, brought suit against the EPA in 1981 to attempt to force it to revoke the interim RMCL. The EPA, in response, promised to rule on the issue when its studies were complete. South Carolina sued again in 1984, seeking faster action from the EPA, and this led to issuance of a consent decree in January 1985.[41]

Eventually the EPA settled this seemingly irresolvable issue by ducking underneath it. Concluding after its studies that dental fluorosis in the United States was a cosmetic defect rather than a health problem, the EPA proposed an RMCL for F of 4.0 ppm F, on the grounds that this level was sufficiently low to protect against crippling skeletal fluorosis.[42] By late 1986, this RMCL became the *maximum contaminant level* for 4.0 ppm F, meaning that the EPA now had a standard to enforce. The original level of 2.0 ppm F became a secondary standard; that is, it

was a nonenforceable recommended maximum, in effect a guideline. This secondary standard was justified on the grounds that "2 mg/L would prevent the majority of cases of water-related cosmetically objectionable dental fluorosis while still allowing for the beneficial effects of F (prevention of dental caries)."[43]

Although some aspects of this debate resembled a Gilbert and Sullivan operetta, it raised the serious question of whether control of dental fluorosis should be a subject for national standards or whether the issue should be left to states or localities to handle. State dental directors have to carry much of the regulatory load, and many are unhappy with the requirement that local communities must be notified when their F levels are between 2 and 4 ppm, especially since the EPA mandates that the word *contaminant* (again!) must appear in the letters of notification.[44]

Standards of this sort quite properly need reexamination from time to time. In 1992, the EPA requested the National Research Council to review the issue of primary and secondary standards for F in drinking water. An expert committee whose members had a variety of backgrounds (most were from outside dentistry) worked for more than a year and concluded that there was no current evidence to justify a change in the standards.[90] The committee recommended that the issue of the relationship of F exposure to health be revisited at regular intervals because new evidence was appearing continuously. Following this report, the EPA decided in late 1993 not to change what was then called the *maximum contaminant level goal* of 4.0 ppm F.[45] This standard still holds.[46]

CARIES REDUCTIONS FROM FLUORIDATION

For many years, the statement that "water fluoridation reduces dental caries experience by half" was hardly questioned within dentistry. At a time when drinking water was the only significant source of F, that statement was probably true enough. Its basis was Dean's 21 cities epidemiologic study of naturally fluoridated areas,[29,31] supplemented by the results of the initial four controlled fluoridation projects begun in 1945-46. A summary of the results of these four pioneering studies is presented in

Table 25-3 Decayed, missing, and filled (DMF) teeth per child ages 12-14 years and missing teeth per child at the end of the study term in four pioneer fluoridation communities[5]

Community	Year	Mean DMF Teeth per Child	Percent Difference	Missing Teeth per Child	Percent Difference
Grand Rapids (F)	1944-45	9.58	55.5	0.84	65.6
	1959	4.26		0.29	
Evanston (F)	1946	9.03	48.4	0.19	68.4
	1959	4.66		0.06	
Sarnia (non-F)	1959	7.46		0.75	
Brantford (F)	1959	3.23	56.7	0.22	70.7
Kingston* (non-F)	1960	12.46		0.92	
Newburgh* (F)	1960	3.73	70.1	0.10	89.1

Note: Fluoridated communities are designated by F, nonfluoridated by non-F, after city name.
*Children in Kingston and Newburgh were ages 13-14 years.

Table 25-3. The table shows that after 13-15 years of fluoridation, DMF (decayed, missing, and filled) scores in 12- to 14-year-old permanent-resident children favored fluoridation by 48% to 70%. In absolute terms, average DMF levels in the fluoridated communities dropped from 7-9 teeth at the start of the studies to 3-4 teeth per child after 13-15 years.

Since those studies, exposure to F from toothpaste, other dental products, and food and drink has become universal. As a result, water fluoridation has moved from being the sole F exposure, as it was in those early days, to one of a number of F exposures. Caries status overall has continued to improve, and overall F exposure has to take much of the credit for that. Another reason for the inability to attribute 50% reductions in caries to water fluoridation today is that the effects of F in drinking water diffuse into surrounding communities and raise the baseline. Nonetheless, 12-year-old children living in states where more than half of the communities have fluoridated water have 26% fewer decayed tooth surfaces per year than 12-year-old children living in states where less than one quarter of the communities are fluoridated.[61] A rigorous systematic review in Britain, carried out by an expert group at the University of York, concluded that the median increase in the proportion of persons with DMFT score (number of decayed, missing, and filled permanent teeth) of 0 attributable to water fluoridation was 15%.[85] Because the review had strict criteria for inclusion and exclusion of studies, this conclusion was reached from a fairly small number of studies. (One of the conclusions of

the systematic review was that the large body of literature on the effectiveness of water fluoridation was generally of poor quality, as was the literature claiming harm from fluoridation.)

It would thus be unreasonable to expect continuation of 50% reductions in caries levels from fluoridated water alone; the generally reduced caries levels we enjoy are today a result of total F exposure from all sources. The continuing importance of water fluoridation as a cornerstone of public policy, however, is indicated by the fact that the CDC lists it as one of the top 10 public health achievements of the twentieth century.[124]

Reducing the Disparities

Disparities refers to the differences in health status between favored and unfavored groups in our society, usually racial-ethnic groups and those of different socioeconomic status (SES). Disparities are a complex and persistent problem, with economic costs as well as political and moral overtones. Fluoridation has the major social advantage of benefiting children in lower SES areas relatively more than those in higher SES areas.[10,19,57,73,97,100] An example is shown in Fig. 25-1, which presents data from the most recent clinical examinations in the Newburgh-Kingston studies in New York. When caries levels found in 7- to 14-year-old poor and nonpoor children in the 1995 examinations were compared, the greatest disparity was seen between the poor and nonpoor in nonfluoridated Kingston rather than between poor groups in the two cities. Reducing the disparities in health status between high- and low-SES

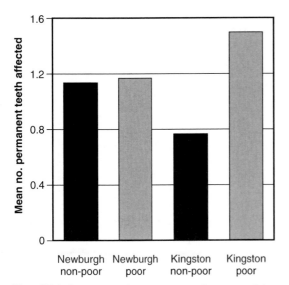

Fig. 25-1 Caries experience, expressed as covariate-adjusted mean decayed, missing and filled surfaces per child in 7- to 14-year-old children in Newburgh and Kingston, New York, by poverty status ("poor" children were defined as those participating in the school lunch program).[77] (From Burt BA: Fluoridation and Social Equity. J Public Health Dent 2002; 62:195–200. *Reproduced by permission of the Journal of Public Dentistry.*)

areas is a United States national health objective for 2010, and fluoridation does its part to help achieve this goal.

The most searching assessment of fluoridation's effectiveness, including its effectiveness in reducing disparities between groups, came with the systematic review carried out by the Centre for Reviews and Dissemination at the University of York in Britain in 2000 and referred to earlier.[85] This review is the most rigorous scrutiny of existing data on fluoridation yet carried out. It has been criticized by both proponents and opponents of fluoridation because the stringent inclusion and exclusion criteria led to the omission of many reports from consideration. One of the aims of this exhaustive review was to determine if fluoridation reduced the disparity in caries experience between higher and lower SES groups. Most of the 15 papers selected to examine this question reported data for 5-year-old children. The review found no difference between fluoridated and nonfluoridated areas in the magnitude of the disparities between children of different SES groups when caries *prevalence* was measured. However, a favorable reduction in differences between social groups was seen

when caries *severity* was the measure. Data for ages other than 5 years were too limited to permit conclusions.

Caries Reductions in Children

Studies of the effectiveness of fluoridation in reducing caries experience in children far outnumber studies of its effectiveness in adults. The many fluoridation studies conducted in different parts of the world have varied in quality of design and operation, but their results have still been remarkably uniform. Differences in oral health between fluoridated and nonfluoridated areas are easier to demonstrate when there are relatively few fluoridated areas, so that the diffusion effect (see earlier) has less impact. In Britain, where water fluoridation is not widespread, reductions of around 50% are still found in primary and mixed dentitions.[15,47,58,74,116,120] Similar results have been reported in Brazil[27]; in Australia, where comparisons were based on school dental service data for groups of 9000 or more children[111,112]; in New Zealand[121]; and in Ireland.[93]

Where fluoridation is widespread, as in the United States, differences in caries experience between children in fluoridated and nonfluoridated communities are now estimated to be more on the order of 18%-35%.[17,26] However, how much of F's benefits is due to water fluoridation, rather than to overall F exposure, really cannot be estimated with any precision now for the following reasons:

- The development and almost universal use of fluoridated toothpaste and other dental products containing F, plus the presence of F in food and beverages processed with fluoridated water, means that there are many different F exposures for the average American.
- The extreme mobility of the U.S. population means that most people have had varied exposures to fluoridated water at different times of life. When this is added to the diffusion effect (described earlier), it is clear that there is no way of finding true control subjects in the United States.
- History of exposure to fluoridation is difficult to document in research studies. There are no biomarkers for lifetime exposure, and interview data can be unreliable.

Caries Reductions in Adults

The caries-inhibitory effects of F are not confined to childhood. Contrary assumptions were surprisingly common in light of the evidence in Chapter 24 and stemmed from beliefs that (1) the primary cariostatic action of F was preeruptive, and (2) caries was a disease of childhood. Neither of these beliefs is viewed as true today. Over a lifetime, fluoridation reduces coronal and root caries.[60,91]

Studies of fluoridation's effects in adulthood began early with McKay's recognition that 45-year-old adults benefitted from consuming fluoridated water.[86] Adults born and raised in naturally fluoridated Colorado Springs were found to have 60% lower mean DMF scores than their counterparts in nonfluoridated Boulder. Residents of Colorado Springs also had far fewer teeth missing.[104,106] Similar findings among adults came from Aurora, Illinois, a city with 1.2 ppm F naturally occurring in its drinking water.[39] Both the Colorado Springs and the Aurora studies went to considerable lengths to confine the analysis to permanent residents, to assess lifetime effects of exposure to fluoridated water. In light of today's questions about preeruptive and posteruptive cariostatic effects of F, it is a pity that the deliberate exclusion of study subjects who moved into the fluoridated areas after childhood precluded any consideration of this issue. It is also unfortunate that neither study assessed the SES of the people concerned. In fairness, sensitivity to the impact of SES on health status (see Chapters 20 and 21) was not as sharp at the time of these studies as it is today, but the net effect is to diminish their value in the perspective of history.

A later study did use more detailed statistical analysis in evaluating data from Lordsburg (3.5 ppm F) and Deming (0.7 ppm F), New Mexico. SES status was higher in Deming. Results still favored the community with the higher F level. After other important variables were controlled for, Deming adults were found to have two more restored teeth per person than did those in Lordsburg, although fluorosis was naturally more severe in Lordsburg.[36] The DMFT data for these two communities are shown in Fig. 25-2.

Root caries is also less prevalent in fluoridated areas than in nonfluoridated areas.[21,115] This finding is important, because with increas-

ing tooth retention in an aging population the amount of root caries would otherwise be expected to increase and become a greater treatment problem in the future. It is not yet clear whether F's protective effect against root caries is due to topical action on exposed root surfaces, to incorporation of F into cementum before root exposure in the oral cavity, or to a combination of both.

Prenatal Benefits

The policy issue of whether prenatal exposure to F actively promotes caries resistance in the infant is related to the use of supplements and is discussed in Chapter 26. F ingested by the mother crosses the placenta and enters the fetal circulation.[94,114] The fetal plasma F level is correlated with the maternal level, although it is somewhat lower, probably because much of the F is taken up by the rapidly mineralizing skeleton and teeth of the fetus.[94] The pertinent question is whether the developing primary dentition has enhanced resistance to caries because of this additional F.

Some support for a prenatal exposure benefit came from the Evanston fluoridation study, in which children who were exposed to fluoridated water in utero as well as postnatally were reported to have fewer carious lesions than those who received it only postnatally.[11] Other authorities, however, did not find this effect.[8,67] A comprehensive 1981 review concluded that there was probably no benefit in prenatal F exposure, though it was not ruled out completely.[34] If the offspring derives any benefit at all from prenatal F exposure, such benefit would be slight.

The absence of prenatal exposure benefits is a part of the discussion of preeruptive versus posteruptive effects in determining how F works. Benefits or lack of them aside, it is clear that fluoridation is quite safe for the developing fetus. No special precautions are therefore necessary for expectant mothers in fluoridated areas.

Effects on the Primary Dentition

Early fluoridation studies reported caries reductions in the primary dentition of about the same range as was found in the permanent dentition.[5,66,119] More recent British data show that this range of caries reduction attributable to

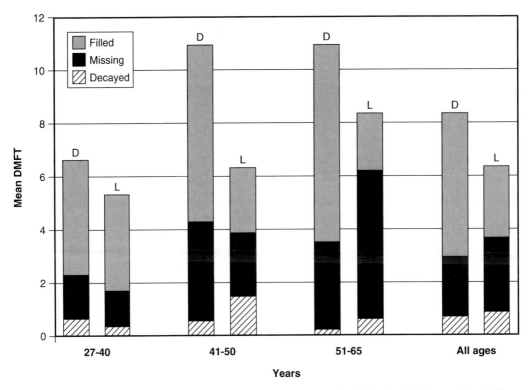

Fig. 25-2 Decayed, missing, and filled teeth (DMFT) in adults ages 27-65 in Deming (D; 0.7 ppm F in drinking water) and Lordsburg (L; 3.5 ppm F in drinking water), New Mexico.[36]

fluoridation is being maintained.[15,24,25,35,50,72,89] The primary dentition clearly benefits from exposure to fluoridated drinking water.

Partial Exposure to Fluoridation

A concentration of about 1.0 ppm F is regarded as optimum for caries prevention in a moderate climate. What happens in those communities with water naturally fluoridated at suboptimum levels, such as 0.4-0.7 ppm F? Dental benefits still are found and are generally proportional to the F concentration. A decision as to whether fluoridation is worthwhile in a community whose water contains, say, 0.6 ppm F is not easily made, for it is not certain whether the cost of fluoridating is worth the additional dental benefits expected.

The United States and Canada are highly mobile societies. Many people have therefore spent part of their lives in a fluoridated area and part in a nonfluoridated area. The benefit of partial exposure to fluoridated water in adulthood has not been documented, but there is evidence that partial exposure in childhood reduces caries experience in proportion to the length of exposure.[5,6] In nonfluoridated Coldwater, Michigan, children who had moved to Coldwater after some residence in a fluoridated area had lower caries experience than did those who had lived in Coldwater all their lives.[20] A British study demonstrated a 27% reduction in caries incidence over 4 years among children who were 12 years old when fluoridation began in their community, relative to the incidence in control children in nonfluoridated areas.[64]

The evidence regarding partial exposure to fluoridated water indicates that a cariostatic benefit will be received that is more or less proportional to the extent of the exposure. Maximum benefit naturally comes with lifetime exposure.

Caries Patterns When Fluoridation Ceases

At the time when drinking water was the only important source of F, there was evidence from four communities in which fluoridation was started and stopped some years later that caries diminished with fluoridation and then increased again after fluoridation stopped. Two of these four communities were in Scotland, one was in Germany, and one in Wisconsin.[32,78,81,117] In Wick, Scotland, there was a particularly noticeable increase in caries prevalence after fluoridation ceased in 1979.[117]

More recent instances of caries patterns following the cessation of fluoridation, all in the modern era of multiple exposures to F, have given rather different results. In British Columbia, Canada, caries in a high-SES city continued to decline after fluoridation ended, a finding largely attributed to the anticariogenic effects of other F sources.[84] Similar patterns have been reported in Europe, both in the permanent dentition[79,107] and in the primary dentition,[108] and these patterns are consistent with those of the Tiel-Culemborg study (see Fig. 25-3). In the

United States, cessation of fluoridation for 11 months led to no discernible change in caries patterns. Again, this was in a high-SES community in which regular use of F toothpaste was the norm.[22]

Fluoridation ended in 1973 in Tiel, the test city in the landmark Tiel-Culemborg study in the Netherlands. At the time, caries experience was far more favorable in fluoridated Tiel than in Culemborg. But 15 years after fluoridation ended in Tiel, the caries experience of Culemborg children looked better.[75] This finding illustrates the importance of constant exposure to F (in this case through fluoridated water) for full dental benefits, as well as the effectiveness of other F exposures, most notably the widespread use of F toothpaste since the mid-1970s. (Because Culemborg was of higher SES than Tiel, it would be expected that use of F toothpaste among its inhabitants would be greater.) These changes in caries among children in Tiel and Culemborg, relative to fluoridation and subsequent exposure to F toothpaste, are shown in Fig. 25-3. Had water fluoridation continued in Tiel, we would expect caries experience in that city still to be better than that in Culemborg, but we will never really know.

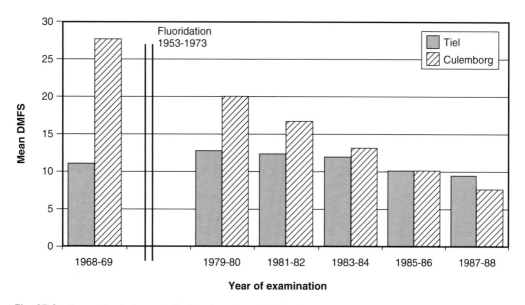

Fig. 25-3 Decayed, missing, and filled tooth surfaces (DMFS) in 15-year-old children in Tiel and Culemborg, the Netherlands, before fluoridation ended in Tiel and for 15 years thereafter. The drinking water of Tiel was fluoridated between 1953 and 1973.[75]

The continued decline in caries experience after fluoridation ceases would be expected in communities in which there is regular and frequent exposure to F from toothpaste and other sources, whereas a caries increase would be expected if drinking water were the only F source. These findings emphasize yet again that regular exposure to low-concentration F is what leads to reduced caries experience, not necessarily exposure to any one F vehicle. Water fluoridation is the most efficient way to bring F to a community, but other exposure methods work as well.

FLUORIDATION IN THE AGE OF MULTIPLE FLUORIDE EXPOSURE

With caries levels at their lowest ever and F available from a variety of sources, the question arises of whether water fluoridation is still needed. The answer is clearly, "Yes, it is." Although overall caries experience in the populations of the United States, Canada, western European nations, Australia, and New Zealand continues to diminish, we have noted that the caries-preventive effects directly attributable to water fluoridation are not as high as they once were. The pioneering four studies reported caries reductions of 50%-70% (see Table 25-3), whereas more recent studies of fluoridation's effects produce less clearcut differences.[33,70,82] The prime reason that effects attributable to water fluoridation are reduced while overall caries experience still continues to decline is that an increase has occurred in exposure to F from other sources. The main such source is F toothpaste, but there are also possibly significant amounts of F in processed foods and beverages. The rise in the prevalence of fluorosis (see Chapter 22) also attests to a broad increase in F exposure.

On the other hand, some recent studies of fluoridation's effects in Britain and Australia have yielded results that still show caries experience to be significantly lower in fluoridated communities.[38,47,101,111] One theory put forward to explain these mixed results is that the clear benefits of water fluoridation tend to be seen more in places where fluoridation is less common, which thus reduces the diffusion effects[61] and emphasizes the impact from water fluoridation. The standard method of measuring exposure to fluoridated water has traditionally been ecologic: that is, if you live in a fluoridated community you drink fluoridated water; if you live in a nonfluoridated community you do not. This may have been adequate in earlier days, but in today's world of high mobility, heavy consumption of soft drinks and bottled water, extensive use of water softeners (which can take F from water), and high consumption of processed foods, the ecologic approach becomes increasingly questionable in research design.

With differences in caries levels between fluoridated and nonfluoridated communities becoming increasingly blurred, the decision to fluoridate a water supply is not always as automatic as it once was. It can be argued that, when caries experience is already low, good F exposure comes from other sources, and the economic cost of installing fluoridation is high, then fluoridation is unnecessary. However, there are two good reasons to argue for fluoridation except in the most exceptional circumstances. One is the cost effectiveness of the measure compared to other methods of caries control (discussed in the next section), and the second is the social equity benefits of fluoridation. Alone among caries control strategies, fluoridation reaches everyone in a community, and as described earlier it has been shown to reduce the strong SES gradient (see Chapter 20) usually seen in caries distribution. Caries is still more prevalent and severe in lower SES groups than in higher SES groups in fluoridated communities, but the differences are much less marked than they are in nonfluoridated communities (see Fig. 25-1). This factor of social equity alone is a strong argument for fluoridating a community's drinking water.

ECONOMICS OF FLUORIDATION

People look at the costs of fluoridation in different ways. A city manager will be concerned about the impact of equipment and operating costs on the city's budget—a subject that can make any city council nervous. Proponents of fluoridation stress the impressive cost effectiveness of the measure over the long term. Dental practitioners usually support fluoridation because it is the right thing to do, even though some have had reservations about diminished practice income as a result. People opposed to fluoridation may claim that "costs" include social costs such as alleged ill health and environmental damage. An economic analysis of water fluoridation, under modern conditions of widespread availability of fluorides, found that under typical conditions the annual per person cost *savings* in fluoridated communities ranged from $15.95 in small communities (fewer than 5000) to nearly $18.62 in larger communities (more than 20,000). This analysis took into account the costs of installing and maintaining necessary equipment and operating water plants, the expected effectiveness of fluoridation, estimates of expected cavities in nonfluoridated communities, cost of treatment of cavities, and time lost visiting the dentist for treatment.[62]

A 1989 workshop found that per capita cost was affected by the following:
- The size of the community: the bigger the population to be reached, the lower the per capita cost
- The number of F injection points required in the water system
- The amount and type of equipment used
- The amount and type of F chemical used, its price, and the cost of transportation and storage
- Probably the expertise of water plant personnel[99]

Although city managers may well be impressed by the low per capita cost, they will be more immediately interested in the total front-end expenditures. This information will best come from the state health department's water supply division, because each community has its own characteristics. The CDC can also help. Per capita cost is generally inversely proportional to the size of the population to be served, although total expenditures on equipment and material are naturally greater in larger communities.

F compounds used in fluoridation are sodium fluoride and sodium silicofluoride, both solids, and hydrofluosilicic acid, a liquid. The availability, and hence price, of all three is highly variable, and prices can also be greatly affected by fluctuations in transportation costs. If a water system has several sources, such as a river plus a number of wells, a separate set of fluoridation equipment may be required for each. Where natural F content is relatively high, less F needs to be added, which thus reduces the cost of supplies.

Although additional personnel costs for fluoridation at a water treatment plant are virtually negligible in a large city, they can be a significant factor in the running costs of fluoridation in a small community. The CDC recommends that water plant operators receive at least 1 day/year of training to allow them to remain efficient and up-to-date. This training may be provided through the CDC's technical assistance program or may be given by health department water supply personnel or university faculty.

Savings in Treatment Costs

Data have been available for years to show that the costs of restorative care for children are sharply reduced by fluoridation. In the Newburgh-Kingston study, initial dental care for 6-year-old children cost 58% less in fluoridated Newburgh than in nonfluoridated Kingston.[3] These savings came from the reduction in the number of extractions and restorations needed, and the smaller proportion of complex restorations required. Comparable findings in British studies, which reported a savings of 49% for children ages 4-5 and 54% for children ages 11-12, have been maintained even after the caries decline was recognized.[7]

Some caveats are required, however, in interpreting these findings on cost savings. First, whereas restorative costs for children are certainly decreased, the effect of fluoridation on the costs of adult dental care is less clear. It could be hypothesized, for example, that dollar savings achieved early in life are lost in later life, because greater tooth retention increases the need for periodontal treatment and the placement of crowns and bridges in later years. The greater the degree of tooth retention, the more dental services may be needed in the later years of life. (Of course, this argument applies to monetary expenditures only: the worth of a healthy dentition throughout life will vary from one individual to another—virtually beyond price for some, of little value to others.)

A second caveat concerns the provision of diagnostic and preventive services to children in a fluoridated area. If many of these services are only marginally necessary, supplying them will add to the cost of services without providing much in the way of benefits. With declining caries and the associated diminished need for restorations, diagnosis and prevention assume a greater proportion of the total cost of dental care. Children with an obviously low caries attack rate in a fluoridated area do not need to visit the dentist as often as they used to, and they require bitewing radiographs less frequently. Data have also shown that F gel applications in an insured population, most of whom lived in a fluoridated area, bore no relation to caries experience.[37] If dentists continue to see such children twice a year and apply the full battery of diagnostic and preventive services each time (all in the name of "good preventive dentistry"), the substantial savings that can be realized in the cost of restorative treatment will be drastically reduced.[18]

POLITICS OF FLUORIDATION

Despite the powerful evidence in favor of water fluoridation as public policy, its implementation has been sporadic in the United States and even slower in most other countries. Frequently it has been the subject of vigorous opposition. Although the major arguments of opponents have varied down the years, opposition remains a persistent fact of life.

Whose job is it to see that fluoridation is implemented in a community in which the conditions are right for it? The ultimate decision is made by mayors, town councils, state legislatures, or the electorate. But these decisions do not just happen by themselves. Dental professionals must make the main commitment to promoting fluoridation, for without their support the issue will almost certainly fail. However, the inherent problem is that this commitment can demand a kind of leadership with which dental professionals are often not comfortable: political action, public speaking, and a level of visibility that can have troubling ethical undertones. Dental and dental hygiene schools do not train their graduates for political action. The detailed role of dental professionals in promoting fluoridation is discussed in Chapter 5.

Public Attitudes and Knowledge

Polls of public opinion down the years have shown that the majority of Americans support water fluoridation; opposition to fluoridation is reported by 10%-20% of the U.S. population. For example, a national Gallup poll in 1991 found that 78% approved of fluoridation, although the sample was confined to parents.[92] The 1990 National Health Interview Survey found that 76% of those with more than 12 years of education knew what water fluoridation was for, compared to 36% of those with less than 12 years of education.[56] Approval ratings vary considerably in different regions and communities, often according to whether fluoridation has been a recent local issue or not. Although national and local studies find that opponents of fluoridation constitute a minority,[49] history has shown repeatedly that even a small single-issue group, when dedicated and well organized, can sway political decisions. Many of those who say they are in favor are really passively so, and a sizable proportion of people polled in public opinion surveys are just not particularly interested in fluoridation one way or the other. This factor immediately evens out the numbers in most political campaigns.

Social scientists were first attracted to the fluoridation issue because of the community conflict it generated, and much of their research dates from the 1960s. Since then the volume of social science research has diminished. That is to be regretted, for common sense tells us that some issues that dictate today's attitudes toward fluoridation, such as environmental concerns, must have changed since the 1960s.

Some of this social science research attempted to "profile" antifluoridationists, the rationale being that opposition could then be predicted and countered during promotional efforts. Unfortunately, the infinite complexities of human beliefs and behavior resulted in a picture that is anything but clear. Some of the studies on the attitudes of persons who voted against fluoridation in referenda, for example, concluded that opponents felt a sense of deprivation or powerlessness, and that they held a grudge against "them," the people whom they saw to be directing society. In this view, a general discontent with society at large can be conveniently expressed by opposing fluoridation.[59,63,96,110]

Although opponents of fluoridation have been characterized as more likely to be older, childless people of lower than median income and education, a referendum can also fail in a young, high-income, and highly educated community.[109] The prevailing image of the profluoridationist from the 1960s research is one of a younger married person with small children and with above-median income and education. Even at that time, however, this image was blurred by a finding of support in all SES groups[55] and by a Californian study that found greater opposition to fluoridation among non-manual than among manual workers.[63]

This confused picture of attitudes to fluoridation still pertained in more recent times. A study in Norway, where there is no water fluoridation, found a 20% rise in public opposition to fluoridated water between 1973 and 1983. Pinpointing the cause was difficult, but it was thought to stem from a perception that dental health was improving anyway so that fluoridation was an unnecessary risk.[102] In a Massachusetts study 60% of the state's voters said they favored fluoridation in a telephone survey, but this figure was at odds with the fact that 61% voted against it in a referendum.[129]

Some have always opposed fluoridation on the basis of freedom of choice[71]; that is, they believe that the dichotomous nature of fluoridation (the community either fluoridates its water or it does not) removes individual choice. This issue remains alive and well, as some would argue it should in a healthy society. However one looks at it, the evidence is that public attitudes toward fluoridating water have become more accepting since opinions were first measured in the 1950s.

Opposition to Fluoridation

The dichotomous nature of fluoridation ensures that there will be organized political opposition to its adoption. Even apart from specific arguments on effectiveness and health effects, skilled opponents can easily exploit the issues of "over-regulation," increasing environmental sensitivity, and cynicism about governmental policies and officials.

Tactics of those opposed to fluoridation have become more sophisticated in recent years. Opponents, though small in number, have learned how to exploit society's concerns about health, whether real or imagined, and how to work effectively with legislatures and city councils. Most states have small "pure water councils," loosely affiliated with each other, which

spring to life to oppose fluoridation when the question arises in a community. There is also a handful of PhDs, physicians, and dentists, who tend to appear anywhere in the country (or in the world, for that matter) to support a local antifluoridation group.

Court Decisions on Fluoridation

Many communities that have begun water fluoridation have had legal suits brought against them in an effort to stop it. Although lower courts have ruled against fluoridation in a few of these many suits, fluoridation has never been ruled against in appellate court. Lower courts that have found against fluoridation have usually done so on the basis of personal liberty and religious beliefs.[14,23,118]

By as early as 1965 state supreme courts had upheld the legality and constitutionality of fluoridation on 13 occasions.[103] By 1984, 13 appeals had reached the U.S. Supreme Court, which on every occasion either dismissed the appeal or refused review.[14] No American court of last resort has ever ruled against fluoridation for any reason.

The most searching courtroom scrutiny of water fluoridation, especially with respect to its impact on human health, occurred in Glasgow, Scotland, in 1983. Known as the Strathclyde case, it was the longest court case in British legal history. The presiding judge, Lord Jauncey, ruled that the evidence for the safety of fluoridation was convincing.[87]

Fluoridation Decisions at the Community Level

Unless state law dictates otherwise, a decision to fluoridate is made by the local entity under whose jurisdiction the water supply falls. This can be a city council, county commission, water board, or board of health. Even when a city provides water to suburban areas and surrounding townships, the decision remains that of the city council, although the issue becomes more complicated in these cases. In locations where the issue is volatile, however, many councils do not want to make the decision without a clear indication of public feeling, and that often means holding a referendum.

The first referendum on fluoridation was in 1950, in Stevens Point, Wisconsin.[88] It lost. McNeil's entertaining description of that campaign shows how quickly fluoridation can flare up into a major issue and how an unprepared dental community, no matter how well intentioned, can make some serious political errors. The outcomes of referenda had not improved much until recent times. It was estimated in 1970 that two-thirds of the first 900 referenda were lost,[76] and 33 of the 41 held in 1980 were also lost.[48] The CDC records show that in 2000-03 referenda were successful 58% of the time, and in cities with more than 150,000 people the figure was closer to 75%. This improvement tells us that dentistry is learning how to act in these situations and that perhaps the idea of fluoridation is not as contentious as it once was in the national consciousness. Perhaps we can even say that water fluoridation has become institutionalized.

THE FUTURE

Chapters 24 and 25 have examined the F issue from many perspectives. It all began with Colorado brown stain and it led to water fluoridation, dentistry's greatest contribution to the public's health. F has changed the face of America (literally!), banished childhood toothache for millions, and raised the prospects of an uneventful lifetime dental history for millions more. Its controlled use has improved the quality of life for all it reaches, and good oral health is primarily a quality-of-life issue. It is the most cost-effective method of bringing F to a community, and it benefits the socially deprived relatively more than the socially advantaged. F has also probably done more to change the nature of dental practice over the last generation than any other single factor.

Despite all those benefits, and despite the fact that fluoridation reaches over 62% of the American population, recent progress has been slow. Society changes and issues that were not considered during the time of Dean and McClure nor during the 1950s and 1960s when steady progress was made in implementing fluoridation have to be dealt with if progress is to continue. Social science research on public acceptance of fluoridation has not moved forward much since the 1960s, and some feel that dental, medical, and social researchers have at least partly failed to carry on from the superb start that the Dean-

McClure generation gave us. Proponents of fluoridation have also made honest mistakes in promoting it. What appeared to some, in retrospect, as arrogance and complacency in past years can still present problems in promoting fluoridation today. In a free society, water fluoridation can only continue as public policy if the public accepts it.

REFERENCES

 1. Arnold FA Jr, Dean HT, Knutson JW. Effect of fluoridated public water supplies on dental caries incidence. Results of the seventh year of study at Grand Rapids and Muskegon, Mich. Public Health Rep 1953;68: 141-8.
 2. Arnold FA Jr, Likins RC, Russell AL, Scott DB. Fifteenth year of the Grand Rapids fluoridation study. J Am Dent Assoc 1962;65:780-5.
 3. Ast DB, Cons NC, Pollard ST, Garfinkel J. Time and cost factors to provide regular periodic dental care for children in a fluoridated and nonfluoridated area: Final report. J Am Dent Assoc 1970;80:770-6.
 4. Ast DB, Finn SB, McCaffrey I. The Newburgh-Kingston caries-fluorine study. I. Dental findings after three years of water fluoridation. Am J Public Health 1950; 40:716-24.
 5. Ast DB, Fitzgerald B. Effectiveness of water fluoridation. J Am Dent Assoc 1962;65:581-7.
 6. Ast DB, Smith DJ, Wachs B, Cantwell KT. The Newburgh-Kingston caries-fluorine study. XIV. Combined clinical and roentgenographic dental findings after ten years of fluoride experience. J Am Dent Assoc 1956;52:314-25.
 7. Attwood D, Blinkhorn AS. Reassessment of the effect of fluoridation on cost of dental treatment among Scottish schoolchildren. Community Dent Oral Epidemiol 1989;17:79-82.
 8. Backer Dirks O. The relation between the fluoridation of water and dental caries experience. Int Dent J 1967;17:582-605.
 9. Backer Dirks O, Houwink B, Kwant GW. The results of 6½ years of artificial drinking water in the Netherlands; the Tiel-Culemborg experiment. Arch Oral Biol 1961;5:284-300.
10. Barsley R, Sutherland J, McFarland L. Water fluoridation and costs of Medicaid treatment for dental decay—Louisiana, 1995-1996. MMWR Morb Mortal Wkly Rep 1999;48:753-7.
11. Blayney JR, Hill IN. Evanston dental caries study. XXIV. Prenatal fluorides: Value of waterborne fluorides during pregnancy. J Am Dent Assoc 1964;69:291-4.
12. Blayney JR, Hill IN. Fluorine and dental caries. J Am Dent Assoc 1967;74(Spec Issue):233-302.
13. Blayney JR, Tucker WH. The Evanston dental caries study. J Dent Res 1948;27:279-86.
14. Block LE. Antifluoridationists persist: The constitutional basis for fluoridation. J Public Health Dent 1986;46:188-98.

15. Booth IM, Mitropoulos CM, Worthington HV. A comparison between the dental health of 3-year-old children living in fluoridated Huddersfield and non-fluoridated Dewsbury in 1989. Community Dent Health 1992;9:151-7.

16. British Fluoridation Society. Fluoridation worldwide, update note, website: http://www.bfsweb.org/extent%20chapter.pdf. Accessed January 23, 2004.

17. Brunelle JA, Carlos JP. Recent trends in dental caries in U.S. children and the effect of water fluoridation. J Dent Res 1990;69(Spec Issue):723-7.

18. Burt BA. Diagnostic and preventive services in a national incremental dental plan for children. J Public Health Dent 1977;37:31-46.

19. Burt BA. Fluoridation and social equity. J Public Health Dent 2002;62:195-200.

20. Burt BA, Eklund SA, Loesche WJ. Dental benefits of limited exposure to fluoridated water in childhood. J Dent Res 1986;61:1322-5.

21. Burt BA, Ismail AI, Eklund SA. Root caries in an optimally fluoridated and a high fluoride community. J Dent Res 1986;65:1154-8.

22. Burt BA, Keels MA, Heller KE. The effects of a break in water fluoridation on the development of dental caries and fluorosis. J Dent Res 2000;79:761-9.

23. Butler HW. Legal aspects of fluoridating community water supplies. J Am Dent Assoc 1962;65:653-8.

24. Carmichael CL, French AD, Rugg-Gunn AJ, Furness JA. The relationship between social class and caries experience in five-year-old children in Newcastle and Northumberland after twelve years' fluoridation. Community Dent Health 1984;1:47-54.

25. Carmichael CL, Rugg-Gunn AJ, Ferrell RS. The relationship between fluoridation, social class and caries experience in 5-year-old children in Newcastle and Northumberland in 1987. Br Dent J 1989;167:57-61.

26. Clark DC, Hann HJ, Williamson MF, Berkowitz J. Effects of lifelong consumption of fluoridated water or use of fluoride supplements on dental caries prevalence. Community Dent Oral Epidemiol 1995;23:20-4.

27. Cortes DF, Ellwood RP, O'Mullane DM, Bastos JR. Drinking water fluoride levels, dental fluorosis, and caries experience in Brazil. J Public Health Dent 1996;56:226-8.

28. Dean HT. The investigation of physiological effects by the epidemiological method. In: Moulton FR, ed: Fluorine and dental health. Washington DC: American Association for the Advancement of Science, 1942:23-31.

29. Dean HT, Arnold FA Jr, Elvove E. Domestic water and dental caries. V. Additional studies of the relation of fluoride domestic waters to dental caries experience in 4,425 white children aged 12-14 years of 13 cities in 4 states. Public Health Rep 1942;57:1155-79.

30. Dean HT, Arnold FA Jr, Jay P, Knutson JW. Studies on mass control of dental caries through fluoridation of the public water supply. Public Health Rep 1950;65:1403-8.

31. Dean HT, Jay P, Arnold FA Jr, Elvove E. Domestic water and dental caries. II. A study of 2,832 white children aged 12-14 years, of eight suburban Chicago communities, including *L. acidophilus* studies of 1,761 children. Public Health Rep 1941;56:761-92.

32. Department of Health and Social Security (Great Britain). The fluoridation studies in the United Kingdom and the results achieved after eleven years. London: Her Majesty's Stationery Office, 1969:33-44.

33. Downer MC, Blinkhorn AS, Holt RD, et al. Dental caries experience and defects of dental enamel among 12-year-old children in north London, Edinburgh, Glasgow, and Dublin. Community Dent Oral Epidemiol 1994;22:283-5.

34. Driscoll WS. Review of clinical research on prenatal fluorides. ASDC J Dent Child 1981;48:109-17.

35. Duxbury JT, Lennon MA, Mitropoulos CM, Worthington HV. Differences in caries levels in 5-year-old children in Newcastle and North Manchester in 1985. Br Dent J 1987;162:457-8.

36. Eklund SA, Burt BA, Ismail AI, Calderone JJ. High-fluoride drinking water, fluorosis and dental caries in adults. J Am Dent Assoc 1987;114:324-8.

37. Eklund SA, Pittman JL, Heller KE. Professionally applied topical fluoride and restorative care in insured children. J Public Health Dent 2000;60:33-8.

38. Ellwood RP, O'Mullane DM. The association between area deprivation and dental caries in groups with and without fluoride in their drinking water. Community Dent Health 1995;12:18-22.

39. Englander HR, Wallace DA. Effects of naturally fluoridated water on dental caries in adults. Public Health Rep 1962;77:887-93.

40. Environmental Protection Agency. Interim primary drinking water regulations. Fed Register 1980 Feb 17;45:57332-57.

41. Environmental Protection Agency. National primary drinking water regulations; fluoride. Fed Register 1985 May 14;50:20164-75.

42. Environmental Protection Agency. National primary drinking water regulations; fluoride. Fed Register 1985 Nov 14;50:47142-71.

43. Environmental Protection Agency. National primary and secondary drinking water regulations: Fluoride; final rule. Fed Register 1986 Apr 18;51:11396-412.

44. Environmental Protection Agency. Drinking water regulations; public notification. Fed Register 1987 Oct 28;52:41534-50.

45. Environmental Protection Agency. Drinking water maximum contaminant level goal; fluoride. Fed Register 1993 Dec 29;58:68826-7.

46. Environmental Protection Agency. Ground water and drinking water: List of drinking water contaminants and MCLs, website: http://www.epa.gov/safewater/mcl.html#mcls. Accessed January 23, 2004.

47. Evans DJ, Rugg-Gunn AJ, Tabari ED. The effect of 25 years of water fluoridation in Newcastle assessed in four surveys of 5-year-old children over an 18-year period. Br Dent J 1995;178:60-4.

48. Faine RC, Collins JJ, Daniel J, et al. The 1980 fluoridation campaigns: A discussion of results. J Public Health Dent 1981;41:138-42.

49. Frazier PJ. Public and professional adoption of certain measures to prevent dental decay. In: Cohen LK, Bryant PS, eds: Social sciences and dentistry. A critical

bibliography. Vol II. London: Quintessence/Fédération Dentaire Internationale, 1984:84-144.

50. French AD, Carmichael CL, Rugg-Gunn AJ, Furness JA. Fluoridation and dental caries experience in 5-year-old children in Newcastle and Northumberland in 1981. Br Dent J 1984;156:54-7.

51. Galagan DJ. Climate and controlled fluoridation. J Am Dent Assoc 1953;47:159-70.

52. Galagan DJ, Lamson GG Jr. Climate and endemic dental fluorosis. Public Health Rep 1953;68:497-508.

53. Galagan DJ, Vermillion JR. Determining optimum fluoride concentrations. Public Health Rep 1957;72:491-3.

54. Galagan DJ, Vermillion JR, Nevitt GA, et al. Climate and fluid intake. Public Health Rep 1957;72:484-90.

55. Gamson WA, Irons PH. Community characteristics and fluoridation outcome. J Soc Issues 1961;17:66-74.

56. Gift HC, Corbin SB, Nowjack-Raymer RE. Public knowledge of prevention of dental disease. Public Health Rep 1994;109:397-404.

57. Gillcrist JA, Brumley DE, Blackford JU. Community fluoridation status and caries experience in children. J Public Health Dent 2001;61:168-71.

58. Gray MM, Davies-Slowik J. Changes in the percentage of 5-year-old children with no experience of decay in Dudley towns since the implementation of fluoridation schemes in 1987. Br Dent J 2001;190:30-2.

59. Green AL. The ideology of anti-fluoridation leaders. J Social Issues 1961;17:13-25.

60. Grembowski D, Fiset L, Milgrom P, et al. Does fluoridation reduce the use of dental services among adults? Med Care 1997;35:454-71.

61. Griffin SO, Gooch BF, Lockwood SA, Tomar SL. Quantifying the diffused benefit from water fluoridation in the United States. Community Dent Oral Epidemiol 2001;29:120-9.

62. Griffin SO, Jones K, Tomar SL. An economic evaluation of community water fluoridation. J Public Health Dent 2001;61:78-86.

63. Hahn HD. Fluoridation and patterns in community politics. J Public Health Dent 1965;25:152-7.

64. Hardwick JL, Teasdale J, Bloodworth G. Caries increments over 4 years in children aged 12 at the start of water fluoridation. Br Dent J 1982;153:217-22.

65. Heller KE, Sohn W, Burt BA, Eklund SA. Water consumption in the United States in 1994-96 and implications for water fluoridation policy. J Public Health Dent 1999;59:3-11.

66. Hill IN, Blayney JR, Wolf W. The Evanston dental caries study. XVI. Reduction in dental caries attack rates in children six to eight years old. J Am Dent Assoc 1956;53:327-33.

67. Horowitz HS, Heifetz SB. Effects of prenatal exposure to fluoridation on dental caries. Public Health Rep 1967;82:297-304.

68. Hutton WL, Linscott BW, Williams DB. The Brantford fluorine experiment. Interim report after five years of water fluoridation. Can J Public Health 1951;42:81-7.

69. Hutton WL, Linscott BW, Williams DB. Final report of local studies on water fluoridation in Brantford. Can J Public Health 1956;47:89-92.

70. Ismail AI. What is the effective concentration of fluoride? Community Dent Oral Epidemiol 1995;23:246-51.

71. Isman R. Public views on fluoridation and other preventive dental practices. Community Dent Oral Epidemiol 1983;11:217-23.

72. Jackson D, James PM, Thomas FD. Fluoridation in Anglesey 1983: A clinical study of dental caries. Br Dent J 1985;158:45-9.

73. Jones CM, Taylor GO, Whittle JG, et al. Water fluoridation, tooth decay in 5 year olds, and social deprivation measured by the Jarman score: Analysis of data from British dental surveys. Br Med J 1997;315:514-7.

74. Jones CM, Worthington H. Water fluoridation, poverty and tooth decay in 12-year-old children. J Dent 2000;28:389-93.

75. Kalsbeek H, Kwant GW, Groeneveld A, et al. Caries experience of 15-year-old children in the Netherlands after discontinuation of water fluoridation. Caries Res 1993;27:201-5.

76. Knutson JW. Water fluoridation after 25 years. J Am Dent Assoc 1970;80:765-9.

77. Kumar JV, Swango PA, Lininger LL, et al. Changes in dental fluorosis and dental caries in Newburgh and Kingston, New York. Am J Public Health 1998;88:1866-70.

78. Künzel W. Effect of an interruption in water fluoridation on the caries prevalence of the primary and secondary dentition. Caries Res 1980;14:304-10.

79. Künzel W, Fischer T, Lorenz R, Bruhmann S. Decline of caries prevalence after the cessation of water fluoridation in the former East Germany. Community Dent Oral Epidemiol 2000;28:382-9.

80. Lalumandier JA, Jones JL. Fluoride concentrations in drinking water. J Am Water Works Assoc 1999;91:42-51.

81. Lemke CW, Doherty JM, Arra MC. Controlled fluoridation: The dental effects of discontinuation in Antigo, Wisconsin. J Am Dent Assoc 1970;80:782-6.

82. Lewis DW, Banting DW. Water fluoridation: Current effectiveness and dental fluorosis. Community Dent Oral Epidemiol 1994;22:153-8.

83. Marshall TA, Levy SM, Broffitt B, et al. Patterns of beverage consumption during the transition stage of infant nutrition. J Am Diet Assoc 2003;103:1350-3.

84. Maupome G, Clark DC, Levy SM, Berkowitz J. Patterns of dental caries following the cessation of water fluoridation. Community Dent Oral Epidemiol 2001;29:37-47.

85. McDonagh M, Whiting P, Bradley M, et al. A systematic review of public water fluoridation 2000, website: http://www.york.ac.uk/inst/crd/fluores.htm. Accessed January 26, 2004.

86. McKay FS. Mass control of dental caries through the use of domestic water supplies containing fluorine. Am J Public Health 1948;38:828-32.

87. McKechnie R. The Strathclyde fluoridation case. Community Dent Health 1985;2:63-8.

88. McNeil DR. The fight for fluoridation. New York: Oxford University Press, 1957.

89. Mitropoulos CM, Lennon MA, Langford JW, Robinson DJ. Differences in dental caries experience in 14-year-old children in fluoridated South Birmingham and in Bolton in 1987. Br Dent J 1988;164:349-50.

90. National Research Council. Health effects of ingested fluoride. Washington DC: National Academy Press, 1993.

91. Newbrun E. Effectiveness of water fluoridation. J Public Health Dent 1989;49(Spec Issue):279-89.

92. Newbrun E. The fluoridation war: A scientific dispute or a religious argument? J Public Health Dent 1996;56(Spec Issue):246-52.

93. O'Mullane DM, Whelton H, Costelloe P, et al. The results of water fluoridation in Ireland. J Public Health Dent 1996;56(Spec Issue):259-64.

94. Parker PR, Bawden JW. Prenatal fluoride exposure: Measurement of plasma levels and enamel uptake in the guinea pig. J Dent Res 1986;65:1341-5.

95. Petersen PE. The world oral health report 2003. Community Dent Oral Epidemiol 2003;31(Suppl 1):3-23.

96. Pinard M. Structural attachments and political support in urban politics: The case of fluoridation referendums. Am J Sociol 1963;68:513-26.

97. Provart SJ, Carmichael CL. The relationship between caries, fluoridation and material deprivation in five-year-old children in County Durham. Community Dent Health 1995;12:200-3.

98. Republic of Ireland, Department of Health. Forum on fluoridation 2002, website: http://www.doh.ie/publications/fluoridation/pdfs/forum.pdf. Accessed February 16, 2004.

99. Results of the workshop. J Public Health Dent 1989;49(Spec Issue):331-7.

100. Riley JC, Lennon MA, Ellwood RP. The effect of water fluoridation and social inequalities on dental caries in 5-year-old children. Int J Epidemiol 1999;28:300-5.

101. Riordan PJ. Dental caries and fluoride exposure in Western Australia. J Dent Res 1991;70:1029-34.

102. Rise J, Kraft P. Opinions about water fluoridation in Norwegian adults. Community Dent Health 1986;3:313-20.

103. Roemer R. Water fluoridation: Public health responsibility and the democratic process. Am J Public Health 1965;55:1337-48.

104. Russell AL. The inhibition of approximal caries in adults with lifelong fluoride exposure. J Dent Res 1953;32:138-43.

105. Russell AL. Dental fluorosis in Grand Rapids during the seventeenth year of fluoridation. J Am Dent Assoc 1962;65:608-12.

106. Russell AL, Elvove E. Domestic water and dental caries. VII. A study of the fluoride-dental caries relationship in an adult population. Public Health Rep 1951;66:1389-401.

107. Seppä L, Hausen H, Karkkainen S, Larmas M. Caries occurrence in a fluoridated and a nonfluoridated town in Finland: A retrospective study using longitudinal data from public dental records. Caries Res 2002;36:308-14.

108. Seppä L, Karkkainen S, Hausen H. Caries in the primary dentition, after discontinuation of water fluoridation, among children receiving comprehensive dental care. Community Dent Oral Epidemiol 2000;28:281-8.

109. Shaw CT. Characteristics of supporters and rejectors of a fluoridation referendum and a guide for other community programs. J Am Dent Assoc 1969;78:339-41.

110. Simmel A. A signpost for research on fluoridation conflicts: The concept of relative deprivation. J Soc Issues 1961;17:26-36.

111. Slade GD, Davies MJ, Spencer AJ, Stewart JF. Associations between exposure to fluoridated drinking water and dental caries experience among children in two Australian states. J Public Health Dent 1995;55:218-28.

112. Slade GD, Spencer AJ, Davies MJ, Stewart JF. Influence of exposure to fluoridated water on socioeconomic inequalities in children's caries experience. Community Dent Oral Epidemiol 1996;24:89-100.

113. Sohn W, Heller KE, Burt BA. Fluid consumption related to climate among children in the United States. J Public Health Dent 2001;61:99-106.

114. Stamm JW. Perspectives on the use of prenatal fluorides: A reactor's comments. ASDC J Dent Child 1981;48:128-33.

115. Stamm JS, Banting DW, Imrey PB. Adult root caries survey of two similar communities with contrasting natural fluoride levels. J Am Dent Assoc 1990;120:143-9.

116. Stephen KW, Macpherson LM, Gilmour WH, et al. A blind caries and fluorosis prevalence study of schoolchildren in naturally fluoridated and nonfluoridated townships of Morayshire, Scotland. Community Dent Oral Epidemiol 2002;30:70-9.

117. Stephen KW, McCall DR, Tullis JI. Caries prevalence in northern Scotland before, and 5 years after, water fluoridation. Br Dent J 1987;163:324-6.

118. Strong GA. Liberty, religion, and fluoridation. J Am Dent Assoc 1968;76:1398-409.

119. Tank G, Storvick CA. Caries experience of children one to six years old in two Oregon communities (Corvallis and Albany). I. Effect of fluoride on caries experience and eruption of teeth. J Am Dent Assoc 1964;69:749-57.

120. Thomas FD, Kassab JY, Jones BM. Fluoridation in Anglesey 1993: A clinical study of dental caries in 5-year-old children who had experienced sub-optimal fluoridation. Br Dent J 1995;178:55-9.

121. Treasure ET, Dever JG. The prevalence of caries in 5-year-old children living in fluoridated and non-fluoridated communities in New Zealand. N Z Dent J 1992;88:9-13.

122. US Public Health Service. Public Health Service drinking water standards 1962. PHS Publication No. 956. Washington DC: Government Printing Office, 1962.

123. US Public Health Service, Maternal and child health library, website: http://www.mchlibrary.info/databases/search.lasso. Accessed February 5, 2004.

124. US Public Health Service, Centers for Disease Control and Prevention. Ten great public health achievements: United States 1900-1999. MMWR Morb Mortal Wkly Rep 1999;48:241-3.

125. US Public Health Service, Centers for Disease Control and Prevention. Oral health resources: Fluoridation statistics 2000; status of water fluoridation in the United States, website: http://www.cdc.gov/OralHealth/factsheets/fl-stats-us2000.htm. Accessed January 23, 2004.

126. US Public Health Service, Centers for Disease Control and Prevention. Preventive health and health services block grant, website: http://www.cdc.gov/nccdphp/blockgrant/index.htm#1d-returnblockgrant. Accessed January 31, 2004.

127. US Public Health Service, Centers for Disease Control and Prevention. Oral health resources: State-by-state reports, cooperative agreements, website: http://www.cdc.gov/oralhealth/state_reports/cooperative_agreements/index.htm. Accessed January 31, 2004.

128. US Public Health Service, Division of Dental Health. Natural fluoride content of community water supplies 1969. Washington DC: Government Printing Office, undated.

129. Weintraub JA, Connolly GN, Lambert CA, Douglass CW. What Massachusetts residents know about fluoridation. J Public Health Dent 1985;240-6.

130. World Health Organization. Fluorides and oral health. WHO Technical Report No. 846. Geneva: WHO, 1994.

26

Other Uses of Fluoride in Caries Prevention

Fluoride (F) was first used to prevent dental caries by adding it to drinking water, but it was not long before alternative methods were put into practice. The result today is that F is used in a variety of ways to control caries in public health programs, individual patient care, and self-care. Dental professionals today must use F with the knowledge that there is extensive background exposure to F through drinking water, toothpaste, mouthrinses, and processed food and drink. We stated in Chapter 24 that F works best to control caries when low ambient levels are constantly present in the oral cavity (in plaque, saliva, enamel surface, soft tissues). Any use of F rinses, professionally applied gels, or F dietary supplements should be aimed toward achieving that condition, either for the individual patient or for the public.

This chapter examines the evidence to support the use of F in salt, school drinking water, milk, dietary supplements, professionally applied gels and varnishes, and F mouthrinses, and makes recommendations for their use. The chapter closes with an assessment of multiple F exposures.

FLUORIDATED SALT

Salt fluoridation is the controlled addition of F to domestic salt (F salt) for the purpose of preventing dental caries. Salt fluoridation follows the same public health principle as water fluoridation: namely, that a small amount of F in a dietary staple serves to inhibit dental caries with little conscious action on the individual's part. The concept of adding F to salt followed the success of iodization of salt, which had been initiated in Switzerland in 1922 to prevent goiter, the thyroid condition endemic to the Swiss Alpine region at the time.

F salt was first used in Switzerland in 1955. There is no water fluoridation in Switzerland, and the nation has only one salt processing and distribution company. Switzerland is a prosperous, highly developed country, and there have been few problems with safety and control of the procedure. The reduction in caries incidence in Swiss communities in which F salt has a good market share, although measured only in before-after designs, appears similar to that found with water fluoridation.[38,110,146] F salt has been well accepted by the Swiss public and now accounts for approximately 80% of the salt market. The effects of salt fluoridation have also been studied in Colombia[65] and Hungary[150] with generally favorable results, and good results have been reported in Jamaica[58,112] and Mexico.[81] Worldwide, it is estimated that approximately 40 million people consume F salt daily.[125]

Although the evidence for the effectiveness of F salt is consistent, it comes from only a limited number of observational studies rather than from clinical trials. The results of the observational studies have been contaminated by the concurrent use of F toothpaste, so that not all of the observed reduction in caries can be attributed to consumption of F salt.[165] In terms of how F salt works to inhibit caries, salivary F concentration has been found to show a small but significant increase for at least 5 minutes after ingestion of the F salt, and these levels return to baseline in 20 minutes.[103] Given the role of salivary F as a reservoir (see Chapter 24), this appears to be how F salt produces its beneficial effects.

The concentration of F in salt is based on estimates of salt consumption and is evaluated by studies of urinary F concentration. The material most commonly used to fluoridate salt is potassium fluoride (KF), although sodium fluoride (NaF) is also used. The early Swiss studies began with salt fluoridated to 90 parts per million (ppm), but it soon became clear that this level was too low. In the early 1970s the concentration was increased to 250 mg KF/kg salt (or 225 mg NaF/kg salt), a level based on estimated adult salt consumption of some 8-10 g/day. Although patterns of salt consumption vary from one country to another,[80] 250 or 350 mg KF/kg salt now appears to be the standard in Switzerland and other countries as well.

Salt fluoridation has political appeal because it gives consumers a choice in a way that water fluoridation does not. In most places using F salt, it appears alongside nonfluoridated salt on the supermarket shelves, and purchasers can make their own choices. The Swiss canton of Vaud, interestingly enough, removes that choice by fluoridating all salt available on the supermarket shelves as well as the salt delivered in bulk to restaurants, bakeries, food processors, hospitals, and other institutions. Oral health

should benefit as a result, although consumer choice is curtailed.

Some concerns have been expressed that use of F salt may promote increased salt consumption with possibly detrimental effects on hypertension, although there is no evidence that this has happened. Nothing in the use of F salt encourages people to consume more salt than usual.

By the mid-1990s use of F salt was established in France, Germany, Belgium, Spain, and the Czech Republic, as well as in Switzerland. In Switzerland the market share is around 80%, and in Germany it is over 60%. In the western hemisphere, F salt use is established in 14 countries of South America and the Caribbean, most notably Costa Rica, Mexico, Colombia, Ecuador, Uruguay, Venezuela, and Jamaica. Further growth in Latin America is planned. F salt has never been used in the United States or Canada, and given the mass distribution of food, the multiple salt production companies, and the extent of water fluoridation, salt fluoridation would not be appropriate in either country.

FLUORIDATED SCHOOL DRINKING WATER

In rural areas in which community water fluoridation is not possible, the approach of fluoridating the schools' drinking water was promoted for some years. The procedure was reported to reduce dental caries among schoolchildren by about 40%,[75] although none of these studies was conducted blind and there were no concurrent controls.

Relative to community water fluoridation, the disadvantages of school water fluoridation are that children do not receive the benefits until they are old enough to begin school, and of course they drink the water only when school is in session. To compensate for this reduced exposure, the recommended concentration is 4.5 times the optimum for community-wide water fluoridation. At its peak, school water fluoridation was introduced in 13 states in the United States. Data reported by states to the Division of Oral Health of the Centers for Disease Control and Prevention (CDC) show that in 1981 school water fluoridation was established in 470 schools serving some 170,000 children. Its current extent is not known but is much lower than the 1981 peak. There is no record of the procedure's being used in countries outside the United States.

Despite the CDC's issuance of safety guidelines, a number of overspill mishaps have occurred, fortunately without lasting ill effects.[3,72,163] The CDC no longer promotes school water fluoridation.

FLUORIDATED MILK

Milk fluoridation is the addition of a measured quantity of F to bottled or packaged milk (F milk) to be drunk by children. The rationale is that this procedure targets F directly to children, and thus it should theoretically be more efficient than fluoridating the drinking water. Having both fluoridated and nonfluoridated milk available also maintains consumer choice.

The mode of action seems to be from salivary return of F to the oral cavity.[160] Salivary F levels are raised 45 minutes after ingestion,[26] and plaque F levels are raised threefold over resting levels for up to 4 hours after ingestion.[57,126] Urinary F levels in children are similar to those found in a community with water fluoridated at 1 ppm.[88]

Only one randomized double-blind trial has been conducted to test the efficacy of consumption of F milk,[147] although a test of F milk readily fits the randomized design. Other studies examining the efficacy of milk fluoridation have been seriously flawed. A few public health programs using fluoridated milk have become established, such as in Bulgaria[119] and in St. Helens, near Liverpool.[97] However, it is hard to recommend further research into milk fluoridation for the United States in view of the large number of F vehicles available today.

DIETARY FLUORIDE SUPPLEMENTS

Because the assumption in the 1940s was that the effect of fluoridated water was mainly preeruptive, dietary supplements were intended to mimic the observed action of fluoridated water. F supplements in the form of tablets, lozenges, drops, liquids, and F-vitamin preparations have been used around the world since the 1940s.

F supplements have F quantities of 1 mg, 0.5 mg, or 0.25 mg. They were originally made

as a 1-mg F pill to be dissolved in a liter of the infant's drinking water, an approach which in time gave way to the simpler once-a-day ingestion of the tablet. Later, chewable tablets and lozenges were manufactured for older children, to be chewed or sucked 1-2 minutes before swallowing, the intent here being to obtain both topical and systemic effects. Most tablets contain neutral NaF, although acidulated phosphate F (APF) tablets have been tested. There are also F-vitamin drops for infants, often prescribed by pediatricians.

Caries Prevention by Fluoride Supplementation

Early studies of the preeruptive caries-preventive effects of F supplementation in children were often seriously deficient and thus yielded questionable results. Some of the highest caries reductions, around 80% over several years, were reported by American studies in the mid-1970s,[1,105] but flaws in these studies included self-selection into test and control groups or the absence of concurrent controls, high attrition rates, and nonblinded examiners. The association that practitioners have observed between conscientious use of F supplements and freedom from caries also cannot be taken as evidence of efficacy, because compliance with the F supplementation regimen is naturally higher among dentally aware people who also have other good oral health habits.

Evidence to favor a preeruptive benefit from F supplementation remains limited to retrospective analyses. Positive results have been reported retrospectively,[5,32,40,41,60,108,166,167] but self-selection bias was evident in all of these studies. Other retrospective studies found no difference in caries experience between those children who reported using F supplements and those who did not.[14,17,64,74,86,155]

Although the evidence for preeruptive benefits from F supplementation is weak, well-conducted randomized clinical trials using placebos and blinded examiners have shown that it can have posteruptive benefits in school-age children. Studies in which the supplements were chewed, swished, and swallowed under supervision have reported caries reductions of 20%-28% over 3-6 years.[43,50] Caries reductions of 81% were reported in a Glasgow study in which children from lower socioeconomic groups who were initially 5.5 years of age sucked a 1-mg F tablet or a placebo under supervision in schools every school day for 3 years.[148]

In summary, F supplements have a posteruptive effect because they meet the goal of maintaining ambient F in the oral cavity. However, there is no good evidence to demonstrate a preeruptive benefit.

Dosing Schedules

To obtain F supplements in the United States and Canada, a prescription by a dentist or physician is required; both the American Dental Association (ADA) and the American Academy of Pediatrics (AAP) maintain schedules of recommended doses of F supplements. However, before 1979 the two schedules did not coincide: the AAP first recommended 0.5 mg/day[6] for children under 2 years of age, whereas the ADA recommended 0.25 mg/day. The AAP altered its earlier recommendations[7] in 1979 to bring them into line with those of the ADA and reaffirmed these new recommendations in 1986.[8]

As the dosing schedules for F supplements are revised periodically, the trend has been to make them ever more conservative. In response to the growing evidence that use of F supplements is a risk factor for fluorosis, the ADA revised its schedule in 1994 to reduce the amount of F ingested by young children, and the AAP accepted this schedule a year later.[9] The current ADA-recommended schedule, based on the age of the child and the concentration of F in the water supply, is shown in Table 26-1. The thinking in Europe is similarly conservative: a European Community group recommended that a supplement of 0.5 mg F be used only for "at-risk" individuals from the age of 3 years onward. This group also declared that F supplementation had no place as a public health measure.[34]

Table 26-1 Recommended dosage levels of supplemental fluoride as established by the American Dental Association in 1994 (in mg F/day)[12]

Age	Concentration of Fluoride in Water (ppm)		
	<0.3	0.3-0.7	>0.7
6 mo–3 yr	0.25	—	—
3–6 yr	0.50	0.25	—
6–16 yr	1.00	0.50	—

Fluorosis Risk From Fluoride Supplementation

Reduction of the early AAP recommendation of 0.5 mg/day for children under 2 years of age was overdue, for this dosage probably led to a considerable degree of fluorosis. One study in the Boston area that used the old AAP schedule, for example, was successful in terms of caries reduction, but 67% of the children developed very mild or mild fluorosis.[2] Excess F ingestion in infancy and early childhood through inappropriate prescription of F supplements is unfortunately more common than it should be. A 1980 national survey of pediatricians found that around 20% of them who practiced in fluoridated areas were prescribing F supplements for child patients who lived in the same communities,[104] a clearly inappropriate action that increases the risk of dental fluorosis. Things were no better 15 years later.[124] These studies have emphasized the need for continuing education of both physicians and dentists. If supplements are to be prescribed at all, they should certainly not be prescribed for patients who consume fluoridated water.

The major concern now associated with supplement use is that of dental fluorosis. Although fluorosis can develop at any preeruptive stage, late secretion and early maturation have been identified as the developmental times when dental enamel is especially sensitive to ingested F.[42,59,95] Although some studies found no association between supplement use and the development of fluorosis,[15,171] considerably more have reported a clear association.[2,39-41,74,86,94,96,133,153,155,169,170] A series of excellent case-control studies has provided strong evidence for a cause-and-effect relation between use of F supplements and dental fluorosis,[121-123] and a comprehensive meta-analysis also concluded that use of F supplements is a risk factor for fluorosis.[83]

The weight of evidence is that F supplements, when ingested prior to tooth eruption, are a risk factor for dental fluorosis in both fluoridated and nonfluoridated areas.

Appropriate Use of Fluoride Supplements

Although F supplements are reportedly used by some 16% of American children under 2 years of age,[117] their continued prescription in North America needs to be thoughtfully reviewed. As often is the case in public health, their use requires trade-off decisions: F supplements have some beneficial impact on oral health, but there is also the hazard of fluorosis when they are used in an era of wide exposure to F. The reasons why prescription of F supplements for infants and young children needs to be considered carefully can be spelled out as follows:

- Evidence to support a preeruptive anticariogenic effect for F supplementation is weak.
- F supplementation has been identified as a risk factor for dental fluorosis, and the prevalence of fluorosis is increasing.
- The prevalence of caries continues to decline, which reduces the need to pursue a strategy that carries documented risks with little counterbalancing benefit.[30]

In light of the advantages and disadvantages of F supplements in a time of widespread F exposure, calls have been made for a reevaluation of their use among young children.[14,82,132] They have a place when used to achieve a posteruptive effect in children older than 7 years, and it is likely that they would be useful in the growing population of older dentate people who are at risk of both coronal and root caries, although this issue has not yet been studied. At the very least, when F supplements are prescribed for infants and young children, parents or guardians should be informed of the fluorosis risk that accompanies the limited cariostatic benefits.

Prenatal Fluoride Supplementation

The question of whether to prescribe F supplements for an expectant woman to increase caries resistance in the offspring has been debated for years. In light of the discussion on dietary F supplements in general, it is not surprising that current views are that any enhanced resistance to caries will be only minor at best. The only prospective randomized trial of prenatal F supplementation found no significant difference in the caries experience of the offspring.[100] Therefore use of prenatal supplements is not recommended.

F can cross the placental barrier and enter the fetal circulation.[31,120] Fetal plasma F levels are correlated with maternal levels, although gener-

ally they are lower. F is taken up in the mineralizing tissues of the fetus; fetal enamel levels go up with an increase in maternal plasma F levels.[120] The most critical time for F uptake in enamel, as noted earlier, is the late secretion and early maturation phase. As a result, prenatal F exposure will have little effect, especially since mineralization of even primary teeth is not far advanced at birth.

Collectively the research evidence suggests that prenatal F administration cannot be supported. As long ago as 1966, the U.S. Food and Drug Administration banned advertisements which claimed that prenatal F administration would increase the caries resistance of offspring.[161] No convincing research has emerged since then to change that picture, and hence the ban still pertains. Although there is nothing to suggest that prenatal F supplementation will harm either fetus or mother, no evidence exists to support claims of prenatal benefit.

PROFESSIONALLY APPLIED FLUORIDE GELS

The F compounds that dental professionals routinely use in tray applications are highly concentrated, and careful attention to technique and to the amounts used is required. Table 26-2 lists the quantities and concentrations of the F compounds most frequently used in dental practice, as well as those used in public health programs and self-applied by individuals. Box 26-1 is a guide to estimating the amounts of F in dental products, and Box 26-2 brings together the information on toxic exposure to F.

Early work on professionally applied F began even before the first water fluoridation projects[21,91] and within a few years the Knutson technique was developed.[90] In this method, a 2% solution of NaF is applied in a series of four treatments over a period of several days, following an initial prophylaxis. In the 1950s the annual application of 8% stannous fluoride (SnF_2) was reported to give beneficial results similar to those achieved with NaF. But staining problems were reported, and the material had an unpleasant taste. Since the early 1960s, APF has become the most widely used F compound for professional application. This material has a pH of about 3.0 and was developed after experimental work showed that the topical uptake of

Table 26-2 Concentration and quantity of fluoride in commonly used topical fluoride compounds

Compound	Concentration (ppm)	Quantity
Topically applied agents		
2% NaF	9050	45 mg in 5 ml*
1.23% APF solution, gel, or prophylactic paste	12,300	62 mg in 5 g
8% SnF$_2$ solution	19,363	97 mg in 5 ml
0.4% SnF$_2$ gel	968	4.9 mg in 5 g
5% NaF varnish (2.26% F)	22,600	51 mg in 5 ml
Mouthrinses		
0.2% NaF—weekly	905	9 mg in 10 ml†
0.05% NaF—daily	226	2 mg in 10 ml
0.1% SnF—daily	242	2 mg in 10 ml
APF rinse (0.1% fluoride)—weekly	1000	10 mg in 10 ml
APF rinse (0.022% fluoride)—daily	200	2 mg in 10 ml
		1 mg in 5 ml of oral rinse supplement (rinse and swallow)
Toothpastes		
0.76% Na$_2$FPO$_3$	1000	1 mg/g‡
0.243% NaF	1105	1.1 mg/g
1.14% NaF	1500	1.5 mg/g
0.4% NaF	966	1 mg/g
0.4% Na$_2$FPO$_3$	526	0.5 mg/g
0.304% Na$_2$FPO$_3$	401	0.4 mg/g

Note: Some figures are rounded.
APF, Acidulated phosphate fluoride.
*A topical application or prophylactic treatment uses about 5 ml or 5 g of material.
†Amounts of 5 and 10 ml are used in supervised mouthrinsing.
‡An average load of toothpaste on the brush is about 1 g.

F by enamel was greater in an acidic environment.[28] The agent has been tested in several concentrations, the most common being 1.23% F, usually as NaF, in orthophosphoric acid. The material is nonirritating and nonstaining, will tolerate the addition of flavorings, and is well accepted by patients.

Procedures for the professional application of F agents were originally developed on the assumption that the F would form a fluorapatite in the crystalline structure of the enamel. A prophylactic treatment was thus considered mandatory before the application of the F to maximize this reaction. Subsequent research, however, shows that high-concentration F such as that in APF gels tends to form a "calcium fluoride–like" material on the enamel surface[46] and thus serves as a reservoir of F that becomes available for remineralization when pH drops.

The nature of this calcium fluoride–like material is still debated by scientists, but as a result of its formation, a prophylaxis before a professional F application is unnecessary because it is no more beneficial than toothbrushing and flossing by the patient.[79,134,137] This finding allows a considerable time savings in office F applications. Professional gel-tray applications have long been considered not to be cost effective for public health programs, although they might be a reasonable approach for highly susceptible special groups in targeted programs.[99]

F-containing prophylactic pastes are widely used in dentistry; the reasoning behind their development was that the prophylaxis and the professional F application could be carried out at the same time. However, results from clinical trials that tested this procedure were disappointing. When a prophylactic paste is to

---

BOX 26-1   How To Estimate the Amount of Fluoride in a Dental Product

Basic information

$$1 \text{ oz} = 28.4 \text{ g}$$

"Percent" means g or ml per 100 g or ml; e.g., 2% NaF solution means 2 g NaF per 100 ml water

Atomic weights: Na = 23; F = 19, Sn = 119; P = 31; O = 16

Fluoride compounds most often used are NaF, SnF_2, Na_2FPO_3

Example 1: How much F is in 10 ml of 0.05% NaF mouthrinse?

The mouthrinse has 0.05 g of NaF per 100 ml of rinse

= 50 mg of NaF, or 5 mg of NaF per 10 ml

Amount of F = $5 \times 19/42$ = 2.26 mg

Example 2: How much F is in a 6.4-oz tube of Colgate MFP toothpaste? (6.4 oz = 181.8 g)

Colgate with sodium monofluorophosphate (MFP) is 0.76% Na_2FPO_3, so it has 0.76 g of MFP per 100 ml of toothpaste

Grams of Na_2FPO_3 in a 6.4-oz tube = $0.76 \times 181.8/100$ = 1.38 g, which is 1380 mg Na_2FPO_3

Amount of F in the tube = $1380 \times 19/144$ = 182.1 mg

Example 3: How much F is in an 8.2-oz tube of Crest toothpaste? (8.2 oz = 232.9 g)

Crest contains 0.243% NaF, so it has 0.243 g of NaF per 100 ml of toothpaste

Grams of NaF in an 8.2-oz tube = $0.243 \times 232.9/100$ = 0.566 g, which is 566 mg NaF

Amount of F in the tube = $566 \times 19/42$ = 256 mg

BOX 26-2   Data on Toxic Fluoride Intake Levels in Humans[29,69]

- Certainly lethal dose (CLD) = 32-64 mg F/kg body weight.
- Death is likely in a child who ingests more than 15 mg F/kg body weight.
- Probably toxic dose (PTD), defined as the minimum dose that could cause toxic signs and symptoms, including death, and the ingestion of which should trigger immediate intervention and hospitalization = 5 mg F/kg body weight.

The 10th and 90th percentiles of weight for children at various ages are as follows:

Age	Weight
1 year	8-12 kg
2 years	10-15 kg
3 years	12-17 kg
4 years	14-20 kg
6 years	17-27 kg
8 years	22-34 kg

So for a child about 7 years of age, who would weight approximately 20 kg, the PTD would be around 100 mg F.

be used it should routinely be an F-containing paste, but such use is not by itself a substitute for a professional F gel application.

FLUORIDE VARNISHES

F varnish is not intended to be as permanent as a fissure sealant (see Chapter 27); rather it is a vehicle for holding F in close contact with the tooth for a period of time. A theoretical advantage for varnishes over other methods of professional F application is that varnishes are adhesive and hence should maximize F contact with the tooth surface. Varnishes are a way of using high F concentrations in small amounts of material. F varnishes are widely used in Europe and Canada, and were accepted for use in the United States in 1994.

Early European clinical trials on the efficacy of F varnishes gave mixed results,[73,93,116] and a large clinical trial in Quebec, which ran for nearly 5 years in communities chosen for their high caries experience, reported only moderate efficacy.[33] As with most modern clinical trials in North America, the study was conducted in an environment of extensive F exposure from toothpaste, which always makes the impact of any one F vehicle difficult to discern. Later studies in Europe demonstrated the efficacy of F varnishes.[37,71] They have been shown to slow the progression of existing enamel lesions[127] and to be at least as effective as APF gel when applied semiannually.[142] A systematic review found that there was a substantial caries-preventive effect from F varnishes, although this conclusion was based mostly on studies that used no concurrent controls.[106]

Varnishes must be reapplied at regular intervals to maintain their cariostatic effect,[141] and investigations continue into the optimum application frequency. Varnishes are clearly effective, although as a professionally applied agent they are inherently more expensive than self-applied preventives. It is not yet clear whether varnishes can be most efficiently used in clinical programs in high-caries populations or whether their use is best reserved for treatment of individual patients on an ad hoc basis. In any event, they are a useful addition to the dental practitioner's F armamentarium for use in caries-susceptible patients. They have, for example, been found effective in pre-

venting decalcification beneath orthodontic bands.[4]

Several interesting public health programs in the United States use F varnish to bridge the gap between dental and medical practice. One program is working to bring appropriate use of F varnish into the medical school curriculum,[66] whereas in another, physicians in most of North Carolina use F varnish to prevent early childhood caries in their at-risk young patients.[139] This latter program is premised on the fact that a much higher proportion of infants visit a physician's office than visit a dental office (see Chapter 2). Contrary to some expectations, the physicians and their staff have reacted positively, which offers exciting prospects for the prevention of this distressing condition, as well as closer cooperation between the professions.

FLUORIDE MOUTHRINSES

The idea of preventing caries by rinsing the mouth with dilute F solutions has been around for decades,[21] but it was some years before F mouthrinsing became a standard procedure in preventive dentistry. A Swedish report in 1965 that found a nearly 50% reduction in caries increment over 2 years[157] naturally sparked interest in the procedure. Since then, NaF rinses have been extensively tested; other rinses tested to a lesser extent include those containing APF, SnF_2, ammonium fluoride, and amine fluoride. NaF rinses became the most widely used of these products because of lower expense and better taste.

NaF formulations have been tested as a weekly rinse at 0.2% F and as a daily rinse at 0.05% F. School-based programs have found the weekly regimen to be the most convenient, whereas daily rinsing is most appropriate for individual use. The caries reductions from daily rinsing are only slightly greater than those from weekly rinsing,[52,70] and the slight differences do not compensate for the greater practicality and lower cost of weekly rinsing in a school-based program. For home use, dentists can advise patients to buy an F mouthrinse from the drugstore or supermarket. Products come and go; a list of current products with ADA approval can be found on the ADA's website (http://www.ada.org/ada/seal/sealsrch.asp).

Most studies testing the efficacy of NaF rinses date from the 1970s. Collectively they showed that regular use of NaF mouthrinses reduces caries increments in children by 20%-35% over periods of 2-3 years.[23,44,63,76,136,140] Positive benefits were also reported in the primary dentition.[136] APF rinse-and-swallow rinse is also beneficial,[1] although given the potential for fluorosis from systemic absorption, this product should be prescribed with caution in younger children. A limited number of tests with 0.1% SnF_2 rinse have demonstrated positive caries reductions,[111,128] and SnF_2 has also demonstrated antibacterial properties not possessed by NaF.[154,156] Continuing caries reductions over long-term use of 10 years or so were reported,[22] and retained benefits have also been found in children some years after they completed a school rinsing program.[67,98]

F mouthrinsing became established as a major caries-preventive public health program in the United States, Canada, and other countries during the 1970s. According to the CDC, 3.25 million American schoolchildren were in F mouthrinsing programs in 1988, spread over 11,000 sites. This number has dropped considerably since then because cost effectiveness is hard to maintain with declining caries levels.

Despite all these seemingly favorable results, a systematic review found that there were not enough high-quality trials from which to reach a conclusion on the efficacy of F mouthrinses.[16] However, it was the National Preventive Dentistry Demonstration Program (NPDDP), a large program conducted in 10 U.S. cities during 1976-81 to compare the costs and effectiveness of a series of preventive mechanisms, that raised most doubts about F mouthrinsing as a public health procedure.

The NPDDP found that the effectiveness of F mouthrinsing was poor, both in overall results[89] and in separate assessments of first-grade children with high and low caries increments.[48] Earlier reviews by the NPDDP researchers had reported serious flaws in the conduct of many earlier studies that did not use concurrent control groups[25] and in some of the economic analyses that led to the assumption of cost effectiveness.[145] Quite strong criticism was also leveled at the way in which the National Institute of Dental and Craniofacial Research had used its data to promote the use of

F mouthrinses in public health programs.[47] At the same time, the NPDDP itself was criticized on the grounds of faulty design and analysis.[61] The atmosphere of uncertainty was dissipated to some extent at a workshop on the cost effectiveness of preventive procedures in 1989, where it was concluded that F mouthrinsing is a reasonable procedure to use in high-risk individuals or groups, though of questionable cost effectiveness as a population-based strategy.[99]

This debate emphasizes the need for clinical trials to be conducted with due regard for the principles of experimental studies (see Chapter 13) and the dangers in extrapolating data from demonstrations and other noncontrolled projects to public policy. F mouthrinsing continues to be used in public health projects, although program directors are taking more care in the selection of communities in which to conduct them: for example, such projects are no longer promoted in fluoridated communities. F mouthrinsing is now seen as appropriate for high-risk groups rather than as a population strategy.

FLUORIDE TOOTHPASTES

Toothpastes without active ingredients, meaning those that contain abrasive and flavoring agents only and thus are intended for oral hygiene and cosmetic benefits, have no anti-caries action by themselves. But because toothbrushing is a social norm in high-income countries, a variety of preventive and therapeutic agents (both known and hypothetical) have been added to toothpastes over the years. Early efforts to produce anticariogenic toothpastes included the addition of ammonia, antibiotics, chlorophyll, and various other agents to toothpastes. None of these agents was effective. To date, F is the only nonprescription toothpaste additive that has been shown to prevent caries.

The earliest attempts to add F to toothpaste were unsuccessful because of the incompatible abrasives used in the products, which bound the F and thus made it biologically unavailable. The first successful clinical trials of an F additive used SnF_2 with a calcium pyrophosphate abrasive.[115] These positive results were replicated during the 1960s in other American and British studies using the same formulation, and caries reductions in children in the 15%-30% range over 2-3 years were reported.[77,84,85,114,144] Clinical trials of F toothpastes in fluoridated areas have demonstrated an additive effect,[101,109,164] and there is some evidence that use of F toothpaste prevents root caries in older adults.[18]

In all, more than 90 clinical trials have been conducted with various F compounds as the active ingredient: SnF_2, NaF, sodium monofluorophosphate (MFP), and amine fluoride have all been successfully tested.[35] Even more compatible abrasives have been developed and tried: insoluble metaphosphate, sodium trimetaphosphate, hydrated silica gel, calcium carbonate, dicalcium dihydrate, and calcium pyrophosphate are the main ones. New formulations are constantly under investigation and are soon marketed when found effective.

There is some laboratory evidence that toothpastes with NaF are more efficacious than those with MFP, although clinical data on this subject are hard to interpret. Analyses of data available in the early 1990s were split on the issue, with discussion often becoming pedantic. Subsequent clinical trials that gave a slight edge to NaF required very large groups to show statistical significance,[107,149] and another trial found no difference between NaF and MFP products.[45] Given the size of the market, this sort of dueling is likely to continue, although it seems unlikely that there will be a serious difference between the products at the population level.

Serious marketing of F toothpastes was underway by the early 1970s, and public acceptance was immediate in virtually all of the high-income nations. By the 1990s, F toothpastes accounted for well over 90% of the toothpaste market in the United States, Canada, and many other countries. Their use in low-income countries, where F toothpastes could potentially fill an important preventive role, is inhibited by their relatively high cost and poor distribution, and often by the relative absence of oral hygiene methods that are taken for granted in the developed world. The FDI World Dental Federation is looking for ways to develop affordable F toothpastes (http://www.fdiworldental.org), but progress is slow. The development of affordable F toothpaste for the low-income world is a challenge to the manufacturers and to dentistry in general.

Quality of the Fluoride Toothpaste Trials

It must be stated at this point that many of the clinical trials for F toothpaste are among the most elegant trials to be found in dentistry, or in all of biomedicine for that matter, to demonstrate the efficacy of a product. All of the essential features of the best clinical trials (see Chapter 13) can be found in many of these studies: randomized groups, double-blind designs, placebo controls, meticulous procedural protocols. Because the water fluoridation field trials have inherent design limitations (see Chapter 25), opponents of fluoridation can attack their validity. But if the issue is the efficacy of F exposure, the F toothpaste trials collectively include many studies that meet the gold standard for such trials. Taken together, the toothpaste trials provide the strongest evidence we have that F exposure is efficacious in controlling caries.

Fluoride Concentrations in Toothpastes

The F toothpastes that first became widely marketed contained about 1000-1100 ppm F. When introduced into the oral cavity, F in toothpaste is taken up directly by demineralized enamel,[129,152] although its retention on sound enamel is thought to be of relatively minor importance. It also increases the F concentration in dental plaque,[54,55,143] thus leaving a store of F available for remineralization when pH drops. Salivary F levels, normally low in resting saliva, rise 100- or even 1000-fold after toothbrushing with F toothpaste.[138] This level drops over the next few hours, with some of the salivary F being taken up by plaque. Postbrushing levels of intraoral F are affected by the amount and vigor of rinsing after brushing[53]; the best advice for adults is to rinse gently after brushing.

Because laboratory studies showed that the uptake of F into demineralized enamel and into plaque was proportional to the concentration of F in the toothpaste, a natural next step was the testing of toothpastes with higher concentrations. Toothpastes with 1500 ppm F have been found slightly more efficacious than the 1000-ppm F products.[36,62,118] A review of the action of these higher-concentration toothpastes concluded that an MFP toothpaste with 1500 ppm F reduced the caries increment by another 12% over that achieved by the standard F toothpastes with 1000-1100 ppm F,[134] although the results of studies with toothpastes containing mixed F compounds were more equivocal. Clinical trials have also been conducted with toothpastes of 2500 ppm F or more with mixed results. Studies in Scotland, testing several products, found that caries reductions were proportional to the F concentration in the toothpastes,[149] but two North American studies found no difference between the 2500-ppm F MFP products and standard-strength F toothpastes.[102,135]

At the other end of the spectrum, concerns about the fluorosis risk from the swallowing of toothpaste by children have led to the testing of toothpastes with lower than standard levels of F for use by children. The first clinical trials compared products with 250 ppm F against those with 1000 ppm F and yielded conflicting results.[92,113] Findings from later studies of 500- to 550-ppm F products, however, suggested that they may be no less efficacious than 1000-ppm F toothpastes.[159,168] Because children can swallow between 0.12 and 0.38 mg of toothpaste per brushing,[20] the marketing of lower-F toothpastes is likely to reduce the risk of fluorosis while substantially retaining caries-preventive benefits. Toothpastes containing 400 ppm F have been available in Europe, Australia, and New Zealand for years, although these 400-ppm F products have not been tested in clinical trials. They are not available in the United States and Canada, despite strong calls to market these child-strength toothpastes in North America.

Use of F toothpastes has just about been institutionalized in the United States and in many other countries. It is hard to find a toothpaste that does not contain F, and manufacturers no longer bother to use F content as part of their advertising. Further research can be expected to focus on determining the most favorable formulations of F plus abrasive and the most appropriate F concentrations. A welcome development, alluded to already, would be the marketing of children's toothpastes of 500-550 ppm F separately from adult-strength products, which might be 1500-2500 ppm F. The principal reason for the absence of adult-strength F toothpastes is that the swallowing of F toothpaste by children is a risk factor for fluorosis (see Chapter 22); thus, if children swallow

higher-F toothpaste, then the prevalence and severity of fluorosis may get worse. On the other hand, higher-F toothpastes are likely to be more beneficial in preventing coronal and root caries in adults than the first-generation products. Perhaps the market could manage both forms of toothpaste with appropriate color coding and warning labels on the high-F products.

Standards for Toothpaste Efficacy

The toothpaste market is a multibillion-dollar industry in the United States, so competition between major manufacturers is keen. Companies incur much research and development expense to secure the ADA's seal of approval for their products; the logo on the package improves marketing and is a guide for consumers as well. Because of the multitude of formulations of F plus abrasive available, the ADA developed guidelines for use in judging applications for its seal of approval for F toothpastes.[10] With newer formulations replacing earlier products and advertising claims being made of superiority over rival products, the ADA went further in 1988, conducting a workshop to determine what evidence would be adequate to substantiate claims of equivalency or superiority of a particular formulation (i.e., F ingredient with compatible abrasives) relative to other formulations.[11] The workshop determined that such claims always had to be backed by rigorous clinical trials in human populations and that such trials required the use of the rival product as a positive control. The trials had to be designed to show a 10% difference in caries increment with a power of 80% (see Chapter 13). The ADA's seal of approval goes to particular formulations rather than to products. The list of toothpastes that carry the seal, which can be found on the ADA website, is now quite long and seems to be constantly growing.

Global Impact of Fluoride Toothpastes

The impact of F toothpaste use on global caries experience has been profound. F exposure is accepted as the main reason for the decline of dental caries over recent years, and most authorities believe that F toothpaste has been the most important F vehicle on a global scale.[27] The caries reductions of 15%-30% achieved in most clinical trials may appear modest compared to those attributed to water fluoridation, but it must be remembered that these were trials of 2-3 years' duration, whereas water fluoridation studies usually measured lifetime exposure. Because, as we know, F works most effectively to prevent caries when small amounts are in the oral cavity at all times, there is no reason why regular lifetime use of F toothpaste should not give results that are similar to those of lifetime use of fluoridated water.

MULTIPLE FLUORIDE EXPOSURES

The majority of clinical trials of F products test only a single agent. In the modern world, however, exposure to multiple sources of F is the rule rather than the exception. People who live in fluoridated areas brush their teeth with F toothpastes and are periodically given professional F applications by their dentists. F mouthrinsing is used in public health programs, and some cosmetic mouthwashes contain F. Then there are dietary supplements, whether used appropriately or not, as well as the poorly quantified F exposures from food and drink. When these are added together, it becomes readily apparent that people in most high-income countries are being exposed to much more F than they used to be.

This phenomenon of multiple F exposures can be viewed from several perspectives. In one way it is beneficial because, with the several different anticaries actions of F (see Chapter 24), fuller advantage is being taken of F's potential. On the other hand, the increasing prevalence of fluorosis (see Chapter 22) is almost certain to be a product of these multiple and poorly controlled F exposures. Dentistry's goal, though not an easy one to achieve for either an individual patient or the community, is to maximize the benefits from F exposure while avoiding an unacceptable level of the undesirable side effects.

Multiple F therapies, whether in fluoridated or nonfluoridated areas, are clearly beneficial for patients who are unusually susceptible to caries. For example, excellent results in preventing caries were achieved in patients who had received radiation treatment for oral cancer, a treatment that can produce dysfunction of the salivary glands and hence loss of salivary buffering capacity. The therapy included F gel-tray applications, daily F mouthrinsing, and routine use of F toothpaste.[49]

Caries reductions above those expected from fluoridated water alone have been found among children in fluoridated areas who (1) underwent annual topical applications of SnF_2,[76] (2) received F mouthrinses and gel-tray applications in combination,[68] or (3) performed intensive self-application of F using custom-made trays.[56] An 11-year demonstration project, begun by the National Institute of Dental Research in 1972, provided F supplements, F mouthrinses, and F toothpastes to children in a poor rural area. The intention was to show that school-based combined F programs could reduce caries experience in rural areas.[78] Cohorts of 1983 participants had MF (decayed, missing, and filled) scores that were 65% lower than those in baseline cohorts in 1972. The demonstration was unfortunately not designed to permit identification of the individual effects of the different F regimens, and the absence of concurrent controls made interpretation of the caries reductions uncertain.

In the context of cost effectiveness, the data on the use of F mouthrinses in fluoridated areas are worth examining in detail: Table 26-3 presents these data for five North American studies. A beneficial effect can be seen in each case, although even in the earlier studies the effects were limited in terms of absolute caries reductions. A later study of multiple F exposures measured the comparative impact of F tablets and F rinses.[51] After 8 years children who both ingested the F tablets (after chewing) and rinsed weekly with neutral 0.2% NaF solution had a caries increment that was 33% lower than that for children who rinsed only and 15% lower than that for those who took the supplements only. However, in the age of low caries experience the largest absolute difference between groups was only 1.17 DMFS (decayed, missing, or filled tooth surfaces) over the 8 years. Cost-effectiveness issues arise given results such as these: when a new F program is instituted among children who already have some F exposure and low caries experience, is the additional benefit worth the cost?

The last two lines of Table 26-3 showing data from the NPDDP provoked the subsequent criticisms of F mouthrinsing mentioned earlier in this chapter. Table 26-4 gives the results of studies in which supervised brushing with an

Table 26-3   Summarized results of studies of fluoride mouthrinses in fluoridated areas

Material	Age-Groups	Duration	% Reduction	DMFS Reduction	Reference
0.1% SnF$_2$ daily	8-13 yr	20 mo	33.1*	1.00	Radike et al[128]
			43.3†	1.22	
0.05% NaF daily	12 yr	30 mo	27.9*	0.72	Driscoll et al[52]
			49.7*	0.94	
0.2% NaF weekly	12 yr	30 mo	22.1*	0.57	Driscoll et al[52]
			55.0†	1.04	
0.2% NaF weekly	9 yr	24 mo	33.8	0.52	Kawall et al[87]
0.2% NaF weekly	Grades 1-2	48 mo	Not given‡	0.29	Bell et al[19]
	Grade 5	24 mo	Not given‡	0.03	

DMFS, Decayed, missing, and filled tooth surfaces.
*First of two examiners.
†Second of two examiners.
‡Could not be determined from the data provided.

Table 26-4   Summarized results of studies of additive effects of fluoride mouthrinsing and supervised brushing with fluoride toothpastes DMFS Increments

Age-Groups	Duration	F Rinse*	F Toothpaste†	Rinse + Toothpaste‡	Placebo	Reference
Approximately 13 yr	24 mo	4.81 (13.1%)§	4.44 (17.9%)§	4.12 (22.7%)§	5.61	Ashley et al[13]
11 yr	30 mo	4.79 (23.4%)§	5.14 (17.8%)§	5.30 (15.2%)§	6.51	Ringelberg et al[131]
10-13 yr	30 mo	None	6.30	5.60 (11.1%)¶	None	Triol et al[158]
11-12 yr	36 mo	4.72 (24.5%)§	4.60 (26.3%)§	4.76 (26.8%)§	6.25	Blinkhorn et al[24]

DMFS, Decayed, missing, and filled tooth surfaces.
*0.05% NaF daily at school.
†0.76% Sodium monofluorophosphate except for Ringelberg et al[79] (0.4% stannous fluoride, unsupervised).
‡All conducted supervised rinse immediately after brushing.
§Percentage reduction compared to placebo control.
¶Percentage reduction compared to sodium monofluorophosphate toothpaste alone.

F toothpaste was combined with supervised daily F mouthrinsing at school, and the results were compared with those for each procedure alone. The results for the combined procedures are, at best, only slightly superior to the use of either alone. Scandinavian studies, not included in Table 26-4 because they tested weekly or fortnightly rinsing and unsupervised home use of an F toothpaste, also reported little added benefit from the rinsing programs at school.[15]

Because caries experience in North American children has generally reached lower levels than those at which the results in Tables 26-3 and 26-4 were produced, it is hard to argue for the cost effectiveness of F mouthrinsing in fluoridated

areas, especially where frequent use of F toothpaste is common. This conclusion was confirmed at the 1989 workshop on cost effectiveness of preventive programs.[130]

Cost effectiveness is a less important issue for the private patient than for public health programs, but selection of a preventive regimen for an individual patient should still take into account the likely added benefit of multiple exposures. To illustrate, professional F applications are of dubious additional value to the individual patient in a fluoridated area who brushes daily with F toothpaste and who has little caries problem. However, even in a fluoridated area, more caries-susceptible patients may get reasonable additional benefit from professional F gel applications or prescribed daily use of F mouthrinses. In these decisions, the clinical judgment should always be guided by experimental data and can be enhanced by attention to the CDC recommendations on F use.[162] As we have said already, however, broad exposure to multiple sources of F is the norm in North America today. When introducing a new F program in a community, therefore, a public health administrator must assess whether the program will produce benefits beyond those already being provided by other F exposures. The evidence just cited shows that additional benefits will probably accrue, but the bigger public health question is whether the extra benefits will be worth the cost of the program.

REFERENCES

1. Asendin R, depula PF, Brudevold F. Effects of daily rinsing and ingestion of fluoride solutions upon dental caries and enamel fluoride. Arch Oral Biol 1972; 17:1705-14.
2. Aasenden R, Peebles TC. Effects of fluoride supplementation from birth on deciduous and permanent teeth. Arch Oral Biol 1974;19:321-6.
3. Acute fluoride poisoning—North Carolina. MMWR Morb Mortal Wkly Rep 1974;23:199.
4. Adriaens ML, Dermaut LR, Verbeeck RM. The use of "Fluor Protector," a fluoride varnish, as a caries prevention method under orthodontic molar bands. Eur J Orthod 1990;12:316-9.
5. Allmark C, Green HP, Linney AD, et al. A community study of fluoride tablets for school children in Portsmouth. Results after six years. Br Dent J 1982; 153:426-30.
6. American Academy of Pediatrics, Committee on Nutrition. Fluoride as a nutrient. Pediatrics 1972;49: 456-9.
7. American Academy of Pediatrics, Committee on Nutrition. Fluoride supplementation: Revised dosage schedule. Pediatrics 1979;63:150-2.
8. American Academy of Pediatrics, Committee on Nutrition. Fluoride supplementation. Pediatrics 1986; 77:758-61.
9. American Academy of Pediatrics, Committee on Nutrition. Fluoride supplementation for children: Interim policy recommendations. Pediatrics 1995;95: 777.
10. American Dental Association, Council on Dental Therapeutics. Guidelines for the acceptance of fluoride-containing dentifrices. J Am Dent Assoc 1985;110: 545-7.
11. American Dental Association, Council on Dental Therapeutics. Report of workshop aimed at defining guidelines for caries clinical trials: Superiority and equivalency claims for anticaries dentifrices. J Am Dent Assoc 1988;117:663-5.
12. American Dental Association, Council on Dental Therapeutics. New fluoride schedule adopted; therapeutics council affirms workshop outcome. ADA News 1994 May 16;25:12, 14.
13. Ashley FP, Mainwaring PJ, Emslie RD, Naylor MN. Clinical testing of a mouthrinse and a dentifrice containing fluoride. Br Dent J 1977;143:333-8.
14. Awad MA, Hargreaves JA, Thompson GW. Dental caries and fluorosis in 7-9 and 11-14 year old children who received fluoride supplements from birth. J Can Dent Assoc 1994;60:318-22.
15. Axelsson P, Paulander J, Nordkvist K, Karlsson R. Effect of fluoride containing dentifrice, mouthrinsing, and varnish on approximal dental caries in a 3-year clinical trial. Community Dent Oral Epidemiol 1987;15: 177-80.
16. Bader JD, Shugars DA, Bonito AJ. A systematic review of selected caries prevention and management methods. Community Dent Oral Epidemiol 2001;29:399-411.
17. Bagramian RA, Narendran S, Ward M. Relationship of dental caries and fluorosis to fluoride supplement history in a non-fluoridated sample of schoolchildren. Adv Dent Res 1989;3:161-7.
18. Baysan A, Lynch E, Ellwood R, et al. Reversal of primary root caries using dentifrices containing 5,000 and 1,100 ppm fluoride. Caries Res 2001;35:41-6.
19. Bell RM, Klein SP, Bohannan HM, et al. Treatment effects in the National Preventive Dentistry Demonstration Program. Rand Corporation Report No. R-3072-RWJ. Santa Monica CA: Rand, 1984.
20. Beltran ED, Szpunar SM. Fluoride in toothpastes for children: Suggestion for change. Pediatr Dent 1988; 10:185-8.
21. Bibby BG, Zander HA, McKellegaet M, Labunsky B. Preliminary reports on the effect on dental caries of the use of sodium fluoride in a prophylactic cleaning mixture and in a mouthwash. J Dent Res 1946;25: 207-11.
22. Birkeland JM, Broch L, Jorkjend L. Benefits and prognoses following 10 years of a fluoride mouthrinsing program. Scand J Dent Res 1977;85:31-7.
23. Birkeland JM, Torell P. Caries-preventive fluoride mouthrinses. Caries Res 1978;12(Suppl 1):38-51.
24. Blinkhorn AS, Holloway PJ, Davies TG. Combined effects of a fluoride dentifrice and mouthrinse on the incidence of dental caries. Community Dent Oral Epidemiol 1983;11:7-11.
25. Bohannan HM, Graves RC, Disney JA, et al. Effect of secular decline in caries on the evaluation of preventive dentistry demonstrations. J Public Health Dent 1985; 45:83-9.
26. Boros I, Keszler P, Banoczy J. Fluoride concentrations of unstimulated whole and labial gland saliva in young adults after fluoride intake with milk. Caries Res 2001;35:167-72.
27. Bratthall D, Hänsel Petersson G, Sundberg H. Reasons for the caries decline: What do the experts believe? Eur J Oral Sci 1996;104:416-22.
28. Brudevold F, Savory A, Gardner DE, et al. A study of acidulated fluoride solutions. I. In vitro effects on enamel. Arch Oral Biol 1963;8:179-82.

29. Burt BA. The changing patterns of systemic fluoride intake. J Dent Res 1992;71:1228-37.

30. Burt BA. The case for eliminating the use of dietary fluoride supplements for young children. J Public Health Dent 1999;59:269-74.

31. Caldera R, Chavinie J, Fermanian J, et al. Maternal-fetal transfer of fluoride in pregnant women. Biol Neonate 1988;54:263-9.

32. Clark DC, Hann HJ, Williamson MF, Berkowitz J. Effects of lifelong consumption of fluoridated water or use of fluoride supplements on dental caries prevalence. Community Dent Oral Epidemiol 1995;23:20-4.

33. Clark DC, Stamm JW, Tessier C, Robert G. The final results of the Sherbrooke-Lac Megantic fluoride varnish study. J Can Dent Assoc 1987;53:919-22.

34. Clarkson J. A European view of fluoride supplementation. Br Dent J 1992;172:357.

35. Clarkson JE, Ellwood RP, Chandler RE. A comprehensive summary of fluoride dentifrice caries clinical trials. Am J Dent 1993;6(Spec Issue):S59-S106.

36. Conti AJ, Lotzkar S, Daley R, et al. A 3-year clinical trial to compare efficacy of dentifrices containing 1.14% and 0.76% sodium monofluorophosphate. Community Dent Oral Epidemiol 1988;16:135-8.

37. de Bruyn H, Arends J. Fluoride varnishes—a review. J Biol Buccale 1987;15:71-82.

38. De Crousaz P, Marthaler TM, Weisner V, et al. Caries prevalence of children after 12 years of salt fluoridation in a canton of Switzerland. Helv Odontol Acta 1985; 29:21-31.

39. de Liefde B, Herbison GP. Prevalence of developmental defects of enamel and dental caries in New Zealand children receiving different fluoride supplementation. Community Dent Oral Epidemiol 1985;13:164-7.

40. de Liefde B, Herbison GP. The prevalence of developmental defects of enamel and dental caries in New Zealand children receiving differing fluoride supplementation, in 1982 and 1985. N Z Dent J 1989;85:2-8.

41. D'Hoore W, Van Nieuwenhuysen JP. Benefits and risks of fluoride supplementation: Caries prevention versus dental fluorosis. Eur J Pediatr 1992;151:613-6.

42. DenBesten PK, Thariani H. Biological mechanisms of fluorosis and level and timing of systemic exposure to fluoride with respect to fluorosis. J Dent Res 1992; 71:1238-43.

43. DePaola PF, Lax M. The caries-inhibiting effect of acidulated phosphate-fluoride chewable tablets: A two-year double-blind study. J Am Dent Assoc 1968;76:554-7.

44. DePaola PF, Soparkar P, Foley S, et al. Effect of high-concentration ammonium and sodium fluoride rinses in dental caries in schoolchildren. Community Dent Oral Epidemiol 1977;5:7-14.

45. DePaola PF, Soparkar PM, Triol C, et al. The relative anticaries effectiveness of sodium monofluorophosphate and sodium fluoride as contained in currently available dentifrice formulations. Am J Dent 1993; 6(Spec Issue):S7-S12.

46. Dijkman TG, Arends J. The role of "CaF2-like" material in topical fluoridation of enamel in situ. Acta Odontol Scand 1988;46:391-7.

47. Disney JA, Bohannan HM, Klein SP, Bell RM. A case study in contesting the conventional wisdom: School-based fluoride mouthrinse programs in the USA. Community Dent Oral Epidemiol 1990;18:46-54.

48. Disney JA, Graves RC, Stamm JW, et al. Comparative effects of a 4-year fluoride mouthrinse program on high and low caries forming grade 1 children. Community Dent Oral Epidemiol 1989;17:139-43.

49. Dreizen S, Brown LR, Daly TE, Drane JB. Prevention of xerostomia-related dental caries in irradiated dental patients. J Dent Res 1977;56:99-104.

50. Driscoll WS, Heifetz SB, Korts DC. Effect of chewable fluoride tablets on dental caries in schoolchildren: Results after six years of use. J Am Dent Assoc 1978;97:820-4.

51. Driscoll WS, Nowjack-Raymer R, Selwitz RH, Li SH. A comparison of the caries-preventive effects of fluoride mouthrinsing, fluoride tablets, and both procedures combined: Final results after eight years. J Public Health Dent 1992;52:111-6.

52. Driscoll WS, Swango PA, Horowitz AM, Kingman A. Caries-preventive effects of daily and weekly fluoride mouthrinsing in a fluoridated community: Final results after 30 months. J Am Dent Assoc 1982;105:1010-3.

53. Duckworth RM, Knoop DT, Stephen KW. Effect of mouthrinsing after toothbrushing with a fluoride dentifrice on human salivary fluoride levels. Caries Res 1991;25:287-91.

54. Duckworth RM, Morgan SN. Oral fluoride retention after use of fluoride dentifrices. Caries Res 1991;25: 123-9.

55. Duckworth RM, Morgan SN, Burchell CK. Fluoride in plaque following use of dentifrices containing sodium monofluorophosphate. J Dent Res 1989;68:130-3.

56. Englander HR, Sherrill LT, Miller BG, et al. Incremental rates of dental caries after repeated topical sodium fluoride applications in children with lifelong consumption of fluoridated water. J Am Dent Assoc 1971;82:354-8.

57. Engstrom K, Petersson LG, Twetman S. Fluoride concentration in supragingival dental plaque after a single intake or habitual consumption of fluoridated milk. Acta Odontol Scand 2002;60:311-4.

58. Estupinan-Day SR, Baez R, Horowitz H, et al. Salt fluoridation and dental caries in Jamaica. Community Dent Oral Epidemiol 2001;29:247-52.

59. Evans RW, Stamm JW. An epidemiologic estimate of the critical period during which human maxillary central incisors are most susceptible to fluorosis. J Public Health Dent 1991;51:251-9.

60. Fanning EA, Cellier KM, Somerville CM. South Australian kindergarten children: Effects of fluoride tablets and fluoridated water on dental caries in primary teeth. Aust Dent J 1980;25:259-63.

61. Fleiss JL. A dissenting opinion on the National Preventive Dentistry Demonstration Program. Am J Public Health 1986;76:445-7.

62. Fogels HR, Meade JJ, Griffith J, et al. A clinical investigation of a high-level fluoride dentifrice. ASDC J Dent Child 1988;55:210-5.

63. Forsman B. The caries preventing effect of mouthrinsing with 0.025 percent sodium fluoride solution in Swedish children. Community Dent Oral Epidemiol 1974;2:58-65.

64. Friis-Haché E, Bergmann J, Wenzel A, et al. Dental health status and attitudes to dental care in families participating in a Danish fluoride tablet program. Community Dent Oral Epidemiol 1984;12:303-7.

65. Gillespie GM, Roviralta G, eds. Salt fluoridation. Scientific Publication No. 501. Washington DC: Pan American Health Organization (WHO-AMRO), 1985.

66. Graham E, Negron R, Domoto P, Milgrom P. Children's oral health in the medical curriculum: A collaborative intervention at a university-affiliated hospital. J Dent Educ 2003;67:338-47.

67. Haugejorden O, Lervik T, Riordan PJ. Comparison of caries prevalence 7 years after discontinuation of school-based fluoride rinsing or toothbrushing in Norway. Community Dent Oral Epidemiol 1985;13: 2-6.

68. Heifetz SB, Franchi GJ, Mosley GW, et al. Combined anticariogenic effect of fluoride gel-trays and fluoride mouthrinsing in an optimally fluoridated community. Clin Prev Dent 1979;6:21-8.

69. Heifetz SB, Horowitz HS. Amounts of fluoride in self-administered dental products: Safety considerations for children. Pediatrics 1986;77:876-82.

70. Heifetz SB, Meyers R, Kingman A. A comparison of the anticaries effectiveness of daily and weekly rinsing with sodium fluoride solutions: Findings after two years. Pediatr Dent 1980;3:17-20.

71. Helfenstein U, Steiner M. Fluoride varnishes (Duraphat): A meta-analysis. Community Dent Oral Epidemiol 1994;22:1-5.

72. Hoffman R, Mann J, Calderone J, et al. Acute fluoride poisoning in a New Mexico elementary school. Pediatrics 1980;65:897-900.

73. Holm AK. Effect of fluoride varnish (Duraphat) in pre-school children. Community Dent Oral Epidemiol 1979;7:241-5.

74. Holm AK, Andersson R. Enamel mineralization disturbances in 12-year-old children with known early exposure to fluorides. Community Dent Oral Epidemiol 1982;10:335-9.

75. Horowitz HS. School fluoridation for the prevention of dental caries. Int Dent J 1973;23:346-53.

76. Horowitz HS, Heifetz SB. Evaluation of topical applications of stannous fluoride to teeth of children born and reared in a fluoridated community; final report. ASDC J Dent Child 1969;36:65-71.

77. Horowitz HS, Law FE, Thompson MB, Chamberlin SR. Evaluation of a stannous fluoride dentifrice for use in dental public health programs. I. Basic findings. J Am Dent Assoc 1966;72:408-22.

78. Horowitz HS, Meyers RJ, Heifetz SB, et al. Combined fluoride, school-based program in a fluoride-deficient area: Results of an 11-year study. J Am Dent Assoc 1986;112:621-5.

79. Houpt M, Koeningsberg S, Shey Z. The effect of prior toothcleaning on the efficacy of topical fluoride treatment: Two-year results. Clin Prev Dent 1983;5(4): 8-10.

80. Intersalt Cooperative Research Group. Intersalt: An international study of electrolyte excretion and blood pressure. Results for 24 hour urinary sodium and potassium excretion. Br Med J 1988;297:319-28.

81. Irigoyen ME, Sanchez-Hinojosa G. Changes in dental caries prevalence in 12-year-old students in the State of Mexico after 9 years of salt fluoridation. Caries Res 2000;34:303-7.

82. Ismail AI. Fluoride supplements: Current effectiveness, side effects, and recommendations. Community Dent Oral Epidemiol 1994;22:164-72.

83. Ismail AI, Bandekar RR. Fluoride supplements and fluorosis: A meta-analysis. Community Dent Oral Epidemiol 1999;27:48-56.

84. James PMC, Anderson RJ. Clinical testing of a stannous fluoride-calcium pyrophosphate dentifrice in Buckinghamshire school children. Br Dent J 1967; 123:33-9.

85. Jordan WA, Peterson JK. Caries inhibiting value of a dentifrice containing stannous fluoride: Final report of a two-year study. J Am Dent Assoc 1959;58:42-4.

86. Kalsbeek H, Verrips E, Backer Dirks O. Use of fluoride tablets and effect on prevalence of dental caries and dental fluorosis. Community Dent Oral Epidemiol 1992;20:241-5.

87. Kawall K, Lewis DW, Hargreaves JA. The effect of a fluoride mouthrinse in an optimally fluoridated community: Final two year results [abstract]. J Dent Res 1981;60:471.

88. Ketley CE, Cochran JA, Lennon MA, et al. Urinary fluoride excretion of young children exposed to different fluoride regimes. Community Dent Health 2002;19: 12-7.

89. Klein SP, Bohannan HM, Bell RM, et al. The cost and effectiveness of school-based preventive dental care. Am J Public Health 1985;75:382-91.

90. Knutson JW. Sodium fluoride solutions: Technique for application to the teeth. J Am Dent Assoc 1948;36: 37-9.

91. Knutson JW, Armstrong WD. Effect of topically applied sodium fluoride on dental caries experience. Public Health Rep 1943;58:1701-15.

92. Koch G, Petersson LG, Kling E, Kling L. Effect of 250 and 1000 ppm fluoride dentifrice on caries. A three-year clinical study. Swed Dent J 1982;6:233-8.

93. Koch G, Petersson LG, Ryden H. Effect of fluoride varnish (Duraphat) treatment every six months compared with weekly mouthrinses with 0.2 percent NaF solution on dental caries. Swed Dent J 1979;3:39-44.

94. Larsen MJ, Kirkegaard E, Poulsen S, Fejerskov O. Dental fluorosis among participants in a non-supervised fluoride tablet program. Community Dent Oral Epidemiol 1989;17:204-6.

95. Larsen MJ, Richards A, Fejerskov O. Development of dental fluorosis according to age at start of fluoride supplementation. Caries Res 1985;19:519-27.

96. Lalumandier JA, Rozier RG. The prevalence and risk factors of fluorosis among patients in a pediatric dental practice. Pediatr Dent 1995;17:19-25.

97. Lennon MA, Jones S, Woodward SM. Some operational aspects of school-milk fluoridation in St. Helens, Merseyside, UK. Adv Dent Res 1995;9:118-9.

98. Leske GS, Ripa LW, Green E. Posttreatment benefits in a school-based fluoride mouthrinsing program. Final results after 7 years of rinsing by all participants. Clin Prev Dent 1986;8(5):19-23.

99. Leverett DH. Effectiveness of mouthrinsing with fluoride solutions in preventing coronal and root caries. J Public Health Dent 1989;49(Spec Issue):310-6.

100. Leverett DH, Adair SM, Vaughan BW, et al. Randomized clinical trial of the effect of prenatal fluoride supplements in preventing dental caries. Caries Res 1997;31:174-9.

101. Lind OP, Von der Fehr FR, Joost Larsen M, Moller IJ. Anticaries effect of a 2% Na_2PO_3F-dentifrice in a Danish fluoride area. Community Dent Oral Epidemiol 1976;4:7-14.

102. Lu KH, Ruhlman CD, Chung KL, et al. A three-year clinical comparison of a sodium monofluorophosphate dentifrice with sodium fluoride dentifrices on dental caries in children. ASDC J Dent Child 1987;54:241-4.

103. Macpherson LM, Stephen KW. The effect on human salivary fluoride concentration of consuming fluoridated salt–containing baked food items. Arch Oral Biol 2001;46:983-8.

104. Margolis FJ, Burt BA, Schork MA, et al. Fluoride supplements for children: A survey of physicians' prescription practices. Am J Dis Child 1980;134:865-8.

105. Margolis FJ, Reames HR, Freshman E, et al. Fluoride: Ten-year prospective study of deciduous and permanent dentition. Am J Dis Child 1975;130:794-800.

106. Marinho VC, Higgins JP, Logan S, Sheiham A. Fluoride varnishes for preventing dental caries in children and adolescents. Cochrane Database Syst Rev 2002(3): CD002279.

107. Marks RG, Conti AJ, Moorhead JE, et al. Results from a three-year caries clinical trial comparing NaF and SMFP fluoride formulations. Int Dent J 1994;44 (3 Suppl 1):275-85.

108. Marthaler TM. Caries inhibiting effect of fluoride tablets. Helv Odontol Acta 1969;13:1-13.

109. Marthaler TM. Caries inhibition by an amine fluoride dentifrice: Results after 6 years in children with low caries activity. Helv Odontol Acta 1974;18:35-44.

110. Marthaler TM, Steiner M, Menghini G, de Crousaz P. DMF teeth in schoolchildren after 18 years of collective salt fluoridation. Caries Res 1989;23:48.

111. McConchie JM, Richardson AS, Hole LW, et al. Caries-preventive effect of two concentrations of stannous fluoride mouthrinse. Community Dent Oral Epidemiol 1977;5:278-83.

112. Meyer-Lueckel H, Satzinger T, Kielbassa AM. Caries prevalence among 6- to 16-year-old students in Jamaica 12 years after the introduction of salt fluoridation. Caries Res 2002;36:170-3.

113. Mitropoulos CM, Holloway PJ, Davies TG, Worthington HV. Relative efficacy of dentifrices containing 250 or 1000 ppm F^- in preventing dental caries—report of a 32-month clinical trial. Community Dent Health 1984;1:193-200.

114. Muhler JC. Effect of a stannous fluoride dentifrice on caries reduction in children during a three-year study period. J Am Dent Assoc 1962;64:216-24.

115. Muhler JC, Radike AW, Nebergall WH, Day HG. Comparison between the anticariogenic effects of dentifrices containing stannous fluoride and sodium fluoride. J Am Dent Assoc 1955;51:556-9.

116. Murray JJ, Winter GB, Hurst CP. Duraphat fluoride varnish: A 2-year clinical trial in 5-year-old children. Br Dent J 1977;143:11-7.

117. Nourjah P, Horowitz AM, Wagener DK. Factors associated with the use of fluoride supplements and fluoride dentifrice by infants and toddlers. J Public Health Dent 1994;54:47-54.

118. O'Mullane DM, Kavanagh D, Ellwood RP, et al. A three-year clinical trial of a combination of trimetaphosphate and sodium fluoride in silica toothpastes. J Dent Res 1997;76:1776-81.

119. Pakhomov GN, Ivanova K, Møller IJ, Vrabcheva M. Dental caries-reducing effects of a milk fluoridation project in Bulgaria. J Public Health Dent 1995;55: 234-7.

120. Parker PR, Bawden JW. Prenatal fluoride exposure: Measurement of plasma levels and enamel uptake in the guinea pig. J Dent Res 1986;65:1341-5.

121. Pendrys DG, Katz RV. Risk of enamel fluorosis associated with fluoride supplementation, infant formula, and fluoride dentifrice use. Am J Epidemiol 1989; 130:1199-208.

122. Pendrys DG, Katz RV, Morse DE. Risk factors for enamel fluorosis in a fluoridated population. Am J Epidemiol 1994;140:461-71.

123. Pendrys DG, Katz RV, Morse DE. Risk factors for enamel fluorosis in a nonfluoridated population. Am J Epidemiol 1996;143:808-15.

124. Pendrys DG, Morse DE. Fluoride supplement use by children in fluoridated communities. J Public Health Dent 1995;55:160-4.

125. Petersen PE. The world oral health report 2003. Community Dent Oral Epidemiol 2003;31(Suppl 1):3-23.

126. Petersson LG, Arvidsson I, Lynch E, et al. Fluoride concentrations in saliva and dental plaque in young children after intake of fluoridated milk. Caries Res 2002;36:40-3.

127. Peyron M, Matsson L, Birkhed D. Progression of approximal caries in primary molars and the effect of Duraphat treatment. Scand J Dent Res 1992;100: 314-8.

128. Radike AW, Gish CW, Peterson JK, et al. Clinical evaluation of stannous fluoride as an anticaries mouthrinse. J Am Dent Assoc 1973;86:404-8.

129. Reintsema H, Schuthof J, Arends J. An in vivo investigation of the fluoride uptake in partially demineralized human enamel from several different dentifrices. J Dent Res 1985;64:19-23.

130. Results of the workshop. J Public Health Dent 1989;49(Spec Issue):331-7.

131. Ringelberg ML, Webster DB, Dixon DO, LeZotte DC. The caries-preventive effect of amine fluorides and inorganic fluorides in a mouthrinse or dentifrice after 30 months of use. J Am Dent Assoc 1979; 98:202-8.

132. Riordan PJ. Fluoride supplements in caries prevention: A literature review and proposal for a new dosage schedule. J Public Health Dent 1993;53:174-89.

133. Riordan PJ, Banks JA. Dental fluorosis and fluoride exposure in Western Australia. J Dent Res 1991; 70:1022-8.

134. Ripa LW. Clinical studies of high-potency fluoride dentifrices: A review. J Am Dent Assoc 1989;118:85-91.

135. Ripa LW, Leske GS, Forte F, Varma A. Caries inhibition of mixed NaF–Na$_2$PO$_3$F dentifrices containing 1,000 and 2,500 ppm F: 3-year results. J Am Dent Assoc 1988;116:69-73.

136. Ripa LW, Leske GS, Sposato AL, Rebich T Jr. Supervised weekly rinsing with a 0.2% neutral NaF solution: Results after 5 years. Community Dent Oral Epidemiol 1983;11:1-6.

137. Ripa LW, Leske GS, Sposato A, Varma A. Effect of prior toothcleaning on bi-annual professional acidulated phosphate fluoride topical fluoride gel-tray treatments. Caries Res 1985;18:457-64.

138. Rölla G, Ekstrand J. Fluoride in oral fluids and dental plaque. In: Fejerskov O, Ekstrand J, Burt BA, eds: Fluoride in dentistry. 2nd ed. Copenhagen: Munksgaard, 1996:215-20.

139. Rozier RG, Sutton BK, Bawden JW, et al. Prevention of early childhood caries in North Carolina medical practices: Implications for research and practice. J Dent Educ 2003;67:876-85.

140. Rugg-Gunn AJ, Holloway PJ, Davies TGH. Caries prevention by daily fluoride mouthrinsing. Br Dent J 1973;135:353-60.

141. Seppä L. Studies of fluoride varnishes in Finland. Proc Finn Dent Soc 1991;87:541-7.

142. Seppä L, Leppanen T, Hausen H. Fluoride varnish versus acidulated phosphate fluoride gel: A 3-year clinical trial. Caries Res 1995;29:327-30.

143. Sidi AD. Effect of brushing with fluoride toothpastes on the fluoride, calcium, and inorganic phosphorus concentrations in approximal plaque of young adults. Caries Res 1989;23:268-71.

144. Slack GL, Berman DS, Martin WJ, Hardie JM. Clinical testing of a stannous fluoride-calcium pyrophosphate dentifrice in Essex school girls. Br Dent J 1967;123: 26-32.

145. Stamm JW, Bohannan HM, Graves RC, Disney JA. The efficiency of caries prevention with weekly fluoride mouthrinses. J Dent Educ 1984;48:617-26.

146. Steiner M, Menghini G, Marthaler TM. The caries incidence in schoolchildren in Canton of Glarus 13 years after the introduction of highly fluoridated salt. Schweiz Monatsschr Zahnmed 1989;99:897-901.

147. Stephen KW, Boyle IT, Campbell D, et al. Five-year double-blind fluoridated milk study in Scotland. Community Dent Oral Epidemiol 1984;12:223-9.

148. Stephen KW, Campbell D. Caries reduction and cost benefit after 3 years of sucking fluoride tablets daily at school. A double-blind trial. Br Dent J 1978;144: 202-6.

149. Stephen KW, Creanor SL, Russell JI, et al. A 3-year oral health dose-response study of sodium monofluorophosphate dentifrices with and without zinc citrate: Anti-caries results. Community Dent Oral Epidemiol 1988;16:321-5.

150. Stephen KW, Macpherson LM, Gorzo I, Gilmour WH. Effect of fluoridated salt intake in infancy: A blind caries and fluorosis study in 8th grade Hungarian pupils. Community Dent Oral Epidemiol 1999;27:210-5.

151. Stephen KW, McCall DR, Gilmour WH. Incisor enamel mottling in child cohorts which had or had not taken fluoride supplements from 0-12 years of age. Proc Finn Dent Soc 1991;87:595-605.

152. Stookey GK, Schemehorn BR, Cheetham BL, et al. In situ fluoride uptake from fluoride dentifrices by carious enamel. J Dent Res 1985;64:900-3.

153. Suckling GW, Pearce EI. Developmental defects of enamel in a group of New Zealand children: Their prevalence and some associated etiological factors. Community Dent Oral Epidemiol 1984;12:177-84.

154. Svanberg M, Rölla G. *Streptococcus mutans* in plaque and saliva after mouthrinsing with SnF$_2$. Scand J Dent Res 1982;90:292-8.

155. Thylstrup A, Fejerskov O, Bruun C, Kann J. Enamel changes and dental caries in 7-year-old children given fluoride tablets from shortly after birth. Caries Res 1979;13:265-76.

156. Tinanoff N, Klock B, Camosci DA, Manwell MA. Microbiologic effects of SnF$_2$ and NaF mouthrinses in subjects with high caries activity: Results after one year. J Dent Res 1983;62:907-11.

157. Torell P, Ericsson Y. Two-year clinical tests with different methods of local caries-preventive fluorine application in Swedish school-children. Acta Odontol Scand 1965;23:287-322.

158. Triol CW, Kranz SM, Volpe AR, et al. Anticaries effect of a sodium fluoride rinse and an MFP dentifrice in a nonfluoridated water area: A thirty-month study. Clin Prev Dent 1980;9(2):13-5.

159. Triol CW, Mandanas BY, Juliano GF, et al. A clinical study of children comparing anticaries effect of two fluoride dentifrices. A 31-month study. Clin Prev Dent 1987;9(2):22-4.

160. Twetman S, Nederfors T, Petersson LG. Fluoride concentration in whole saliva and separate gland secretions in schoolchildren after intake of fluoridated milk. Caries Res 1998;32:412-6.

161. US Department of Health, Education, and Welfare, Food and Drug Administration. Oral prenatal drugs containing fluorides for human use. Fed Register 1966 Oct 20;31:13537.

162. US Public Health Service, Centers for Disease Control and Prevention. Recommendations for using fluoride to prevent and control dental caries in the United States. MMWR Recomm Rep 2001;50(RR-14):1-42.

163. Vogt RL, Witherell L, LaRue D, Klaucke DN. Acute fluoride poisoning associated with an on-site fluoridator in a Vermont elementary school. Am J Public Health 1982;72:1168-9.

164. Von der Fehr FR, Möller IJ. Caries-preventive fluoride dentifrices. Caries Res 1978;12(Suppl 1):31-7.

165. Warpeha R, Beltran-Aguilar E, Baez R. Methodological and biological factors explaining the reduction in dental caries in Jamaican school children between 1984 and 1995. Pan Am J Public Health 2001;10: 37-44.

166. Widenheim J, Birkhed D. Caries-preventive effect on primary and permanent teeth and cost-effectiveness of an NaF tablet preschool program. Community Dent Oral Epidemiol 1991;19:88-92.

167. Widenheim J, Birkhed D, Granath L, Lindgren G. Preeruptive effect of NaF tablets on caries in children from 12 to 17 years of age. Community Dent Oral Epidemiol 1986;14:1-4.

168. Winter GB, Holt RD, Williams BF. Clinical trial of a low-fluoride toothpaste for young children. Int Dent J 1989;39:227-35.

169. Woltgens JH, Etty EJ, Nieuwland WM. Prevalence of mottled enamel in permanent dentition of children participating in a fluoride programme at the Amsterdam dental school. J Biol Buccale 1989;17:15-20.

170. Woolfolk MW, Faja BW, Bagramian RA. Relation of sources of systemic fluoride to prevalence of dental fluorosis. J Public Health Dent 1989;49:78-82.

Fissure Sealants

A fissure sealant is a plastic, professionally applied material used to occlude the pits and fissures of teeth. The purpose is to provide a physical barrier to the impaction of substrate for cariogenic bacteria in those crevices and hence to prevent caries from developing. Sealants also can halt the carious process after it has begun and can be used as a form of treatment for early lesions. All sealants are applied to the tooth in liquid form and polymerize (or "cure") in place a short time later.

The correct name for this group of materials is *pit-and-fissure sealants*, but they are more commonly referred to as *fissure sealants*, or just *sealants* (the term we will use). This chapter discusses the use of sealants in caries prevention, examines the issue of their cost effectiveness, and makes recommendations for their use.

HISTORICAL DEVELOPMENT

The idea of physically occluding pits and fissures is hardly new, for as long ago as 1923 Hyatt suggested a technique he called "prophylactic odontotomy."[52] Developed in an age of severe and seemingly universal caries, Hyatt's technique involved minimal operative preparation of sound fissures and restoration with amalgam. The idea was not fully accepted even before the days of modern preventive

dentistry,[58] but it led to widespread use of the "preventive restoration," meaning a full Black's cavity restoration with "extension for prevention" in sound fissures, placed on the grounds that without intervention such areas would soon decay anyway. For many years, this type of restoration was considered good preventive practice, and perhaps it was when there were few other preventive options. Although we have no way of knowing just how much caries this method "prevented," the extensive use of the preventive restoration served to artificially inflate DMF (decayed, missing, and filled) scores (see Chapter 15).[55]

In the prefluoride era, various chemicals were painted onto the tooth surface in an effort to prevent caries, but none proved successful.[11,57] Even after fluoride entered dental practice, interest in a specific preventive agent for pit-and-fissure caries persisted, but it proved difficult to find a material that adhered successfully to enamel in the oral environment. The breakthrough came in 1955 with Buonocore's development of the acid-etch technique.[21] By the mid-1960s cyanoacrylates had been used as sealant materials with some success,[30] but their production was not continued.[91] In the late 1960s the "bis-GMA" formulation (a sealant that is the reaction product of bisphenol A and glycidyl methacrylate with a methyl methacrylate monomer) was developed and proved successful in a feasibility trial.[22] The bis-GMA formulation became the basis of a number of other products that soon came onto the market. The American Dental Association (ADA) issued provisional acceptance of the first bis-GMA material, Nuva-Seal, in 1972[4] and full acceptance in 1976.[5] The number and types of accepted materials have grown steadily since then and will likely continue to grow in the future. Currently, the most widely used sealant materials are either bis-GMA resin or urethane based.[109] There is also considerable interest in the potential use of glass ionomer–based materials and fluoride-containing varnishes as sealant materials, but the research literature to date shows their retention to be inferior to that of the conventional sealant materials.[9,16,17,56,69-71,96,97,105,116]

RATIONALE FOR SEALANTS

It has been recognized for years that fissured occlusal surfaces are the most vulnerable to caries. With the continuing caries decline among children, caries is more and more a disease of the fissured surfaces as the rate of interproximal caries development continues to decline faster than the overall rate of caries experience.[13,99] Occlusal surfaces are also those least protected by fluorides,[12] so the case for sealant application as a complementary procedure to fluoride use is even stronger. As of the early 1990s, at least 83% of all decayed or filled surfaces in the permanent teeth of 5- to 17-year-olds were in pit-and-fissure surfaces.[19] In fact, the appropriate delivery of fluorides and sealants together, in theory at least, presents the prospect of controlling caries to low levels previously unimaginable.

SEALANT PRODUCTS AND PROCEDURES

The original bis-GMA materials, now referred to as first-generation sealants, polymerized under ultraviolet (UV) light, a procedure that required a bulky UV light source in the oral cavity. Second-generation sealants are chemically polymerized; that is, when they are mixed, the operator has a fixed time to apply the sealant before it hardens. A number of such sealants are

currently available. Third-generation sealants are those cured by visible light, which gives the operator the advantage of curing the sealant only when satisfied that it is all correctly in place. That advantage also applied to first-generation UV-cured sealants, but the visible light sources are far more compact and less expensive than the original UV light sources. Some second- and third-generation sealants are colored or opaque to make them more visible at clinical examination.

It should also be noted that in 1996 a research report from Spain concluded that, shortly after placement of sealants, bisphenol A and bisphenol A dimethacrylate monomers could be detected in saliva and that these monomers showed estrogen-like activity when tested in in vitro cultures of human breast cell tumors.[68] This effect is of concern, because it theoretically could result in increased tumor cell growth. To date there is no evidence that the transient amounts of these chemicals in saliva represent an important exposure in humans. In addition, none of the sealants that currently carries the ADA seal of acceptance produces detectable levels of bisphenol A.[1] However, the Spanish finding does point out that any material used in dentistry must be thoroughly evaluated for potential risk and that, regardless of how safe it appears to be, practitioners must take care to use any procedure or material only when the patient is likely to benefit from it. The ADA provides continual updates on these and related matters on its website (http://www.ada.org/prof/resources/positions/statements/index.asp).

Sealant application is a simple though meticulous procedure that requires attention to all details of technique, especially moisture control. Even slight moisture contamination during sealant application and curing will result in failure. When applying a sealant, the operator begins by washing and drying the tooth surface, then etching with acid to demineralize the surface layers of enamel in and around the fissures. The etchant is supplied as either a liquid or a gel; 35%-37% orthophosphoric acid is the most commonly used agent.[109] Acid etching dissolves out some of the inorganic fraction of the enamel, which subsequently allows "tags" of sealant to penetrate and thus enhances retention. Some of these tags can extend up to

100 μm into enamel, although tags of 15-20 μm are more common.[92] After etching, the tooth surface is again washed and dried thoroughly, and the liquid sealant is applied and worked into the fissures and pits. The sealant is then polymerized (by visible light or by self-curing) and trimmed if necessary. Detailed descriptions of the application process are available.[109]

By the early twenty-first century, the application of sealants as a purely caries-preventive procedure was merging into the popularity of conservative restoration procedures, many of which also used the acid-etch technique. The trend was stimulated by the caries decline, which meant that practitioners increasingly had to manage small, slowly developing lesions rather than large cavities, and by the rapid developments in composite materials. Dentistry began moving away from placement of amalgams in traditionally prepared Black's cavities with extension for prevention and toward minimum-preparation restorations, which were far less invasive, lasted longer, and were more esthetic.[35] The preventive resin and sealed composite restoration,[49,63,110] sealed glass ionomer restoration,[46] "tunnel" restoration for small proximal restorations,[28] and even sealed amalgams[63,64] are changing the face of restorative dentistry. The distinction between a purely preventive sealant placed on a sound tooth, sealant placed on an incipient lesion, and a minimum-preparation sealed restoration is becoming increasingly blurred. The challenge is to understand the indications for each and to use each appropriately.

SEALANT CLINICAL TRIAL DESIGN

The initial clinical trials for testing the efficacy of sealants necessarily differed from the classical model (see Chapter 13) in several respects:
- The study design was usually "half-mouth," in which the analytic unit is a contralateral pair of teeth, usually first or second molars. Because test and control teeth are in the same mouth, the required number of study subjects (see Chapter 13) could be reduced.
- There was no placebo sealant; the control tooth of each pair in these earlier trials was simply left untreated (a passive control).

- Examiners could not be blinded in a trial with a passive control, for they could see the sealant on the test tooth.

Because of the overwhelming weight of the evidence for the efficacy of sealants, recent trials testing new products now most commonly apply an accepted sealant as a positive control on the control tooth or individual dentition. Because positive controls are used in comparative studies, the examiners should be blind as to which sealant is the test product and which is the positive control. Because differences in efficacy between the test product and the control are expected to be small, the numbers of subjects needed is fairly high.

SEALANT EFFICACY

A large number of well-conducted sealant studies have been carried out, which allows conclusions on their efficacy to be stated with some confidence. The panel at the National Institutes of Health Consensus Conference on dental sealants in 1983, one of the relatively few such conferences held on dental procedures, concluded that sealants were highly efficacious.[67] The panel also noted, however, that practitioners were slow to adopt their use and that insurance carriers were also hesitant about adding sealant application to their list of benefits. The Medicaid programs in all 50 states now cover sealant application, and although precise numbers are unavailable, the number of privately insured groups with sealant coverage continues to grow.

The first clinical sealant studies in the 1960s yielded spectacular results, with caries reductions of 99% reported.[22] These initial studies, however, carefully selected both the patients and the teeth to be sealed. By the end of the 1970s, there was clear evidence from numerous clinical trials in different populations that sealants were highly efficacious when applied correctly.[76] Studies since then using second- and third-generation sealants have almost all yielded results highly favoring their use; reviews of what is now an extensive literature have all reached highly favorable conclusions regarding their efficacy.[77,78,100,113] Well-controlled clinical trials have shown good results after 5 years,[48] 7 years,[65] and 10 years[78]; and 10-year and 15-year retrospective reports also showed encouraging results.[94,95] The favorable evidence has led the ADA to strongly support the appropriate use of sealants in general practice.[2,3]

Evidence for the efficacy of sealant application in private practice, although scanty, also appears favorable. In an observational study in Canada, sealed first permanent molars had a 75% lower incidence of new restorations than originally sound but unsealed molars.[53] The authors acknowledged that use of sealants was more common in caries-free children and in children whose parents had higher levels of education, which could account for some of the lower caries increment, but the differences in caries experience were so large that sealants had to have played a substantial role. It is nevertheless important to be cautious in interpreting outcomes from observational studies in which patients are not randomly assigned to receive or not to receive sealants. As has been pointed out in a study of the use of sealants in a Medicaid program, the children who actually received sealants tended to be at lower risk; that is, they were more likely to have been caries free initially and were more likely to have been classified by the study examiners as not needing sealants.[80] The authors pointed out that this pattern of nonrandom use of sealants in the least caries-prone children could lead to overestimates of sealant effectiveness. Nevertheless, there is ample reason to think that, with appropriate patient selection, sealant application is highly effective in private practice.

Findings from the earlier clinical studies of sealants that have been supported by later research include the following:

- Sealant is generally retained better on mandibular than on maxillary molars. This is attributed to better accessibility and more favorable tooth morphology.
- Sealants are better retained when placed in older children. This is thought to be due to the ability to achieve better isolation in more completely erupted teeth and the ability of the older child to cooperate in maintaining a dry field.
- Retention seems better on bicuspids than on molars. This too is likely to come from better accessibility, plus the fact that in studies in which children have had bicuspids sealed they were obviously older than children who had only their first molars available for sealing.

- Retention of sealant is synonymous with freedom from caries. An early concern was how the caries status of a tooth could be judged beneath intact sealant, but subsequent clinical research has shown that caries does not progress beneath intact sealant.
- Loss of sealant is greatest in the first 6 months after application. The sealant is probably lost very early in that period, however, because the data suggest that the rapidly lost sealants are those that never properly adhered in the first place. The most likely reason for this kind of failure is moisture contamination. A properly placed sealant will gradually wear down after a period of years, but protection from caries seems to remain, perhaps because of the sealant tags. The quickly lost sealant almost certainly has no tags, so the tooth concerned becomes vulnerable again.

These results demonstrated unequivocally the considerable efficacy of sealants; they also gave hints of the more recent realization that sealants are more difficult to successfully apply and maintain on the very teeth that are most vulnerable, that is, the early-erupting molars in caries-prone children. On the other hand, sealants seem to be retained best on teeth that are least caries prone (e.g., bicuspids) and in children with low caries risk.[18] This realization is part of what has lead to efforts to target sealant use to the most susceptible groups, individuals, and teeth, an issue discussed later in this chapter.

Later studies of sealant efficacy have led to four additional conclusions that have an important bearing on the way sealants are used in clinical practice. These conclusions are discussed in the following sections.

All ADA-Approved Sealant Types Have Similar Efficacy

With the evolution of sealant systems and the large number of brands now available, it is logical for dentists to ask which type is best. The response from clinical studies is that all accepted sealants are effective when applied properly. Results of numerous trials have demonstrated that the retention of the light-cured sealants is equivalent to that of the chemically polymerized products.[50,81,102,117]

No UV-cured sealants have been among the list of ADA-approved sealants for a number of years, because they have been superseded by the chemically polymerized and visible light–cured sealants. The dental practitioner's choice thus comes down to personal taste: an autopolymerized sealant hardens a specified time after preparation, just like many other products used in dentistry. The visible light–cured resins require the handling of an extra piece of equipment, the light source, but setting time is controlled by the operator.

Sealants Can Be Safely Placed over Incipient Caries

A conclusion of the National Institutes of Health consensus panel in 1983 was that evidence supported the use of sealants to arrest the progress of incipient lesions.[67] Nothing has occurred since then to alter that conclusion.

Modern sealants were developed as a primary preventive procedure—that is, to be placed on sound surfaces—but shades of Hyatt's philosophy soon emerged. Given that sealants occluded the fissures, it was logical to question whether caries could progress beneath a sealant. The answer, after a number of studies, is now clear. When a sealant is placed over an incipient carious lesion, meaning a stained fissure in which softness at the base can be detected but in which cavitation has not yet occurred, caries does not progress provided the sealant remains intact. Sealant is retained on the carious teeth just as well as on sound teeth,[42] and neither lesion depth nor microbiologic counts progresses under intact sealant.[41,66] Reviews of these and other studies have concluded that the evidence is strong that caries-active lesions become caries inactive beneath intact sealant.[38,103] As restorative philosophy continues to evolve toward increasingly conservative cavity preparations, more recent reports confirm that even carious dentin, when isolated under a minimal restoration and sealant, does not progress.[63] These results provide further assurance that the clinician need not fear the placement of sealant over incipient caries. Indeed, as discussed later in this chapter, consensus is developing that the placement of sealants over incipient lesions is one of their most effective uses.

Sealants Are of Uncertain Value on Primary Teeth

Some early research showed poorer retention of sealant on primary tooth enamel, although results were better in some later studies.[75,93] The different enamel structure of primary teeth was thought to be a possible reason, although moisture contamination may also have been greater with younger children. Subsequent laboratory studies have shown that a short etch time is effective for primary enamel,[106] and sealant retention on primary molars in a large Head Start program in Tennessee was equivalent to that on permanent molars.[43] What is not clear, however, is whether the usual caries pattern in primary molars is compatible with optimal sealant effectiveness, despite retentive success. In many children, the occlusal surfaces of primary molars are not highly fissured and thus are not especially caries prone. Further, when caries is a problem in primary molars, the first lesion is often interproximal. Sealants are not effective in these circumstances.

Sealants Are an Important Part of Public Health Programs

With the decline of dental caries among children, especially interproximal caries, sealant programs are becoming more appropriate choices in public caries prevention programs for children. Although many dental public health initiatives are directed toward encouraging the use of sealants in private practice, there is also considerable activity in the development of projects to actually place sealants in public programs. In 2002 29 states reported having school-based or school-linked sealant programs, serving 193,000 children.[108] These programs operate either in schools, usually with portable equipment, or in community clinics. How effective these programs can be both in increasing sealant prevalence and in reducing racial disparities in sealant use is demonstrated by the data in Fig. 27-1. In the Ohio sealant programs, the overall prevalence of sealants in third-grade students was approximately twice as high in schools with a sealant program as in those without such a program, and the absolute and relative racial disparities also diminished.[107] The philosophy behind these public sealant programs is almost always to bring this

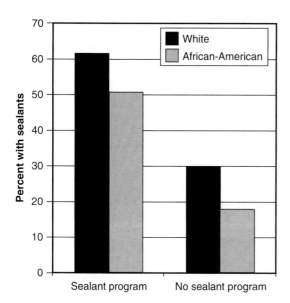

Fig. 27-1 Dental sealant prevalence in third-grade children in Ohio, in schools with and without a dental sealant program, 1998-99.[107]

preventive procedure to children who otherwise would be unlikely to receive comprehensive dental care. School-based and school-linked programs are targeted to schools with a high proportion of children from low-income families or schools with a high number of children with untreated dental needs, or to areas in which there is a shortage of dentists.[10]

SEALANTS IN PUBLIC PROGRAMS

Research has shown that trained auxiliaries can apply sealant just as successfully as can dentists.[25,61] This is an important finding in public health, for the cost effectiveness of sealant programs virtually depends on deployment of auxiliaries.[23] It is unfortunate that regulations in some states do not permit auxiliaries to apply sealant, a provision that is hard to defend as being in the public interest. The on-site presence of a dentist will obviously add to the cost of a public program without necessarily improving its outcome. Several public health sealant programs have managed to deal with these problems and have subsequently flourished. One is in New Mexico, which required revision of its dental practice act to permit auxiliaries to apply sealant in the state-administered program.[87] The New Mexico program, which uses mobile teams with portable equipment,

found 67% retention of one-time sealant applications after 6 years. In sixth-graders who had received sealants on their first molars in grades 1, 2, or 3, only 5.6% of those surfaces subsequently become carious, compared with 26.9% of the same surfaces in children who were not in the sealant program.[24] Even allowing for some self-selection bias, those figures are impressive. In the Canadian province of Saskatchewan, 79% of sealants applied by dental therapists were retained 3 years later, and sealed teeth developed 46% less caries than their unsealed counterparts after 4 years.[54] In Canada's Prince Edward Island program, there is annual resealing when needed. In that province, 85% of sealants were successful after 8-10 years,[83] similar to results reported for a 10-year study in Sweden.[115]

In addition to providing geographic targeting (see Chapter 4) of sealant programs to schools in more deprived communities, most public sealant programs also treat only children at specific stages of dental development (i.e., soon after eruption of the first and second molars). In the United States, where children begin school at age 6, grades 1-2 are the best times for sealing first molars, and grades 6-7 for sealing second molars.[14,59] Sealing of bicuspids and primary teeth is not usually a part of public programs because far fewer bicuspids decay than do molars,[6,33] and a primary molar that is sound in grade 1 will probably stay that way. A good body of experience in the operation of programs with sealant teams has now accumulated,[24,53] and excellent guides to the development and operation of public sealant programs are available.[26,72]

We referred earlier in this chapter to the prospect of using sealants and fluoride together to reduce caries-associated problems to lower levels than could even have been imagined only a few decades ago. Sealant placement is an obvious adjunct to water fluoridation; a comprehensive 1989 review found that sealants were more effective in fluoridated areas than in nonfluoridated areas, although the difference was slight.[113] Sealants also have been tested in combination with fluoride mouthrinsing. In a New York study, after 2 years the 84 children in grades 2-3 with sealants had an increment of only 0.03 DMFS (decayed, missing, and filled surfaces), compared with an increment of 0.47 DMFS in the control group. In the 84 children in the sealant-rinse group, there were only 3 new decayed or filled surfaces over the 2 years, 2 of them occlusal, whereas in the 51 controls, there were 24 new decayed or filled surfaces, 15 of them occlusal.[79] In another study that used a sequential cross-sectional comparison group, a 23% decline in occlusal caries over a 4-year period in 14- to 17-year-olds was attributed to the addition of sealant placement to an ongoing school-based fluoride program.[85] These data suggest that nearly complete prevention of caries at levels that require invasive restorations is indeed theoretically possible, but its achievement might be costly. As we saw with topical fluoride application in Chapter 26, there comes a point at which the underlying risk of caries in some individuals is so low that additional fluoride exposure is not warranted. The same is likely to be true for sealant placement. In those individuals (and teeth, in the case of sealants) in whom the risk of occlusal caries is very low, the cost of placing and maintaining sealants may outweigh the potential benefit that sealants can be expected to provide. This is the biggest question a public health administrator has to deal with when considering sealant programs: can we afford it, and is the benefit from sealants worth the cost?

COST EFFECTIVENESS OF SEALANTS

Questions arose about the cost effectiveness of sealants in public programs almost from their first use. A public health community that considered water fluoridation to be the gold standard in terms of the cost effectiveness of public programs naturally looked askance at this one-on-one procedure, and an early economic assessment was not encouraging.[36] However, in this review dentists, rather than auxiliaries, applied the sealant, and retention of the first-generation sealant was not high.

Cost effectiveness is defined as use of the least expensive way, from among competing alternatives, of meeting a defined objective.[112] It differs from *cost benefit*, which is the ratio of an activity's cost to the monetary benefit it produces, although it is conceptually similar to *efficiency*, which is the return on effort expended.[111] The term *a cost-effective program* is virtually synonymous with *an efficient program*.

The cost-effectiveness issue arises in public dental programs when a dental director whose objective is to reduce caries experience in a child population by a specified amount over a specified time considers the use of water fluoridation, sealant placement, application of fluoride varnish, use of fluoride mouthrinses, or dental health education to meet that objective. The director weighs the costs of each program against the anticipated benefit. (In a fluoridated community in which people routinely use fluoride toothpastes, have high utilization of dental services, and have very low caries levels, introducing no new program might also be a rational alternative.) Thinking in terms of cost effectiveness has moved dentistry away from an attitude of "the more prevention the better" to careful selection of which programs are likely to be the most efficient. Cost effectiveness is also at the root of discussions on targeting preventive programs to the most susceptible groups and individuals rather than applying them across the board (see Chapters 4 and 20).

Are sealants expensive? That depends on what they are compared with. For example, compared to fluoridated water and other types of self-applied fluorides, sealants are a relatively expensive alternative requiring application by a professional. In terms of fees charged by dentists in private practice, the average fee for a sealant application has remained at approximately 50% of the fee for a one-surface amalgam restoration. The ADA's 2001 survey of fees charged by general practitioners in private practice found that the mean fee for sealant application was $31.89 per tooth, whereas the mean fee for placement of a one-surface amalgam in a posterior permanent tooth was $73.21 and for a one-surface composite resin restoration on a posterior tooth was $98.17.[7] In public programs, it has been shown that sealant application can be even less expensive. The average cost of providing a sealant in public programs in the mid-1990s was $8.17 per tooth, well under the average of $24.42 charged in private offices as of 1995.[10] The ability to provide sealants at lower cost in public programs is attributable in part to the economies that are possible through treating large numbers of children in a "captive" setting in schools and through the extensive use of auxiliary personnel to place the sealants.

The other side of expense is effectiveness. The evidence cited earlier shows that sealants are highly effective; their widespread use can have an immediate and substantial impact on the caries experience of a group that would otherwise experience occlusal caries. Although there are few specific studies on the relative cost effectiveness of sealants and other preventive procedures, a 1989 workshop gave sealants a favorable cost-effectiveness review, rating them slightly higher in nonfluoridated areas because of the higher probability of caries attack.[73] This means that sealant application is not only a logical public health program to choose in light of caries distribution in the early twenty-first century, but it may well be one of the more efficient ones as well. However, it must be stated that the cost-effectiveness issue is far from settled and is really wide open for additional research. To illustrate, readers may have noted the vexing conundrum that, whereas sealants may be more effective in fluoridated areas,[113] the 1989 workshop concluded that they are likely to be more cost effective in nonfluoridated areas.[73] This is the case because, although in a fluoridated area a higher *percentage* of carious lesions will be on occlusal surfaces and thus preventable with sealants, in a nonfluoridated area, there will actually be a higher *total number* of occlusal lesions that could potentially be prevented.

In the context of the targeting issue, it follows that sealants would be more cost effective if they could be applied to the teeth with the greatest probability of decaying, so that they would not be "wasted" on teeth that would not decay anyway. Although prediction methods are not yet precise enough to accomplish this for sound teeth, an obvious approach with sealants is to take advantage of their demonstrated efficacy when applied to early lesions. The cost advantage of this approach was demonstrated more than 20 years ago[62]: sealant application showed a benefit-cost ratio of only 0.3:1 in caries-inactive subjects but of 1.02:1 in caries-active subjects. In another study, the most favorable cost-effectiveness ratios were found when sealant placement was limited to children who already had restorations in one or more first permanent molars.[114] In yet another school-based study, although sealants were effective overall, their effect was especially striking on surfaces that were initially diagnosed as having incipient lesions.[45] Table 27-1 summarizes some of the data from that report. These data

indicate that, over a 5-year period, in surfaces that were initially diagnosed as sound, 8.1% of those that were sealed and 12.5% of those that were not sealed became carious. On the other hand, of those teeth initially diagnosed as having incipient caries (i.e., they had dark staining or a chalky appearance, or caused a slight "stick" of the explorer but had no visible enamel surface defect), 10.8% of those that were sealed became carious, compared with 51.8% of those that were not sealed. Similarly, interim results from a clinical trial[44] in which teeth determined not to require restorations were randomly assigned to receive or not receive sealants showed the same type of gradient according to baseline diagnosis. Fig. 27-2 shows that, after an average of 26 months of enrollment in the study, 3% of the sealed teeth that were initially diagnosed as sound required restorations, whereas 6% of sound teeth not sealed required restorations. In the case of teeth initially rated as having a questionable area, 20% of the sealed teeth required restoration, whereas 41% of such teeth that were unsealed required restorations. Of those diagnosed as having incipient, noncavitated lesions, 39% and 60% of sealed and unsealed teeth, respectively, required restoration. Finally, in a retrospective study of an insured population, which was necessarily an observational study, it was found that, in the 5 years after eruption, both first and second molars that were sealed were restored slightly over one-half as often as unsealed teeth (Fig. 27-3).[31]

Taken together, the data from these various studies show two things very clearly: first, that initial diagnosis makes a very large difference, at least in the short term, with regard to the value of

Table 27-1 Percentage of surfaces (absolute numbers in parentheses) becoming carious after 5 years in sealed and unsealed first permanent molars, by initial diagnosis[45]

	Initial Diagnosis	
	Sound	Incipient
Sealed	8.1% (24/297)	10.8% (41/380)
Nonsealed	12.5% (8/64)	51.8% (29/56)

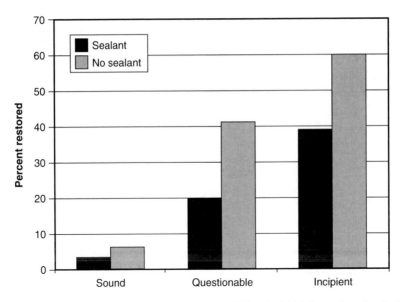

Fig. 27-2 Requirement for restoration of permanent molars in children by initial diagnosis and sealant placement, after 26 months of enrollment in the study.[44]

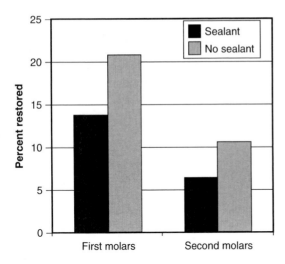

Fig. 27-3 Restoration prevalence after 5 years in sealed and unsealed first and second permanent molars in an insured population.[31]

sealants; and, second, that in the "real world" sealants are not successful 100% of the time. Although the placement of a sealant reduced the risk that a subsequent restoration would be required in all cases, some risk of needing a future restoration still existed, especially when the initial diagnosis was of a questionable or incipient lesion. These observations are also in agreement with the findings of a simulation and sensitivity analysis[40] that compared the likely costs and out-comes of three sealant strategies: sealing all, none, or a targeted subset of permanent molars. In this analysis, if caries increments were high and sealant costs were low, a strategy of sealing all would be most cost effective. On the other hand, if caries levels were low and sealant costs were high, a targeted strategy would be preferable.

These results suggest strongly that applying sealants only to those teeth with early lesions or to the teeth of children with a history of caries is likely to be much more efficient than a blanket sealing of all potentially at-risk teeth. It is worth remembering, too, that if caries incidence continues to decline, the need for selective use of sealant in this way becomes even greater if the material is to be used efficiently. Use of sealant only on incipient lesions is, in effect, using it as an early restoration rather than as primary prevention, an approach that may require a different mindset in prevention-oriented dentists. It also further blurs the distinction between the use of sealants as primary preventive agents and their various uses in minimal-preparation restorations, as discussed earlier.

There are cost-effectiveness issues in private practice too, although they differ from those in public programs.[2,6] After all, the value of preventive care eventually depends on what the individual thinks it is worth. A dentist is probably justified in sealing a number of teeth in a patient who wants prevention at any price, even if the dentist believes, for example, that the bicuspids being sealed are unlikely to decay. The more pertinent issue facing a practitioner is whether to seal or restore a deeply fissured molar with a suspicious fissure. Is it valid to compare these two options on a cost-effectiveness basis? Some commentators have said no, because one is a preventive procedure and the other is restorative.[47,77,98] Perhaps, but if a sealant is viewed as a noninvasive restoration, then it becomes a valid comparison. One study directly compared the costs of sealing a caries-free molar with the costs of restoring the carious contralateral molar with amalgam. When all maintenance care was taken into consideration, including necessary replacements of both sealant and amalgam, the average cumulative time to place and maintain a sealant over 7 years was 10 minutes 45 seconds; for an amalgam it was 14 minutes 26 seconds.[101] Another small-scale follow-up of 12 pairs of children concluded that treatment costs in children who did not receive sealant was 1.64 times greater than the costs in a group who had sealant maintained over the period.[94] Although these data are not conclusive, collectively they suggest that appropriate use of sealants on early lesions is efficacious, conserves tooth structure, and is likely to be cost effective. As caries experience continues to decline, the use of sealants is likely to be focused even more on the early lesion rather than the totally sound tooth.

PUBLIC AND PROFESSIONAL ATTITUDES TOWARD SEALANTS

The slow adoption of sealants by practitioners, despite the excellent results in many studies, has been puzzling. Even the main pediatric dental organizations in the United States did not adopt policies to encourage the use of sealants until 1983.[8] In a series of conferences and symposia in the early 1980s that addressed the slow adoption of sealants, the reasons given for dentists' hesitancy included skepticism about efficacy, fear of "sealing in decay," and failure of many third-party carriers to cover sealant application. Virtually identical reasons were still given by dentists who were not using sealants as recently as 1992.[90] Many dentists also expressed a sublime faith in the longevity of amalgams, a faith that research shows is seriously misplaced.[6]

Even though the trend to more widespread use of sealants has developed slowly, it is consistent. Some growth in the numbers of dentists using sealants was evident through the 1980s,[29,51,82] and by the early 1990s several states reported that more than 90% of general dentists were using sealants.[15,39,90] Growing acceptance of the use of sealants over incipient lesions was also evident. In a 1985 survey in Washington state, only 18% of dentists who used sealants reported doing so over incipient lesions,[27] but in 1992 more than 77% of Ohio dentists reported a willingness to seal over incipient caries, at least under some circumstances.[90] This trend toward more widespread use of sealants is likely to continue, because the dentists most likely to use sealants are the younger, more recent dental school graduates,[90] and the acceptance of sealants by patients appears to be heavily influenced by the recommendations of their dentists.[60,84,90]

Data on the prevalence of sealants in national surveys also show that their use is increasing. Data from the 1986-87 national survey of U.S. schoolchildren ages 5-17 years indicated that 7.6% had one or more dental sealants on permanent teeth.[20] By 1991, however, the results from the first part of the third National Health and Nutrition Examination Survey (NHANES III) showed that this proportion had risen to 18.5%.[86] Although this increase is encouraging and is likely to continue, a note of caution is in order because this higher level of sealant application will be most helpful if the sealants are being placed in children who are most likely to develop carious lesions.[89] For maximum benefit, it is important that dentists in private practice, as well as those in charge of public programs, target their sealant applications to the patients most likely to profit from them.

The evidence is also consistent regarding the characteristics of patients who receive sealants. Higher levels of parental education and income, and enrollment in a dental insurance program repeatedly have been shown to be associated with sealant use.[60,84,104] These characteristics are associated with greater use of virtually all forms of dental care.

Lack of dental insurance coverage has been cited as a major factor in the slow acceptance of sealants,[37,67,90] although this situation, too, appears to be improving. By 1994 all 50 states had included sealant placement as a benefit in their Medicaid programs,[88] and although exact numbers are unavailable, it is evident that an increasing proportion of private insurers are including sealant placement as a benefit. However, the economic picture for insurers is not clear, because adding sealant placement to a benefit package usually requires an increase in premiums, especially because caries experience, and thus the need for restorations, continues to fall.[32,34]

Although it is evident that dentists and patients are becoming increasingly comfortable with the use of sealants, it is also true that the view as to their most appropriate use continues to evolve. In the earliest days, sealants were thought of almost exclusively as a material to be used on sound pit-and-fissure surfaces to prevent the development of a carious lesion. As the technology has developed and the overall caries pattern has changed, there has been an evolution in thinking. It is now widely accepted that not all children nor all teeth need sealants. Caries-free children, in the absence of other indications of risk, are not good candidates for sealant placement. A key criterion is that the fissured surface must be at significant risk for disease. This also has led to the view that sealant placement is appropriate for older children and adults in selected cases.[2,74,89] In this regard, sealants are increasingly seen as part of a trend toward much more conservative restorations.[63] Timely placement of sealant on a tooth with an incipient lesion, with a conservative restoration if necessary, is increasingly viewed as the most appropriate care, regardless of the age of the patient.

As must any other tool in the dental armamentarium, sealants must be used appropriately, in a way that is (1) compatible with the properties of the material, (2) consistent with the nature of the condition that they are meant to prevent or treat, and (3) acceptable in terms of cost to the provider and patient. Sealants and the associated composite products are among the most exciting technologic developments in dentistry. The technology and the standards for sealant use will undoubtedly continue to progress. At the same time, optimal use of sealants is also likely to remain somewhat different in public health programs than in private practice. In public programs, sealants should continue to be highly effective in reducing the burden of caries in high-risk children. This is because the children are selected on the basis of untreated disease and limited access to routine dental care, and large numbers of children can be treated under the traditional approach of sealing large numbers of teeth, including many that are sound. On the other hand, for patients who are available for regular care in private practice, the trend is toward a more selective, individual approach to sealant use. Here the decision to treat is made on the basis of the expected risk for the individual child and tooth surface, and with the knowledge that sealants are part of a conservative approach to restorative care. The role of sealants and the related restorative materials in improving the oral health of the public is substantial. The challenge for the practitioner is to be alert for the inevitable evolution of the recommendations for the most appropriate use of these materials.

REFERENCES

1. American Dental Association. ADA positions and statements: Estrogenic effects of bisphenol A lacking in dental sealants, updated June 05, 2002, website: http://www.ada.org/prof/resources/positions/statements/seal_est.a Accessed June 21, 2004.
2. American Dental Association, Council on Access, Prevention and Interprofessional Relations; Council on Scientific Affairs. Dental sealants. J Am Dent Assoc 1997;128:485-8.
3. American Dental Association, Council on Dental Health and Health Planning, Council on Dental Materials, Instruments, and Equipment. Pit and fissure sealants. J Am Dent Assoc 1987;114:671-2.
4. American Dental Association, Council on Dental Materials and Devices. Nuva-Seal pit and fissure sealant classified as provisionally accepted. J Am Dent Assoc 1972;84:1109.
5. American Dental Association, Council on Dental Materials and Devices. Pit and fissure sealants. J Am Dent Assoc 1976;93:134.
6. American Dental Association, Council on Dental Research. Cost-effectiveness of sealants in private practice and standards for use in prepaid dental care. J Am Dent Assoc 1985;110:103-7.
7. American Dental Association, Survey Center. Survey of dental fees 2001. Chicago: ADA, 2002.
8. American Society of Dentistry for Children, American Academy of Pedodontics. Rationale and guidelines for pit and fissure sealants. ASDC J Dent Child 1983; 50:156.

9. Aranda M, Garcia-Godoy F. Clinical evaluation of the retention and wear of a light-cured pit and fissure glass ionomer sealant. J Clin Pediatr Dent 1995;19:273-7.

10. Association of State and Territorial Dental Directors. School-based and school-linked public health dental sealant programs in the United States, 1992-93. Columbus OH: ASTDD, 1997.

11. Ast DB, Bushel A, Chase HC. A clinical study of caries prophylaxis with zinc chloride and potassium ferrocyanide. J Am Dent Assoc 1950;41:437-42.

12. Backer Dirks O. The benefits of water fluoridation. Caries Res 1974;8(Suppl 1):2-15.

13. Bohannan HM. Caries distribution and the case for sealants. J Public Health Dent 1983;43:200-4.

14. Bohannan HM, Disney JA, Graves RC, et al. Indications for sealant use in a community-based preventive dentistry program. J Dent Educ 1984;48(Suppl 2): 45-55.

15. Bowman PA, Fitzgerald CM. Utah dentists' sealant usage survey. ASDC J Dent Child 1990;57:134-8.

16. Bravo M, Garcia-Anilo I, Baca P, Llodra JC. A 48-month survival analysis comparing sealant (Delton) with fluoride varnish (Duraphat) in 6- to 8-year-old children. Community Dent Oral Epidemiol 1997;25: 247-50.

17. Bravo M, Llodra JC, Baca P, Oserio E. Effectiveness of visible light fissure sealant (Delton) versus fluoride varnish (Duraphat): 24-month clinical trial. Community Dent Oral Epidemiol 1996;24:42-6.

18. Bravo M, Oserio E, Garcia-Anillo I, et al. The influence of dft index on sealant success: A 48-month survival analysis. J Dent Res 1996;75:768-74.

19. Brown LJ, Kaste LM, Selwitz RH, Furman LJ. Dental caries and sealant usage in U.S. children, 1988-1991. J Am Dent Assoc 1996;127:335-43.

20. Brunelle JA. Prevalence of dental sealants in U.S. schoolchildren [abstract]. J Dent Res 1989;68(Spec Issue):183.

21. Buonocore MG. A simple method of increasing the adhesion of acrylic filling materials to enamel surfaces. J Dent Res 1955;34:849-53.

22. Buonocore MG. Caries prevention in pits and fissures sealed with an adhesive resin polymerized by ultraviolet light: A two-year study of a single adhesive application. J Am Dent Assoc 1971;82:1090-3.

23. Burt BA. Fissure sealants: Clinical and economic factors. J Dent Educ 1984;48:96-102.

24. Calderone JJ, Davis JM. The New Mexico sealant program: A progress report. J Public Health Dent 1987;47:145-9.

25. Calderone JJ, Mueller LA. The cost of sealant application in a state dental disease prevention program. J Public Health Dent 1983;43:249-54.

26. Carter NL. Seal America: The prevention intervention. Cincinnati: American Association of Community Dental Programs, Cincinnati Health Department, 1995, ca 100 pp, 1 videotape (4:30 minutes, VHS).

27. Chapko MK. A study of the intentional use of pit and fissure sealants over carious lesions. J Public Health Dent 1987;47:139-42.

28. Christiansen GJ. Preventive restorative dentistry. Int Dent J 1990;40:259-66.

29. Cohen L, LaBelle A, Romberg E. The use of pit and fissure sealants in private practice: A national survey. J Public Health Dent 1988;48:26-35.

30. Cueto EL, Buonocore MG. Sealing of pits and fissures with an adhesive resin: Its use in caries prevention. J Am Dent Assoc 1967;75:121-8.

31. Dennison JB, Straffon LH, Smith RC. Effectiveness of sealant treatment over five years in an insured population. J Am Dent Assoc 2000;131:597-605.

32. Eklund SA. Factors affecting the cost of fissure sealants: A dental insurer's perspective. J Public Health Dent 1986;46:133-40.

33. Eklund SA, Ismail AI. The development of occlusal and proximal lesions: Implications for fissure sealants. J Public Health Dent 1986;46:114-21.

34. Eklund SA, Pittman JL, Smith RC. Trends in dental care among insured Americans: 1980 to 1995. J Am Dent Assoc 1997;128:171-8.

35. Elderton RJ. Restorations without conventional cavity preparations. Int Dent J 1988;38:112-8.

36. Foch CB. The costs, effects, and benefits of preventive dental care: A literature review. Rand Report No. N-1732-RWJF. Santa Monica CA: Rand, 1981.

37. Glasrud PH, Frazier PJ, Horowitz AM. Insurance reimbursement for sealants in 1986: Report of a survey. ASDC J Dent Child 1987;54:81-8.

38. Going RE. Sealant effect on incipient caries, enamel maturation, and future caries susceptibility. J Dent Educ 1984;48:35-41.

39. Gonzales CD, Frazier PJ, Messer LB. Sealant use by general practitioners: A Minnesota survey. ASDC J Dent Child 1991;58:38-45.

40. Griffin SO, Griffin PM, Gooch BF, Barker LK. Comparing the costs of three sealant delivery strategies. J Dent Res 2002;81:641-5.

41. Handelman SL, Leverett DH, Espeland MA, Curzon JA. Clinical radiographic evaluation of sealed carious and sound tooth surfaces. J Am Dent Assoc 1986;113:751-4.

42. Handelman SL, Leverett DH, Espeland M, Curzon J. Retention of sealants over carious and sound tooth surfaces. Community Dent Oral Epidemiol 1987;15: 1-5.

43. Hardison JR, Collier DR, Sprouse LW, et al. Retention of pit and fissure sealant on the primary molars of 3- and 4-year-old children after 1 year. J Am Dent Assoc 1987;114:613-5.

44. Heller K, Eklund S, Lubwama R, Fisher M. Sealing of sound, questionable, and incipient caries surfaces. Presented at: International Association for Dental Research, 80th general session, 8 March 2002, San Diego CA. Abstract 2767.

45. Heller KE, Reed SG, Bruner FW, et al. Longitudinal evaluation of sealing molars with and without incipient dental caries in a public health program. J Public Health Dent 1995;55:148-53.

46. Henry RJ, Jerrell RG. The glass ionomer rest-a-seal. ASDC J Dent Child 1989;56:283-7.

47. Horowitz HS. Pit and fissure sealants in private practice and public health programmes: Analysis of cost-effectiveness. Int Dent J 1980;30:117-26.

48. Horowitz HS, Heifetz SB, Poulsen S. Retention and effectiveness of a single application of an adhesive

sealant in preventing occlusal caries, final report after five years of study in Kalispell, Montana. J Am Dent Assoc 1977;95:1133-9.

49. Houpt M, Eidelman E, Shey Z, et al. Occlusal composite restorations: 4-year results. J Am Dent Assoc 1985;110: 351-3.

50. Houpt M, Fuks A, Shapira J, et al. Autopolymerized versus light-polymerized fissure sealant. J Am Dent Assoc 1987;115:55-6.

51. Hunt RJ, Kohout FJ, Beck JD. The use of pit and fissure sealants in private dental practices. ASDC J Dent Child 1984;51:29-33.

52. Hyatt TP. Prophylactic odontotomy. Dent Cosmos 1923;65:234-41.

53. Ismail AI, Gagnon P. A longitudinal evaluation of fissure sealants applied in dental practices. J Dent Res 1995;74:1583-90.

54. Ismail AI, King W, Clark DC. An evaluation of the Saskatchewan pit and fissure sealant program: A longitudinal followup. J Public Health Dent 1989;49: 206-11.

55. Jackson D. Caries experience in English children and young adults during the years 1947-1972. Br Dent J 1974;137:91-8.

56. Karlzen-Reuterving G, van Dijken JWV. A three-year follow-up of glass ionomer cement and resin fissure sealants. ASDC J Dent Child 1995;62:108-10.

57. Klein H, Knutson JW. Studies on dental caries. Effect of ammoniacal silver nitrate on caries in the first permanent molars. J Am Dent Assoc 1942;29:1420-6.

58. Klein H, Palmer CE. "Therapeutic odontotomy" and "preventive dentistry." J Am Dent Assoc 1940;27: 1054-5.

59. Kuthy RA, Ashton JJ. Eruption pattern of permanent molars: Implications for school-based dental sealant programs. J Public Health Dent 1989;49:7-14.

60. Lang WP, Weintraub JA, Choi C, Bagramian RA. Fissure sealant knowledge and characteristics of parents as a function of their child's sealant status. J Public Health Dent 1988;48:132-7.

61. Leske GS, Pollard S, Cons N. The effectiveness of dental hygienist teams in applying a pit and fissure sealant. J Prev Dent 1976;3:33-6.

62. Leverett DH, Handelman SL, Brenner CM, Iker HP. Use of sealants in the prevention and early treatment of carious lesions: Cost analysis. J Am Dent Assoc 1983; 106:39-42.

63. Mertz-Fairhurst EJ, Adair SM, Sams DR, et al. Cariostatic and ultraconservative sealed restorations: Nine-year results among children and adults. ASDC J Dent Child 1995;62:97-107.

64. Mertz-Fairhurst EJ, Call-Smith KM, Shuster GS, et al. Clinical performance of sealed composite restorations placed over caries compared with sealed and unsealed amalgam restorations. J Am Dent Assoc 1987;115: 689-94.

65. Mertz-Fairhurst EJ, Fairhurst CW, Williams JE, et al. A comparative clinical study of two pit and fissure sealants: 7-year results in Augusta, GA. J Am Dent Assoc 1984;109:252-5.

66. Mertz-Fairhurst EJ, Schuster GS, Fairhurst CW. Arresting caries by sealants: Results of a clinical study. J Am Dent Assoc 1986;112:194-7.

67. National Institutes of Health Consensus Development Conference Statement. Dental sealants in the prevention of tooth decay. J Dent Educ 1984;48:126-31.

68. Olea N, Pulgar R, Perez P, et al. Estrogenicity of resin-based composites and sealants used in dentistry. Environ Health Perspect 1996;104:298-305.

69. Pardi V, Pereira AC, Mailhe FL, et al. A 5-year evaluation of two glass-ionomer cements used as fissure sealants. Community Dent Oral Epidemiol 2003;31: 386-91.

70. Pereira AC, Pardi V, Mailhe FL, et al. A 3-year clinical evaluation of glass-ionomer cements used as fissure sealants. Am J Dent 2003;16:23-7.

71. Poulsen S, Beiruti N, Sadat N. A comparison of retention and the effect on caries of fissure sealing with a glass-ionomer and resin-based sealant. Community Dent Oral Epidemiol 2001;29:298-301.

72. Proceedings of the workshop on guidelines for sealant use. J Public Health Dent 1995;5:257-313.

73. Results of the workshop. J Public Health Dent 1989;49(Spec Issue):331-7.

74. Richardson PS, McIntyre IG. Susceptibility of tooth surfaces to carious attack in young adults. Community Dent Health 1996;13:163-8.

75. Ripa LW. Sealant retention on primary teeth: A critique of clinical and laboratory studies. J Pedod 1979;3: 275-90.

76. Ripa LW. Occlusal sealants: Rationale and review of clinical trials. Int Dent J 1980;30:127-39.

77. Ripa LW. Occlusal sealants: An overview of clinical studies. J Public Health Dent 1983;43:216-25.

78. Ripa LW. Sealants revisited: An update of the effectiveness of pit and fissure sealants. Caries Res 1993; 27(Suppl 1):77-82.

79. Ripa LW, Leske GS, Forte F. The combined use of pit and fissure sealants and fluoride mouthrinsing in second and third grade children: Final clinical results after two years. Pediatr Dent 1987;9:118-20.

80. Robison VA, Rozier RG, Weintraub JA, Koch GG. The relationship between clinical tooth status and receipt of sealants among child Medicaid recipients. J Dent Res 1997;76:1862-8.

81. Rock WP, Weatherill S, Anderson RJ. Retention of three fissure sealant resins. The effects of etching agent and curing method. Results over 3 years. Br Dent J 1990; 168:323-5.

82. Romberg E, Cohen LA, LaBelle AD. A national survey of sealant use by pediatric dentists. ASDC J Dent Child 1988;55:257-64.

83. Romcke RG, Lewis DW, Maze BD, Vickerson RA. Retention and maintenance of fissure sealants over 10 years. J Can Dent Assoc 1990;56:235-7.

84. Selwitz RH, Colley BJ, Rozier RG. Factors associated with parental acceptance of dental sealants. J Public Health Dent 1992;52:137-45.

85. Selwitz RH, Nowjack-Raymer R, Driscoll WS, Li S-H. Evaluation after 4 years of the combined use of fluoride and dental sealants. Community Dent Oral Epidemiol 1995;23:30-5.

86. Selwitz RH, Winn DM, Kingman A, Zion GR. The prevalence of dental sealants in the US population: Findings from NHANES III, 1988-91. J Dent Res 1996; 75:652-60.

87. Siegal MD, Calderone JJ. Controversy over the supervision of dental hygienists: Impact on a community-based sealant program. J Public Health Dent 1986;46:156-60.

88. Siegal MD. Promotion and use of pit and fissure sealants: An introduction to the special issue. J Public Health Dent 1995;55:259-60.

89. Siegal MD, Farquhar CL, Bouchard JM. Dental sealants: Who needs them? Public Health Rep 1997; 112:98-106.

90. Siegal MD, Garcia AI, Kandray DP, Giljahn LK. The use of dental sealants by Ohio dentists. J Public Health Dent 1996;56:12-21.

91. Silverstone LM. Operative measures for caries prevention. Caries Res 1978;12(Suppl 1):103-12.

92. Silverstone LM. State of the art on sealant research and priorities for further research. J Dent Educ 1984;48: 107-18.

93. Simonsen RJ. Fissure sealants in primary molars: Retention of colored sealants with variable etch times, at twelve months. ASDC J Dent Child 1979;46:382-4.

94. Simonsen RJ. Retention and effectiveness of a single application of white sealant after 10 years. J Am Dent Assoc 1987;115:31-6.

95. Simonsen RJ. Retention and effectiveness of dental sealant after 15 years. J Am Dent Assoc 1991;122(11): 34-42.

96. Simonsen RJ. Glass ionomer as fissure sealant—a critical review. J Public Health Dent 1996;56:146-9.

97. Songpaisan Y, Bratthal D, Phantumvanit P, Somridhivej Y. Effects of glass ionomer cement, resin-based pit and fissure sealant and HF applications on occlusal caries in a developing country field trial. Community Dent Oral Epidemiol 1995;23:25-9.

98. Stamm JW. The use of fissure sealants in public health programs: A reactor's comments. J Public Health Dent 1983;43:243-6.

99. Stamm JW. Is there a need for dental sealants? Epidemiological indications in the 1980s. J Dent Educ 1984;48:9-17.

100. Stephen KW, Strang R. Fissure sealants: A review. Community Dent Health 1985;2:149-56.

101. Straffon LH, Dennison JB. Clinical evaluation comparing sealant and amalgam after 7 years: Final report. J Am Dent Assoc 1988;117:751-5.

102. Sveen OB, Jensen OE. Two-year clinical evaluation of Delton and Prisma-Shield. Clin Prev Dent 1986; 8(5):9-11.

103. Swift EJ Jr. The effect of sealants on dental caries: A review. J Am Dent Assoc 1988;116:700-4.

104. Taichman LS, Eklund SA, Selwitz RH. Sealant coverage and the use of sealants among insured children. Presented at: International Association for Dental Research, 82nd general session, 11 March 2004, Honolulu HI. Abstract 0687.

105. Taifour D, Frenken JE, van't Hof MA, et al. Effects of glass ionomer sealants in newly erupted molars after 5 years: A pilot study. Community Dent Oral Epidemiol 2003;31:314-9.

106. Tandon S, Kumari R, Udupa S. The effect of etch-time on the bond strength of a sealant and on the etch-pattern in primary and permanent enamel: An evaluation. ASDC J Dent Child 1989;56:186-90.

107. US Department of Health and Human Services, Centers for Disease Control and Prevention. Impact of targeted, school-based dental sealant programs in reducing racial and economic disparities in sealant prevalence among schoolchildren—Ohio, 1998-1999. MMWR Morb Mortal Wkly Rep 2001;50:736-8.

108. US Department of Health and Human Services, Centers for Disease Control and Prevention. Oral health resources: Preventing dental caries, October 31, 2002, website: http://www.cdc.gov/OralHealth/factsheets/dental_caries.htm. Accessed June 30, 2004.

109. Waggoner WF, Siegal M. Pit and fissure sealant application: Updating the technique. J Am Dent Assoc 1996;127:351-61.

110. Walker JD, Jensen ME, Pinkham JR. A clinical review of preventive resin restorations. ASDC J Dent Child 1990;57:257-9.

111. Warner KE. Issues in cost effectiveness in health care. J Public Health Dent 1989;49(Spec Issue):272-8.

112. Warner KE, Luce BR. Cost-benefit and cost-effectiveness analysis in health care. Ann Arbor MI: Health Administration Press, 1982:46-50.

113. Weintraub JA. The effectiveness of pit and fissure sealants. J Public Health Dent 1989;49:317-30.

114. Weintraub JA, Stearns SC, Burt BA, et al. A retrospective analysis of the cost-effectiveness of dental sealants in a children's health center. Soc Sci Med 1993; 36:1483-93.

115. Wendt LK, Koch G. Fissure sealant in permanent first molars after 10 years. Swed Dent J 1988;12:181-5.

116. Winkler TM, Deschepper EJ, Dean JA, et al. Using a resin-modified glass ionomer as an occlusal sealant: A one-year clinical study. J Am Dent Assoc 1996;127: 1508-14.

117. Wright GZ, Friedman CS, Plotzke O, Feasby WH. A comparison between autopolymerizing and visible-light-activated sealants. Clin Prev Dent 1988;10(1): 14-7.

Diet and Plaque Control

Probably more effort has been expended over the years in trying to prevent caries by dietary control and toothbrushing than by any other method. These efforts have been a major part of traditional dental health education, and they are aimed at changing personal behavior by exhorting people to voluntarily restrict their consumption of sugars and to brush faithfully. America's response is to eat more sugar than ever, although oral hygiene is also probably better than ever.

The ingestion of sugars and other highly refined carbohydrates is a necessary condition for dental caries to begin (see Chapter 20). Although mass education to restrict sugar consumption clearly has not worked, restriction of dietary sugars remains an appropriate part of the strategy for controlling caries in a caries-susceptible patient. Development of low- and noncariogenic sugar substitutes also provides a few more options for these patients.

Sugars as a risk factor for dental caries were discussed in Chapter 20. This chapter takes a critical look at the role of dietary approaches to preventing oral disease, at the potential for caries control through the use of sugar substitutes, and at the most appropriate place for oral hygiene in caries control.

NUTRITION AND ORAL DISEASES

Diet refers to the food and drink that pass through the mouth, whereas nutrition is concerned with the absorption and metabolism of nutrients from dietary sources. We stated in Chapter 20 that there is little evidence to show that nutritional deficiencies, either during tooth development or subsequently, cause dental caries. Similarly, in Chapter 21 we discussed how periodontitis cannot be treated as a nutritional disorder. Malnourishment is unusual in the well-fed societies of North America, although it is occasionally seen among some who live in deprived circumstances and among individuals with eating disorders. Where malnutrition is more widespread, as it is in some low-income countries, there is a potential link between malnutrition and the oral diseases, as was discussed in Chapters 20 and 21.

Despite the infrequency of nutritional disturbances among North Americans, some well-meaning dentists have extolled the virtues of controlling dental caries and periodontal diseases through nutritional counseling. In cases of rare metabolic diseases that can disrupt the immune system, oral conditions may be improved when the patient's nutritional status is improved, but in healthy, well-nourished patients there is no basis for treating existing dental disease through nutritional (as distinct from dietary) counseling.

The nutritional status of a patient is rightly the concern of the attending dental professional, and all dentists and hygienists should be sensitive to the signs of nutritional disturbances. When a nutritional disturbance or eating disorder is suspected, referral to a physician or nutritionist is the correct course of action. Even when such a patient is treated successfully for the nutritional problem, improvement in oral status is likely to follow as a consequence only in the most severe cases.

WHAT IS MEANT BY A CARIOGENIC FOOD?

The sugars or other readily fermentable carbohydrates (Box 28-1) in any food can be metabolized by cariogenic bacteria in plaque. Food with this property is termed *acidogenic*. Acidogenesis is a necessary, though not sufficient, condition for the development of caries. The ubiquity of sugars in processed foods means that a wide range of foods and drinks are acidogenic. Whether an acidogenic food is cariogenic or not will depend greatly on a number of factors specific to the individual who eats it, factors such as predominant bacterial flora, flow rate and buffering capacity of saliva, fluoride availability, and individual immune factors. Whether caries develops or not also depends on how much of the food is eaten and how frequently it is consumed, whether it is eaten in isolation or with other foods, and the nature of any accompanying foods. We therefore cannot be certain whether a particular acidogenic food is cariogenic or not for a particular patient, even if the risk seems high. However, we can be confident about the converse: because acidogenesis is a necessary condition for caries, a nonacidogenic food must also be a noncariogenic food.

The concept of a cariogenic food was too broad to be of practical use in caries control, so attempts were made to determine the *cariogenic potential* of a food, defined as the food's ability to foster caries in humans under conditions conducive to caries formation.[49] The underlying idea in defining cariogenic potential was to draw up a rank order of cariogenic foods, but a 1986 workshop on food cariogenicity concluded that this approach was unproductive. Although efforts to identify cariogenic foods were not followed up because that category was so broad, the workshop agreed that there was value in identifying nonacidogenic foods, which by definition have no cariogenic potential.[30] Such foods can then be confidently recommended to patients who need a sugar-restricted diet.

BOX 28-1 What Are Cariogenic Foods?

Sugars and other fermentable carbohydrates are part of the etiologic chain in dental caries. The phrase *other fermentable carbohydrates* is used a lot in the literature, and it sounds both broad and vague. What are these "other fermentable carbohydrates"? The term refers to the cooked or milled starches in the refined flours used in making cookies, biscuits, sweet rolls, croissants, and other processed foods. Their dental significance is that as simple carbohydrates they can be broken down further by the salivary enzyme amylase while still in the mouth and then metabolized by cariogenic bacteria just as sugars are. For that reason these simple carbohydrates are considered potentially cariogenic. Some evidence suggests that starch-sugar mixtures are more cariogenic than sugars alone.[19,20,35,71]

Starch is a branched or unbranched polysaccharide chain of glucose molecules. The term usually refers to the complex, large-molecule carbohydrates such as those found in potatoes, broccoli, other fruits and vegetables, and whole grains. These are all carbohydrates that have long been viewed as essentially noncariogenic because they break down very little in the oral cavity.[60,75] These sugars are part of the structure of fruits, vegetables, and milk, and as such are called *intrinsic* sugars. Intrinsic sugars are considered virtually noncariogenic when eaten in moderate amounts. Added sugars, sometimes called *extrinsic* sugars, are held to be the sugars that are metabolized by cariogenic plaque bacteria and trigger the events that lead to demineralization. Some of the literature on this subject expands the term *sugars* to *nonmilk extrinsic sugars*.

There is no important difference in cariogenicity between refined sugars and brown sugar. Despite the earlier comment on intrinsic sugars, adherence to a high-fruit diet does not necessarily protect from caries.[41] However, as an after-school snack, fruits have considerably more nutritional value than the average candy bar.

A diet that is generous in vegetables and fruits and is light in processed food is recognized universally as compatible with general health. It is also compatible with dental health.

The cariogenic potential of a single food cannot be satisfactorily tested in human studies because of the "background noise" from other uncontrolled consumption of food components in a normal mixed diet.[24] As one example, studies to determine whether the consumption of presweetened breakfast cereals increased caries incidence were unable to control for other crucial variables.[26] The 1986 workshop suggested guidelines for testing the cariogenic potential of foods using a combination of several testing regimens, including animal models and in vitro procedures.[30] These protocols were intended to identify foods with no cariogenic potential, especially snack foods, but they have not received much attention.

The Swiss government has been testing the cariogenic potential of snack foods since 1982 and has permitted snack foods there to be labeled *Zahnfreundlich* (which means "tooth-friendly" and implies nonerosiveness as well) if they do not lower the pH of interdental plaque below 5.7 for up to 30 minutes after consumption.[48] Under this well-accepted program, tests of food products are carried out telemetrically with a plaque electrode. Accepted products are usually confectionery items sweetened with the sugar alcohols xylitol, sorbitol, mannitol, or maltitol, or with Lycasin, a hydrogenated starch derivative. Fructose does not pass the test.

The impact of this program on the dental health of the Swiss people is difficult to document, however. It is likely to be positive because a high proportion of Swiss children and adults have learned to recognize the "tooth-friendly" logo and to understand that it indicates oral health benefits.[74] The concept has spread to a number of other countries, including the United States, where the Food and Drug Administration (FDA) in 1996 permitted the claim "does not promote tooth decay" to be made for sugar-free foods that met specified test conditions.[46]

SOFT DRINKS

We noted in Chapter 20 that soft drink consumption is associated with caries and that high consumption of soft drinks increases the risk of caries.[50] Therefore caries control calls for modest consumption of soft drinks, but in the current social environment it is difficult to

promote that message. One obstacle is America's insatiable thirst for carbonated soft drinks and the nonstop advertising that goes along with it. Even though soft drink consumption has leveled out in the United States over recent years, it averaged 54.2 gallons per person in 2002.[18] For years all of this sugar consumption was seen as a matter of no concern, but more recently the high consumption of soft drinks has been linked with the global obesity epidemic,[67] an epidemic that is well recognized in the United States. One response to such a problem should be promotion of good nutrition in infancy, but instead the trend in recent years has gone the other way, with juices and soft drinks replacing breast milk, formula, and cow's milk. This change generally is not beneficial,[68] and too many children are already overweight when they begin school. Soft drink companies have been aggressively marketing their products by contracting with cash-poor school districts for the exclusive right to stock the vending machines in the schools, known as "pouring rights." This, too, is a trend that is not in the public health interest, and it has been vigorously opposed by the American Academy of Pediatrics.[4]

When we discussed health promotion in Chapter 5 we talked about the necessity for an environment in which people could choose to be healthy. Aggressive marketing of soft drinks, together with what to a child's eyes is the apparent blessing that school districts give to unrestricted consumption of a particular brand of soft drink, threatens that environment. Health professionals in general agree that soft drinks have little, if any, place in the infant's diet and should be consumed only moderately in later childhood. This is an issue on which it is logical for dental professionals to join their medical and public health colleagues in promoting healthy diets for children, for clearly both dental and general health concerns are involved.

In view of these issues, it came as a surprise in 2003 when the American Academy of Pediatric Dentistry (AAPD) received a grant from the Coca-Cola Company for research into dental decay.[5] Among the concerns raised by this action, the main one is that this alliance will be seen as an endorsement of soft drink consumption in early childhood by the AAPD. This action also puts the AAPD at odds with its medical colleagues in the American Academy of Pediatrics, which has a clear policy of asking schools to reconsider these pouring-rights contracts in the interests of children's health.[4] The AAPD liaison with Coca-Cola also is contrary to the long-standing policy of the American Dental Association to oppose promotion of low-nutrient foods and drinks to children.[6]

CONSUMPTION OF SUGARS

The material known by the lay term *sugar* is sucrose, a disaccharide that is the most common form of sugar consumed by humans. Sucrose and other sugars, both monosaccharides and disaccharides, are added to a wide variety of processed foods; labels on supermarket staples like canned soups, salad dressings, and processed meats frequently put sugars high on the list of ingredients. The ingredients on a label are listed in order of relative proportions, so the higher on the list an ingredient appears, the more of it there is in the product.

Consumption of sugars in all forms has continued to rise in the United States for many years. It exceeded 120 pounds (54.5 kg) per capita per year in the 1920s[8] and has risen steadily since then. Fig. 28-1 graphs data from the U.S. Department of Agriculture for 1972-2002 to show that, although average consumption of all sugars rose steadily over that period, sucrose consumption declined through 1984 and has leveled out since then. Consumption of monosaccharides continues to increase. Average per capita consumption of all sugars in the United States reached 146.1 pounds (66.4 kg) in 2002, one of the highest levels of national consumption in the world. For contrast, some international values for consumption of sucrose (not necessarily of total sugars) are shown in Fig. 28-2. These data do not include the monosaccharides that account for more than half of consumption in the United States, although monosaccharides are a much smaller fraction of the sugars consumed in other countries.

Most monosaccharide now consumed in the United States is high-fructose corn syrup (HFCS), widely used in place of sucrose in processed foods and soft drinks. HFCS consists mostly of fructose, glucose, and other oligosaccharides. It is used by food manufacturers

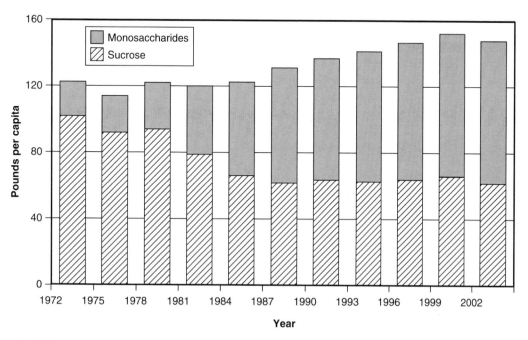

Fig. 28-1 Mean annual consumption of total sugars, sucrose, and high-fructose corn syrup plus other monosaccharides in the United States, 1972-2002.[94]

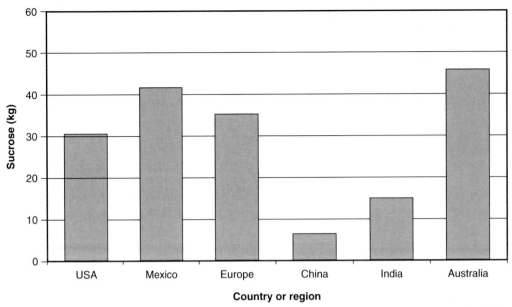

Fig. 28-2 Mean annual consumption of sucrose in the United States, Europe, and four other countries in 1996. (Data are for sucrose only and do not include consumption of high-fructose corn syrup and other monosaccharides.)[93]

instead of sucrose because it is cheaper and is produced domestically, so that it is available from a stable market. Corn is a cheap and abundant crop in the United States. But sucrose has such a variety of desirable characteristics from the food manufacturer's point of view that it is difficult to replace. Not only does it have a sweet taste, but sucrose can be baked and boiled without losing its desirable properties of adding body, luster, and texture to a food product, promoting the emulsification of fats, and acting as a preservative. When HFCS is used instead of sucrose in processed foods, the other desirable qualities of sucrose must come from additives, the use of which arouses anxiety in many people. To complicate the potential health issues, sucrose can be more harmful to human health than was once thought because evidence exists that it contributes directly to the global epidemic of obesity.[67]

A caveat regarding the data in Figs. 28-1 and 28-2 is that they are all "disappearance" data (i.e., they are derived from the amount of sugar that is produced and then distributed from storage warehouses). Disappearance data do not account for industrial use, wastage, and other losses. Just how much of the "disappeared" sugars actually is consumed by humans is a matter of speculation, but disappearance figures by

themselves most likely overestimate human consumption. Still, these data are collected in the same way from year to year, so the trends represented are accurate enough, even if the absolute amounts should not be taken too literally.

In addition to the considerable shift from sucrose to HFCS and other syrups in processed food, two other major changes have taken place in sugar consumption patterns since the early twentieth century[28]:

- The proportion of energy intake from carbohydrate foods has swung from a preponderance obtained from complex starches (bread, potatoes, whole grain cereals) to a preponderance obtained from simple carbohydrates (principally sugars).
- The main use of sugars has changed from discretionary consumption (i.e., from the sugar bowl on the table) to consumption by way of processed foods, the "hidden sugars." By the mid-1970s, three quarters of all sugars consumed came from processed foods.

CARIOGENICITY OF DIFFERENT SUGARS

Sucrose for years was billed as the "archcriminal" of dental caries because it was considered to be so much more cariogenic than other sugars.[72] However, later research has suggested that the differences between sucrose and the various monosaccharides in terms of cariogenic potential are less than originally believed.[48,59] This is a difficult issue to study in humans because of the variability of the human diet, so views are based principally on extrapolations from animal studies and laboratory research. One study in Sweden involving a small number of preschool children found that those consuming invert sugar (a mixture of glucose and fructose) in place of sucrose had a lower caries increment over 2 years,[36] although the differences did not reach statistical significance. However, one could speculate whether America's reduced consumption of sucrose (see Fig. 28-1) has been a factor in the sharp reduction in approximal and smooth surface caries relative to the overall caries decline (see Chapter 20). This speculation is based on the fact that the production of extracellular polysaccharides in plaque depends on sucrose[73] and that smooth surface caries will only develop with plaque that adheres by means of extracellular polysaccharides.

NONCARIOGENIC SUGAR SUBSTITUTES

The development of noncaloric sugar substitutes, marketed for weight control, is big business in the United States. Commercial development of these products, from the laboratory to marketing, is time consuming and expensive. This is mainly because manufacturers must meet stringent FDA requirements for demonstrated safety before such products go to market. However, despite the sometimes formidable costs involved, sugar substitutes continue to be developed. Some, such as the noncaloric saccharin, have been in common use in the United States and elsewhere for years. Aspartame, a dipeptide composed of two naturally occurring amino acids, became available in the United States in 1982.

Research into the dental applications of sugar substitutes goes back several decades. The rationale is that *Streptococcus mutans* and *Streptococcus sobrinus* emerge in plaque flora when sugar substrate is plentiful but can be suppressed when the diet is low in sugars. A widely used group of sugar substitutes are the caloric

sweeteners known as the sugar alcohols. The most commonly used sugar alcohol in the United States has been sorbitol, which is the standard sweetener in several "sugarless" chewing gums and over-the-counter medicines. The advantage of sorbitol over sugars, in terms of cariogenesis, is that in small amounts it does not lower the pH of plaque to the point at which enamel demineralization occurs.[21] Sorbitol is considered to have low cariogenicity rather than to be noncariogenic, however, because when larger amounts are consumed both the acid production in plaque and the number of sorbitol-fermenting microorganisms can increase.[22] Cariogenic microorganisms "learn" to metabolize sorbitol when their sugar supply is restricted, a form of adaptation to sorbitol that has also been demonstrated in animals.[34] Several clinical trials of sorbitol chewing gum, however, have shown that these problems do not occur when consumption levels are low, around two sticks of gum per day. Use of sorbitol gum at this level at least does not promote caries[39] and may help to reverse early demineralization of a lesion.[32,58,62]

The sugar alcohol that has received most research attention is xylitol. Xylitol, like other sugar alcohols, is caloric but has been shown to be noncariogenic and to possess the properties of a marketable sweetener. In the late 1960s and early 1970s, xylitol was the subject of interesting experiments in the Finnish city of Turku, known as the Turku sugar studies.[86] In the first of the Turku studies, a small group of volunteer adults made virtually complete substitution of xylitol for sucrose in their diets, a change made possible by having food manufacturers prepare special nonsucrose, xylitol-sweetened foods for the 2 years of the study. A second test group consumed fructose-sweetened foods under the same protocol, and a third group acted as controls by consuming a conventional sucrose-containing diet. By necessity, this study deviated from the requirements of an ideal clinical trial in that the participants were self-selected and were aware of their group assignment. Still, the magnitude of the differences among the groups in new caries experience was impressive. Over 2 years there were practically no new carious lesions in the xylitol group, whereas there were more than seven per person in the group eating the usual sucrose diet and four per person in the fructose-consuming group. Lesions in the adult test subjects, whose average age was 27.5 years, were almost all of the "white spot" variety (i.e., reversible early demineralization) on smooth surfaces.[84] The quantity of plaque formed in the xylitol group was also significantly lower.[86]

In a separate 1-year clinical trial in Turku, young adult subjects consumed an average of four sticks a day of xylitol-sweetened chewing gum, with no other changes in conventional diet. Control group subjects consumed the same amount of sucrose-sweetened gum. After a year the test group subjects averaged 0.3 new DMF (decayed, missing, or filled) surfaces compared with nearly 4 surfaces in the sucrose group.[85] The lesions were again mostly white spots, which is why the caries incidence appears high.

Subsequent field trials of xylitol-sweetened gum and confectionery products have continued to give impressive results.[2,10,52,56] Other field studies, in one instance with fluoride added to xylitol gum, have yielded acceptable positive results only slightly clouded by questionable study design and data analysis. [15,55,83] In comparisons between sorbitol and xylitol, xylitol has yielded better results, probably because of its antibacterial properties.[31,37,45] Maternal consumption of xylitol has also been shown to block the transmission of mutans streptococci from mother to child.[51,88]

Xylitol cannot be metabolized by cariogenic microorganisms[16,40] and thus does not reduce the pH of plaque. The counts of salivary *S. mutans* drop as a consequence of consistent use of xylitol gum, probably because replacement of sucrose by xylitol in plaque starves the cariogenic microorganisms. Further analysis of data from the Turku studies,[77,78] in addition to the results of laboratory studies,[87] suggests that xylitol may promote remineralization, and there are also reports that xylitol can arrest established dentin caries.[66] This evidence has led to the possibility that xylitol may be more than noncariogenic and may actually be therapeutic or anticariogenic. Although these claims require further confirmation before they can be accepted, research supports the conclusion that even partial substitution of xylitol for sucrose, such as in confectionery products, is an effective means of caries prevention at the public health level.[82]

In terms of general health consequences, some of the earlier xylitol studies reported some mild laxative effects in some study participants, but this was not reported in more recent trials when lower dosages were used. Xylitol has been approved for "special dietary use" in the United States since 1963, although it remains hard to find in chewing gums and other snack products. Xylitol is much more expensive than sucrose, however, and because it is destroyed by heat it cannot be used in cooked food products. Thus its use may be restricted to products such as chewing gum that require only small amounts of sweetener. With the FDA's acceptance of the "tooth-friendly" logo,[46] it is hoped that more xylitol-sweetened products will be seen in the United States. Currently xylitol is much more common in chewing gum in Canada and Europe.

"CLEANSING" AND "PROTECTIVE" FOODS

As discussed in Chapter 20, long-held and strenuously asserted beliefs about the anticariogenic properties of "cleansing" foods have little substance. The thinking here was that chewing a fibrous food (apple, carrot, celery) would clean plaque from tooth surfaces and thus prevent caries; however, research has long since shown that chewing fibrous foods does not remove plaque. Of course, there is obvious nutritional merit in snacking on fresh fruits and vegetables rather than on candy bars: more fiber, more vitamins and minerals, less fat. But unless the sugar intake of persons eating fibrous snacks is drastically reduced in addition, which as stated earlier is difficult to do without a radical move away from processed foods, the impact on caries will be minimal. Even that very symbol of oral health, the apple, has been shown to lower plaque pH soon after ingestion[38] and to induce caries in rats when eaten ad libitum.[91]

One food with reported protective factors is cheese; there is evidence in humans to show that finishing a meal with cheese reduces the acidity of plaque[79] and therefore presumably its cariogenicity. Animal studies, which of course can be more tightly controlled than studies in humans, support this finding.[61]

In addition to fluoride, other dietary trace elements have been associated with caries experience: molybdenum with low disease levels[81] and selenium with high levels.[43] However, evidence for an important etiologic role is weak, and these reports have no practical implications for caries control. Among the various food additives intended to reduce the carious attack, phosphates have probably received most attention. In numerous animal studies phosphates have been shown to reduce caries when added to the diet, but studies in humans have yielded disappointing results.[54,63] The reductions in caries have been too small to be of any significance, and the phosphate tends to give the food an unpleasant taste.

Nutritious and fibrous foods are naturally to be recommended for good general health. Although the impact on oral health of a balanced diet high in unprocessed foods can only be good, it cannot be demonstrated under modern conditions of fluoride exposure that such a diet, by itself, will improve oral health status. Nor is there any evidence to support chewing of carrots, celery, or apples as a means of cleaning plaque from teeth. This form of dietary counseling should not become the centerpiece of dental health education, although dental personnel should always encourage healthy food choices by their patients.

CARIES CONTROL BY DIETARY RESTRICTION

A dietary regimen that involved strict control of carbohydrate intake was developed for caries control in the immediately prefluoride years.[53] Success was based on reducing counts of *Lactobacillus acidophilus*, and this regimen demanded almost total abstinence from all forms of carbohydrate for a short period, with a gradual return to limited carbohydrate intake. This draconian regimen of dietary control was too much for most patients, however, and it had little broad-scale success. Of more concern in today's world, drastic reduction of all forms of carbohydrate, which include fruits and vegetables, is clearly unwise because it could lead either to excessive intake of fat and protein or to energy deprivation. Dietary guidelines from the U.S. Department of Agriculture urge the consumption of more unrefined carbohydrates (e.g., fruits, vegetables, and whole grains) but retain the recommendation for restrained consumption of refined carbohydrates (sugars and other fermentable carbohydrates).[92]

In Chapter 20 we discussed how the Vipeholm study[42] influenced dental health education and how application of the results of that landmark study may have become misdirected. In normal-living populations, there is no epidemiologic evidence that consumption of sticky foods is more strongly associated with caries experience than is consumption of sugared drinks, although this conclusion depends on the quantities consumed (i.e., food cariogenicity rather than cariogenic potential). Sugared rinses served very well to demonstrate the *Stephan curve*, the first laboratory demonstration that ingestion of sugars caused an immediate sharp drop in plaque pH, followed by a gradual return to normal pH due to salivary buffering action.[90] The Stephan curve is shown in Fig. 28-3. Sugared rinses were also the basis of experimental caries studies in humans,[96] so advice to "take your sugars in drinks rather than sticky foods" can hardly be recommended given this evidence. Another aspect of this subject is that consumer perceptions of "sticky" foods are poorly related to objective measures of food retention.[57]

We also discussed in Chapter 20 how prospective studies in the 1980s could not demonstrate a relationship between caries experience and frequency of eating among children, and that the conclusion of the Vipeholm study on the importance of frequency of consumption may have been based on a distorted eating pattern that is rarely seen in the general population. Health educators today are advised to concentrate on reducing total intake of sugars by caries-susceptible people rather than to focus on "sticky" foods or details of snacking frequency.

Research studies in humans have identified many people who get little caries even though they consume a lot of sugars[25,80]; extensive dietary counseling for such individuals is clearly not time well spent. The philosophy behind extensive effort to obtain major reductions in such individuals' consumption of sugars to prevent a small amount of disease must be seriously questioned. Patients who are more susceptible to caries, however, can benefit considerably. Therefore extensive dietary counseling in the dental office should be concentrated on patients who show an obvious susceptibility to caries.

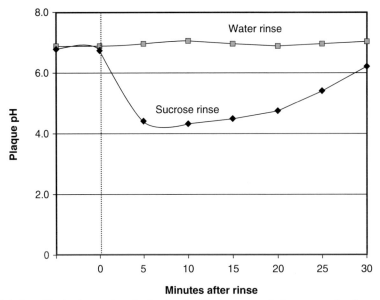

Fig. 28-3 Data from Stephan's experiments showing the Stephan curve. In the group using the sucrose rinse, a sharp and immediate drop in plaque pH was seen; in the control group using a water rinse, no change occurred.[90]

On a community level, dietary advice in dental health education should be linked with general efforts to educate the public regarding wise food choices for healthy living and judicious use of the national dietary guidelines. High-sugar foods are often high-fat foods as well, so dentally oriented advice is completely in harmony with broad advice to enhance the public health. Drastic reductions in sugar consumption, even if feasible in the United States, may or may not have much impact on caries levels but would likely lead to replacement of lost energy by consumption of fat.[27] This would clearly not be a move to enhance the public health.

PLAQUE CONTROL

Dietary restriction has historically been used in conjunction with frequent plaque removal to prevent caries. From the time of Miller in the 1880s, caries was seen as theoretically preventable by regular and careful oral hygiene procedures to remove plaque. Countless hours of dental health education have been devoted to promoting that end, based on the adage that "a clean tooth never decays." This approach to controlling caries by focusing on oral hygiene is based on the "nonspecific plaque hypothesis," which in turn was based on the incorrect assumption that all bacteria in plaque are of

equal cariogenicity and should therefore be removed. It also stems from the pioneering work of Stephan in the 1940s (see Fig. 28-3), which quickly became the basis for dental health education aimed at promoting brushing immediately after eating to neutralize the impact of "acid attacks."

Even with all the knowledge gained from modern research, however, the relation between caries incidence and level of oral hygiene can still be confusing. Plaque harbors cariogenic and periodontopathogenic bacteria, but it also is the main intraoral repository of fluoride and other remineralizing substances. Presumably the human race evolved plaque for some beneficial purpose, although one would doubt it from the message given out by most dental health education materials.

Despite historically mixed research evidence linking oral hygiene to caries incidence,[7,17,69] interest in stringent oral hygiene was piqued by a series of reports in the 1970s which concluded that caries incidence in children could be virtually eliminated by meticulous plaque removal carried out by trained dental auxiliaries at frequent intervals.[11-13,64] These reports are known collectively as the Karlstad studies after the Swedish county in which they were conducted. Intervals between professional cleanings were 2 weeks in younger children, whereas in older children spectacular results were maintained when the time between cleanings was extended to 8 weeks after an initial 2 years at 2-week intervals.[65] The procedures involved in the professional cleaning of children's teeth are detailed in Chapter 29.

Benefits of this protocol probably came from a combination of (1) plaque control, (2) intensive use of topical fluoride paste, and (3) dental health education and oral hygiene practices at home, although the researchers concluded that most benefit came from the oral hygiene procedures.[12] Caries reductions of 98% were reported over 2 years,[11] although attempts by others to replicate the Karlstad regimen were not able to achieve the same level of success.[1,9,14,44] More recently, studies on the Danish island of Bornholm have reported great caries-preventive success through rigorous control of plaque deposits on erupting first molars.[29] Like the Karlstad regimen, the Bornholm approach is resource intensive, so much so that it is of doubtful utility in places that do not have Scandinavian-level resources in a school dental services.

Studies carried out by Scandinavian researchers with small groups of children continue to relate good oral hygiene to low caries experience.[3,23,47,70] Poor oral hygiene is also a clear risk factor for root caries in older people.[89,95] On the other hand, despite extensive improvements in the caries status of Quebec children between 1977 and 1990, no improvement in oral hygiene could be found,[76] and oral hygiene levels were not associated with the progression of white spots to dentinal lesions.[33] Even if a poor level of oral hygiene *does* promote caries, extensive professional care to clean up a dirty mouth may not be time well spent if the underlying reasons for poor oral hygiene are not addressed.

Good oral hygiene is so clearly a desirable goal for social and periodontal reasons (see Chapter 29) that education or treatment to achieve it cannot be simply dismissed. The question, however, is one of cost effectiveness, of the best use of a professional's time. The intensity of the Karlstad protocol, in education and home care as well as in the professional treatments themselves, demands a high investment in equipment and personnel and absorbs some 3 hours of chair time per child each year.[9] The cost

of the Karlstad approach therefore makes it unrealistic for most public services; caries prevention efforts are far better channeled into fluoride and sealant programs. The main purpose of regular toothbrushing, in terms of caries prevention, is to introduce fluoride into the mouth regularly via the toothpaste. The plaque-removal effect appears secondary in caries prevention, although it can have primary benefits in controlling gingivitis (see Chapter 29). Regular toothbrushing with a fluoride toothpaste should be encouraged as a regular daily routine for all people, whether susceptible to caries or not.

REFERENCES

1. Agerbaek N, Poulsen S, Melsen B, Glavind L. Effect of professional toothcleaning every third week on gingivitis and dental caries in children. Community Dent Oral Epidemiol 1978;6:40-1.
2. Alanen P, Isokangas P, Gutmann K. Xylitol candies in caries prevention: Results of a field study in Estonian children. Community Dent Oral Epidemiol 2000;28:218-24.
3. Aleksejuniene J, Arneberg P, Eriksen HM. Caries prevalence and oral hygiene in Lithuanian children and adolescents. Acta Odontol Scand 1996;54:75-80.
4. American Academy of Pediatrics. AAP says soft drinks in schools should be restricted, website: http://www.aap.org/advocacy/releases/jansoftdrinks.htm. Accessed February 4, 2004.
5. American Academy of Pediatric Dentistry. Partnership to promote pediatric dental health, website: http://www.aapd.org/hottopics/news.asp?NEWS_ID=210. Accessed February 4, 2004.
6. American Dental Association. Oral health topics A–Z: Diet and oral health, website: http://www.ada.org/public/topics/softdrink_faq.asp#1. Accessed March 4, 2004.
7. Andlaw RJ. Oral hygiene and dental caries; a review. Int Dent J 1978;28:1-6.
8. Antar MA, Ohlson MA, Hodges RE. Changes in retail market food supplies in the United States in the last seventy years in relation to the incidence of coronary heart disease, with special reference to dietary carbohydrates and essential fatty acids. Am J Clin Nutr 1964;14:169-78.
9. Ashley FP, Sainsbury RH. The effect of a school-based plaque control programme on caries and gingivitis. Br Dent J 1981;150:41-5.
10. Autio JT. Effect of xylitol chewing gum on salivary *Streptococcus mutans* in preschool children. ASDC J Dent Child 2002;69:81-6.
11. Axelsson P, Lindhe J. The effect of a preventive programme on dental plaque, gingivitis and caries in school children. Results after one and two years. J Clin Periodontol 1974;1:126-38.
12. Axelsson P, Lindhe J. Effect of fluoride on gingivitis and dental caries in a preventive program based on plaque

control. Community Dent Oral Epidemiol 1975;3: 156-60.

13. Axelsson P, Lindhe J, Waseby J. The effect of various plaque control measures on gingivitis and caries in schoolchildren. Community Dent Oral Epidemiol 1976;4:232-9.

14. Badersten A, Egelberg J, Koch G. Effect of monthly prophylaxis on caries and gingivitis in schoolchildren. Community Dent Oral Epidemiol 1975;3:1-4.

15. Barmes D, Barnaud J, Khambonanda S, Infirri JS. Field trials of preventive regimens in Thailand and French Polynesia. Int Dent J 1985;35:66-72.

16. Beckers HJ. Influence of xylitol on growth, establishment, and cariogenicity of *Streptococcus mutans* in dental plaque of rats. Caries Res 1988;22:166-73.

17. Bellini HT, Arneberg P, von der Fehr FR. Oral hygiene and caries: A review. Acta Odontol Scand 1981;39:257-65.

18. Beverage Marketing Corporation. 2003 soft drink top 10 review, website: http://beverageworld.com/beverageworld/images/pdf/soft-drink_sponsor_splenda_bw_303.pdf. Accessed February 3, 2004.

19. Bibby BG. The cariogenicity of snack foods and confections. J Am Dent Assoc 1975;90:121-32.

20. Bibby BG. Diet, nutrition, and oral health: A rational approach for the dental practice. J Am Dent Assoc 1984;109:30.

21. Birkhed D, Edwardsson S, Kalfas S, Svensater G. Cariogenicity of sorbitol. Swed Dent J 1984;8:147-54.

22. Birkhed D, Svensater G, Edwardsson S. Cariological studies of individuals with long-term sorbitol consumption. Caries Res 1990;24:220-3.

23. Bjertness E. The importance of oral hygiene on variation in dental caries in adults. Acta Odontol Scand 1991;49:97-102.

24. Bowen WH. Food components and caries. Adv Dent Res 1994;8:215-20.

25. Burt BA, Eklund SA, Morgan KJ, et al. The effects of sugars intake and frequency of ingestion on dental caries increment in a three-year longitudinal study. J Dent Res 1988;67:1422-9.

26. Burt BA, Ismail AI. Diet, nutrition, and food cariogenicity. J Dent Res 1986;65(Spec Issue):1475-84.

27. Burt BA, Szpunar SM. The Michigan Study: The relationship between sugars intake and dental caries over three years. Int Dent J 1994;44:230-40.

28. Cantor SM. Patterns of use. In: National Academy of Sciences. Sweeteners: Issues and uncertainties. Academy forum, fourth of a series. Washington DC: National Academy of Sciences, 1975:19-29.

29. Carvalho JC, Thylstrup A, Ekstrand KR. Results after 3 years of non-operative caries treatment of erupting permanent first molars. Community Dent Oral Epidemiol 1992;20:187-92.

30. DePaola DP. Executive summary. J Dent Res 1986; 65(Spec Issue):1540-3.

31. Edgar WM. Sugar substitutes, chewing gum and dental caries—a review. Br Dent J 1998;184:29-32.

32. Edgar WM, Geddes DA. Chewing gum and dental health—a review. Br Dent J 1990;168:173-7.

33. Etty EJ, Henneberke M, Gruythuysen RJ, Woltgens JH. Influence of oral hygiene on early enamel caries. Caries Res 1994;28:132-6.

34. Firestone AR, Navia JM. In vivo measurements of sulcal plaque pH after topical applications of sorbitol and sucrose in rats fed sorbitol or sucrose. J Dent Res 1986;65:1020-3.

35. Firestone AR, Schmid R, Muhlemann HR. Effect on the length and number of intervals between meals on caries in rats. Caries Res 1984;18:128-33.

36. Frostell G, Birkhed D, Edwardsson S, et al. Effect of partial substitution of invert sugar for sucrose in combination with Duraphat treatment on caries development in preschool children: The Malmö study. Caries Res 1991;25:304-10.

37. Gales MA, Nguyen TM. Sorbitol compared with xylitol in prevention of dental caries. Ann Pharmacopother 2000;34:98-100.

38. Geddes DA, Edgar WM, Jenkins GN, Rugg-Gunn AJ. Apples, salted peanuts and plaque pH. Br Dent J 1977;142:317-9.

39. Glass RL. A two-year clinical trial of sorbitol chewing gum. Caries Res 1983;17:365-8.

40. Grenby TH, Phillips A, Mistry M. Studies of the dental properties of lactitol compared with five other bulk sweeteners in vitro. Caries Res 1989;23:315-9.

41. Grobler SR. The effect of a high consumption of citrus fruit and a mixture of other fruits on dental caries in man. Clin Prev Dent 1991;13(4):13-7.

42. Gustaffson BE, Quensel CE, Lanke LS, et al. The Vipehölm dental caries study. The effect of different levels of carbohydrate intake on caries activity in 436 individuals observed for five years. Acta Odontol Scand 1954;11:232-364.

43. Hadjimarkos DM. Selenium: A caries-enhancing trace element. Caries Res 1969;3:14-22.

44. Hamp SE, Johansson LA, Karlsson R. Clinical effects of preventive regimens for young people in their early and middle teens in relation to previous experience with dental prevention. Acta Odontol Scand 1984;42:99-108.

45. Hayes C. The effect of non-cariogenic sweeteners on the prevention of dental caries: A review of the evidence. J Dent Educ 2001;65:1106-9.

46. Health claims: Dietary sugar alcohols and dental caries. Fed Register 1996;61(165):43446-7.

47. Holst A, Martensson I, Laurin M. Identification of caries risk children and prevention of caries in pre-school children. Swed Dent J 1997;21:185-91.

48. Imfeld T, Mühlemann HR. Evaluation of sugar substitutes in preventive cariology. J Prev Dent 1977;4:8-14.

49. Integration of methods—working group consensus report. J Dent Res 1986;65(Spec Issue):1537-9.

50. Ismail AI, Burt BA, Eklund SA. The cariogenicity of soft drinks in the United States. J Am Dent Assoc 1984; 109:241-5.

51. Isokangas P, Soderling E, Pienihakkinen K, Alanen P. Occurrence of dental decay in children after maternal consumption of xylitol chewing gum, a follow-up from 0 to 5 years of age. J Dent Res 2000;79:1885-9.

52. Isokangas P, Tiekso J, Alanen P, Makinen KK. Long-term effect of xylitol chewing gum on dental caries. Community Dent Oral Epidemiol 1989;17:200-3.

53. Jay P. The reduction of oral *Lactobacillus acidophilus* counts by the periodic restriction of carbohydrate. Am J Orthod Oral Surg 1947;33:162-84.

54. Jenkins GN. Current concepts concerning the development of dental caries. Int Dent J 1972;22:350-62.

55. Kandelman D, Bar A, Hefti A. Collaborative WHO xylitol field study in French Polynesia. I. Baseline prevalence and 32-month caries increment. Caries Res 1988;22:55-62.

56. Kandelman D, Gagnon G. A 24-month clinical study of the incidence and progression of dental caries in relation to consumption of chewing gum containing xylitol in school preventive programs. J Dent Res 1990; 69:1771-5.

57. Kashket S, Van Houte J, Lopez LR, Stocks S. Lack of correlation between food retention on the human dentition and consumer perception of food stickiness. J Dent Res 1991;70:1314-9.

58. Kashket S, Yaskell T, Lopez LR. Prevention of sucrose-induced demineralization of tooth enamel by chewing sorbitol gum. J Dent Res 1989;68:460-2.

59. Koulourides T, Bodden S, Keller S, et al. Cariogenicity of nine sugars tested with an intraoral device in man. Caries Res 1976;10:427-41.

60. Krasse B. Oral effect of other carbohydrates. Int Dent J 1982;32:24-32.

61. Krobicka A, Bowen WH, Pearson S, Young DA. The effects of cheese snacks on caries in desalivated rats. J Dent Res 1987;66:1116-9.

62. Leach SA, Lee GT, Edgar WM. Remineralization of artificial caries-like lesions in human enamel in situ by chewing sorbitol gum. J Dent Res 1989;68:1064-8.

63. Lilienthal B. Phosphates and dental caries. Monogr Oral Sci 1977;6:1-107.

64. Lindhe J, Axelsson P. The effect of proper oral hygiene and topical fluoride application on caries and gingivitis in Swedish schoolchildren. Community Dent Oral Epidemiol 1973;1:9-16.

65. Lindhe J, Axelsson P, Tollskog G. The effect of proper oral hygiene on gingivitis and dental caries in schoolchildren. Community Dent Oral Epidemiol 1975;3: 150-5.

66. Makinen KK, Makinen P-L, Pape H Jr, et al. Stabilisation of rampant caries: Polyol gums and arrest of dentine caries in two long-term cohort studies in young subjects. Int Dent J 1995;45:93-107.

67. Mann J. Sugar revisited—again [editorial]. Bull World Health Organ 2003;81:552.

68. Marshall TA, Levy SM, Broffitt B, et al. Patterns of beverage consumption during the transition stage of infant nutrition. J Am Diet Assoc 103:1350-3.

69. Mascarenhas AK. Oral hygiene as a risk indicator of enamel and dentin caries. Community Dent Oral Epidemiol 1998;26:331-9.

70. Mathiesen AT, Ogaard B, Rölla G. Oral hygiene as a variable in dental caries experience in 14-year-olds exposed to fluoride. Caries Res 1996;30:29-33.

71. Mundorff SA, Featherstone JDB, Bibby BG, et al. Cariogenic potential of foods. I. Caries in the rat model. Caries Res 1990;24:344-55.

72. Newbrun E. Sucrose, the arch criminal of dental caries. Odontol Revy 1967;18:373-86.

73. Newbrun E. Sucrose in the dynamics of the carious process. Int Dent J 1982;32:13-23.

74. Newbrun E. The potential role of alternative sweeteners in caries prevention. Isr J Dent Sci 1990;2: 200-13.

75. Newbrun E, Hoover C, Mettraux C, Graf H. Comparison of dietary habits and dental health of subjects with hereditary fructose intolerance and control subjects. J Am Dent Assoc 1980;101:619-26.

76. Payette M, Brodeur JM. Comparison of dental caries and oral hygiene indices for 13- to 14-year-old Quebec children between 1977 and 1989-1990. J Can Dent Assoc 1992;58:921-2, 926-9, 932-3.

77. Rekola M. Changes in buccal white spots during 2-year consumption of dietary sucrose or xylitol. Acta Odontol Scand 1986;44:285-90.

78. Rekola M. Correlation between caries incidence and frequency of chewing gum sweetened with sucrose or xylitol. Proc Finn Dent Soc 1989;85:21-4.

79. Rugg-Gunn AJ, Edgar WM, Geddes DA, Jenkins GN. The effect of different meal patterns upon plaque pH in human subjects. Br Dent J 1975;139:351-6.

80. Rugg-Gunn AJ, Hackett AF, Appleton DR, et al. Relationship between dietary habits and caries increment assessed over two years in 405 English school children. Arch Oral Biol 1984;29:983-92.

81. Schamschula RG, Adkins BL, Barmes DE, et al. WHO study of dental caries etiology in Papua, New Guinea. WHO Offset Publication No. 40. Geneva: World Health Organization, 1978.

82. Scheinin A. Field studies on sugar substitutes. Int Dent J 1985;35:195-200.

83. Scheinin A, Banoczy J, Szoke J, et al. Collaborative WHO xylitol field studies in Hungary. I. Three-year caries activity in institutionalized children. Acta Odontol Scand 1985;43:327-47.

84. Scheinin A, Makinen KK. Turku sugar studies; an overview. Acta Odontol Scand 1976;34:405-8.

85. Scheinin A, Makinen KK, Tammisalo E, Rekola M. Turku sugar studies. XVIII. Incidence of dental caries in relation to 1-year consumption of xylitol chewing gum. Acta Odontol Scand 1975;33:269-78.

86. Scheinen A, Makinen KK, Ylitalo K. Turku sugar studies. V. Final report on the effect of sucrose, fructose, and xylitol diets on the caries incidence in man. Acta Odontol Scand 1976;34:179-216.

87. Smits MT, Arends J. Influence of extraoral xylitol and sucrose dippings on enamel demineralization in vivo. Caries Res 1988;22:160-5.

88. Soderling E, Isokangas P, Pienihakkinen K, Tenovuo J. Influence of maternal xylitol consumption on acquisition of mutans streptococci by infants. J Dent Res 2000;79:882-7.

89. Steele JG, Sheiham A, Marcenes W, et al. Clinical and behavioural risk indicators for root caries in older people. Gerodontology 2001;18:95-101.

90. Stephan RM. Changes in hydrogen-ion concentration on tooth surfaces and in carious lesions. J Am Dent Assoc 1940;27:718-23.

91. Stephan RM. Effect of different types of human foods on dental health in experimental animals. J Dent Res 1966;45:1551-61.

92. US Department of Agriculture. Food guide pyramid, website: http://www.nal.usda.gov/fnic/etext/000023.html#xtocid2381818. Accessed July 2, 2004.

93. US Department of Agriculture, Economic Research Service. Sugar and sweetener; situation and outlook report. SSS-220, June 1997.

94. US Department of Agriculture, Economic Research Service. Per capita consumption of sugars in the United States, 1972-2002, website: http://www.ers.usda.gov/briefing/sugar/data/table50.xls. Accessed February 2, 2004.

95. Vehkalahti MM, Vrbic VL, Peric LM, Matvoz ES. Oral hygiene and root caries occurrence in Slovenian adults. Int Dent J 1997;47:26-31.

96. Von der Fehr FR, Loe H, Theilade E. Experimental caries in man. Caries Res 1970;4:131-48.

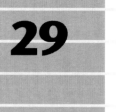

29　Prevention of Periodontal Diseases

Although our understanding of periodontal conditions is growing rapidly (see Chapter 21), prevention and control of periodontal conditions still must be based on the periodic removal of plaque and calculus, whether by the individual or by a dental professional. There is no parallel in prevention of periodontal diseases to a public health measure such as water fluoridation.

Our current understanding that only some 5%-15% of the population suffers from serious periodontitis has led some to downplay the importance of prevention; this is the view that "periodontal disease doesn't matter anymore." This view is clearly faulty, because this level of prevalence still means that some 30 million Americans suffer from serious periodontitis. Based on the data given in Chapter 21, eight times that number have moderate adult periodontitis, much of which requires treatment and could probably be prevented. Prevention of periodontitis still is clearly a worthwhile public health endeavor; the problems and the frustrations come with our limitations in how to accomplish it. Even though our understanding of periodontitis has expanded greatly over recent years, the only practical approach to pre-

vention of periodontitis (as opposed to its control through clinical treatment) is to prevent and control gingivitis.

RATIONALE FOR PLAQUE CONTROL

The rationale for controlling periodontal conditions by regular plaque removal is based on the premise that supragingival plaque, if undisturbed, will become subgingival plaque,[92] and subgingival plaque has the potential to be colonized by periodontopathogenic bacteria. Although relatively few gingivitis sites progress to periodontitis (see Chapter 21), we still cannot identify those sites that will. Accordingly, the principle for prevention has not changed for years: the regular and consistent control of plaque buildup, supragingival and subgingival, soft and mineralized (calculus), on the teeth and in the gingival crevices. This approach is bacteriologically nonspecific, for it seeks to control the buildup of *all* plaque. It also depends strongly on individual motivation for success. Plaque control is therefore unlikely ever to be completely effective in preventing periodontal diseases in a population, although individual success is common. Until research produces methods of controlling periodontal infection, enhancing host response, and identifying susceptible individuals, however, mass plaque control by personal, professional, or chemical means is the best we can do.

This chapter deals with methods for controlling the deposition of dental plaque, an approach that can effectively prevent gingivitis. As was detailed in Chapter 21, however, the role of plaque in periodontitis is not so straightforward. Plaque deposits may be a necessary condition for periodontitis, but clearly they are not sufficient. In other words, susceptible people may have to be stringent about oral hygiene, but there are millions of people with poor oral hygiene who do not have serious periodontitis. There is an analogy here with the role of consumption of sugars in the development of caries: caries-susceptible persons have to restrict their intake of sugars, but there are many people who consume a lot of sugars but have little or no caries as a consequence.

NATURE OF DENTAL PLAQUE

Although dental plaque is commonly depicted as the root cause of both caries and periodontitis, one should remember that it must have evolved in humans for some purpose. Commercial advertising would have us believe that oral health depends on the complete removal of all plaque at all times, but clearly that is not only not possible but also not desirable. Dental plaque forms naturally on the teeth and benefits the host by helping to prevent intraoral colonization by exogenous species.[88] Plaque's role in promoting remineralization of demineralized lesions was described in Chapter 20.

Dental plaque is a natural biofilm that forms on the tooth surface and consists of a diverse microbial community embedded in a polymer matrix of bacterial and salivary origin.[89] After a tooth surface is cleaned, the pellicle, a conditioning film of proteins and glycoproteins, is adsorbed rapidly onto the tooth surface. The interactions between pellicle and early bacterial colonizers are the first steps in plaque formation. Secondary bacterial colonizers adhere to these early colonizers through specific molecular interactions, a process that contributes to the pattern of bacterial succession. The biofilm character of plaque allows the survival of a diverse bacterial flora.[24] Although microbial adhesion is how plaque formation begins, microbial multiplication is thought to be the dominant factor in the buildup of dental plaque, and the nature of this microbial proliferation is highly dependent on the local environment. Because environmental conditions vary from place to place within the oral cavity, each site with plaque represents its own distinct ecosystem, and the dominant microbial composition at the site depends on the outcome of numerous host-microbe and microbe-microbe interactions.[106]

The clinical picture of all this activity has been well described. After plaque has been completely removed, it re-forms slowly on the supragingival tooth surface for about 3 days, and then if left undisturbed it increases rapidly to reach a maximum bulk after 7 days. The various microbial interactions actually keep the bacterial composition of plaque relatively stable, but when this homeostasis breaks down, the shifts in microbial balance can set up conditions for caries or gingivitis to begin. Plaque accumulation around the gingival margin leads to an inflammatory host response and an increased flow of gingival crevicular fluid.[88] Few bacteria can be isolated from around healthy gingival tissue, although with gingivitis there is a considerable increase in the numbers and complexity of bacteria as the lesion develops.[92] Subgingival plaque microflora shift from being predominantly gram positive to including increased levels of anaerobic gram-negative organisms; the character of subgingival plaque is thus quite different from that of supragingival plaque. Specifically, the gram-negative anaerobes *Porphyromonas gingivalis* and *Bacteroides forsythus* in subgingival plaque have been associated with both loss of periodontal attachment and bone loss.[48,49] Frequent professional supragingival cleaning, added to good personal oral hygiene, has a beneficial effect with regard to subgingival microbiota in moderately deep pockets.[54,120] Subgingival plaque is also characterized by oral spirochetes, whose role in periodontitis is still not clear, although their presence in the subgingival plaque is seen as a marker for disease.[118]

Calculus was formerly viewed only as an "irritating factor" in the development of periodontitis[64] and did not get much research attention. Today, however, calculus is recognized as a calcified matrix that can harbor periodontopathogenic bacteria, and subgingival calculus is closely associated with gingivitis and periodontitis.[33] Therefore, the initial formation and continued presence of both supragingival and subgingival calculus are to be prevented to the extent possible. The only known method is to control the initial formation of supragingival plaque and calculus.

APPROACHES TO PLAQUE CONTROL

Because plaque has some identifiable health functions and because disease comes more from an upset in the homeostatic balance than from infection with exogenous organisms, disease prevention should be geared more toward plaque control than plaque eradication. This concept is referred to as the *ecologic plaque hypothesis.*[87] The goal in preventing periodontitis is to prevent fresh plaque from becoming *established* plaque, which permits the growth of specific periodontopathogenic bacteria,[102,123] and to prevent supragingival plaque from becoming established subgingivally.

Several approaches to plaque control can be quickly ruled out as having no scientific basis: rinsing with water and chewing a fibrous food (e.g., remove loose food debris but do not affect plaque). There is no evidence to alter the long-held view that preventive benefits cannot be achieved by changes in diet or nutrition,[74,110] although, given the importance of the host response in periodontitis and the fact that nutrition is a vital part of the immune reaction, the role of nutrition in periodontitis should continue to be studied.

Primary prevention of gingivitis requires consistent, thorough control of plaque accumulation on a lifetime basis. The rationale is to prevent plaque from reaching the stage of maturity at which gingivitis begins. Some people are capable of maintaining an adequate oral hygiene status largely by their own efforts, but many are not. The dental professional will consistently see some level of gingivitis in the latter patients and may become frustrated in the effort to eliminate gingivitis entirely. For these patients, the dental professional's goal should be to maintain the gingivitis at as low a level as possible. As long as the lowest possible level of

gingivitis can be maintained over time, subsequent loss of periodontal support is likely to be minimized. This is true for the majority of patients who are at low risk of severe periodontitis. It is less the case for those patients with aggressive periodontitis who fit the compromised host model described in Chapter 21. Prevention of disease in these patients is difficult because we do not yet have the means of influencing the deficient host response to a periodontal challenge.

As long as plaque accumulation remains supragingival, it can be controlled by mechanical or chemotherapeutic means.[101] Once plaque becomes established subgingivally, however, the individual patient cannot remove it by self-care, and professional intervention is necessary. The goal of prevention of periodontal conditions through plaque control by the individual is to keep supragingival plaque from accumulating.

There are essentially three approaches to preventing the build-up of dental plaque, each of which is assessed in turn. They are:
- Mechanical plaque removal by the individual
- Mechanical plaque removal by the dental professional
- Chemotherapeutic methods of plaque control

MECHANICAL PLAQUE REMOVAL BY THE INDIVIDUAL

Self-care is a fundamental part of periodontal health. Unless the individual is able to maintain at least a reasonable level of oral cleanliness by regular and consistent home care, the benefits of treatment by dental professionals will be limited. Individual effort means mechanical plaque removal with a toothbrush and aids such as dental floss, an interproximal brush, and wood points.

Although individual oral hygiene practices are fundamental to the promotion of oral health, it is surprising how little is really known about such basic things as the most efficient type of toothbrush and how often the teeth should be brushed. Research studies in these areas have often been run for only short periods and with atypical populations, such as dental or dental hygiene students. Long-term effects and the validity of projecting results to the general population are thus difficult to assess.

Frequency of Toothbrushing

The limited information that is available indicates that a thorough oral cleansing should be carried out at 24- to 48-hour intervals.[61,66] Considering the time needed for plaque to mature bacteriologically, brushing after every meal, which was usually impractical anyway, is unnecessary to prevent gingivitis. But because toothbrushing with a fluoride toothpaste is also a major source of fluoride exposure for caries prevention, it is best carried out at least twice per day to maintain oral health. Brushing in the morning and evening fits with most peoples' daily routines and should be the basis for education of the public and dental patients. Of course, patients who have received treatment for periodontitis are likely to be at high risk for further disease, and more stringent home care regimens may be required for them.[120]

Type of Toothbrush

Little research has been carried out on the best type of toothbrush; what evidence there is suggests that it really does not matter much. Children clearly should use a smaller brush, and the dentist or hygienist may want to recommend different sizes and degrees of softness, depending on each patient's manual dexterity, enthusiasm, and oral health. Soft brushes generally are preferred to minimize gingival damage with enthusiastic brushing. Manufacturers are constantly coming out with new designs, so anyone can find a toothbrush that is comfortable and efficient. However, these recommendations are based on common sense rather than on firm evidence.

Electric toothbrushes with a rotary action have been found to be more effective plaque removers in closely supervised clinical trials,[117] although it is uncertain how well these findings reflect everyday effectiveness. Both manual and power-driven toothbrushes are effective if used properly; differences between individuals' brushing efficiency are likely to be much greater than inherent differences between types of toothbrushes. New versions of power-driven brushes are constantly being marketed, some with heavy advertising, and most have not been subjected to rigorous testing. Power brushes may be particularly useful for handicapped persons or others with low manual dexterity.

Toothbrushing Methods

A variety of toothbrushing methods, some requiring a lot of manual gymnastics, have been described in the dental literature down the years. Proponents of one method or another have traditionally been vehement in the defense of their method's efficacy, a good example of the rule that the level of passion that people have about an issue is inversely proportional to its scientific basis. In fact there is little difference between the various methods in their ability to remove dental plaque.[42,52,100,103] From these studies, limited though some of them are, the scrub method emerges as the simplest technique available and one that is no less effective than any other. It requires minimal manual dexterity and patient concentration, and generally seems best for most persons.

Interdental Cleaning

The rationale for supplementing toothbrushing with use of dental floss, interdental brushes, or wood points to clean below the contact areas is that even assiduous use of the toothbrush usually cannot penetrate these areas efficiently. There is some limited evidence that interdental cleaning, by floss or interdental brushes, reduces interdental gingivitis and plaque more than toothbrushing alone.[27,78]

Many dental health education materials extol the efficacy of dental floss: "brush and floss" long ago replaced the exhortation to just "brush." There is still little evidence, however, to show that flossing, as practiced by the individual with normal interdental spaces, adds much to the efficiency of brushing,[55,100,107] nor are the limited research studies able to find a difference between waxed and unwaxed floss in cleaning efficiency.[22,30,40,78] In cases in which papillae have diminished to leave open interdental spaces, interdental brushes are superior to floss.[23,32] Many people prefer wood points to floss because floss can break and become stuck in awkward contact areas, and wood points can be effective interdental cleaners.

Individual Motivation

The individual practice of regular, thorough, and consistent oral hygiene procedures depends largely on the interest of the individual in his or her oral health. Dentally conscious people have this interest already, but many others do not. Oral hygiene practices must fit into the lifestyle of each individual, and lifestyles are rarely changed by exhortation. To illustrate the lifestyle issue, a British study found that schoolchildren who reported more frequent toothbrushing also reported more frequent bathing, use of deodorant, and hand washing after visiting the toilet.[85] Information like this comes as no surprise.

Knowledge is usually thought to precede action, although a study of periodontal patients in North Carolina found poor correlation between knowledge of the disease process and periodontal health.[16] Carefully thought-out and well-organized motivational programs aimed at schoolchildren have produced poor results in the United States.[53,56] A typical finding came from a study of supervised daily toothbrushing by schoolchildren in Sweden: gingivitis was reduced for the duration of the program, but the improvement disappeared when the supervision ended.[70,71] Although compliance with periodontitis treatment instructions is related to health beliefs,[65] the effects of individual chairside instruction are usually weak.[115,122] Doubts are thus raised about what motivational programs really do; they may succeed only in reinforcing existing favorable attitudes and not in altering negative ones.[90] A Danish longitudinal study found that oral hygiene behavior in youth was found to predict periodontal health in adulthood,[73] a finding which confirms that attitudes and oral health behavior are principally determined by factors outside the dental office. (Issues in health promotion are discussed more fully in Chapter 5.)

For dental professionals who try to induce individual patients to improve their daily oral hygiene performance, greatest success may come from a personal and common sense approach by the dentist or hygienist. Some patients will respond better than others. Objective monitoring by measurement of gingival bleeding, pocket depth, periodontal attachment levels, calculus deposits, and plaque is important because subjective impressions of progress can be misleading. Reinforcement of simple messages and constant encouragement

of the individual's efforts seem to be important factors. Oral health professionals must work within the limitations of the individual patient, and within their own limitations too.

Oral hygiene in the United States is considered by most experts to be constantly improving, a trend thought to result from heightened awareness, heavy advertising, and constantly improving oral hygiene products. Public health education programs intended to produce mass improvement in oral hygiene have had little measurable impact on this trend.[43,53] Time given to this form of education in public health programs, especially in populations bombarded by television commercials about oral hygiene, could probably be much better spent on primary prevention or on providing dental care to needy people. This may not be the case, however, in a low-income country, where basic knowledge of oral hygiene may be lacking. "Toothbrush drills" are quite properly a common part of dental public health education in such countries, whereas they may be unnecessary in high-income nations.

MECHANICAL PLAQUE REMOVAL BY THE DENTAL PROFESSIONAL

Professional care is necessary to remove subgingival plaque and calculus; the patient cannot remove plaque from deep pockets. The benefits of professional plaque removal have been shown in studies of children and adults who were in reasonable periodontal health to begin with, as well as in studies of adults receiving treatment for advanced disease.

Karlstad Studies

The discussion of the Karlstad studies in Chapter 28 was related principally to caries; this section discusses the studies in relation to periodontal diseases. Among children, spectacular success in preventing gingivitis was reported by the Axelsson-Lindhe group in their investigations in Karlstad, Sweden.[10,11,13,69] Studying children ages 7-14 years, this research group set out to show that a regimen of intensive prophylactic procedures that went considerably beyond routine prophylaxis would be effective in preventing both caries and gingivitis. The detailed protocol for the Karlstad regimen is given in Box 29-1.

BOX 29-1 Protocol for the Oral Cleaning Carried Out in the Children Ages 7-14 Who Participated in the Karlstad Studies[10,69]

- Detailed initial explanations of oral disease etiology and purpose of treatment by the dentist or auxiliary carrying out the treatment. Involvement of the family was considered integral to the program's success.
- Identification of plaque in the patient's mouth by disclosing tablet, then demonstration of correct toothbrushing technique for removing the stain. The patient then used dental floss under supervision. These oral hygiene instructions were repeated throughout the course of treatment as necessary.
- Rubber cup cleaning of accessible surfaces and use of engine-mounted pointed bristle to clean fissures in occlusal surfaces. A fluoride-containing prophylactic paste was used for these procedures.
- Interdental cleaning, again by the dentist or auxiliary providing the treatment, with dental floss and reciprocating interproximal tips. Again, the fluoridated prophylactic paste was forced interdentally and kept in close contact with the proximal surfaces by the floss and the tips.

These procedures were carried out by professionals every 2 weeks over a 2-year period. In the third year, the time between these "professional cleanings," as the Karlstad researchers called them, was extended to 4 weeks for the 7- to 11-year-olds and to 8 weeks for the 13- to 14-year-olds. The continuing good results with this reduced frequency of cleaning was attributed to the background effects of the first 2 years. These researchers were firm in their contention that professional cleanings five to eight times per year are still not enough by themselves to control gingivitis.

Other European groups who carried out studies using the Karlstad protocols also achieved good results, although none of them quite reached the Karlstad heights.[1,7,17,62] A British study followed up its participants a year after the study ended, and it is probably not surprising that the 3-year reduction in plaque mass of 54% had by then declined to 26%.[8]

No studies of the Karlstad regimen have been carried out in the United States or Canada because the expense of this personnel-intensive regimen is beyond the capacity of public health agencies. In addition, the implied paternalism of the regimen probably cuts against the North American cultural grain of individualism. One study in the United States found that performing prophylactic procedures twice per year in children ages 10-11 produced neither beneficial reductions in gingivitis nor improvements in oral hygiene levels,[99] although this schedule is much less intense than the Karlstad regimen. Another study of a Karlstad-type regimen in young Brazilians found that the intensive preventive care did not slow down the progression of periodontitis when compared to either routine oral hygiene instruction or to no instruction.[3] The authors speculated that they may have been dealing with a compromised host type of periodontitis (see Chapter 21). Periodontitis would not be expected to respond much to even intensive oral hygiene if the cause lies in a deficient host response, whereas periodontitis caused by local factors would show a response.

Prophylactic Treatment for Adults

Routine prophylactic care of nondiseased adults is discussed here, rather than the treatment of patients with periodontitis, which is a different issue. Patients, by definition, are either susceptible to periodontitis or not, so all clinical studies showing the value of maintenance prophylactic care in treated patients are carried out in susceptible populations.[96,97]

Studies that examined the value of routine prophylaxis in adult populations in the community (i.e., in adults who were not patients) are now many years old. Qualified success from routine prophylactic treatments in adults (on a less intense schedule than the Karlstad regimen) was reported in Norway.[84] For 5 years factory workers received a prophylactic treatment plus oral hygiene instruction at 6-month intervals, or at 3-month intervals for "more severely affected" individuals. The greatest benefits were gained by persons whose oral hygiene status was best to begin with, and least success was achieved among those with initially poor oral hygiene. This difference in results emphasizes the importance of self-care and the limitations of professional cleaning without it.

In Axelsson and Lindhe's study of adults in Karlstad over 15 years, the professional cleanings were carried out every 2-3 months for the first 6 years, and one or two times per year for a subsequent 9 years for most participants.[14]

A small subgroup of persons who had developed caries or further loss of attachment during the study were retained on a more intensive professional cleaning regimen for the entire 15 years. All participants exhibited almost no further loss of periodontal attachment during this period. In line with the philosophy of these researchers, intensive oral hygiene instruction for self-care accompanied the professional cleanings. The authors concluded that self-performed oral hygiene (with a fluoride toothpaste of course) together with a stringent regimen of professional treatment maintained oral health. The stringency of the regimen was increased for patients considered to be at greater risk for periodontitis.

In the United States a study involving office workers in California found that a professional prophylactic treatment plus intensive oral hygiene instruction every 2-4 months reduced levels of plaque and gingivitis relative to a control group and greatly slowed the rate of loss of attachment.[111] A separate study of young men found a tendency toward improved gingival health accompanying greater frequency of prophylactic procedures, although differences resulting from prophylactic treatments at 12-month, 6-month, and 4-month intervals were not pronounced.[113] An Air Force study[68] found that beneficial results were proportional to the frequency of the prophylactic treatment received; best results were achieved in the group that received four prophylactic treatments per year plus oral hygiene instruction at each appointment. None of these American studies achieved Karlstad-type results, but they did not test nearly so intensive a regimen. Collectively, they demonstrated modest across-the-board results. In light of our current views, it would have been helpful if the authors had reported their results in terms of distributional patterns; it is likely that, as other similar studies have shown, best results were achieved in those patients who were best motivated to begin with.

PROFESSIONAL PLUS PERSONAL CARE

The studies just described have some limitations, but collectively they indicate that professional prophylactic treatment can help with plaque control in many people. It must be reemphasized, however, that the best results were obtained when excellent personal oral hygiene status was maintained by the individual, which raises questions about the value of regular professional prophylactic treatments for periodontally healthy adults with good oral hygiene.

The conclusions from these studies suggest that a thorough professional prophylactic procedure at 2- to 4-month intervals (longer in some patients), combined with a high level of individual oral hygiene, is enough to prevent the destructive periodontal disease that leads to tooth loss. It might also be overtreatment. Whether the same results could be achieved in periodontally healthy adults without the professional intervention is an open question. Questions also arise in view of the epidemiologic studies in untreated populations (see Chapter 21), which show that some people with virtually no oral hygiene practices, and hence extensive gingivitis, develop little serious periodontitis. It could be concluded that persons susceptible to periodontitis may need frequent professional maintenance care, but the need for such care for nonsusceptible persons is by no means so clear.

CHEMOTHERAPEUTIC METHODS OF PLAQUE CONTROL

The inability of many persons to remove their own dental plaque consistently results from insufficient knowledge, poor mechanical dexterity, or lack of opportunity or motivation. The idea of a chemical method of plaque removal, a mouthrinse or toothpaste that does it all, is therefore highly attractive. Research over many years has led to the development of products that show some plaque-control success in specific circumstances. Commercial competition in the marketing of plaque-preventive products is keen, so much so that the American Dental Association (ADA) has established guidelines for conducting clinical trials of products claiming to control plaque to support their acceptance by the Council on Dental Therapeutics.[4] These guidelines are listed in Box 29-2, and they conform well to the requirements of acceptable clinical trials given in Chapter 13. If consistently applied, they will serve professionals as well as the public in their choice of both prescription

BOX 29-2 Criteria for Clinical Studies To Test Efficacy of Products Claiming To Control Plaque Formation To Support Their Acceptance by the American Dental Association[4]

- Characteristics of the study population should represent those of typical product users.
- Active products should be used in a normal regimen and compared with placebo control or, where applicable, an active control.
- Crossover or parallel design studies are acceptable.
- Studies should last a minimum of 6 months.
- Two studies conducted by independent investigators are required.
- Microbiologic sampling should estimate plaque qualitatively to complement indexes that measure plaque quantitatively.
- Plaque and gingivitis scoring and microbiologic sampling should be conducted at baseline, at 6 months, and at an intermediate period.
- Microbiologic profile should demonstrate that pathogenic or opportunistic microorganisms do not develop over the course of the study.
- The toxicologic profile of products should include the results of carcinogenicity and mutagenicity assays in addition to generally recognized tests for drug safety.

and over-the-counter oral hygiene products. These testing guidelines do not, however, apply to those toothpastes marketed as "anticalculus" products, because the ADA considers the action of these toothpastes in inhibiting the re-formation of supragingival calculus after a prophylactic treatment (discussed later) to be cosmetic rather than therapeutic.

Day-to-day plaque control in the healthy individual must be separated from the use of antibiotics or other medications in the treatment of established disease. Antibiotics have no place in prophylactic control.

Chlorhexidine

Chlorhexidine gluconate (CHX) has been used effectively in the form of a mouthrinse (10 ml 0.2%, once or twice daily), a topical gel applied by dental professionals (1.0% to 2.0% daily), a toothpaste (0.4% to 1.0%), a chewing gum with xylitol,[108] a spray,[34] and a direct injection into

periodontal pockets. When introduced into the oral cavity, CHX adheres to anionic substrates and is released over 8-12 hours. Mucosal and gingival penetration is minimal, and it is poorly absorbed from the gastrointestinal tract.[46] CHX has a wide range of bactericidal action, and its selective effect against *Streptococcus mutans* makes it of value in caries control in patients with special problems.[28,124,125]

Early short-term studies found that CHX rinses inhibited the formation of plaque almost completely.[81,82] However, because these initial studies were conducted with periodontally healthy dental students who ceased routine oral hygiene procedures for the study duration, the generalizability of these findings is doubtful. Results of short-term studies by other researchers using CHX in gels and toothpastes were less clear-cut and revealed some undesirable side effects.[19,38] Staining of teeth and restorations, for example, was a persistent problem.

Results of longer-term studies, conducted over 2 years, showed that the routine use of CHX was not appropriate. One study found no changes in plaque and gingivitis levels among the dental students who were the test subjects, although again their initial excellent oral hygiene status could have masked any beneficial effects of the CHX.[59] Another found reduced levels of plaque and gingivitis in a 2-year study (also involving dental and medical students), although one perplexing finding was that supragingival calculus deposition increased in the test group.[83] Other 6-month studies have also reported increased deposition of supragingival calculus,[50,67] although in both studies it was considered of no clinical consequence.

By the end of the 1970s, the limitations in the routine use of CHX were widely accepted, although it was clear that CHX could play a useful role in plaque control. The side effect of staining, plus the chance that resistant organisms could develop, were enough to produce warnings from leading periodontists against the indiscriminate use of CHX.[80] In addition, CHX does not affect subgingival plaque, which means that its preventive effect in periodontal diseases is limited to preventing the deposition of supragingival plaque after a professional cleansing. Subsequent research has confirmed these earlier findings. European and American studies of 6 months' duration confirmed that use of CHX, whether as a twice-daily rinse with a 0.12% formulation or applied in other forms and concentrations, reduced gingivitis, gingival bleeding, and plaque deposits.[2,12,50,67]

CHX has been used for years in much of Europe as an antiseptic rinse before oral surgery, to improve plaque control up to 3-4 weeks after periodontal surgery, and as an oral hygiene aid for patients with immobilized jaws recovering from fractures. This limited and selective application of CHX, because of its well-documented undesirable side effects, is also its recommended role in the United States and Canada.

CHX is marketed in the United States under the brand name of Peridex. It has been accepted by the ADA[6] as a safe and effective antiplaque agent under the 1986 ADA guidelines (see Box 29-2). Its use should be restricted to patients with periodontitis, and it has no public health applications.

Other Antibacterial Compounds

In short-term studies, alexidine dihydrochloride mouthrinse (10-15 ml, 0.035%-0.05%) has yielded results similar to those found for CHX. Reductions in plaque and gingivitis were recorded,[36,77,119] although some reductions were of little clinical importance.[29,109] Mild staining was also reported in all of these studies. Mouthrinses using octenidine[94] and cetylpyridinium chloride[9] have been tested with mixed results; sanguinarine has been tested with some reported success.[47,63,116] The over-the-counter mouthrinse Listerine, in which essential oils are the active ingredients, as been accepted by the ADA as a safe and effective antiplaque rinse[5] under its 1986 guidelines. Mouthrinses combining CHX and essential oils are also effective.[104]

Stannous fluoride also seems to have antiplaque properties, probably because it affects the growth and adherence of bacteria rather than because it exerts a direct bactericidal action. Stabilization of stannous fluoride in an anhydrous formulation, instead of in an aqueous preparation, has increased its efficacy.[91] Stabilized stannous fluoride at 0.454% in a toothpaste reduces gingivitis, although this product was found to be no better than a control toothpaste (with sodium fluoride only)

in restricting the buildup of supragingival plaque.[20,95]

Toothpastes with baking soda and peroxide (together) are marketed as plaque inhibitors, but clinical trials and in vivo testing have provided no evidence for efficacy in reducing plaque buildup and gingivitis following a prophylactic treatment.[15,21,114] The performance of a baking soda and peroxide toothpaste was notably inferior to that of a stabilized stannous fluoride product in the same test.[21]

Anticalculus ("Tartar-Control") Toothpastes

Efforts to find a toothpaste ingredient that prevents the formation of calculus on teeth go back a long way,[57,112] and until recently they were not successful. However, research during the 1960s found that pyrophosphate prevented calcification by interfering with the conversion of amorphous calcium phosphate to hydroxyapatite.[41] When this was added to the finding that the concentration of pyrophosphate in the plaque of low calculus formers was higher than in the plaque of high calculus formers,[37] the stage was set for testing the anticalculus effect of pyrophosphate in toothpaste.[86] Commercially marketed anticalculus toothpastes mostly contain a mix of soluble pyrophosphates at 3.3% concentration, with or without additional ingredients. These compounds are not part of the abrasive system of the toothpaste, and they are independent of the fluoride added for caries control.

A number of studies have demonstrated that pyrophosphates can effectively inhibit the formation of supragingival calculus after it has been removed by a prophylactic procedure.[26,31,75,76,79,121] These studies were all of fairly similar design. They ran for 2-6 months in groups of adult subjects, mostly selected for their propensity to form calculus quickly. All subjects received a thorough prophylactic treatment to remove all calculus and were then randomly allocated to test and control groups. In all of the studies, test subjects exposed to the pyrophosphates were found to have considerably less supragingival calculus formation than was seen in the control subjects.

Triclosan is an antibacterial agent that inhibits plaque buildup by adsorbing to the tooth surface and perhaps by exerting direct antiinflammatory effects on mediators of gingival inflammation.[45] It has been shown to be highly effective at preventing plaque deposition after a professional prophylactic treatment and reducing gingival bleeding, especially when it is combined with a copolymer of methoxyethylene and maleic acid.[44] Studies have shown the efficacy of triclosan (compared to a toothpaste with only sodium fluoride as an active ingredient) when used as a mouthrinse at 0.1% or 0.2%,[58] or at 0.3% concentration in a toothpaste with 2% copolymer.[25,60,93,98] Efficacy of the triclosan-copolymer formulation is independent of the type of fluoride used in the toothpaste, and it is more effective than a fluoride-only dentifrice at reducing existing plaque and gingivitis.[72] Studies of triclosan-copolymer and other ingredients such as pyrophosphates and zinc citrate have given generally positive results,[18,35,39,51,105] and work on these formulations is continuing.

What these anticalculus toothpastes do and do not do must be noted. They inhibit the deposition of new supragingival calculus after a professional cleaning, and do so without adverse tissue reaction. Triclosan-copolymer has been shown to reduce existing plaque and gingivitis.[72] These toothpastes do not remove existing supragingival calculus, and they have no effect on existing subgingival calculus. The ADA's website lists a number of toothpastes that have been accepted as being tartar-control as well as anticavity products, and the number is likely to continue growing.

The marketing of constantly more effective plaque-control toothpastes that otherwise do not affect the oral ecology can only lead to further improvements in oral hygiene and reduction in gingivitis. It is reasonable to assume that adult periodontitis should also be reduced in time, although there is no evidence yet to show that this happens. We also do not yet know if these products have any impact on aggressive periodontitis, although because of the compromised host etiology of that condition they are likely to be less effective in such cases.

COMMUNITY-BASED CONTROL OF PERIODONTAL DISEASES

Until some means can be found to enhance the host response of susceptible persons, there will always be a minority of individuals who are at special risk of losing teeth from periodontitis. Oral hygiene is especially important in such individuals, even though periodontal infections may represent only part of the disease problem (compromised host response is the rest of it and is little affected by oral hygiene).

Public programs of dental health education aimed at improving general standards of oral hygiene have long been a mainstay of dental public health. Their effectiveness is hard to demonstrate, even though it is likely that public standards of oral hygiene are continuing to improve. Because oral hygiene is of high cultural value, extensive and sophisticated commercial advertising must have made a strong impact on public oral hygiene behavior. As a result, the potential additional impact of organized programs of oral hygiene education need to be carefully thought through before such programs are launched. They are likely to be of most value when directed at populations that have little exposure to commercial advertising or that do not espouse the middle-class values of oral hygiene assumed by media advertising. Public education in oral hygiene is useful in many developing countries, although the programs should always be monitored periodically for effectiveness.

REFERENCES

1. Agerbaek N, Poulsen S, Melsen B, Glavind L. Effect of professional toothcleansing every third week on gingivitis and dental caries in children. Community Dent Oral Epidemiol 1978;6:40-1.
2. Ainamo J, Asikainen S, Paloheimo L. Gingival bleeding after chlorhexidine mouthrinses. J Clin Periodontol 1982;9:337-45.
3. Albandar JM, Buischi YA, Oliveira LB, Axelsson P. Lack of effect of oral hygiene training on periodontal disease progression over 3 years in adolescents. J Periodontol 1995;66:255-60.
4. American Dental Association, Council on Dental Therapeutics. Guidelines for acceptance of chemotherapeutic products for the control of supragingival dental plaque and gingivitis. J Am Dent Assoc 1986;112:529-32.
5. American Dental Association, Council on Dental Therapeutics. Council on Dental Therapeutics accepts Listerine. J Am Dent Assoc 1988;117:515-6.
6. American Dental Association, Council on Dental Therapeutics. Council on Dental Therapeutics accepts Peridex. J Am Dent Assoc 1988;117:516-7.
7. Ashley FP, Sainsbury RH. The effect of a school-based plaque control programme on caries and gingivitis. Br Dent J 1981;150:41-5.

8. Ashley FP, Sainsbury RH. Post-study effects of a school-based plaque control programme. Br Dent J 1982;153:337-8.

9. Ashley FP, Skinner A, Jackson PY, Wilson RF. Effect of a 0.1% cetylpyridinium chloride mouthrinse on the accumulation and biochemical composition of dental plaque in young adults. Caries Res 1984;18:465-71.

10. Axelsson P, Lindhe J. The effect of a preventive programme on dental plaque, gingivitis and caries in school children. Results after one and two years. J Clin Periodontol 1974;1:126-38.

11. Axelsson P, Lindhe J. Effect of fluoride on gingivitis and dental caries in a preventive program based on plaque control. Community Dent Oral Epidemiol 1975;3:159-60.

12. Axelsson P, Lindhe J. Efficacy of mouthrinses in inhibiting dental plaque and gingivitis in man. J Clin Periodontol 1987;14:205-12.

13. Axelsson P, Lindhe J, Waseby J. The effect of various plaque control measures on gingivitis and caries in schoolchildren. Community Dent Oral Epidemiol 1976;4:232-9.

14. Axelsson P, Lindhe J, Wystrom B. On the prevention of caries and periodontal disease. Results of a 15-year longitudinal study in adults. J Clin Periodontol 1991;18:182-9.

15. Bacca LA, Leusch M, Lanzalaco AC, et al. A comparison of intraoral antimicrobial effects of stabilized stannous fluoride dentifrice, baking soda/peroxide dentifrice, conventional NaF dentifrice and essential oil mouthrinse. J Clin Dent 1997;8(Spec Issue):54-61.

16. Bader JD, Rozier RG, McFall WT Jr, Ramsey DL. Association of dental health knowledge with periodontal conditions among regular patients. Community Dent Oral Epidemiol 1990;18:32-6.

17. Badersten A, Egelberg J, Koch G. Effect of monthly prophylaxis on caries and gingivitis in schoolchildren. Community Dent Oral Epidemiol 1975;3:1-4.

18. Banoczy J, Sari K, Schiff T, et al. Anticalculus efficacy of three dentifrices. Am J Dent 1995;8:205-8.

19. Bassiouny MA, Grant AA. The tooth-brush application of chlorhexidine. Br Dent J 1975;139:323-7.

20. Beiswanger BB, Doyle PM, Jackson RD, et al. The clinical effect of dentifrices containing stabilized stannous fluoride on plaque formation and gingivitis—a six-month study with ad libitum brushing. J Clin Dent 1995;6(Spec No.):46-53.

21. Beiswanger BB, McClanahan SF, Bartizek RD, et al. The comparative efficacy of stabilized stannous fluoride dentifrice, peroxide/baking soda dentifrice and essential oil mouthrinse for the prevention of gingivitis. J Clin Dent 1997;8(Spec Issue):46-53.

22. Bergenholtz A, Brithon J. Plaque removal by dental floss or toothpicks. An intraindividual comparative study. J Clin Periodontol 1980;7:516-24.

23. Bergenholtz A, Olsson A. Efficacy of plaque-removal using interdental brushes and waxed dental floss. Scand J Dent Res 1984;92:198-203.

24. Bernimoulin JP. Recent concepts in plaque formation. J Clin Periodontol 2003;30(Suppl 5):7-9.

25. Bolden TE, Zambon JJ, Sowinski J, et al. The clinical effect of a dentifrice containing triclosan and a copolymer in a sodium fluoride/silica base on plaque formation and gingivitis: A six-month clinical study. J Clin Dent 1992;3:125-31.

26. Bollmer BW, Sturzenberger OP, Vick V, Grossman E. Reduction of calculus and Peridex stain with Tartar-Control Crest. J Clin Dent 1995;6:185-7.

27. Bouwsma O, Caton J, Polson A, Espeland M. Effect of personal oral hygiene on bleeding interdental gingiva. Histologic changes. J Periodontol 1988;59:80-6.

28. Bowden GH. Mutans streptococci, caries, and chlorhexidine. J Can Dent Assoc 1996;62:700, 703-7.

29. Carlson HC, Porter K, Alms TH. The effect of an alexidine mouthwash on dental plaque and gingivitis. J Periodontol 1977;48:216-8.

30. Carr MP, Rice GL, Horton JE. Evaluation of floss types for interproximal plaque removal. Am J Dent 2000;13:212-4.

31. Chitke UM, Rudolph MJ, Reinach SG. Anti-calculus effects of dentifrice containing pyrophosphate compared with control. Clin Prev Dent 1992;14(4):29-33.

32. Christou V, Timmerman MF, Van der Velden U, Van der Weijden FA. Comparison of different approaches of interdental oral hygiene: Interdental brushes versus dental floss. J Periodontol 1998;69:759-64.

33. Christersson LA, Grossi SG, Dunford RG, et al. Dental plaque and calculus: Risk indicators for their formation. J Dent Res 1992;71:1425-30.

34. Clavero J, Baca P, Junco P, Gonzalez MP. Effects of 0.2% chlorhexidine spray applied once or twice daily on plaque accumulation and gingival inflammation in a geriatric population. J Clin Periodontol 2003;30:773-7.

35. Cohen S, Schiff T, McCool J, et al. Anticalculus efficacy of a dentifrice containing potassium nitrate, soluble pyrophosphatase, PVM/MA copolymer, and sodium fluoride in a silica base: A twelve-week clinical study. J Clin Dent 1994;5(Spec No.):93-6.

36. Deasy MJ, Formicola AJ, Johnson DH, Howe EG. Inhibitory effects of an alexidine mouthrinse on dental plaque formation. Clin Prev Dent 1979;1(2):6-9.

37. Edgar WM, Jenkins GN. Inorganic pyrophosphate in human parotid saliva and dental plaque. Arch Oral Biol 1972;17:219-23.

38. Emilson CG, Fornell J. Effect of toothbrushing with chlorhexidine gel on salivary microflora, oral hygiene, and caries. Scand J Dent Res 1976;84:308-19.

39. Fairbrother KJ, Kowolik MJ, Curzon ME, et al. The comparative clinical efficacy of pyrophosphate/triclosan, copolymer/triclosan and zinc citrate/triclosan dentifrices for the reduction of supragingival calculus formation. J Clin Dent 1997;8(Spec No.):62-6.

40. Finkelstein P, Grossman E. The effectiveness of dental floss in reducing gingival inflammation. J Dent Res 1979;58:1034-9.

41. Fleisch H, Russell GG, Bisaz S, et al. Influence of pyrophosphate on the transformation of amorphous to crystalline calcium phosphate. Calcif Tissue Res 1968;2:49-59.

42. Frandsen AM, Barbano JP, Suomi JD, et al. A comparison of the effectiveness of the Charters', scrub, and roll methods of toothbrushing in removing plaque. Scand J Dent Res 1972;80:267-71.

43. Frazier PJ. A new look at dental health education in community programs. Dent Hyg 1978;52:176-86.
44. Gaffar A, Afflitto J, Nabi N, et al. Recent advances in plaque, gingivitis, tartar and caries prevention technology. Int Dent J 1994;44(Suppl 1):63-70.
45. Gaffar A, Scherl D, Afflito J, Coleman EJ. The effect of triclosan on mediators of gingival inflammation. J Clin Periodontol 1995;22:480-4.
46. Greenstein G, Berman C, Jaffin R. Chlorhexidine: An adjunct to periodontal therapy. J Periodontol 1986;57:370-7.
47. Grenby TH. The use of sanguinarine in mouthwashes and toothpaste compared with some other antimicrobial agents. Br Dent J 1995;178:254-8.
48. Grossi SG, Genco RJ, Machtei EE, et al. Assessment of risk for periodontal disease. II. Risk indicators for alveolar bone loss. J Periodontol 1995;66:23-9.
49. Grossi SG, Zambon JJ, Ho AW, et al. Assessment of risk for periodontal disease. I. Risk indicators for attachment loss. J Periodontol 1994;65:260-7.
50. Grossman E. Chlorhexidine efficacy on gingivitis tested. J Periodontal Res 1986;21:33-43.
51. Grossman E, Hou L, Bollmer BW, et al. Triclosan/pyrophosphate dentifrice: Dental plaque and gingivitis effects in a 6-month randomized controlled clinical study. J Clin Dent 2002;13:149-57.
52. Hansen F, Gjermo P. The plaque-removing effect of four toothbrushing methods. Scand J Dent Res 1971;79:502-6.
53. Heifetz SB, Bagramian RA, Suomi JD, Segreto VA. Programs for the mass control of plaque; an appraisal. J Public Health Dent 1973;33:91-5.
54. Hellstrom MK, Ramberg P, Krok L, Lindhe J. The effect of supragingival plaque control on the subgingival microflora in human periodontitis. J Clin Periodontol 1996;23:934-40.
55. Hill HC, Levi PA, Glickman I. The effects of waxed and unwaxed dental floss on interdental plaque accumulation and interdental gingival health. J Periodontol 1973;44:411-3.
56. Horowitz AM. Oral hygiene measures. J Can Dent Assoc 1980;46:43-6.
57. Jackson D. The efficacy of 2 percent sodium ricinoleate in toothpaste to reduce gingival inflammation. Br Dent J 1962;112:487-93.
58. Jenkins S, Addy M, Newcombe RJ. A dose-response study of triclosan mouthrinses on plaque regrowth. J Clin Periodontol 1993;20:609-12.
59. Johansen JR, Gjermo P, Eriksen HM. Effect of 2 years' use of chlorhexidine-containing dentifrices on plaque, gingivitis, and caries. Scand J Dent Res 1975;83:288-92.
60. Kanchanakamol U, Umpriwan R, Jotikasthira N, et al. Reduction of plaque formation and gingivitis by a dentifrice containing triclosan and copolymer. J Periodontol 1995;66:109-12.
61. Kelner RM, Wohl BR, Deasy MJ, Formicola AJ. Gingival inflammation as related to frequency of plaque removal. J Periodontol 1974;45:303-7.
62. Kjaerheim V, von der Fehr FR, Poulsen S. Two-year study on the effect of professional toothcleaning on schoolchildren in Oppergord, Norway. Community Dent Oral Epidemiol 1980;8:401-6.
63. Kopczyk RA, Abrams H, Brown AT, et al. Clinical and microbiological effects of a sanguinaria-containing mouthrinse and dentifrice with and without fluoride during 6 months of use. J Periodontol 1991;62:617-22.
64. Kreshover SJ, Russell AL. Periodontal disease. J Am Dent Assoc 1958;56:625-9.
65. Kuhner MK, Raetzke PB. The effect of health beliefs on the compliance of periodontal patients with oral hygiene instructions. J Periodontol 1989;60:51-6.
66. Lang NP, Cumming BR, Loe H. Toothbrushing frequency as it relates to plaque development and gingival health. J Periodontol 1973;44:396-405.
67. Lang NP, Hotz P, Graf H, et al. Effects of supervised chlorhexidine mouthrinses in children; a longitudinal clinical trial. J Periodontal Res 1982;17:101-11.
68. Lightner LM, O'Leary TJ, Drake RB, et al. Preventive periodontic treatment procedures: Results over 46 months. J Periodontol 1971;42:555-61.
69. Lindhe J, Axelsson P, Tollskog G. The effect of proper oral hygiene on gingivitis and dental caries in schoolchildren. Community Dent Oral Epidemiol 1975;3:150-5.
70. Lindhe J, Koch G. The effect of supervised oral hygiene on the gingiva of children. Progression and inhibition of gingivitis. J Periodontal Res 1966;1:260-7.
71. Lindhe J, Koch G. The effect of supervised oral hygiene on the gingiva of children. Lack of prolonged effect of supervision. J Periodontal Res 1967;2:215-20.
72. Lindhe J, Rosling B, Socransky SS, Volpe AR. The effect of a triclosan-containing dentifrice on established plaque and gingivitis. J Clin Periodontol 1993;20:327-34.
73. Lissau I, Holst D, Friis-Haasche E. Dental health behaviors and periodontal disease indicators in Danish youths. A 10-year epidemiological follow-up. J Clin Periodontol 1990;17:42-7.
74. Listgarten MA. Prevention of periodontal disease in the future. J Clin Periodontol 1979;6:32-6.
75. Lobene RR. A clinical study of the anticalculus effect of a dentifrice containing soluble pyrophosphate and sodium fluoride. Clin Prev Dent 1986;8(3):5-7.
76. Lobene RR. A clinical comparison of the anticalculus effect of two commercially-available dentifrices. Clin Prev Dent 1987;9(4):3-8.
77. Lobene RR, Soparkar PM. The effect of an alexidine mouthwash on plaque and gingivitis. J Am Dent Assoc 1973;87:848-51.
78. Lobene RR, Soparkar PM, Newman MB. Use of dental floss; effect on plaque and gingivitis. Clin Prev Dent 1982;4(1):5-8.
79. Lobene RR, Soparkar PM, Newman MB, Kohut BE. Reduced formation of supragingival calculus with use of fluoride-zinc chloride dentifrice. J Am Dent Assoc 1987;114:350-2.
80. Löe H. Principles and progress in the prevention of periodontal diseases. In: Lehner T, Cimasoni G, eds: The borderland between caries and periodontal disease. II. New York: Grune and Stratton, 1980:255-68.
81. Löe H, Rindom Schiott C. The effect of suppression of the oral microflora upon the development of dental plaque and gingivitis. In: McHugh WD, ed: Dental plaque. Edinburgh: Livingston, 1970:247-55.

82. Löe H, Rindom Schiott C. The effects of mouthrinses and topical application of chlorhexidine on the development of dental plaque and gingivitis in man. J Periodontal Res 1970;5:79-83.

83. Löe H, Rindom Schiott C, Glavind L, Karring T. Two years' oral use of chlorhexidine in man. I. General design and clinical effects. J Periodontal Res 1976;11: 135-44.

84. Lovdal A, Arno A, Schei O, Waerhaug J. Combined effect of subgingival scaling and controlled oral hygiene on the incidence of gingivitis. Acta Odontol Scand 1961;19:537-55.

85. Macgregor IDM, Balding JW. Toothbrushing frequency and personal hygiene in 14-year-old schoolchildren. Br Dent J 1987;162:141-4.

86. Mallatt ME, Beiswanger BB, Stookey GK, et al. Influence of soluble pyrophosphate on calculus formation in adults. J Dent Res 1985;64:1159-62.

87. Marsh PD. Microbial ecology of dental plaque and its significance in health and disease. Adv Dent Res 1994;8:263-71.

88. Marsh PD. Plaque as a biofilm: Pharmacological principles of drug delivery and action in the sub- and supragingival environment. Oral Dis 2003;9(Suppl 1):16-22.

89. Marsh PD, Bradshaw DJ. Dental plaque as biofilm. J Ind Microbiol 1995;15:169-75.

90. Melsen B, Agerbaek N. Effect of an instructional motivation program on oral health in Danish adolescents after 1 and 2 years. Community Dent Oral Epidemiol 1980;8:72-8.

91. Miller S, Truong T, Heu R, et al. Recent advances in stannous fluoride technology: Antibacterial efficacy and mechanism of action towards hypersensitivity. Int Dent J 1994;44(Suppl 1):83-98.

92. Page RC, Offenbacher S, Schroeder HE, et al. Advances in the pathogenesis of periodontitis: Summary of developments, clinical implications and future directions. Periodontol 2000 1997;14:264-48.

93. Palomo F, Wantland L, Sanchez A, et al. The effect of three commercially available dentifrices containing triclosan on supragingival plaque formation and gingivitis: A six month clinical study. Int Dent J 1994;44(Suppl 1):75-81.

94. Patters MR, Anerud K, Trummel CL, et al. Inhibition of plaque formation in humans by octenidine mouthrinse. J Periodontal Res 1983;18:212-9.

95. Perlich MA, Bacca LA, Bollmer BW, et al. The clinical effect of a stabilized stannous fluoride dentifrice on plaque formation, gingivitis and gingival bleeding: A six-month study. J Clin Dent 1995;6(Spec No.): 54-8.

96. Pihlstrom BL, Ortiz-Campos C, McHugh RB. A randomized four-year study of periodontal therapy. J Periodontol 1981;52:227-42.

97. Ramfjord SP, Knowles JW, Nissle RR, et al. Longitudinal study of periodontal therapy. J Periodontol 1973;44: 66-77.

98. Renvert S, Birkhed D. Comparison between 3 triclosan dentifrices on plaque, gingivitis and salivary microflora. J Clin Periodontol 1995;22:63-70.

99. Ripa LW, Berenie JT, Leske GS. The effect of professionally administered bi-annual prophylaxes on the oral hygiene, gingival health and caries scores of school children. Two-year study. J Prev Dent 1976;3:22-6.

100. Robinson E. A comparative evaluation of the scrub and Bass methods of toothbrushing with flossing as an adjunct. Am J Public Health 1976;66:1078-81.

101. Robinson PJ. Gingivitis: A prelude to periodontitis? J Clin Dent 1995;6(Spec No.):41-5.

102. Russell RR. Control of specific plaque bacteria. Adv Dent Res 1994;8:285-90.

103. Sangnes G, Zachrisson B, Gjermo P. Effectiveness of vertical and horizontal brushing techniques in plaque removal. ASDC J Dent Child 1972;39:94-7.

104. Santos A. Evidence-based control of plaque and gingivitis. J Clin Periodontol 2003;30(Suppl 5):13-6.

105. Saxton CA, Huntington E, Cummins D. The effect of dentifrices containing triclosan on the development of gingivitis in a 21-day experimental gingivitis study. Int Dent J 1993;43(Suppl 1):423-9.

106. Scheie AA. Mechanisms of dental plaque formation. Adv Dent Res 1994;8:246-53.

107. Schmid MO, Balmelli OP, Saxer UP. Plaque removing effect of toothbrush, dental floss, and a toothpick. J Clin Periodontol 1976;3:157-65.

108. Simons D, Brailsford S, Kidd EA, Beighton D. The effect of chlorhexidine acetate/xylitol chewing gum on the plaque and gingival indices of elderly occupants in residential homes. J Clin Periodontol 2001;28:1010-5.

109. Spolsky VW, Bhatia HL, Forsythe A, Levin BS. The effect of an antimicrobial mouthwash on dental plaque and gingivitis in young adults. J Periodontol 1975;46:685-90.

110. Suomi JD. Prevention and control of periodontal disease. J Am Dent Assoc 1971;83:1271-87.

111. Suomi JD, Greene JC, Vermillion JC, et al. The effect of controlled oral hygiene procedures on the progression of periodontal disease in adults. Results after third and final year. J Periodontol 1971;42:152-60.

112. Suomi JD, Horowitz HS, Barbano JP, et al. A clinical trial of a calculus-inhibitory dentifrice. J Periodontol 1974;45:139-45.

113. Suomi JD, Smith LW, Chang JJ, Barbano JP. Study of the effect of different prophylaxis frequencies on the periodontium of young adult males. J Periodontol 1973;44:406-10.

114. Taller SH. The effect of baking soda/hydrogen peroxide dentifrice (Mentadent) and 0.12 percent chlorhexidine gluconate mouthrinse (Peridex) in reducing gingival bleeding. J N J Dent Assoc 1993;64: 23-5, 27.

115. Tan HH, Saxton CA. Effect of a single dental health care instruction and prophylaxis on gingivitis. Community Dent Oral Epidemiol 1978;6:172-5.

116. Tenenbaum H, Dahan M, Soell M. Effectiveness of a sanguinarine regimen after scaling and root planing. J Periodontol 1999;70:307-11.

117. Walmsley AD. The electric toothbrush: A review. Br Dent J 1997;182:209-18.

118. Wardle HM. The challenge of growing oral spirochaetes. J Med Microbiol 1997;46:104-16.

119. Weatherford TW, Finn SB, Jamison HC. Effects of an alexidine mouthwash on dental plaque and gingivitis

in humans over a six-month period. J Am Dent Assoc 1977;94:528-36.

120. Westfelt E. Rationale of mechanical plaque control. J Clin Periodontol 1996;23(3 Part 2):263-7.

121. Zacherl WA, Pfeiffer HJ, Swancar JR. The effect of soluble pyrophosphates on dental calculus in adults. J Am Dent Assoc 1985;110:737-8.

122. Zaki HA, Bandt CL. The effective use of a self-teaching oral hygiene manual. J Periodontol 1974;45: 491-5.

123. Zambon JJ. Principles of evaluation of the diagnostic value of subgingival bacteria. Ann Periodontol 1997;2:138-48.

124. Zickert I, Emilson CG, Krasse B. Effect of caries preventive measures in children highly infected with the bacterium *Streptococcus mutans*. Arch Oral Biol 1982;27:861-8.

125. Zickert I, Emilson CG, Krasse B. Microbial conditions and caries increment 2 years after discontinuation of controlled antimicrobial measures in Swedish teenagers. Community Dent Oral Epidemiol 1987;15:241-4.

30 Restricting the Use of Tobacco

PREVALENCE OF TOBACCO USE
PATHOLOGIC EFFECTS OF SMOKELESS
  TOBACCO
RESTRICTING TOBACCO USE

Restricting Cigarette Smoking
Restricting Smokeless Tobacco
  Use
WHAT DENTAL PROFESSIONALS CAN DO

Tobacco use is a major risk factor for many diseases, and it is the leading cause of preventable mortality.[34] The bare statistics are brutal: more than 430,000 deaths occur each year attributable to tobacco use in the United States, and some 3000 children and adolescents become new smokers every day. More than 10 million Americans lost their lives prematurely to tobacco-caused diseases during the twentieth century.[54] The annual global death toll was over 4 million in 1998, and at current rates will exceed 8 million by 2020.[62] There is some hope that tobacco control measures will be having an effect by then, because in 2003 the World Health Organization (WHO) concluded a remarkable worldwide Framework Convention on Tobacco Control. This convention calls for health promotional activities among member nations to control tobacco use by a variety of methods.[63]

Controlling exposure to tobacco is a public health issue that involves all health professionals. Dentists and hygienists stand together with their medical colleagues to do what they can to reduce exposure to tobacco, including engaging in health promotional activities on the political front and counseling patients one to one. With regard to oral effects, tobacco use of all kinds is a major risk factor for oral cancer (see Chapter 23), and the degree of risk is proportional to the extent of use. It is also a major risk factor for periodontitis (see Chapter 21), so much so that it may have been a major reason for high levels of periodontitis throughout much of the twentieth century.[30] Estimates are that tobacco use is

responsible for half of the periodontitis and three quarters of the oral cancer seen in the United States.[58] Even dental caries in children has been associated with exposure to secondhand smoke.[4]

Political action to reduce exposure to tobacco is not easy because the tobacco industry is a formidable opponent. Likewise, inducing patients to change established tobacco habits is difficult because tobacco addictions are powerful and there are usually strong social or psychological reasons why a tobacco habit was adopted in the first place. However, as described here, programs are in place that can help.

In this chapter, we do not detail the pathologic effects of cigarette smoking because this information is readily available elsewhere. For example, the most recent of four reports on the health consequences of tobacco from the Surgeon General of the United States describes the ills that come with tobacco use in remorseless detail (http://www.surgeongeneral.gov/library/smokingconsequences). However, we do review the evidence for the pathologic effects of smokeless tobacco, because these have not received the same degree of research attention. This chapter describes the prevalence of smoking and smokeless tobacco use and then looks at the various initiatives that aim to reduce exposure to tobacco in all its forms. These include the programs that dental professionals can use in their practices to help patients quit. Attention is also given to the specific public health issue of reducing the use of smokeless tobacco among young people. The abbreviation

ST is used for smokeless tobacco products; readers can take it as standing for either "smokeless tobacco" or "spit tobacco," according to taste.

PREVALENCE OF TOBACCO USE

Prevalence of cigarette smoking in the United States is now around 23% among adults and has remained around that figure for some years.[52] Smoking prevalence has been cut in half since the first Surgeon General's report on smoking and health in 1964, and this progress is rightly considered one of the 10 greatest public health achievements of the twentieth century.[56] The sobering aspect of this achievement is that most of those who intend to quit have probably already done so, and those who are left are the hard-core smokers, plus the 3000 new young people who start smoking each day. (It is a fair bet that few current smokers in the United States have even heard of WHO's framework convention.) Data on smoking in the United States are presented in Box 30-1. The report is mixed, with the main concerns now centered on youth smoking and the concentration of tobacco use in lower socioeconomic groups.

Heavy marketing of ST products, principally targeted to adolescent and young adult males, has coincided with the national decline in cigarette smoking. Marketing of ST seems to have been successful; consumption of ST products in the United States almost tripled between 1972 and 1991.[49] It was estimated from a national survey that, in 1991, 5.3 million American adults (2.9% of the population) were using ST: 4.8 million men and 533,000 women.[49] This percentage had risen slightly to 3.2% of the population by 1999.[53]

The concerns about ST's appeal to youth seem well founded: 1995 national survey data revealed that 11.4% of high school students had used ST within the previous 30 days, 19.7% of males and 2.4% of females. ST use among whites was 14.5%, among African-Americans 2.2%, and among Hispanic students 4.4%.[31] The 1991 national survey found that 8.2% of males ages 18-24 years were regular ST users, the highest proportion of any age-group. Even if there is some overreporting,[15] presumably by individuals who wish to appear more "macho," these figures are high. Among adults 45 years of age or older, however, ST use was more common among African-Americans than among whites.[21] Usage of ST is highest in the South, in rural areas, and declines with increasing education.[49] Women users of ST are predominantly in the South.[59]

Use of ST is extensive in the military[8,26] and is particularly heavy among Native Americans; a study conducted in seven western states found that 56% of Native Americans in the ninth and tenth grades reported that they were regular users,[11] as were 28.1% of sixth-graders.[7] ST use among Native American women is substantially above the national rate for women.[44] Native Americans emerge as the ethnic group with the heaviest relative use of ST and the only one in which there is almost equivalent use among males and females.[11,61] In one study of Navajo adolescents, over 25% of ST users were found to have leukoplakia, compared to only 4% of nonusers. The duration and frequency of use were highly significant risk factors for leukoplakia.[61]

Prevalence of ST use is also widespread among highly visible professional baseball players; surveys carried out with major and minor league teams found that 39%-46% of players were regular users.[19,60] Another study of baseball players in 1988 found that ST users had 60 times the risk of developing leukoplakia compared with nonusers.[25]

The remarkably high occurrence of oral cancer in India (see Chapter 23) is thought to result from the high prevalence of tobacco chewing in several forms. Because the rate of conversion of leukoplakia and other precancerous lesions to oral cancer is no higher in India than elsewhere,[45] it seems to be the high exposure to tobacco, rather than any inherent characteristics of Indian people, that leads to the high prevalence of leukoplakia, and subsequently oral cancer, in that country.

Since the pathologic effects of cigarette smoking are now extensively documented, tobacco marketing aims to foster the perception that ST is a less risky substitute for cigarettes. However, ST is far from harmless.

PATHOLOGIC EFFECTS OF SMOKELESS TOBACCO

ST is a particularly worrisome form of tobacco, because its current use by young people has the potential to increase the incidence of

---

BOX 30-1   Facts on Smoking Prevalence in the United States, 2001[54]

- In 2001, 46.2 million adults (22.8%) in the United States were current smokers: 25.2% of men and 20.7% of women.
- Among racial and ethnic groups, smoking prevalence was highest among American Indians and Alaskan natives (32.7%) and lowest among Hispanics (16.7%) and Asians (12.4%).
- Among income groups, smoking prevalence was higher among adults living below the poverty level (31.4%) than among those at or above the poverty level (23%).
- Smoking prevalence was highest among those ages 18-24 (26.9%) and 25-44 (25.8%) and lowest among those age 65 and older (10.1%).
- Among current adult smokers, 37.8 million (81.8%) smoked every day, and 8.4 million (18.2%) smoked some days.
- An estimated 44.7 million adults were former smokers in 2001, representing 49.2% of all those who had ever smoked. An estimated 15.3 million adult smokers had stopped smoking for at least 1 day during the preceding 12 months because they were trying to quit.
- Adults who had earned a General Educational Development (GED) diploma (47.8%) and those with a grade 9-11 education (34.3%) showed the highest prevalence of smoking; those with master's, professional, and doctoral degrees showed the lowest prevalence (9.5%).
- Smoking prevalence data for combined years 1965-66 through 2000-01 indicate a slow but steady decrease among both African-Americans and whites.

- In 2000-01, for the first time, smoking prevalence among African-American men was similar to that among white men. Since 1970-74, prevalence has declined more rapidly among African-American men than among white men.
- In 2000-01, smoking prevalence also declined more rapidly among African-American women than among white women. Prevalence among African-American women has been generally lower than among white women since 1993-95. Before 1993-95, prevalence of current smoking generally was comparable among African-American and white women.
- The overall decline in cigarette smoking prevalence in the adult U.S. population is not occurring at a rate that will meet the national health objective for 2010 of 12%.
- In 2000, the Surgeon General concluded that the 2010 objective could be attained only if comprehensive approaches to tobacco control were implemented. Sustained or increasing implementation of comprehensive tobacco-control programs to meet the funding levels recommended by the Centers for Disease Control and Prevention are necessary to attain the 2010 national objective.
- Comprehensive programs that focus on reducing tobacco use among those in different socioeconomic strata, those in different racial and ethnic populations, and groups with different educational levels could help reduce cigarette smoking and tobacco use in general and reduce the extensive morbidity, mortality, and economic costs associated with tobacco use.

---

oral cancer in the future.[40] The American Dental Association (ADA) has firmly stated policies opposing any use of ST, and the ADA clearly rejects ST as a substitute for regular tobacco.[5]

ST is sold in several forms. The main concern is with snuff, a powdered tobacco product, which is used by placing a "dip" between the cheek and gum. Dry snuff contains high concentrations of N-nitrosamines[2,27]; evidence is strong that compounds in this group are carcinogens, especially for oral cancers.[27,39] The N-nitroso compounds found in snuff are DNA-damaging agents in cancers of the aerodi-

gestive tract.[35] A consensus panel of the National Institutes of Health found strong evidence that use of snuff causes oral cancers,[38] a conclusion for which there was ample support at the time[47,57] and subsequently.[3,17,27,29] Nicotine is absorbed from ST in amounts similar to those absorbed from cigarette smoke,[9] which makes ST a potential risk factor for the same diseases that result from smoking. That could be why ST users face a relative risk of 2.1 for cardiovascular disease compared to nonusers. The relative risk for smokers compared to nonsmokers in the same study was 3.2.[10]

The continued use of snuff leads to localized tissue changes, most commonly the development of leukoplakia, which is characterized by the appearance of white, wrinkled mucosa at the site where the snuff is placed. Leukoplakia can become cancerous in 3%-5% of cases,[45] although there is also evidence that these lesions can be reversed if the ST habit is ended.[22,33] With regard to oral conditions other than precancerous soft tissue changes, no good evidence exists that ST can cause caries and periodontal diseases. Gingival recession at the site where the quid or dip is placed is common, however. It has also been found that poor oral hygiene among ST users contributes to the formation of nitrosamines in the oral cavity.[35]

Further evidence for the carcinogenic potential of chewing tobacco comes from studies of women smokers and dippers in the South[59] which found that the relative risk of developing cancer of the gums and buccal mucosa was 4.6 for smokers (i.e., smokers developed oral cancer at 4.6 times the frequency of nonsmokers). However, for users of ST the relative risk was 13-48, with higher risk found in those with longer ST use.

RESTRICTING TOBACCO USE
Restricting Cigarette Smoking

There are good reasons why the early twenty-first century is a good time for a national campaign for smoking cessation (Box 30-2). Funding for such a program looked promising in 1998, when the Master Settlement Agreement with the tobacco companies seemed to ensure seemingly infinite funding to the states for cessation programs.[24] At a time when court actions against the tobacco industry were accumulating, the Master Settlement Agreement was negotiated between the tobacco industry, on the one hand, and a group of state attorneys general, private lawyers, and public health advocates on the other. Under the terms of the settlement, the tobacco industry would get relief from present and future litigation payments, and in exchange would accept some additional regulation of advertising and would make substantial cash payments to state governments. These payments were intended to be used for tobacco control programs, although few states have used these funds for that purpose—because of many states' budgetary problems soon after the settlement, the funds were diverted to become a general-purpose emergency revenue stream.[23] Among other funding problems, in only 36 states do Medicaid programs pay for smoking cessation treatment, including pharmacotherapy, nicotine nasal sprays, nicotine inhalers, nicotine patches, and nicotine gum.[28] This is despite the fact that a higher proportion of Medicaid recipients smoke than do members of the general population.[42]

Despite these stumbling blocks, progress continues to be made on tobacco control. Smoke-free indoor air, especially in bars and restaurants, has been mandated in many local communities and even at the state level in six cases (California, Connecticut, Delaware,

---

BOX 30-2 Reasons Why the Early Twenty-First Century Is an Ideal Time for Bold Steps To Reduce Tobacco Use in the United States[20]

- Although health care funding is scarce, tobacco-related diseases cost $150 billion each year.
- Although numerous effective tobacco-dependence treatments exist, millions of tobacco users are unable to obtain or afford such treatments.
- A major funding source, the 1998 Master Settlement Agreement between the states and the tobacco companies, is being used to plug states' budgetary shortfalls rather than to promote smoking cessation.
- Although the devastating impact of tobacco use on health has been exhaustively documented, the tobacco industry continues to lure adolescents and adults into tobacco dependence through an $11 billion advertising and promotional effort.

Florida, Maine, and New York). Although the Master Settlement Agreement is not working as its backers intended, the public discussions it sparked have served to increase public knowledge and awareness.

The research attention devoted to smoking has lead to development of some effective interventions.[50] These have been put into program plans, intended for both private practice and public health applications, that are built on the tobacco-related objectives of *Healthy People 2010* (see Chapter 5). One plan for community interventions came from the Task Force on Community Preventive Services, an independent (though Centers for Disease Control and Prevention–supported) group of health experts that is developing a guide to community services on a variety of health issues. The task force goals were to direct interventions toward (1) reducing overall exposure to environmental tobacco smoke, (2) reducing tobacco use initiation, and (3) increasing the cessation of tobacco use.[48] The Task Force has conducted a series of systematic reviews to identify the most effective interventions, and its work is continuing. Strongly recommended interventions to date include establishment of smoking bans and restrictions, increase in the unit price for tobacco products, and mass media education.[48]

Restricting Smokeless Tobacco Use

Preventive efforts against the diseases that come with ST use are based principally on public and individual education to convince people to drop the habit or, preferably, not to begin in the first place. The public health efforts of the various professions involved received a boost with the passage of Public Law 99-252, the Comprehensive Smokeless Tobacco Health Education Act, in February 1986. The most relevant details of this legislation are shown in Box 30-3.

Ironically, this national legislation was supported by the tobacco industry, which was spurred to do so because of the likelihood that a majority of states would pass more severe laws of their own.[13] The growth of public concern about the marketing of ST was stimulated by the publicity generated by the 1985 case of *Marsee v US Tobacco Company*. Sean Marsee, a top high school athlete, died of oral cancer at age 19 after years of ST use. The suit was brought by Sean's mother, who charged that the tobacco company engaged in misleading advertising and failed to place warnings on its products.[13] Although Ms. Marsee's suit was not successful, the case engendered a great deal of sympathy and concern.

Voluntarily breaking the ST habit, given that nicotine addiction is involved, seems to be no easier than breaking the cigarette habit. Of 25 adolescent habitual ST users who participated in an intensive program of ST cessation, only 4 had remained successful in quitting 3 months after the program.[18] On the other hand, in another intervention study the number of young male ST users who quit was 50% above the normal rate when participants viewed a 9-minute videotape, were given a self-help

---

BOX 30-3   Major Provisions of Public Law 99-252, the Comprehensive Smokeless Tobacco Health Education Act (February 1986)[32]

- Development and implementation of health education programs and materials to inform the public of health risks resulting from the use of smokeless tobacco products.
- Inclusion of health warning labels on all smokeless tobacco products and advertisements, except those on outdoor billboards.
- Prohibition of radio and television advertising, beginning in August 1986.

- Disclosure to the Secretary of Health and Human Services of the ingredients used in the production of smokeless tobacco as well as the quantity of nicotine in such products.
- Technical assistance in public health education for the states.
- Authorization of research on the effects of smokeless tobacco.

manual, and received an explanation of the risks and "unequivocal advice" to quit.[46]

With this mixed evidence on quitting, strategy should be aimed at preventing young people from starting to use ST, although it is obvious that health education programs need to go well beyond the admonition to "just say no" if they are to be successful. In the 1991 national survey, 22.9% of current ST users reported that they currently smoked, and another 33.3% had formerly smoked.[49] Many ST users report using ST concurrently with alcohol, cigarettes, and marijuana, and peer pressure is a strong influence in getting started.[6] The relationship between cigarette smoking and ST use, as well as other correlates of the habit, is complex and needs further study if education to discourage commencement of either habit is to be successful.[43] Ignorance of the health consequences is common. A Pennsylvania study reported that nearly half the males in grades 7-12 did not believe that ST was harmful.[14] As in any health education for adolescents, the immediately negative effects of ST use (stained teeth, bad breath) can make a greater impression than the long-term health hazards.[16]

Multifaceted strategies were needed to implement the provisions of Public Law 99-252 (see Box 30-3), and a leading role was played by state and local public health agencies.[12] Some states established programs of media advertising and school health education aimed specifically at discouraging the start of ST use. Monitoring the impact of these educational efforts requires considerable survey effort. The monitoring process is proceeding through a series of institutionalized surveys,[21,31] but progress toward reducing ST use is slow. Trends in ST use in Indiana, Iowa, Montana, and West Virginia between 1988 and 1993 showed little change over that period, a finding attributed to increased advertising and promotion by the tobacco industry, despite the existence of Public Law 99-252.[37] Minors still seem to have relatively little trouble obtaining ST, even in states where such sales are prohibited by law.[1]

WHAT DENTAL PROFESSIONALS CAN DO

Dental professionals obviously have a potentially major role to play in educating patients about the hazards of ST use and in helping patients who are already addicted to quit. The task sounds daunting, but it can be done. The National Cancer Institute, one of the National Institutes of Health, funds the National Dental Tobacco-Free Steering Committee, a broadly based group whose mission is to promote tobacco use cessation activities through the dental office. Oral Health America sponsors the National Spit Tobacco Education Program (NSTEP; http://www.nstep.org/nstep.shtml), funded largely by the Robert Wood Johnson Foundation, a group that achieved national prominence largely through its charismatic, highly visible national honorary chairman, baseball legend Joe Garagiola. Mr. Garagiola hammers the message that ST use is not a traditional part of the great American pastime, no matter how the tobacco companies try to make it appear so.

For practitioners helping a patient to quit smoking, there is the clinical practice guideline *Treating Tobacco Use and Dependence* sponsored by the U.S. Public Health Service in collaboration with an array of governmental agencies, educational associations, and practitioner groups.[51] The initial recommendations of this group are shown in Box 30-4, and the website provides a highly detailed approach to working with patients in their attempts to quit (http://www.surgeongeneral.gov/tobacco/clin-pack.html). The clinical practice guideline is interactive and constantly being updated as new research is completed. The National Cancer Institute has a special website devoted entirely to providing a wealth of how-to-quit information that both health professionals and patients can use.[36] An abundance of information on interventions at both the individual and community levels can also be found in *The Guide to Community Preventive Services*.[55] The ADA, with assistance from some grant funding, has also committed a lot of resources to training dentists in tobacco use cessation techniques. When protocols are finalized, these training sessions should become readily available to all dentists.

Use of these sources of information should be part of the routines of every dental office, for tobacco use cessation must be seen as the first treatment priority for almost any oral disease. After all, tobacco use is a serious matter—in fact, it is a matter of life and death.

BOX 30-4 Conclusions and Recommendations on Ways Health Professionals Can Help Patients Stop Smoking[51]

1. Tobacco dependence is a chronic condition that often requires repeated intervention. However, effective treatments exist that can produce long-term or even permanent abstinence.
2. Because effective tobacco dependence treatments are available, every patient who uses tobacco should be offered at least one of these treatments:
   a. Patients *willing* to try to quit tobacco use should be provided with treatments identified as effective in this guideline.
   b. Patients *unwilling* to try to quit tobacco use should be provided with a brief intervention designed to increase their motivation to quit.
3. It is essential that clinicians and health care delivery systems (including administrators, insurers, and purchasers) institutionalize the consistent identification, documentation, and treatment of every tobacco user seen in a health care setting.
4. Brief tobacco dependence treatment is effective, and every patient who uses tobacco should be offered at least brief treatment.
5. There is a strong dose-response relation between the intensity of tobacco dependence counseling and its effectiveness. Treatments involving person-to-person contact (via individual, group, or proactive telephone counseling) are consistently effective, and their effectiveness increases with treatment intensity (e.g., minutes of contact).
6. Three types of counseling and behavioral therapies have been found to be especially effective and should be used with all patients attempting tobacco cessation:
   a. Provision of practical counseling (problem-solving and skills training);
   b. Provision of social support as part of treatment (intratreatment social support); and
   c. Help in securing social support outside of treatment (extratreatment social support).
7. Numerous effective pharmacotherapies for smoking cessation now exist. Except in the presence of contraindications, these should be used with all patients attempting to quit smoking.
   a. Five *first-line* pharmacotherapies have been identified that reliably increase long-term smoking abstinence rates:
      (1) Bupropion sustained release
      (2) Nicotine gum
      (3) Nicotine inhaler
      (4) Nicotine nasal spray
      (5) Nicotine patch
   b. Two *second-line* pharmacotherapies have been identified as efficacious and may be considered by clinicians if first-line pharmacotherapies are not effective:
      (1) Clonidine
      (2) Nortriptyline
   c. Over-the-counter nicotine patches are effective when compared to placebo, and their use should be encouraged.
8. Tobacco dependence treatments are both clinically effective and cost effective relative to other medical and disease prevention interventions. Because of this, insurers and purchasers should ensure that the following occur:
   a. All insurance plans include as a reimbursed benefit the counseling and pharmacotherapeutic treatments identified as effective in this guideline; and
   b. Clinicians are reimbursed for providing tobacco dependence treatment just as they are reimbursed for treating other chronic conditions.

REFERENCES

1. Accessibility to minors of smokeless tobacco products—Broward County, Florida, March-June 1996. MMWR Morb Mortal Wkly Rep 1996;45:1079-82.
2. Adams JD, Owens-Tucciarone P, Hoffmann D. Tobacco-specific N-nitrosamines in dry snuff. Food Chem Toxicol 1987;25:245-6.
3. Ahmed HG, Idris AM, Ibrahim SO. Study of oral epithelial atypia among Sudanese tobacco users by exfoliative cytology. Anticancer Res 2003;23:1943-9.
4. Aligne CA, Moss ME, Auinger P, Weitzman M. Association of pediatric dental caries with passive smoking. JAMA 2003;289:1258-64.
5. American Dental Association. ADA positions and statements: CAPIR statement opposing the use of smokeless tobacco as a smoking cessation technique, website: http://www.ada.org/prof/resources/positions/statements/smokeless.asp. Accessed February 8, 2004.
6. Ary DV, Lichtenstein E, Severson HH. Smokeless tobacco use among male adolescents: Patterns, correlates,

predictors, and the use of other drugs. Prev Med 1987;16:385-401.

7. Backinger CL, Bruerd B, Kinney MB, Szpunar SM. Knowledge, intent to use, and use of smokeless tobacco among sixth grade schoolchildren in six selected U.S. sites. Public Health Rep 1993;108:637-42.

8. Ballweg JA, Bray RM. Smoking and tobacco use by U.S. military personnel. Mil Med 1989;154:165-8.

9. Benowitz NL, Jacob P 3rd, Yu L. Daily use of smokeless tobacco: Systemic effects. Ann Intern Med 1989; 111:112-6.

10. Bolinder G, Alfredsson L, Englund A, de Faire U. Smokeless tobacco use and increased cardiovascular mortality among Swedish construction workers. Am J Public Health 1994;84:399-404.

11. Bruerd B. Smokeless tobacco use among Native American school children. Public Health Rep 1990;105:196-201.

12. Capwell EM. P.L. 99-252 and the roles of state and local governments in decreasing smokeless tobacco use. J Public Health Dent 1990;50:70-6.

13. Chen MS Jr. Evaluating the impact of P.L. 99-252 on decreasing smokeless tobacco use. J Public Health Dent 1990;50:65-9.

14. Cohen RY, Sattler J, Felix MR, Brownell KD. Experimentation with smokeless tobacco and cigarettes by children and adolescents: Relationship to beliefs, peer use, and parental use. Am J Public Health 1987;77:1454-6.

15. Cohen SJ, Katz BP, Drook CA, et al. Overreporting of smokeless tobacco use by adolescent males. J Behav Med 1988;11:383-93.

16. Colborn JW, Cummings KM, Michalek AM. Correlates of adolescents' use of smokeless tobacco. Health Educ Q 1989;16:91-100.

17. Dikshit RP, Kanhere S. Tobacco habits and risk of lung, oropharyngeal and oral cavity cancer: A population-based case-control study in Bhopal, India. Int J Epidemiol 2000;29:609-14.

18. Eakin E, Severson H, Glasgow RE. Development and evaluation of a smokeless tobacco cessation program: A pilot study. NCI Monogr 1989;(8):95-100.

19. Ernster VL, Grady DG, Greene JC, et al. Smokeless tobacco use and health effects among baseball players. JAMA 1990;264:218-24.

20. Fiore MC, Croyle RT, Curry SJ, et al. Preventing 3 million premature deaths and helping 5 million smokers quit: A national action plan for tobacco cessation. Am J Public Health 2004;94:205-10.

21. Giovino GA, Schooley MW, Zhu BP, et al. Surveillance for selected tobacco-use behaviors—United States 1900-1994. MMWR Surveill Summ 1994 Nov 18;43: 1-43.

22. Giunta JL, Connolly G. The reversibility of leukoplakia caused by smokeless tobacco. J Am Dent Assoc 1986;113:50-2.

23. Givel M, Glantz SA. State tobacco settlement funds not being spent on vigorous tobacco control efforts. Oncology 2002;16:152-7.

24. Givel M, Glantz SA. The "Global Settlement" with the tobacco industry: 6 years later. Am J Public Health 2004;94:218-24.

25. Grady D, Greene J, Daniels TE, et al. Oral mucosal lesions found in smokeless tobacco users. J Am Dent Assoc 1990;121:117-23.

26. Grasser JA, Childers E. Prevalence of smokeless tobacco use and clinical oral leukoplakia in a military population. Mil Med 1997;162:401-4.

27. Gupta PC, Murti PR, Bhonsle RB. Epidemiology of cancer by tobacco products and the significance of TSNA. Crit Rev Toxicol 1996;26:183-98.

28. Halpin HA, Keeler CL, Orleans CT, Husten CG. State Medicaid coverage for tobacco-dependence treatments—United States, 1994-2002. MMWR Morb Mortal Wkly Rep 2004;53:54-7.

29. Hashibe M, Sankaranarayanan R, Thomas G, et al. Alcohol drinking, body mass index and the risk of oral leukoplakia in an Indian population. Int J Cancer 2000;88:129-34.

30. Hujoel PP, Bergstrom J, del Aguila MA, DeRouen TA. A hidden chronic periodontitis epidemic during the 20th century? Community Dent Oral Epidemiol 2003;31:1-6.

31. Kann L, Warren CW, Harris WA, et al. Youth risk behavior surveillance—United States, 1995. MMWR CDC Surveill Summ 1996;45(SS-4):1-84.

32. Malvitz DM. Introduction. J Public Health Dent 1990;50:64.

33. Martin GC, Brown JP, Eifler CW, Houston GD. Oral leukoplakia status six weeks after cessation of smokeless tobacco use. J Am Dent Assoc 1999;130:945-54.

34. McGinnis JM, Foege WH. Actual causes of death in the United States. JAMA 1993;270:2207-12.

35. Nair J, Ohshima H, Nair UJ, Bartsch H. Endogenous formation of nitrosamines and oxidative DNA-damaging agents in tobacco users. Crit Rev Toxicol 1996; 26:149-61.

36. National Institutes of Health, National Cancer Institute. Smokefree.gov, website: http://smokefree.gov/. Accessed March 5, 2004.

37. Nelson DE, Tomar SL, Mowery P, Siegel PZ. Trends in smokeless tobacco use among men in four states, 1988 through 1993. Am J Public Health 1996;86: 1300-3.

38. NIH Consensus Development Panel. National Institutes of Health consensus statement. Health implications of smokeless tobacco use. Biomed Pharmacother 1988;42:93-8.

39. Preston-Martin S, Correa P. Epidemiological evidence for the role of nitroso compounds in human cancer. Cancer Surv 1989;8:459-73.

40. Projected smoking-related deaths among youth—United States. MMWR Morb Mortal Wkly Rep 1996;45:971-4.

41. Rodu B. An alternative approach to smoking control [editorial]. Am J Med Sci 1994;308:32-4.

42. Schauffler HH, Mordavsky J, Barker D, Orleans CT. State Medicaid coverage for tobacco-dependence treatments—United States, 1998 and 2000. MMWR Morb Mortal Wkly Rep 2001;50:979-82.

43. Severson HH. Psychosocial factors in the use of smokeless tobacco and their implications for Public Law 99-252. J Public Health Dent 1990;50:90-7.

44. Spangler JG, Dignan MB, Michielutte R. Correlates of tobacco use among Native American women in western North Carolina. Am J Public Health 1997;87:108-11.

45. Squier CA. Smokeless tobacco and oral cancer: A cause for concern? CA Cancer J Clin 1984;34:242-7.

46. Stevens VJ, Severson H, Lichtenstein E, et al. Making the most of a teachable moment: A smokeless-tobacco cessation intervention in the dental office. Am J Public Health 1995;85:231-5.

47. Stockwell HG, Lyman GH. Impact of smoking and smokeless tobacco on the risk of cancer of the head and neck. Head Neck Surg 1986;9:104-10.

48. Task Force on Community Preventive Services. Strategies for reducing exposure to environmental tobacco smoke, increasing tobacco-use cessation, and reducing initiation in communities and health care systems. MMWR Recomm Rep 2000;49(RR-12):1-20, website: http://www.cdc.gov/mmwr/preview/mmwrhtml/rr4912a1.htm. Accessed October 18, 2004.

49. Use of smokeless tobacco among adults—United States 1991. MMWR Morb Mortal Wkly Rep 1993;42:263-6.

50. US Public Health Service. Treating tobacco use and dependence—a systems approach, website: http:// www.surgeongeneral.gov/tobacco/systems.htm. Accessed February 9, 2004.

51. US Public Health Service. Clinician's packet: Treating tobacco use and dependence, website: http://www.surgeongeneral.gov/tobacco/clinpack.html. Accessed February 11, 2004.

52. US Public Health Service, Centers for Disease Control and Prevention. Behavioral Risk Factor Surveillance System: Trends data, website: http://apps.nccd.cdc.gov/brfss/Trends/trendchart.asp. Accessed February 9, 2004.

53. US Public Health Service, Centers for Disease Control and Prevention. Behavioral Risk Factor Surveillance System: Prevalence data, website: http://apps.nccd. cdc.gov/brfss/display. asp?cat=ST&yr=1999&qkey= 6000&state=US. Accessed February 9, 2004.

54. US Public Health Service, Centers for Disease Control and Prevention. Cigarette smoking among adults— United States, 2001, website: http://www.cdc.gov/tobacco/research_data/adults_prev/mmwr_highlights_5240.htm. Accessed February 9, 2004.

55. US Public Health Service, Centers for Disease Control and Prevention. The Guide to community preventive services: Tobacco use prevention and control, website: http://www.cdc.gov/tobacco/comguide.htm. Accessed March 5, 2004.

56. US Public Health Service, Centers for Disease Control and Prevention. Ten great public health achievements: United States 1900-1999. MMWR Morb Mortal Wkly Rep 1999;48:241-3.

57. Winn DM. Smokeless tobacco and cancer: The epidemiologic evidence. CA Cancer J Clin 1988;38:236-43.

58. Winn DM. Tobacco use and oral disease. J Dent Educ 2001;65:306-12.

59. Winn DM, Blot WJ, Shy CM. Snuff dipping and oral cancer among women in the southern United States. N Engl J Med 1981;304:745-9.

60. Wisniewski JF, Bartolucci AA. Comparative patterns of smokeless tobacco usage among major league baseball personnel. J Oral Pathol Med 1989;18:322-6.

61. Wolfe MD, Carlos JP. Oral health effects of smokeless tobacco use in Navajo Indian adolescents. Community Dent Oral Epidemiol 1987;15:230-5.

62. World Health Organization. Why is tobacco a public health priority?, website:http://www.who.int/tobacco/health_ impact/en/. Accessed March 5, 2004.

63. World Health Organization. WHO Framework convention on tobacco control (WHO FCTC), website: http://www.who.int/tobacco/fctc/en/. Accessed March 5, 2004.

INDEX

Edwards Brothers Malloy
Thorofare, NJ USA
May 26, 2015